Y0-BYB-377

# HEALTH CARE STATE RANKINGS
# *1993*

## *Health Care in the 50 United States*

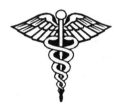

Kathleen O'Leary Morgan,  Scott Morgan and Neal Quitno, Editors

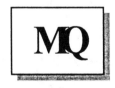

Morgan Quitno Corporation
© Copyright 1993, All Rights Reserved

P.O. Box 1656, Lawrence, KS  66044
800-457-0742 or 913-841-3534

RA407.3
H423
1993

© Copyright 1993 by
Morgan Quitno Corporation
P.O. Box 1656
Lawrence, Kansas  66044

800-457-0742 or 913-841-3534

All Rights Reserved

No part of this book may be reproduced in any form, by photostat, microfilm, xerography, or any other means, or incorporated into any information retrieval system, electronic or mechanical, without the written permission of the copyright owner.  Copyright is not claimed in any material from  U.S. Government sources.  However, its arrangement and compilation along with all other material are subject to the copyright.

ISBN: 0-9625531-4-X
ISSN: 1065-1403

*Health Care State Rankings* sells for $43.95 (we pay shipping).  For those who prefer ranking information tailored to a particular state, we also offer *Health Care State Perspectives*, state-specific reports for each of the 50 states.  These individual guides provide information on a state's data and rank for each of the categories featured in the national *Health Care State Rankings* volume. Perspectives sell for $18.00 , $9.00 if ordered with *Health Care State Rankings*.

First Edition
Printed in the United States of America

**_Printed on recycled paper_**

# PREFACE

We hope you enjoy *Health Care State Rankings 1993*. We think you will find it to be one of the clearest and most comprehensive fact books available on health care in the United States. Our intent is to answer many of the questions that we have ourselves about health care. How many people have insurance? What is the death rate for cancer? How many new cases of lung cancer are expected? How many people have AIDS? What is the birth rate? How much does business spend each year on health care? Which state's citizens drink the most alcohol? How many abortions were performed?

Everyday, health care becomes a more pressing issue in the lives of Americans. This book brings together information from as many reliable sources as possible to paint a statistical portrait of health care in the U.S., both nationally and by state.

This is the first edition of a new series of books by Morgan Quitno providing basic information on a state-by-state basis. This annual takes much from what we learned over the past four years in publishing the comprehensive *State Rankings* reference volume. That book has earned great reviews for simplicity, presentation and clarity. *Health Care State Rankings* is simply a variation on a theme. Our intent is not to present facts in support of one theory or another, but to present the facts and allow the reader to draw his or her own conclusions.

We have made the tables contained in this volume as clear and understandable as possible. Table headings are self-descriptive. However, when additional information is needed, explanatory footnotes are located on the same page. Sources also are clearly noted, again on the same page. Information appearing in this volume is for the most recent year for which comparable data are available from most states.

We have made every effort to simplify the search for data in *Health Care State Rankings 1993*. An extensive table of contents is provided, as well as a detailed index. For added convenience, we have also listed tables for each chapter on chapter break pages. These pages are clearly marked with large tabs. A "thumb index" is located just inside the back cover to speed the search for chapter dividers.

For those among you who have a difficult time translating statistical tables which show data "in millions," "in thousands," etc., we've done your math for you. *Heath Care State Rankings* tables contain all of the necessary "zeroes," so you know right away that Wyoming families spent a total of $660,000,000 on health care in 1991 (table 210).

In all cases, states are ranked on a high-to-low basis. Any ties among the states are listed alphabetically for a given ranking. When a national total is presented, we list each individual state's total and, when applicable, its percentage of the national total. This percentage number is under the heading of a percent sign "%". For example, table 185 shows that New York is home to 7.81% of persons enrolled in HMOs. For further perspective, compare a state's percentage in any given total with its percentage of the nation's population in the population charts provided in the appendix .

The information contained in *Health Care State Rankings* was derived from federal and state government agencies and private organizations. Publications cited as sources sometimes contain additional statistical detail and more comprehensive definitions than can be presented in this volume. More information on the subjects covered may generally be obtained directly from the source. For those readers seeking additional information, a roster of the addresses and telephone numbers of the most commonly cited sources is provided.

Finally, we thank the many individuals, agencies and organizations that provided so much help and information to us in developing this book. It is always encouraging to find how many friendly people there are across this country. The occasional grump just makes everybody else look good.

We always enjoy talking to our growing list of readers. Please call us toll-free at 800-457-0742 or write if you have any questions or suggestions. You will find a postage-paid post card in this book for letting us know what you think. It is only through your input that we can continue to develop truly useful reference books.

THE EDITORS

# WHICH STATE IS HEALTHIEST?

By its nature, a book of rankings lends itself to questions of which is the "best" or "worst." While we do our best to present the data in *Health Care State Rankings 1993* as objectively as possible, we nonetheless found it interesting to take some of the top indicators listed in this book, scramble them in the computer and find out which state is "the healthiest."

For 1993, Utah is winner of our first annual "Good Health State Award." Based on the 22 categories listed on this page, Utah beats out its neighbors, Idaho and Wyoming. Bringing up the rear is Florida, preceded by Delaware in 49th and Missouri in 48th place.

Of course, the categories selected have a lot to do with the outcome of the award. We tried to find statistics that reflect basic health care, access to health care and an overall healthy population. All factors were given equal weight.

Once the factors were determined, we averaged each state's ranking for all 22 categories. Based on these averages, states were then ranked from "most healthy" (lowest average ranking) to "least healthy" (highest average ranking). States with no data available for a given category were assigned a zero for that category and ranked on the remaining factors. In our book, data are listed from highest to lowest. However, for purposes of this award, we inverted rankings for those factors we determined to be "negative." Thus the state with the lowest infant mortality rate in the book (ranking 50th) would be given a number one ranking for this award.

After all the calculating was finished, Utah emerged from the computer as the healthiest. Congratulations to the Beehive State!

THE EDITORS

## 1993 GOOD HEALTH STATE AWARD

| | | | | |
|---|---|---|---|---|
| 1. Utah | 16.27 | 26. Oklahoma | 25.14 |
| 2. Idaho | 18.27 | 27. Oregon | 25.27 |
| 3. Wyoming | 18.55 | 28. Georgia | 25.41 |
| 4. Hawaii | 19.14 | 29. South Carolina | 25.55 |
| 5. Washington | 19.64 | 30. Indiana | 25.73 |
| 6. Minnesota | 19.73 | 31. New Jersey | 26.80 |
| 7. Montana | 20.50 | 32. Illinois | 27.14 |
| 8. North Dakota | 20.91 | 33. Mississippi | 27.36 |
| 9. Colorado | 21.23 | 34. Massachusetts | 27.41 |
| 10. Nebraska | 21.27 | 35. North Carolina | 27.86 |
| 10. South Dakota | 21.27 | 36. New York | 28.00 |
| 12. New Hampshire | 21.55 | 37. Tennessee | 28.05 |
| 13. Maryland | 22.05 | 38. Michigan | 28.14 |
| 14. Texas | 22.14 | 39. Ohio | 28.18 |
| 15. Vermont | 22.36 | 40. Louisiana | 28.36 |
| 16. Alaska | 22.80 | 41. West Virginia | 28.50 |
| 17. Virginia | 23.41 | 42. Nevada | 28.90 |
| 18. Kentucky | 23.59 | 43. Maine | 29.00 |
| 19. Connecticut | 23.76 | 43. Rhode Island | 29.00 |
| 20. Iowa | 23.86 | 45. Pennsylvania | 29.14 |
| 21. Wisconsin | 23.95 | 46. Arkansas | 29.50 |
| 22. New Mexico | 24.18 | 47. Alabama | 30.36 |
| 23. Kansas | 24.25 | 48. Missouri | 30.45 |
| 24. California | 24.52 | 49. Delaware | 32.59 |
| 25. Arizona | 24.64 | 50. Florida | 33.36 |

**POSITIVE (+) AND NEGATIVE (-) FACTORS CONSIDERED:**
1. Birth Rate (Table 2) +
2. Births of Low Birth Weight as a Percent of Live Births (Table 16) -
3. Death Rate (Table 57) -
4. Infant Mortality Rate (Table 63) -
5. Death Rate by AIDS (Table 84) -
6. Estimated Death Rate by Cancer (Table 87) -
7. Death Rate by Suicide (Table 125) -
8. Community Hospitals per 1,000 Square Miles (Table 136) +
9. Beds in Community Hospitals per 100,000 Population (Table 147) +
10. Percent of Population Covered by Health Insurance (Table 179) +
11. Percent Change in Number of Uninsured: 1989 to 1991 (Table 183) -
12. Per Capita Total Health Care Payments (Table 201) -
13. Annual Percent Change in Per Capita Health Care Payments: 1980 to 1991 (Table 206) -
14. Percent of Average Family Income Spent on Health Care (Table 216) -
15. Total Business Health Care Payments per Employee (Table 255) -
16. Percent of Population Enrolled in Medicare Disabled Program (Table 299) -
17. Estimated New Cancer Cases per 100,000 Population (Table 309) -
18. Combined Notifiable Disease Rate (Tables 334, 338-372) -
19. Active Nonfederal Physicians per 100,000 Population (Table 389) +
20. Per Capita Alcohol Consumption (Table 434) -
21. Percent of Adults Who Smoke (Table 447) -
22. Percent of Adults Overweight (Table 449) -

# TABLE OF CONTENTS

## I. Births and Reproductive Health

## II. Deaths

## III. Facilities

## IV. FINANCE

## V. Incidence of Disease

## VI. Personnel

## VII. PHYSICAL FITNESS

## VIII.   Appendix--Population Charts

## IX.   Sources

## X.   Index

# I. BIRTHS AND REPRODUCTIVE HEALTH

# I. BIRTHS AND REPRODUCTIVE HEALTH (continued)

# Births in 1991

## National Total = 4,111,000 Live Births*

| RANK | STATE | BIRTHS | % | RANK | STATE | BIRTHS | % |
|---|---|---|---|---|---|---|---|
| 1 | California | 605,694 | 14.73% | 26 | Colorado | 53,968 | 1.31% |
| 2 | Texas | 325,562 | 7.92% | 27 | Connecticut | 48,282 | 1.17% |
| 3 | New York | 292,400 | 7.11% | 28 | Oklahoma | 47,312 | 1.15% |
| 4 | Florida | 194,457 | 4.73% | 29 | Mississippi | 43,522 | 1.06% |
| 5 | Illinois | 193,987 | 4.72% | 30 | Oregon | 42,807 | 1.04% |
| 6 | Pennsylvania | 168,584 | 4.10% | 31 | Kansas | 37,300 | 0.91% |
| 7 | Ohio | 158,638 | 3.86% | 32 | Iowa | 36,011 | 0.88% |
| 8 | Michigan | 153,359 | 3.73% | 33 | Utah | 35,070 | 0.85% |
| 9 | New Jersey | 117,789 | 2.87% | 34 | Arkansas | 34,588 | 0.84% |
| 10 | Georgia | 110,024 | 2.68% | 35 | New Mexico | 28,160 | 0.68% |
| 11 | North Carolina | 102,442 | 2.49% | 36 | Nebraska | 23,933 | 0.58% |
| 12 | Virginia | 96,610 | 2.35% | 37 | Nevada | 22,973 | 0.56% |
| 13 | Massachusetts | 86,321 | 2.10% | 38 | West Virginia | 22,195 | 0.54% |
| 14 | Indiana | 84,707 | 2.06% | 39 | Hawaii | 20,014 | 0.49% |
| 15 | Maryland | 84,452 | 2.05% | 40 | Idaho | 17,233 | 0.42% |
| 16 | Missouri | 77,991 | 1.90% | 41 | Maine | 16,581 | 0.40% |
| 17 | Washington | 75,734 | 1.84% | 42 | New Hampshire | 16,060 | 0.39% |
| 18 | Louisiana | 74,562 | 1.81% | 43 | Rhode Island | 14,591 | 0.35% |
| 19 | Tennessee | 73,104 | 1.78% | 44 | Montana | 11,544 | 0.28% |
| 20 | Wisconsin | 71,736 | 1.74% | 45 | Alaska | 11,245 | 0.27% |
| 21 | Arizona | 67,656 | 1.65% | 46 | Delaware | 11,175 | 0.27% |
| 22 | Minnesota | 67,020 | 1.63% | 47 | South Dakota | 11,042 | 0.27% |
| 23 | Alabama | 60,513 | 1.47% | 48 | North Dakota | 9,071 | 0.22% |
| 24 | South Carolina | 57,742 | 1.40% | 49 | Vermont | 7,712 | 0.19% |
| 25 | Kentucky | 54,913 | 1.34% | 50 | Wyoming | 6,801 | 0.17% |
| | | | | | District of Columbia | 9,971 | 0.24% |

Source: U.S. Department of Health and Human Services, National Center for Health Statistics
"Monthly Vital Statistics Report" (Vol. 40, No. 13, September 30, 1992)
*Data are provisional estimates by state of residence.

# Birth Rate in 1991

## National Rate = 16.2 Live Births per 1,000 Population*

| RANK | STATE | RATE | | RANK | STATE | RATE |
|------|-------|------|---|------|-------|------|
| 1 | Alaska | 21.1 | | 26 | Missouri | 15.0 |
| 2 | Utah | 20.1 | | 27 | Indiana | 14.9 |
| 3 | California | 19.8 | | 28 | Connecticut | 14.8 |
| 4 | Nevada | 18.8 | | 29 | Kentucky | 14.7 |
| 4 | Texas | 18.8 | | 29 | Nebraska | 14.7 |
| 6 | Arizona | 18.3 | | 29 | Oklahoma | 14.7 |
| 7 | New Mexico | 18.0 | | 32 | Alabama | 14.6 |
| 8 | Hawaii | 17.5 | | 32 | Florida | 14.6 |
| 8 | Maryland | 17.5 | | 32 | Kansas | 14.6 |
| 10 | Louisiana | 17.2 | | 32 | Oregon | 14.6 |
| 11 | Georgia | 16.6 | | 32 | Wyoming | 14.6 |
| 11 | Idaho | 16.6 | | 37 | Massachusetts | 14.5 |
| 11 | Mississippi | 16.6 | | 37 | Rhode Island | 14.5 |
| 14 | Illinois | 16.5 | | 37 | Tennessee | 14.5 |
| 15 | Michigan | 16.4 | | 37 | Wisconsin | 14.5 |
| 16 | New York | 16.2 | | 41 | Ohio | 14.4 |
| 17 | Colorado | 16.1 | | 42 | Montana | 14.3 |
| 18 | Delaware | 16.0 | | 43 | Arkansas | 14.2 |
| 18 | South Carolina | 16.0 | | 44 | North Dakota | 14.0 |
| 20 | South Dakota | 15.4 | | 45 | New Hampshire | 13.9 |
| 20 | Virginia | 15.4 | | 45 | Pennsylvania | 13.9 |
| 22 | North Carolina | 15.2 | | 47 | Maine | 13.2 |
| 22 | Washington | 15.2 | | 47 | Vermont | 13.2 |
| 24 | Minnesota | 15.1 | | 49 | Iowa | 12.6 |
| 24 | New Jersey | 15.1 | | 50 | West Virginia | 12.2 |
| | | | | | District of Columbia | 17.0 |

Source: U.S. Department of Health and Human Services, National Center for Health Statistics
   "Monthly Vital Statistics Report" (Vol. 40, No. 13, September 30, 1992)
*Data are provisional estimates by state of residence.

# Births in 1990

## National Total = 4,179,000 Live Births*

| RANK | STATE | BIRTHS | % | RANK | STATE | BIRTHS | % |
|---|---|---|---|---|---|---|---|
| 1 | California | 617,989 | 14.79% | 26 | Colorado | 52,913 | 1.27% |
| 2 | Texas | 325,752 | 7.79% | 27 | Connecticut | 52,315 | 1.25% |
| 3 | New York | 301,209 | 7.21% | 28 | Oklahoma | 47,250 | 1.13% |
| 4 | Florida | 199,641 | 4.78% | 29 | Oregon | 44,408 | 1.06% |
| 5 | Illinois | 196,107 | 4.69% | 30 | Mississippi | 43,849 | 1.05% |
| 6 | Pennsylvania | 170,888 | 4.09% | 31 | Kansas | 40,074 | 0.96% |
| 7 | Ohio | 164,619 | 3.94% | 32 | Iowa | 39,127 | 0.94% |
| 8 | Michigan | 159,346 | 3.81% | 33 | Utah | 36,216 | 0.87% |
| 9 | New Jersey | 124,082 | 2.97% | 34 | Arkansas | 36,109 | 0.86% |
| 10 | Georgia | 112,899 | 2.70% | 35 | New Mexico | 28,654 | 0.69% |
| 11 | North Carolina | 104,715 | 2.51% | 36 | Nebraska | 24,010 | 0.57% |
| 12 | Virginia | 99,942 | 2.39% | 37 | West Virginia | 22,202 | 0.53% |
| 13 | Massachusetts | 93,222 | 2.23% | 38 | Nevada | 21,255 | 0.51% |
| 14 | Indiana | 85,227 | 2.04% | 39 | Hawaii | 20,413 | 0.49% |
| 15 | Maryland | 83,664 | 2.00% | 40 | New Hampshire | 17,199 | 0.41% |
| 16 | Missouri | 81,157 | 1.94% | 41 | Maine | 16,908 | 0.40% |
| 17 | Washington | 78,106 | 1.87% | 42 | Idaho | 16,594 | 0.40% |
| 18 | Wisconsin | 72,969 | 1.75% | 43 | Rhode Island | 14,963 | 0.36% |
| 19 | Tennessee | 72,747 | 1.74% | 44 | Montana | 11,758 | 0.28% |
| 20 | Louisiana | 71,704 | 1.72% | 45 | Alaska | 11,647 | 0.28% |
| 21 | Arizona | 68,749 | 1.65% | 46 | Delaware | 11,282 | 0.27% |
| 22 | Minnesota | 68,378 | 1.64% | 47 | South Dakota | 10,912 | 0.26% |
| 23 | Alabama | 68,200 | 1.63% | 48 | North Dakota | 9,517 | 0.23% |
| 24 | South Carolina | 59,075 | 1.41% | 49 | Vermont | 8,282 | 0.20% |
| 25 | Kentucky | 57,791 | 1.38% | 50 | Wyoming | 6,984 | 0.17% |
| | | | | | District of Columbia | 10,928 | 0.26% |

Source: U.S. Department of Health and Human Services, National Center for Health Statistics
"Monthly Vital Statistics Report" (Vol. 40, No. 13, September 30, 1992)
*Data are updated, provisional estimates by state of residence.

# Birth Rate in 1990

## National Rate = 16.7 Live Births per 1,000 Population*

| RANK | STATE | RATE | RANK | STATE | RATE |
|---|---|---|---|---|---|
| 1 | Alaska | 22.0 | 26 | Massachusetts | 15.7 |
| 2 | Utah | 21.0 | 26 | Missouri | 15.7 |
| 3 | California | 20.7 | 26 | North Carolina | 15.7 |
| 4 | Texas | 19.0 | 29 | Kentucky | 15.5 |
| 5 | Arizona | 18.9 | 29 | Minnesota | 15.5 |
| 6 | New Mexico | 18.5 | 31 | Oregon | 15.4 |
| 7 | Nevada | 18.2 | 32 | Florida | 15.3 |
| 8 | Hawaii | 18.1 | 33 | New Hampshire | 15.2 |
| 9 | Maryland | 17.6 | 33 | South Dakota | 15.2 |
| 10 | Georgia | 17.3 | 35 | Indiana | 15.1 |
| 11 | Michigan | 17.1 | 36 | Ohio | 15.0 |
| 12 | Illinois | 16.7 | 37 | Arkansas | 14.9 |
| 12 | Mississippi | 16.7 | 37 | Rhode Island | 14.9 |
| 12 | New York | 16.7 | 37 | Wisconsin | 14.9 |
| 15 | South Carolina | 16.6 | 37 | Wyoming | 14.9 |
| 16 | Alabama | 16.5 | 41 | Nebraska | 14.8 |
| 17 | Delaware | 16.4 | 42 | Oklahoma | 14.7 |
| 17 | Louisiana | 16.4 | 43 | Montana | 14.6 |
| 19 | Idaho | 16.2 | 43 | North Dakota | 14.6 |
| 19 | Virginia | 16.2 | 43 | Tennessee | 14.6 |
| 21 | Connecticut | 16.1 | 46 | Vermont | 14.4 |
| 22 | New Jersey | 16.0 | 47 | Pennsylvania | 14.1 |
| 22 | Washington | 16.0 | 48 | Iowa | 13.7 |
| 24 | Colorado | 15.9 | 49 | Maine | 13.6 |
| 25 | Kansas | 15.8 | 50 | West Virginia | 12.1 |
| | | | | District of Columbia | 18.4 |

Source: U.S. Department of Health and Human Services, National Center for Health Statistics
    "Monthly Vital Statistics Report" (Vol. 40, No. 13, September 30, 1992)
*Data are updated, provisional estimates by state of residence.

# Births in 1989

## National Total = 4,040,958 Births*

| RANK | STATE | BIRTHS | % | RANK | STATE | BIRTHS | % |
|---|---|---|---|---|---|---|---|
| 1 | California | 569,992 | 14.11% | 26 | Colorado | 52,711 | 1.30% |
| 2 | Texas | 307,664 | 7.61% | 27 | Connecticut | 49,464 | 1.22% |
| 3 | New York | 291,449 | 7.21% | 28 | Oklahoma | 47,385 | 1.17% |
| 4 | Florida | 193,131 | 4.78% | 29 | Mississippi | 43,047 | 1.07% |
| 5 | Illinois | 190,308 | 4.71% | 30 | Oregon | 41,281 | 1.02% |
| 6 | Pennsylvania | 168,803 | 4.18% | 31 | Iowa | 39,018 | 0.97% |
| 7 | Ohio | 163,952 | 4.06% | 32 | Kansas | 38,737 | 0.96% |
| 8 | Michigan | 148,520 | 3.68% | 33 | Arkansas | 35,911 | 0.89% |
| 9 | New Jersey | 121,841 | 3.02% | 34 | Utah | 35,567 | 0.88% |
| 10 | Georgia | 110,272 | 2.73% | 35 | New Mexico | 27,353 | 0.68% |
| 11 | North Carolina | 102,105 | 2.53% | 36 | Nebraska | 24,216 | 0.60% |
| 12 | Virginia | 96,798 | 2.40% | 37 | West Virginia | 22,163 | 0.55% |
| 13 | Massachusetts | 91,523 | 2.26% | 38 | Nevada | 19,606 | 0.49% |
| 14 | Indiana | 83,469 | 2.07% | 39 | Hawaii | 19,367 | 0.48% |
| 15 | Maryland | 78,265 | 1.94% | 40 | New Hampshire | 17,809 | 0.44% |
| 16 | Missouri | 77,872 | 1.93% | 41 | Maine | 17,466 | 0.43% |
| 17 | Washington | 75,360 | 1.86% | 42 | Idaho | 15,883 | 0.39% |
| 18 | Tennessee | 73,178 | 1.81% | 43 | Rhode Island | 14,768 | 0.37% |
| 19 | Louisiana | 72,752 | 1.80% | 44 | Montana | 11,678 | 0.29% |
| 20 | Wisconsin | 72,002 | 1.78% | 45 | Alaska | 11,666 | 0.29% |
| 21 | Minnesota | 67,518 | 1.67% | 46 | South Dakota | 11,086 | 0.27% |
| 22 | Arizona | 67,196 | 1.66% | 47 | Delaware | 10,730 | 0.27% |
| 23 | Alabama | 62,568 | 1.55% | 48 | North Dakota | 9,570 | 0.24% |
| 24 | South Carolina | 57,330 | 1.42% | 49 | Vermont | 8,494 | 0.21% |
| 25 | Kentucky | 53,424 | 1.32% | 50 | Wyoming | 6,901 | 0.17% |
| | | | | | District of Columbia | 11,789 | 0.29% |

Source: U.S. Department of Health and Human Services, Centers for Disease Control, National Center for Health Statistics
"Monthly Vital Statistics Report" (December 12, 1991)
*By state of residence.

# Births in 1980

## National Total = 3,612,000 Births*

| RANK | STATE | BIRTHS | % | RANK | STATE | BIRTHS | % |
|---|---|---|---|---|---|---|---|
| 1 | California | 403,000 | 11.16% | 26 | Arizona | 50,000 | 1.38% |
| 2 | Texas | 274,000 | 7.59% | 26 | Colorado | 50,000 | 1.38% |
| 3 | New York | 239,000 | 6.62% | 28 | Iowa | 48,000 | 1.33% |
| 4 | Illinois | 190,000 | 5.26% | 28 | Mississippi | 48,000 | 1.33% |
| 5 | Ohio | 169,000 | 4.68% | 30 | Oregon | 43,000 | 1.19% |
| 6 | Pennsylvania | 159,000 | 4.40% | 31 | Utah | 42,000 | 1.16% |
| 7 | Michigan | 146,000 | 4.04% | 32 | Kansas | 41,000 | 1.14% |
| 8 | Florida | 132,000 | 3.65% | 33 | Connecticut | 39,000 | 1.08% |
| 9 | New Jersey | 97,000 | 2.69% | 34 | Arkansas | 37,000 | 1.02% |
| 10 | Georgia | 92,000 | 2.55% | 35 | West Virginia | 29,000 | 0.80% |
| 11 | Indiana | 88,000 | 2.44% | 36 | Nebraska | 27,000 | 0.75% |
| 12 | North Carolina | 84,000 | 2.33% | 37 | New Mexico | 26,000 | 0.72% |
| 13 | Louisiana | 82,000 | 2.27% | 38 | Idaho | 20,000 | 0.55% |
| 14 | Missouri | 79,000 | 2.19% | 39 | Hawaii | 18,000 | 0.50% |
| 15 | Virginia | 78,000 | 2.16% | 40 | Maine | 16,000 | 0.44% |
| 16 | Wisconsin | 75,000 | 2.08% | 41 | Montana | 14,000 | 0.39% |
| 17 | Massachusetts | 73,000 | 2.02% | 41 | New Hampshire | 14,000 | 0.39% |
| 18 | Tennessee | 69,000 | 1.91% | 43 | Nevada | 13,000 | 0.36% |
| 19 | Minnesota | 68,000 | 1.88% | 43 | South Dakota | 13,000 | 0.36% |
| 19 | Washington | 68,000 | 1.88% | 45 | North Dakota | 12,000 | 0.33% |
| 21 | Alabama | 64,000 | 1.77% | 45 | Rhode Island | 12,000 | 0.33% |
| 22 | Kentucky | 60,000 | 1.66% | 47 | Wyoming | 11,000 | 0.30% |
| 22 | Maryland | 60,000 | 1.66% | 48 | Alaska | 10,000 | 0.28% |
| 24 | Oklahoma | 52,000 | 1.44% | 49 | Delaware | 9,000 | 0.25% |
| 24 | South Carolina | 52,000 | 1.44% | 50 | Vermont | 8,000 | 0.22% |
| | | | | | District of Columbia | 9,000 | 0.25% |

Source: U.S. Department of Health and Human Services, Centers for Disease Control, National Center for Health Statistics
"Vital Statistics of the United States, 1980" and "Monthly Vital Statistics Report"
*Live births by state of residence.

# Birth Rate in 1980

## National Rate = 15.9 Births per 1,000 Population*

| RANK | STATE | RATE | RANK | STATE | RATE |
|------|-------|------|------|-------|------|
| 1 | Utah | 28.6 | 24 | Washington | 16.4 |
| 2 | Alaska | 23.7 | 27 | Alabama | 16.3 |
| 3 | Wyoming | 22.5 | 27 | Arkansas | 16.3 |
| 4 | Idaho | 21.4 | 27 | Kentucky | 16.3 |
| 5 | New Mexico | 20.0 | 30 | Indiana | 16.1 |
| 6 | Louisiana | 19.5 | 30 | Missouri | 16.1 |
| 7 | South Dakota | 19.2 | 32 | Wisconsin | 15.9 |
| 7 | Texas | 19.2 | 33 | Delaware | 15.8 |
| 9 | Mississippi | 19.0 | 34 | Michigan | 15.7 |
| 10 | Hawaii | 18.8 | 34 | Ohio | 15.7 |
| 11 | Arizona | 18.4 | 36 | Vermont | 15.4 |
| 11 | North Dakota | 18.4 | 37 | Tennessee | 15.1 |
| 13 | Montana | 18.1 | 37 | West Virginia | 15.1 |
| 14 | Nebraska | 17.4 | 39 | New Hampshire | 14.9 |
| 15 | Colorado | 17.2 | 40 | Virginia | 14.7 |
| 15 | Kansas | 17.2 | 41 | Maine | 14.6 |
| 15 | Oklahoma | 17.2 | 42 | North Carolina | 14.4 |
| 18 | California | 17.0 | 43 | Maryland | 14.2 |
| 19 | Georgia | 16.9 | 44 | New York | 13.6 |
| 20 | Illinois | 16.6 | 45 | Florida | 13.5 |
| 20 | Minnesota | 16.6 | 46 | Pennsylvania | 13.4 |
| 20 | Nevada | 16.6 | 47 | New Jersey | 13.2 |
| 20 | South Carolina | 16.6 | 48 | Rhode Island | 12.9 |
| 24 | Iowa | 16.4 | 49 | Massachusetts | 12.7 |
| 24 | Oregon | 16.4 | 50 | Connecticut | 12.5 |
|  |  |  |  | District of Columbia | 14.7 |

Source: U.S. Department of Health and Human Services, Centers for Disease Control, National Center for Health Statistics
    "Vital Statistics of the United States, 1980" and "Monthly Vital Statistics Report"
* Live births by state of residence.

# Male Births in 1989

## National Total = 2,069,490 Males Born

| RANK | STATE | MALES | % | RANK | STATE | MALES | % |
|---|---|---|---|---|---|---|---|
| 1 | California | 291,386 | 14.08% | 26 | Colorado | 26,923 | 1.30% |
| 2 | Texas | 157,134 | 7.59% | 27 | Connecticut | 25,349 | 1.22% |
| 3 | New York | 149,711 | 7.23% | 28 | Oklahoma | 24,262 | 1.17% |
| 4 | Florida | 99,013 | 4.78% | 29 | Mississippi | 21,976 | 1.06% |
| 5 | Illinois | 97,055 | 4.69% | 30 | Oregon | 21,304 | 1.03% |
| 6 | Pennsylvania | 86,530 | 4.18% | 31 | Kansas | 19,965 | 0.96% |
| 7 | Ohio | 83,883 | 4.05% | 32 | Iowa | 19,955 | 0.96% |
| 8 | Michigan | 76,270 | 3.69% | 33 | Arkansas | 18,408 | 0.89% |
| 9 | New Jersey | 62,446 | 3.02% | 34 | Utah | 18,356 | 0.89% |
| 10 | Georgia | 56,640 | 2.74% | 35 | New Mexico | 14,005 | 0.68% |
| 11 | North Carolina | 52,066 | 2.52% | 36 | Nebraska | 12,520 | 0.60% |
| 12 | Virginia | 49,477 | 2.39% | 37 | West Virginia | 11,289 | 0.55% |
| 13 | Massachusetts | 46,915 | 2.27% | 38 | Nevada | 10,159 | 0.49% |
| 14 | Indiana | 42,904 | 2.07% | 39 | Hawaii | 9,911 | 0.48% |
| 15 | Missouri | 39,962 | 1.93% | 40 | Maine | 9,017 | 0.44% |
| 16 | Maryland | 39,954 | 1.93% | 41 | New Hampshire | 9,008 | 0.44% |
| 17 | Washington | 38,553 | 1.86% | 42 | Idaho | 8,249 | 0.40% |
| 18 | Tennessee | 37,481 | 1.81% | 43 | Rhode Island | 7,581 | 0.37% |
| 19 | Louisiana | 37,303 | 1.80% | 44 | Montana | 5,923 | 0.29% |
| 20 | Wisconsin | 36,829 | 1.78% | 45 | Alaska | 5,878 | 0.28% |
| 21 | Arizona | 34,521 | 1.67% | 46 | South Dakota | 5,718 | 0.28% |
| 22 | Minnesota | 34,435 | 1.66% | 47 | Delaware | 5,515 | 0.27% |
| 23 | Alabama | 32,163 | 1.55% | 48 | North Dakota | 4,891 | 0.24% |
| 24 | South Carolina | 29,250 | 1.41% | 49 | Vermont | 4,371 | 0.21% |
| 25 | Kentucky | 27,519 | 1.33% | 50 | Wyoming | 3,526 | 0.17% |
| | | | | | District of Columbia | 6,031 | 0.29% |

Source: U.S. Department of Health and Human Services, National Center for Health Statistics
Unpublished data (March 4, 1992)

# Female Births in 1989

## National Total = 1,971,468 Females Born

| RANK | STATE | FEMALES | % | RANK | STATE | FEMALES | % |
|---|---|---|---|---|---|---|---|
| 1 | California | 273,606 | 14.13% | 26 | Colorado | 25,788 | 1.31% |
| 2 | Texas | 150,530 | 7.64% | 27 | Connecticut | 24,115 | 1.22% |
| 3 | New York | 141,738 | 7.19% | 28 | Oklahoma | 23,123 | 1.17% |
| 4 | Florida | 94,118 | 4.77% | 29 | Mississippi | 21,071 | 1.07% |
| 5 | Illinois | 93,253 | 4.73% | 30 | Oregon | 19,977 | 1.01% |
| 6 | Pennsylvania | 82,273 | 4.17% | 31 | Iowa | 19,063 | 0.97% |
| 7 | Ohio | 80,069 | 4.06% | 32 | Kansas | 18,772 | 0.95% |
| 8 | Michigan | 72,250 | 3.66% | 33 | Arkansas | 17,503 | 0.89% |
| 9 | New Jersey | 59,395 | 3.01% | 34 | Utah | 17,211 | 0.87% |
| 10 | Georgia | 53,632 | 2.72% | 35 | New Mexico | 13,348 | 0.68% |
| 11 | North Carolina | 50,039 | 2.54% | 36 | Nebraska | 11,696 | 0.59% |
| 12 | Virginia | 47,321 | 2.40% | 37 | West Virginia | 10,874 | 0.55% |
| 13 | Massachusetts | 44,608 | 2.26% | 38 | Hawaii | 9,456 | 0.48% |
| 14 | Indiana | 40,565 | 2.06% | 39 | Nevada | 9,447 | 0.48% |
| 15 | Maryland | 38,311 | 1.94% | 40 | New Hampshire | 8,801 | 0.45% |
| 16 | Missouri | 37,910 | 1.92% | 41 | Maine | 8,449 | 0.43% |
| 17 | Washington | 36,807 | 1.87% | 42 | Idaho | 7,634 | 0.39% |
| 18 | Tennessee | 35,697 | 1.81% | 43 | Rhode Island | 7,187 | 0.36% |
| 19 | Louisiana | 35,449 | 1.80% | 44 | Alaska | 5,788 | 0.29% |
| 20 | Wisconsin | 35,173 | 1.78% | 45 | Montana | 5,755 | 0.29% |
| 21 | Minnesota | 33,083 | 1.68% | 46 | South Dakota | 5,368 | 0.27% |
| 22 | Arizona | 32,675 | 1.66% | 47 | Delaware | 5,215 | 0.26% |
| 23 | Alabama | 30,405 | 1.54% | 48 | North Dakota | 4,679 | 0.24% |
| 24 | South Carolina | 28,080 | 1.42% | 49 | Vermont | 4,123 | 0.21% |
| 25 | Kentucky | 25,905 | 1.31% | 50 | Wyoming | 3,375 | 0.17% |
| | | | | | District of Columbia | 5,758 | 0.29% |

Source: U.S. Department of Health and Human Services, National Center for Health Statistics
   Unpublished data (March 4, 1992)

# Ratio of Males to Females Born in 1989

## National Rate = 1.050 Males Born for Every Female Born*

| RANK | STATE | RATIO | | RANK | STATE | RATIO |
|---|---|---|---|---|---|---|
| 1 | Idaho | 1.081 | | 25 | New Jersey | 1.051 |
| 2 | Nevada | 1.075 | | 27 | Tennessee | 1.050 |
| 3 | Nebraska | 1.070 | | 28 | New Mexico | 1.049 |
| 4 | Maine | 1.067 | | 28 | Oklahoma | 1.049 |
| 4 | Utah | 1.067 | | 30 | Hawaii | 1.048 |
| 6 | Oregon | 1.066 | | 30 | Ohio | 1.048 |
| 7 | South Dakota | 1.065 | | 32 | Iowa | 1.047 |
| 8 | Kansas | 1.064 | | 32 | Washington | 1.047 |
| 9 | Kentucky | 1.062 | | 32 | Wisconsin | 1.047 |
| 10 | Vermont | 1.060 | | 35 | California | 1.046 |
| 11 | Alabama | 1.058 | | 35 | Virginia | 1.046 |
| 11 | Delaware | 1.058 | | 37 | North Dakota | 1.045 |
| 11 | Indiana | 1.058 | | 37 | Wyoming | 1.045 |
| 14 | Arizona | 1.056 | | 39 | Colorado | 1.044 |
| 14 | Georgia | 1.056 | | 39 | Texas | 1.044 |
| 14 | Michigan | 1.056 | | 41 | Maryland | 1.043 |
| 14 | New York | 1.056 | | 41 | Mississippi | 1.043 |
| 18 | Rhode Island | 1.055 | | 43 | South Carolina | 1.042 |
| 19 | Missouri | 1.054 | | 44 | Illinois | 1.041 |
| 20 | Arkansas | 1.052 | | 44 | Minnesota | 1.041 |
| 20 | Florida | 1.052 | | 44 | North Carolina | 1.041 |
| 20 | Louisiana | 1.052 | | 47 | West Virginia | 1.038 |
| 20 | Massachusetts | 1.052 | | 48 | Montana | 1.029 |
| 20 | Pennsylvania | 1.052 | | 49 | New Hampshire | 1.024 |
| 25 | Connecticut | 1.051 | | 50 | Alaska | 1.016 |

| | | | | | District of Columbia | 1.047 |

Source: U.S. Department of Health and Human Services, National Center for Health Statistics
     Unpublished data (March 4, 1992)
*Calculated by the editors.

# White Births in 1989

## National Total = 3,131,991 White Births*

| RANK | STATE | BIRTHS | % | RANK | STATE | BIRTHS | % |
|---|---|---|---|---|---|---|---|
| 1 | California | 448,489 | 14.32% | 26 | Alabama | 40,125 | 1.28% |
| 2 | Texas | 255,070 | 8.14% | 27 | Oregon | 37,498 | 1.20% |
| 3 | New York | 211,904 | 6.77% | 28 | Iowa | 37,032 | 1.18% |
| 4 | Florida | 143,309 | 4.58% | 29 | Oklahoma | 35,589 | 1.14% |
| 5 | Illinois | 139,435 | 4.45% | 30 | South Carolina | 34,214 | 1.09% |
| 6 | Pennsylvania | 138,442 | 4.42% | 31 | Kansas | 33,786 | 1.08% |
| 7 | Ohio | 135,177 | 4.32% | 32 | Utah | 33,250 | 1.06% |
| 8 | Michigan | 114,493 | 3.66% | 33 | Arkansas | 26,787 | 0.86% |
| 9 | New Jersey | 91,675 | 2.93% | 34 | New Mexico | 22,068 | 0.70% |
| 10 | Massachusetts | 78,089 | 2.49% | 35 | Mississippi | 21,970 | 0.70% |
| 11 | Indiana | 72,807 | 2.32% | 36 | Nebraska | 21,941 | 0.70% |
| 12 | Virginia | 69,636 | 2.22% | 37 | West Virginia | 21,113 | 0.67% |
| 13 | Georgia | 68,484 | 2.19% | 38 | New Hampshire | 17,432 | 0.56% |
| 14 | North Carolina | 68,449 | 2.19% | 39 | Maine | 17,080 | 0.55% |
| 15 | Washington | 64,337 | 2.05% | 40 | Nevada | 16,313 | 0.52% |
| 16 | Missouri | 63,185 | 2.02% | 41 | Idaho | 15,157 | 0.48% |
| 17 | Wisconsin | 62,035 | 1.98% | 42 | Rhode Island | 12,825 | 0.41% |
| 18 | Minnesota | 60,638 | 1.94% | 43 | Montana | 9,871 | 0.32% |
| 19 | Arizona | 56,208 | 1.79% | 44 | South Dakota | 9,001 | 0.29% |
| 20 | Tennessee | 54,539 | 1.74% | 45 | Vermont | 8,388 | 0.27% |
| 21 | Maryland | 50,209 | 1.60% | 46 | North Dakota | 8,303 | 0.27% |
| 22 | Kentucky | 47,614 | 1.52% | 47 | Delaware | 7,955 | 0.25% |
| 23 | Colorado | 47,476 | 1.52% | 48 | Alaska | 7,457 | 0.24% |
| 24 | Louisiana | 41,256 | 1.32% | 49 | Wyoming | 6,447 | 0.21% |
| 25 | Connecticut | 41,251 | 1.32% | 50 | Hawaii | 4,477 | 0.14% |
| | | | | | District of Columbia | 1,705 | 0.05% |

Source: U.S. Department of Health and Human Services, Centers for Disease Control, National Center for Health Statistics

"Monthly Vital Statistics Report" (December 12, 1991)

*Race of child, not mother. Live births by state of residence.

# White Births as a Percent of Live Births in 1989

## National Rate = 77.51% of Live Births*

| RANK | STATE | PERCENT | | RANK | STATE | PERCENT |
|------|-------|---------|---|------|-------|---------|
| 1 | Vermont | 98.75 | | 26 | Ohio | 82.45 |
| 2 | New Hampshire | 97.88 | | 27 | Pennsylvania | 82.01 |
| 3 | Maine | 97.79 | | 28 | South Dakota | 81.19 |
| 4 | Idaho | 95.43 | | 29 | Missouri | 81.14 |
| 5 | West Virginia | 95.26 | | 30 | New Mexico | 80.68 |
| 6 | Iowa | 94.91 | | 31 | California | 78.68 |
| 7 | Utah | 93.49 | | 32 | Michigan | 77.09 |
| 8 | Wyoming | 93.42 | | 33 | New Jersey | 75.24 |
| 9 | Oregon | 90.84 | | 34 | Oklahoma | 75.11 |
| 10 | Nebraska | 90.61 | | 35 | Arkansas | 74.59 |
| 11 | Colorado | 90.07 | | 36 | Tennessee | 74.53 |
| 12 | Minnesota | 89.81 | | 37 | Florida | 74.20 |
| 13 | Kentucky | 89.12 | | 38 | Delaware | 74.14 |
| 14 | Indiana | 87.23 | | 39 | Illinois | 73.27 |
| 15 | Kansas | 87.22 | | 40 | New York | 72.71 |
| 16 | Rhode Island | 86.84 | | 41 | Virginia | 71.94 |
| 17 | North Dakota | 86.76 | | 42 | North Carolina | 67.04 |
| 18 | Wisconsin | 86.16 | | 43 | Maryland | 64.15 |
| 19 | Washington | 85.37 | | 44 | Alabama | 64.13 |
| 20 | Massachusetts | 85.32 | | 45 | Alaska | 63.92 |
| 21 | Montana | 84.53 | | 46 | Georgia | 62.10 |
| 22 | Arizona | 83.65 | | 47 | South Carolina | 59.68 |
| 23 | Connecticut | 83.40 | | 48 | Louisiana | 56.71 |
| 24 | Nevada | 83.20 | | 49 | Mississippi | 51.04 |
| 25 | Texas | 82.91 | | 50 | Hawaii | 23.12 |
| | | | | | District of Columbia | 14.46 |

Source: U.S. Department of Health and Human Services, Centers for Disease Control, National Center for Health Statistics
   "Monthly Vital Statistics Report" (December 12, 1991)
*Rates calculated by the editors. Race of child, not mother. Live births by state of residence.

# Black Births in 1989

## National Total = 709,395 Black Births*

| RANK | STATE | BIRTHS | % | RANK | STATE | BIRTHS | % |
|------|-------|--------|---|------|-------|--------|---|
| 1 | New York | 66,286 | 9.34% | 26 | Kentucky | 5,362 | 0.76% |
| 2 | California | 56,631 | 7.98% | 27 | Washington | 3,994 | 0.56% |
| 3 | Florida | 46,617 | 6.57% | 28 | Kansas | 3,734 | 0.53% |
| 4 | Texas | 45,160 | 6.37% | 29 | Colorado | 3,252 | 0.46% |
| 5 | Illinois | 45,085 | 6.36% | 30 | Arizona | 3,097 | 0.44% |
| 6 | Georgia | 40,070 | 5.65% | 31 | Minnesota | 2,951 | 0.42% |
| 7 | Michigan | 30,856 | 4.35% | 32 | Delaware | 2,589 | 0.36% |
| 8 | North Carolina | 30,703 | 4.33% | 33 | Nevada | 2,035 | 0.29% |
| 9 | Louisiana | 29,995 | 4.23% | 34 | Nebraska | 1,546 | 0.22% |
| 10 | Pennsylvania | 27,308 | 3.85% | 35 | Rhode Island | 1,275 | 0.18% |
| 11 | Ohio | 26,836 | 3.78% | 36 | Iowa | 1,260 | 0.18% |
| 12 | New Jersey | 25,164 | 3.55% | 37 | Oregon | 1,204 | 0.17% |
| 13 | Maryland | 24,885 | 3.51% | 38 | Hawaii | 936 | 0.13% |
| 14 | Virginia | 24,104 | 3.40% | 39 | West Virginia | 928 | 0.13% |
| 15 | South Carolina | 22,516 | 3.17% | 40 | New Mexico | 731 | 0.10% |
| 16 | Alabama | 21,850 | 3.08% | 41 | Alaska | 705 | 0.10% |
| 17 | Mississippi | 20,544 | 2.90% | 42 | Utah | 372 | 0.05% |
| 18 | Tennessee | 17,867 | 2.52% | 43 | New Hampshire | 184 | 0.03% |
| 19 | Missouri | 13,360 | 1.88% | 44 | South Dakota | 130 | 0.02% |
| 20 | Indiana | 9,620 | 1.36% | 45 | Maine | 124 | 0.02% |
| 21 | Massachusetts | 9,513 | 1.34% | 46 | North Dakota | 112 | 0.02% |
| 22 | Arkansas | 8,588 | 1.21% | 47 | Wyoming | 99 | 0.01% |
| 23 | Wisconsin | 7,216 | 1.02% | 48 | Idaho | 93 | 0.01% |
| 24 | Connecticut | 7,006 | 0.99% | 49 | Montana | 70 | 0.01% |
| 25 | Oklahoma | 5,523 | 0.78% | 50 | Vermont | 40 | 0.01% |
| | | | | | District of Columbia | 9,269 | 1.31% |

Source: U.S. Department of Health and Human Services, Centers for Disease Control, National Center for Health Statistics
"Monthly Vital Statistics Report" (December 12, 1991)
*Race of child, not mother. Live births by state of residence.

# Black Births as a Percent of Live Births in 1989

## National Rate = 17.56% of Live Births*

| RANK | STATE | PERCENT | RANK | STATE | PERCENT |
|------|-------|---------|------|-------|---------|
| 1 | Mississippi | 47.72 | 26 | Kentucky | 10.04 |
| 2 | Louisiana | 41.23 | 27 | Wisconsin | 10.02 |
| 3 | South Carolina | 39.27 | 28 | California | 9.94 |
| 4 | Georgia | 36.34 | 29 | Kansas | 9.64 |
| 5 | Alabama | 34.92 | 30 | Rhode Island | 8.63 |
| 6 | Maryland | 31.80 | 31 | Nebraska | 6.38 |
| 7 | North Carolina | 30.07 | 32 | Colorado | 6.17 |
| 8 | Virginia | 24.90 | 33 | Alaska | 6.04 |
| 9 | Tennessee | 24.42 | 34 | Washington | 5.30 |
| 10 | Florida | 24.14 | 35 | Hawaii | 4.83 |
| 11 | Delaware | 24.13 | 36 | Arizona | 4.61 |
| 12 | Arkansas | 23.91 | 37 | Minnesota | 4.37 |
| 13 | Illinois | 23.69 | 38 | West Virginia | 4.19 |
| 14 | New York | 22.74 | 39 | Iowa | 3.23 |
| 15 | Michigan | 20.78 | 40 | Oregon | 2.92 |
| 16 | New Jersey | 20.65 | 41 | New Mexico | 2.67 |
| 17 | Missouri | 17.16 | 42 | Wyoming | 1.43 |
| 18 | Ohio | 16.37 | 43 | North Dakota | 1.17 |
| 19 | Pennsylvania | 16.18 | 43 | South Dakota | 1.17 |
| 20 | Texas | 14.68 | 45 | Utah | 1.05 |
| 21 | Connecticut | 14.16 | 46 | New Hampshire | 1.03 |
| 22 | Oklahoma | 11.66 | 47 | Maine | 0.71 |
| 23 | Indiana | 11.53 | 48 | Montana | 0.60 |
| 24 | Massachusetts | 10.39 | 49 | Idaho | 0.59 |
| 25 | Nevada | 10.38 | 50 | Vermont | 0.47 |

District of Columbia          78.62

Source: U.S. Department of Health and Human Services, Centers for Disease Control, National Center for Health Statistics
        "Monthly Vital Statistics Report" (December 12, 1991)
*Rates calculated by the editors.  Race of child, not mother.  Live births by state of residence.

# Births of Low Birth Weight in 1989

## National Total = 284,391 Births of Low Birth Weight*

| RANK | STATE | BIRTHS | % | RANK | STATE | BIRTHS | % |
|---|---|---|---|---|---|---|---|
| 1 | California | 34,764 | 12.22% | 26 | Kentucky | 3,657 | 1.29% |
| 2 | New York | 22,282 | 7.83% | 27 | Connecticut | 3,414 | 1.20% |
| 3 | Texas | 21,462 | 7.55% | 28 | Minnesota | 3,309 | 1.16% |
| 4 | Florida | 14,808 | 5.21% | 29 | Oklahoma | 3,068 | 1.08% |
| 5 | Illinois | 14,645 | 5.15% | 30 | Arkansas | 2,973 | 1.05% |
| 6 | Pennsylvania | 11,943 | 4.20% | 31 | Kansas | 2,370 | 0.83% |
| 7 | Ohio | 11,512 | 4.05% | 32 | Oregon | 2,151 | 0.76% |
| 8 | Michigan | 11,275 | 3.96% | 33 | Iowa | 2,116 | 0.74% |
| 9 | Georgia | 9,202 | 3.24% | 34 | Utah | 2,014 | 0.71% |
| 10 | New Jersey | 8,902 | 3.13% | 35 | New Mexico | 1,896 | 0.67% |
| 11 | North Carolina | 8,270 | 2.91% | 36 | West Virginia | 1,472 | 0.52% |
| 12 | Virginia | 6,872 | 2.42% | 37 | Nevada | 1,410 | 0.50% |
| 13 | Louisiana | 6,626 | 2.33% | 38 | Nebraska | 1,402 | 0.49% |
| 14 | Maryland | 6,260 | 2.20% | 39 | Hawaii | 1,378 | 0.48% |
| 15 | Tennessee | 6,011 | 2.11% | 40 | New Hampshire | 909 | 0.32% |
| 16 | Indiana | 5,488 | 1.93% | 40 | Rhode Island | 909 | 0.32% |
| 17 | Massachusetts | 5,388 | 1.89% | 42 | Idaho | 879 | 0.31% |
| 18 | Missouri | 5,386 | 1.89% | 43 | Maine | 851 | 0.30% |
| 19 | South Carolina | 5,268 | 1.85% | 44 | Delaware | 801 | 0.28% |
| 20 | Alabama | 5,169 | 1.82% | 45 | Montana | 647 | 0.23% |
| 21 | Arizona | 4,262 | 1.50% | 46 | South Dakota | 594 | 0.21% |
| 22 | Washington | 4,219 | 1.48% | 47 | Alaska | 572 | 0.20% |
| 23 | Wisconsin | 4,141 | 1.46% | 48 | Wyoming | 503 | 0.18% |
| 24 | Colorado | 4,088 | 1.44% | 49 | North Dakota | 481 | 0.17% |
| 25 | Mississippi | 4,043 | 1.42% | 50 | Vermont | 462 | 0.16% |
|  |  |  |  |  | District of Columbia | 1,867 | 0.66% |

Source: U.S. Department of Health and Human Services, Centers for Disease Control, National Center for Health Statistics
    "Monthly Vital Statistics Report" (December 12, 1991)
*Less than 2500 grams (5 pounds–8 ounces).  By state of residence.

# Births of Low Birth Weight as a Percent of Live Births in 1989

## National Percent = 7.0% of Live Births*

| RANK | STATE | PERCENT | RANK | STATE | PERCENT |
|------|-------|---------|------|-------|---------|
| 1 | Mississippi | 9.4 | 25 | Kentucky | 6.9 |
| 2 | South Carolina | 9.2 | 25 | Missouri | 6.9 |
| 3 | Louisiana | 9.1 | 28 | Indiana | 6.6 |
| 4 | Georgia | 8.4 | 28 | West Virginia | 6.6 |
| 5 | Alabama | 8.3 | 30 | Oklahoma | 6.5 |
| 5 | Arkansas | 8.3 | 31 | Arizona | 6.3 |
| 7 | Tennessee | 8.2 | 32 | Rhode Island | 6.2 |
| 8 | North Carolina | 8.1 | 33 | California | 6.1 |
| 9 | Maryland | 8.0 | 33 | Kansas | 6.1 |
| 10 | Colorado | 7.8 | 35 | Massachusetts | 5.9 |
| 11 | Florida | 7.7 | 36 | Nebraska | 5.8 |
| 11 | Illinois | 7.7 | 36 | Wisconsin | 5.8 |
| 11 | New York | 7.7 | 38 | Utah | 5.7 |
| 14 | Michigan | 7.6 | 39 | Washington | 5.6 |
| 15 | Delaware | 7.5 | 40 | Idaho | 5.5 |
| 16 | New Jersey | 7.3 | 40 | Montana | 5.5 |
| 16 | Wyoming | 7.3 | 40 | Vermont | 5.5 |
| 18 | Nevada | 7.2 | 43 | Iowa | 5.4 |
| 19 | Hawaii | 7.1 | 43 | South Dakota | 5.4 |
| 19 | Pennsylvania | 7.1 | 45 | Oregon | 5.2 |
| 19 | Virginia | 7.1 | 46 | New Hampshire | 5.1 |
| 22 | New Mexico | 7.0 | 47 | North Dakota | 5.0 |
| 22 | Ohio | 7.0 | 48 | Alaska | 4.9 |
| 22 | Texas | 7.0 | 48 | Maine | 4.9 |
| 25 | Connecticut | 6.9 | 48 | Minnesota | 4.9 |

| | | |
|---|---|---|
| | District of Columbia | 15.9 |

Source: U.S. Department of Health and Human Services, Centers for Disease Control, National Center for Health Statistics
      "Monthly Vital Statistics Report" (December 12, 1991)
*Less than 2500 grams (5 pounds-8 ounces). By state of residence.

# Births of Low Birth Weight in 1980

## National Total = 246,292 Births of Low Birth Weight*

| RANK | STATE | BIRTHS | % | RANK | STATE | BIRTHS | % |
|------|-------|--------|------|------|-------|--------|------|
| 1 | California | 23,734 | 9.64% | 26 | Washington | 3,457 | 1.40% |
| 2 | Texas | 18,959 | 7.70% | 27 | Minnesota | 3,426 | 1.39% |
| 3 | New York | 17,705 | 7.19% | 28 | Arizona | 3,075 | 1.25% |
| 4 | Illinois | 13,716 | 5.57% | 29 | Arkansas | 2,834 | 1.15% |
| 5 | Ohio | 11,401 | 4.63% | 30 | Connecticut | 2,611 | 1.06% |
| 6 | Pennsylvania | 10,323 | 4.19% | 31 | Iowa | 2,408 | 0.98% |
| 7 | Florida | 9,951 | 4.04% | 32 | Kansas | 2,364 | 0.96% |
| 8 | Michigan | 9,909 | 4.02% | 33 | Utah | 2,161 | 0.88% |
| 9 | Georgia | 7,928 | 3.22% | 34 | Oregon | 2,132 | 0.87% |
| 10 | Louisiana | 7,064 | 2.87% | 35 | West Virginia | 1,968 | 0.80% |
| 11 | New Jersey | 6,990 | 2.84% | 36 | New Mexico | 1,643 | 0.67% |
| 12 | North Carolina | 6,696 | 2.72% | 37 | Nebraska | 1,533 | 0.62% |
| 13 | Virginia | 5,849 | 2.37% | 38 | Hawaii | 1,282 | 0.52% |
| 14 | Indiana | 5,530 | 2.25% | 39 | Idaho | 1,075 | 0.44% |
| 15 | Tennessee | 5,524 | 2.24% | 40 | Maine | 1,061 | 0.43% |
| 16 | Missouri | 5,245 | 2.13% | 41 | Nevada | 877 | 0.36% |
| 17 | Alabama | 4,999 | 2.03% | 42 | Montana | 797 | 0.32% |
| 18 | Maryland | 4,905 | 1.99% | 43 | Rhode Island | 769 | 0.31% |
| 19 | South Carolina | 4,479 | 1.82% | 43 | Wyoming | 769 | 0.31% |
| 20 | Massachusetts | 4,410 | 1.79% | 45 | New Hampshire | 738 | 0.30% |
| 21 | Mississippi | 4,148 | 1.68% | 46 | Delaware | 728 | 0.30% |
| 22 | Colorado | 4,094 | 1.66% | 47 | South Dakota | 678 | 0.28% |
| 23 | Kentucky | 4,051 | 1.64% | 48 | North Dakota | 591 | 0.24% |
| 24 | Wisconsin | 4,022 | 1.63% | 49 | Alaska | 511 | 0.21% |
| 25 | Oklahoma | 3,517 | 1.43% | 50 | Vermont | 465 | 0.19% |
| | | | | | District of Columbia | 1,190 | 0.48% |

Source: U.S. Department of Health and Human Services, Centers for Disease Control, National Center for Health Statistics
    "Vital Statistics of the United States, 1980" (Vol. I-Natality, issued 1984)
*Less than 2500 grams (5 pounds-8 ounces). By state of residence.

# Births of Low Birth Weight as a Percent of Live Births in 1980

## National Percent = 6.8% of Live Births*

| RANK | STATE | PERCENT | RANK | STATE | PERCENT |
|------|-------|---------|------|-------|---------|
| 1 | Mississippi | 8.7 | 25 | West Virginia | 6.7 |
| 2 | Georgia | 8.6 | 27 | Missouri | 6.6 |
| 2 | Louisiana | 8.6 | 27 | Nevada | 6.6 |
| 2 | South Carolina | 8.6 | 29 | Maine | 6.5 |
| 5 | Colorado | 8.2 | 29 | Pennsylvania | 6.5 |
| 5 | Maryland | 8.2 | 31 | Indiana | 6.3 |
| 7 | Tennessee | 8.0 | 31 | Rhode Island | 6.3 |
| 8 | Alabama | 7.9 | 33 | Arizona | 6.2 |
| 8 | North Carolina | 7.9 | 34 | Massachusetts | 6.1 |
| 10 | Delaware | 7.7 | 35 | California | 5.9 |
| 11 | Arkansas | 7.6 | 35 | Vermont | 5.9 |
| 11 | Florida | 7.6 | 37 | Kansas | 5.8 |
| 11 | New Mexico | 7.6 | 38 | Montana | 5.6 |
| 14 | Virginia | 7.5 | 38 | Nebraska | 5.6 |
| 15 | New York | 7.4 | 40 | Alaska | 5.4 |
| 16 | Wyoming | 7.3 | 40 | New Hampshire | 5.4 |
| 17 | Illinois | 7.2 | 40 | Wisconsin | 5.4 |
| 17 | New Jersey | 7.2 | 43 | Idaho | 5.3 |
| 19 | Hawaii | 7.1 | 44 | Utah | 5.2 |
| 20 | Michigan | 6.9 | 45 | Minnesota | 5.1 |
| 20 | Texas | 6.9 | 45 | South Dakota | 5.1 |
| 22 | Kentucky | 6.8 | 45 | Washington | 5.1 |
| 22 | Ohio | 6.8 | 48 | Iowa | 5.0 |
| 22 | Oklahoma | 6.8 | 49 | North Dakota | 4.9 |
| 25 | Connecticut | 6.7 | 49 | Oregon | 4.9 |

District of Columbia    12.8

Source: U.S. Department of Health and Human Services, Centers for Disease Control, National Center for Health Statistics
    "Vital Statistics of the United States, 1980" (Vol. I–Natality, issued 1984)
*Less than 2500 grams (5 pounds-8 ounces). By state of residence.

# Ratio of Births to Unmarried Women in 1989

## National Total = 270.8 Births to Unmarried Women per 1,000 Live Births*

| RANK | STATE | RATIO | RANK | STATE | RATIO |
|---|---|---|---|---|---|
| 1 | Mississippi | 393.9 | 26 | New Jersey | 241.0 |
| 2 | Louisiana | 353.1 | 27 | Indiana | 238.4 |
| 3 | New Mexico | 345.4 | 28 | Massachusetts | 238.2 |
| 4 | New York | 319.1 | 29 | Hawaii | 238.0 |
| 5 | Georgia | 316.7 | 30 | Oklahoma | 237.6 |
| 6 | South Carolina | 316.0 | 31 | West Virginia | 235.2 |
| 7 | Illinois | 309.3 | 32 | Nevada | 235.0 |
| 8 | Arizona | 308.2 | 33 | Washington | 234.0 |
| 9 | Florida | 301.9 | 34 | Wisconsin | 233.5 |
| 10 | California | 300.3 | 35 | Kentucky | 225.5 |
| 11 | Alabama | 297.9 | 36 | Maine | 217.9 |
| 12 | Delaware | 291.2 | 37 | South Dakota | 217.8 |
| 13 | Tennessee | 290.8 | 38 | Montana | 217.4 |
| 14 | Maryland | 288.9 | 39 | Colorado | 204.6 |
| 15 | Ohio | 280.1 | 40 | Vermont | 198.4 |
| 16 | Pennsylvania | 279.0 | 41 | Texas | 196.0 |
| 17 | North Carolina | 277.3 | 42 | Kansas | 195.6 |
| 18 | Arkansas | 276.9 | 43 | Minnesota | 194.6 |
| 19 | Missouri | 271.3 | 44 | Iowa | 194.1 |
| 20 | Connecticut | 262.9 | 45 | Nebraska | 192.5 |
| 21 | Oregon | 252.8 | 46 | Wyoming | 184.9 |
| 22 | Virginia | 252.2 | 47 | North Dakota | 168.8 |
| 23 | Rhode Island | 249.5 | 48 | Idaho | 161.2 |
| 24 | Alaska | 245.9 | 49 | New Hampshire | 157.1 |
| 25 | Michigan | 245.4 | 50 | Utah | 126.6 |
|  |  |  |  | District of Columbia | 643.0 |

Source: U.S. Department of Health and Human Services, Centers for Disease Control, National Center for Health Statistics
"Monthly Vital Statistics Report" (December 12, 1991)
*By state of residence.

# Ratio of Births to Unmarried Women in 1980

## National Ratio = 184.3 Births to Unmarried Women per 1,000 Live Births*

| RANK | STATE | RATIO | RANK | STATE | RATIO |
|---|---|---|---|---|---|
| 1 | Mississippi | 280.4 | 25 | Rhode Island | 156.5 |
| 2 | Maryland | 251.5 | 27 | Alaska | 156.2 |
| 3 | Delaware | 241.8 | 28 | Indiana | 155.0 |
| 4 | New York | 238.1 | 29 | Kentucky | 150.5 |
| 5 | Louisiana | 233.6 | 30 | Oregon | 147.9 |
| 6 | Georgia | 231.5 | 31 | Oklahoma | 140.4 |
| 7 | South Carolina | 230.3 | 32 | Wisconsin | 138.7 |
| 8 | Florida | 230.1 | 33 | Maine | 138.6 |
| 9 | Illinois | 225.3 | 34 | Vermont | 137.0 |
| 10 | Alabama | 221.7 | 35 | Washington | 136.0 |
| 11 | California | 213.8 | 36 | Nevada | 134.5 |
| 12 | New Jersey | 210.8 | 37 | South Dakota | 134.1 |
| 13 | Arkansas | 204.8 | 38 | Texas | 133.1 |
| 14 | Tennessee | 198.5 | 39 | West Virginia | 130.5 |
| 15 | Virginia | 191.9 | 40 | Colorado | 130.1 |
| 16 | North Carolina | 190.0 | 41 | Montana | 125.2 |
| 17 | Arizona | 187.1 | 42 | Kansas | 122.5 |
| 18 | Connecticut | 179.4 | 43 | Nebraska | 116.0 |
| 19 | Ohio | 178.1 | 44 | Minnesota | 114.1 |
| 20 | Pennsylvania | 176.9 | 45 | New Hampshire | 109.6 |
| 21 | Missouri | 176.3 | 46 | Iowa | 102.5 |
| 22 | Hawaii | 175.5 | 47 | North Dakota | 92.4 |
| 23 | Michigan | 161.8 | 48 | Wyoming | 82.1 |
| 24 | New Mexico | 160.8 | 49 | Idaho | 78.7 |
| 25 | Massachusetts | 156.5 | 50 | Utah | 62.0 |

|   |   |
|---|---|
| District of Columbia | 564.5 |

Source: U.S. Department of Health and Human Services, Centers for Disease Control, National Center for Health Statistics

"Vital Statistics of the United States, 1980" (Vol. I-Natality, issued 1984)

*By state of residence.

# Ratio of Births to Unmarried White Women in 1989

## National Ratio = 192.2 Births to Unmarried White Women per 1,000 Live Births*

| RANK | STATE | RATIO | | RANK | STATE | RATIO |
|---|---|---|---|---|---|---|
| 1 | New Mexico | 292.9 | | 26 | Tennessee | 163.2 |
| 2 | California | 287.3 | | 27 | Minnesota | 162.2 |
| 3 | Arizona | 267.4 | | 28 | Delaware | 161.7 |
| 4 | Oregon | 240.2 | | 29 | Montana | 161.5 |
| 5 | New York | 231.2 | | 30 | Alaska | 158.1 |
| 6 | West Virginia | 219.0 | | 31 | Kansas | 157.2 |
| 7 | Maine | 216.1 | | 32 | New Hampshire | 156.8 |
| 8 | Rhode Island | 213.4 | | 33 | Idaho | 155.6 |
| 9 | Washington | 213.2 | | 34 | Maryland | 153.6 |
| 10 | Connecticut | 201.6 | | 34 | Nebraska | 153.6 |
| 11 | Massachusetts | 199.5 | | 36 | Arkansas | 152.6 |
| 12 | Vermont | 198.1 | | 37 | New Jersey | 149.5 |
| 13 | Ohio | 197.1 | | 38 | Hawaii | 144.8 |
| 14 | Pennsylvania | 193.5 | | 39 | Texas | 143.1 |
| 15 | Florida | 191.4 | | 40 | Louisiana | 142.7 |
| 16 | Nevada | 190.3 | | 41 | Virginia | 142.4 |
| 17 | Colorado | 186.1 | | 42 | Georgia | 140.0 |
| 18 | Indiana | 181.5 | | 43 | South Carolina | 136.6 |
| 19 | Illinois | 180.1 | | 44 | Michigan | 135.2 |
| 20 | Kentucky | 178.6 | | 45 | South Dakota | 133.5 |
| 21 | Iowa | 177.1 | | 46 | North Carolina | 128.2 |
| 21 | Missouri | 177.1 | | 47 | North Dakota | 126.8 |
| 23 | Wyoming | 174.4 | | 48 | Mississippi | 123.8 |
| 24 | Wisconsin | 170.2 | | 49 | Utah | 116.6 |
| 25 | Oklahoma | 169.7 | | 50 | Alabama | 115.4 |
| | | | | | District of Columbia | 129.8 |

Source: U.S. Department of Health and Human Services, Centers for Disease Control, National Center for Health Statistics
"Monthly Vital Statistics Report" (December 12, 1991)
*By state of residence.

# Ratio of Births to Unmarried Black Women in 1989

## National Ratio = 657.2 Births to Unmarried Black Women per 1,000 Live Births*

| RANK | STATE | RATIO | | RANK | STATE | RATIO |
|------|-------|-------|---|------|-------|-------|
| 1 | Wisconsin | 799.2 | | 26 | Nevada | 636.4 |
| 2 | Pennsylvania | 772.1 | | 27 | New Jersey | 630.3 |
| 3 | Iowa | 767.3 | | 28 | North Carolina | 621.7 |
| 4 | Illinois | 756.3 | | 29 | California | 621.2 |
| 5 | Missouri | 749.8 | | 30 | Arizona | 612.5 |
| 6 | Ohio | 740.4 | | 31 | Massachusetts | 608.2 |
| 7 | Minnesota | 720.2 | | 32 | Kansas | 606.5 |
| 8 | Delaware | 714.3 | | 33 | Virginia | 603.8 |
| 9 | Indiana | 713.0 | | 34 | Maryland | 600.9 |
| 10 | Nebraska | 701.7 | | 35 | South Carolina | 600.3 |
| 11 | Tennessee | 700.9 | | 36 | New Mexico | 558.9 |
| 12 | Oregon | 696.5 | | 37 | Texas | 532.2 |
| 13 | Mississippi | 687.9 | | 38 | Colorado | 532.0 |
| 14 | Arkansas | 682.1 | | 39 | Washington | 530.4 |
| 15 | Michigan | 679.6 | | 40 | Utah | 481.3 |
| 16 | Kentucky | 674.0 | | 41 | Wyoming | 413.3 |
| 17 | Florida | 665.7 | | 42 | Maine | 320.5 |
| 18 | West Virginia | 665.5 | | 43 | Alaska | 296.4 |
| 19 | Connecticut | 661.4 | | 44 | New Hampshire | 283.3 |
| 20 | New York | 657.9 | | 45 | Hawaii | 151.2 |
| 21 | Louisiana | 655.3 | | – | Idaho** | – |
| 22 | Rhode Island | 647.5 | | – | Montana** | – |
| 23 | Alabama | 642.0 | | – | North Dakota** | – |
| 23 | Oklahoma | 642.0 | | – | South Dakota** | – |
| 25 | Georgia | 636.7 | | – | Vermont** | – |

District of Columbia 759.3

Source: U.S. Department of Health and Human Services, Centers for Disease Control, National Center for Health Statistics
    "Monthly Vital Statistics Report" (December 12, 1991)
*By state of residence.
**Insufficient frequency to determine ratio.

# Births to Teenage Mothers in 1989

## National Total = 517,989 Births to Teenage Mothers

| RANK | STATE | BIRTHS | % | RANK | STATE | BIRTHS | % |
|---|---|---|---|---|---|---|---|
| 1 | California | 65,091 | 12.57% | 26 | Wisconsin | 7,269 | 1.40% |
| 2 | Texas | 47,802 | 9.23% | 27 | Arkansas | 7,026 | 1.36% |
| 3 | New York | 27,246 | 5.26% | 28 | Colorado | 5,933 | 1.15% |
| 4 | Florida | 26,947 | 5.20% | 29 | Minnesota | 5,083 | 0.98% |
| 5 | Illinois | 24,947 | 4.82% | 30 | Oregon | 4,927 | 0.95% |
| 6 | Ohio | 22,611 | 4.37% | 31 | Kansas | 4,547 | 0.88% |
| 7 | Michigan | 19,594 | 3.78% | 32 | New Mexico | 4,300 | 0.83% |
| 8 | Pennsylvania | 19,138 | 3.69% | 33 | Connecticut | 4,211 | 0.81% |
| 9 | Georgia | 18,681 | 3.61% | 34 | Iowa | 4,023 | 0.78% |
| 10 | North Carolina | 16,767 | 3.24% | 35 | West Virginia | 3,941 | 0.76% |
| 11 | Tennessee | 12,813 | 2.47% | 36 | Utah | 3,530 | 0.68% |
| 12 | Louisiana | 12,506 | 2.41% | 37 | Nevada | 2,462 | 0.48% |
| 13 | Indiana | 12,019 | 2.32% | 38 | Nebraska | 2,260 | 0.44% |
| 14 | Alabama | 11,421 | 2.20% | 39 | Hawaii | 1,942 | 0.37% |
| 15 | Virginia | 11,368 | 2.19% | 40 | Idaho | 1,890 | 0.36% |
| 16 | Missouri | 10,980 | 2.12% | 41 | Maine | 1,884 | 0.36% |
| 17 | New Jersey | 10,857 | 2.10% | 42 | Rhode Island | 1,496 | 0.29% |
| 18 | South Carolina | 9,773 | 1.89% | 43 | Delaware | 1,377 | 0.27% |
| 19 | Kentucky | 9,362 | 1.81% | 44 | New Hampshire | 1,331 | 0.26% |
| 20 | Mississippi | 9,279 | 1.79% | 45 | South Dakota | 1,215 | 0.23% |
| 21 | Arizona | 9,176 | 1.77% | 46 | Montana | 1,181 | 0.23% |
| 22 | Maryland | 8,571 | 1.65% | 47 | Alaska | 1,169 | 0.23% |
| 23 | Washington | 8,070 | 1.56% | 48 | Wyoming | 853 | 0.16% |
| 24 | Oklahoma | 7,770 | 1.50% | 49 | Vermont | 734 | 0.14% |
| 25 | Massachusetts | 7,742 | 1.49% | 50 | North Dakota | 731 | 0.14% |
| | | | | | District of Columbia | 2,143 | 0.41% |

Source: U.S. Department of Health and Human Services, National Center for Health Statistics
   Unpublished data (November 22, 1991)

# Births to Teenage Mothers as a Percent of Live Births in 1989

## National Rate = 12.82% of Live Births*

| RANK | STATE | PERCENT | RANK | STATE | PERCENT |
|------|-------|---------|------|-------|---------|
| 1 | Mississippi | 21.56 | 26 | Kansas | 11.74 |
| 2 | Arkansas | 19.57 | 26 | Virginia | 11.74 |
| 3 | Alabama | 18.25 | 28 | California | 11.42 |
| 4 | West Virginia | 17.78 | 29 | Pennsylvania | 11.34 |
| 5 | Kentucky | 17.52 | 30 | Colorado | 11.26 |
| 6 | Tennessee | 17.51 | 31 | South Dakota | 10.96 |
| 7 | Louisiana | 17.19 | 32 | Maryland | 10.95 |
| 8 | South Carolina | 17.05 | 33 | Maine | 10.79 |
| 9 | Georgia | 16.94 | 34 | Washington | 10.71 |
| 10 | North Carolina | 16.42 | 35 | Iowa | 10.31 |
| 11 | Oklahoma | 16.40 | 36 | Rhode Island | 10.13 |
| 12 | New Mexico | 15.72 | 37 | Montana | 10.11 |
| 13 | Texas | 15.54 | 38 | Wisconsin | 10.10 |
| 14 | Indiana | 14.40 | 39 | Hawaii | 10.03 |
| 15 | Missouri | 14.10 | 40 | Alaska | 10.02 |
| 16 | Florida | 13.95 | 41 | Utah | 9.92 |
| 17 | Ohio | 13.79 | 42 | New York | 9.35 |
| 18 | Arizona | 13.66 | 43 | Nebraska | 9.33 |
| 19 | Michigan | 13.19 | 44 | New Jersey | 8.91 |
| 20 | Illinois | 13.11 | 45 | Vermont | 8.64 |
| 21 | Delaware | 12.83 | 46 | Connecticut | 8.51 |
| 22 | Nevada | 12.56 | 47 | Massachusetts | 8.46 |
| 23 | Wyoming | 12.36 | 48 | North Dakota | 7.64 |
| 24 | Oregon | 11.94 | 49 | Minnesota | 7.53 |
| 25 | Idaho | 11.90 | 50 | New Hampshire | 7.47 |
| | | | | District of Columbia | 18.18 |

Source: U.S. Department of Health and Human Services, National Center for Health Statistics
      Unpublished data (November 22, 1991)
*Calculated by the editors.

# Births to Teenage Mothers in 1980

## National Total = 562,330 Births

| RANK | STATE | BIRTHS | % | | RANK | STATE | BIRTHS | % |
|---|---|---|---|---|---|---|---|---|
| 1 | California | 56,138 | 9.98% | | 26 | Arkansas | 8,060 | 1.43% |
| 2 | Texas | 50,125 | 8.91% | | 27 | Massachusetts | 7,765 | 1.38% |
| 3 | Illinois | 29,798 | 5.30% | | 28 | Minnesota | 7,048 | 1.25% |
| 4 | New York | 28,206 | 5.02% | | 29 | Colorado | 6,592 | 1.17% |
| 5 | Ohio | 26,567 | 4.72% | | 30 | Kansas | 6,090 | 1.08% |
| 6 | Florida | 24,042 | 4.28% | | 31 | Iowa | 5,962 | 1.06% |
| 7 | Pennsylvania | 22,029 | 3.92% | | 32 | West Virginia | 5,911 | 1.05% |
| 8 | Michigan | 20,401 | 3.63% | | 33 | Oregon | 5,731 | 1.02% |
| 9 | Georgia | 19,137 | 3.40% | | 34 | New Mexico | 4,758 | 0.85% |
| 10 | Louisiana | 16,504 | 2.93% | | 35 | Utah | 4,594 | 0.82% |
| 11 | North Carolina | 16,192 | 2.88% | | 36 | Connecticut | 4,408 | 0.78% |
| 12 | Indiana | 15,331 | 2.73% | | 37 | Nebraska | 3,313 | 0.59% |
| 13 | Tennessee | 13,792 | 2.45% | | 38 | Idaho | 2,645 | 0.47% |
| 14 | Missouri | 13,312 | 2.37% | | 39 | Maine | 2,522 | 0.45% |
| 15 | Alabama | 13,096 | 2.33% | | 40 | Hawaii | 2,085 | 0.37% |
| 16 | Kentucky | 12,559 | 2.23% | | 41 | Nevada | 2,048 | 0.36% |
| 17 | Virginia | 12,138 | 2.16% | | 42 | South Dakota | 1,797 | 0.32% |
| 18 | New Jersey | 11,904 | 2.12% | | 43 | Montana | 1,761 | 0.31% |
| 19 | Mississippi | 11,079 | 1.97% | | 44 | Wyoming | 1,634 | 0.29% |
| 20 | South Carolina | 10,282 | 1.83% | | 45 | Delaware | 1,572 | 0.28% |
| 21 | Oklahoma | 10,206 | 1.81% | | 46 | Rhode Island | 1,502 | 0.27% |
| 22 | Wisconsin | 9,220 | 1.64% | | 47 | New Hampshire | 1,475 | 0.26% |
| 23 | Maryland | 8,885 | 1.58% | | 48 | North Dakota | 1,304 | 0.23% |
| 24 | Washington | 8,495 | 1.51% | | 49 | Alaska | 1,123 | 0.20% |
| 25 | Arizona | 8,235 | 1.46% | | 50 | Vermont | 1,024 | 0.18% |
| | | | | | | District of Columbia | 1,933 | 0.34% |

Source: U.S. Department of Health and Human Services, Centers for Disease Control, National Center for Health Statistics
"Vital Statistics of the United States, 1980" (Vol. I–Natality, issued 1984)

# Births to Teenage Mothers as a Percent of Live Births in 1980

## National Percent = 15.6% of Live Births

| RANK | STATE | PERCENT | | RANK | STATE | PERCENT |
|---|---|---|---|---|---|---|
| 1 | Mississippi | 23.2 | | 26 | Maryland | 14.8 |
| 2 | Arkansas | 21.6 | | 27 | Michigan | 14.0 |
| 3 | Kentucky | 21.1 | | 28 | California | 13.9 |
| 4 | Georgia | 20.7 | | 28 | Pennsylvania | 13.9 |
| 5 | Alabama | 20.6 | | 30 | South Dakota | 13.5 |
| 6 | Louisiana | 20.1 | | 31 | Colorado | 13.3 |
| 6 | West Virginia | 20.1 | | 31 | Oregon | 13.3 |
| 8 | Tennessee | 19.9 | | 33 | Idaho | 13.1 |
| 9 | South Carolina | 19.8 | | 34 | Vermont | 13.0 |
| 10 | Oklahoma | 19.6 | | 35 | Iowa | 12.5 |
| 11 | North Carolina | 19.2 | | 35 | Washington | 12.5 |
| 12 | Texas | 18.3 | | 37 | Montana | 12.4 |
| 13 | Florida | 18.2 | | 38 | New Jersey | 12.3 |
| 13 | New Mexico | 18.2 | | 38 | Rhode Island | 12.3 |
| 15 | Indiana | 17.3 | | 38 | Wisconsin | 12.3 |
| 16 | Missouri | 16.9 | | 41 | Nebraska | 12.1 |
| 17 | Delaware | 16.7 | | 42 | Alaska | 11.8 |
| 18 | Arizona | 16.5 | | 42 | New York | 11.8 |
| 19 | Illinois | 15.7 | | 44 | Hawaii | 11.5 |
| 19 | Ohio | 15.7 | | 45 | Connecticut | 11.4 |
| 21 | Virginia | 15.5 | | 46 | Utah | 11.0 |
| 21 | Wyoming | 15.5 | | 47 | North Dakota | 10.9 |
| 23 | Nevada | 15.4 | | 48 | Massachusetts | 10.7 |
| 24 | Maine | 15.3 | | 48 | New Hampshire | 10.7 |
| 25 | Kansas | 15.0 | | 50 | Minnesota | 10.4 |
| | | | | | District of Columbia | 20.7 |

Source: U.S. Department of Health and Human Services, Centers for Disease Control, National Center for Health Statistics
"Vital Statistics of the United States, 1980" (Vol. I–Natality, issued 1984)

# Births to White Teenage Mothers in 1989

## National Total = 345,102 Births to White Teenage Mothers

| RANK | STATE | BIRTHS | % | RANK | STATE | BIRTHS | % |
|---|---|---|---|---|---|---|---|
| 1 | California | 52,276 | 15.15% | 26 | Oregon | 4,486 | 1.30% |
| 2 | Texas | 37,110 | 10.75% | 27 | South Carolina | 4,424 | 1.28% |
| 3 | New York | 16,778 | 4.86% | 28 | Minnesota | 3,862 | 1.12% |
| 4 | Ohio | 15,866 | 4.60% | 29 | Maryland | 3,760 | 1.09% |
| 5 | Florida | 15,685 | 4.55% | 30 | West Virginia | 3,710 | 1.08% |
| 6 | Illinois | 12,928 | 3.75% | 31 | Iowa | 3,619 | 1.05% |
| 7 | Pennsylvania | 12,760 | 3.70% | 32 | Kansas | 3,596 | 1.04% |
| 8 | Michigan | 11,477 | 3.33% | 33 | New Mexico | 3,530 | 1.02% |
| 9 | Indiana | 9,507 | 2.75% | 34 | Utah | 3,306 | 0.96% |
| 10 | Georgia | 9,163 | 2.66% | 35 | Mississippi | 3,303 | 0.96% |
| 11 | North Carolina | 8,803 | 2.55% | 36 | Connecticut | 2,857 | 0.83% |
| 12 | Tennessee | 8,358 | 2.42% | 37 | Nevada | 1,910 | 0.55% |
| 13 | Kentucky | 7,903 | 2.29% | 38 | Maine | 1,852 | 0.54% |
| 14 | Missouri | 7,492 | 2.17% | 39 | Idaho | 1,808 | 0.52% |
| 15 | Arizona | 7,384 | 2.14% | 40 | Nebraska | 1,790 | 0.52% |
| 16 | Washington | 6,766 | 1.96% | 41 | New Hampshire | 1,311 | 0.38% |
| 17 | Virginia | 6,453 | 1.87% | 42 | Rhode Island | 1,195 | 0.35% |
| 18 | Massachusetts | 6,118 | 1.77% | 43 | Montana | 875 | 0.25% |
| 19 | Alabama | 5,644 | 1.64% | 44 | Wyoming | 790 | 0.23% |
| 20 | New Jersey | 5,523 | 1.60% | 45 | South Dakota | 788 | 0.23% |
| 21 | Oklahoma | 5,479 | 1.59% | 46 | Vermont | 730 | 0.21% |
| 22 | Louisiana | 5,188 | 1.50% | 47 | Delaware | 717 | 0.21% |
| 23 | Colorado | 5,160 | 1.50% | 48 | Alaska | 679 | 0.20% |
| 24 | Wisconsin | 4,825 | 1.40% | 49 | North Dakota | 545 | 0.16% |
| 25 | Arkansas | 4,568 | 1.32% | 50 | Hawaii | 379 | 0.11% |
| | | | | | District of Columbia | 66 | 0.02% |

Source: U.S. Department of Health and Human Services, National Center for Health Statistics
Unpublished data (November 22, 1991)

# Births to White Teenage Mothers as a Percent of White Live Births in 1989

## National Rate = 11.02% of White Live Births*

| RANK | STATE | PERCENT | RANK | STATE | PERCENT |
|------|-------|---------|------|-------|---------|
| 1 | West Virginia | 17.57 | 26 | Kansas | 10.64 |
| 2 | Arkansas | 17.05 | 27 | Washington | 10.52 |
| 3 | Kentucky | 16.60 | 28 | Michigan | 10.02 |
| 4 | New Mexico | 16.00 | 29 | Utah | 9.94 |
| 5 | Oklahoma | 15.40 | 30 | Iowa | 9.77 |
| 6 | Tennessee | 15.32 | 31 | Rhode Island | 9.32 |
| 7 | Mississippi | 15.03 | 32 | Illinois | 9.27 |
| 8 | Texas | 14.55 | 32 | Virginia | 9.27 |
| 9 | Alabama | 14.07 | 34 | Pennsylvania | 9.22 |
| 10 | Georgia | 13.38 | 35 | Alaska | 9.11 |
| 11 | Arizona | 13.14 | 36 | Delaware | 9.01 |
| 12 | Indiana | 13.06 | 37 | Montana | 8.86 |
| 13 | South Carolina | 12.93 | 38 | South Dakota | 8.75 |
| 14 | North Carolina | 12.86 | 39 | Vermont | 8.70 |
| 15 | Louisiana | 12.58 | 40 | Hawaii | 8.47 |
| 16 | Wyoming | 12.25 | 41 | Nebraska | 8.16 |
| 17 | Oregon | 11.96 | 42 | New York | 7.92 |
| 18 | Idaho | 11.93 | 43 | Massachusetts | 7.83 |
| 19 | Missouri | 11.86 | 44 | Wisconsin | 7.78 |
| 20 | Ohio | 11.74 | 45 | New Hampshire | 7.52 |
| 21 | Nevada | 11.71 | 46 | Maryland | 7.49 |
| 22 | California | 11.66 | 47 | Connecticut | 6.93 |
| 23 | Florida | 10.94 | 48 | North Dakota | 6.56 |
| 24 | Colorado | 10.87 | 49 | Minnesota | 6.37 |
| 25 | Maine | 10.84 | 50 | New Jersey | 6.02 |
|  |  |  |  | District of Columbia | 3.87 |

Source: U.S. Department of Health and Human Services, National Center for Health Statistics
    Unpublished data (November 22, 1991)
*Calculated by the editors.

# Births to Black Teenage Mothers in 1989

## National Total = 157,259 Births to Black Teenage Mothers in 1989

| RANK | STATE | BIRTHS | % | RANK | STATE | BIRTHS | % |
|------|-------|--------|---|------|-------|--------|---|
| 1 | Illinois | 11,795 | 7.50% | 26 | Oklahoma | 1,288 | 0.82% |
| 2 | Florida | 11,049 | 7.03% | 27 | Kansas | 841 | 0.53% |
| 3 | Texas | 10,372 | 6.60% | 28 | Delaware | 653 | 0.42% |
| 4 | New York | 10,140 | 6.45% | 29 | Minnesota | 638 | 0.41% |
| 5 | Georgia | 9,424 | 5.99% | 30 | Colorado | 596 | 0.38% |
| 6 | California | 9,207 | 5.85% | 31 | Arizona | 589 | 0.37% |
| 7 | Michigan | 7,835 | 4.98% | 32 | Washington | 584 | 0.37% |
| 8 | North Carolina | 7,543 | 4.80% | 33 | Nevada | 454 | 0.29% |
| 9 | Louisiana | 7,197 | 4.58% | 34 | Nebraska | 373 | 0.24% |
| 10 | Ohio | 6,625 | 4.21% | 35 | Iowa | 323 | 0.21% |
| 11 | Pennsylvania | 6,228 | 3.96% | 36 | West Virginia | 227 | 0.14% |
| 12 | Mississippi | 5,908 | 3.76% | 37 | Rhode Island | 220 | 0.14% |
| 13 | Alabama | 5,745 | 3.65% | 38 | Oregon | 206 | 0.13% |
| 14 | South Carolina | 5,317 | 3.38% | 39 | New Mexico | 105 | 0.07% |
| 15 | New Jersey | 5,240 | 3.33% | 40 | Alaska | 64 | 0.04% |
| 16 | Virginia | 4,813 | 3.06% | 41 | Hawaii | 53 | 0.03% |
| 17 | Maryland | 4,696 | 2.99% | 42 | Utah | 35 | 0.02% |
| 18 | Tennessee | 4,422 | 2.81% | 43 | New Hampshire | 14 | 0.01% |
| 19 | Missouri | 3,388 | 2.15% | 44 | Maine | 11 | 0.01% |
| 20 | Indiana | 2,462 | 1.57% | 45 | Wyoming | 9 | 0.01% |
| 21 | Arkansas | 2,425 | 1.54% | 46 | North Dakota | 7 | 0.00% |
| 22 | Wisconsin | 2,072 | 1.32% | 47 | Idaho | 6 | 0.00% |
| 23 | Kentucky | 1,430 | 0.91% | 48 | Montana | 5 | 0.00% |
| 24 | Massachusetts | 1,354 | 0.86% | 48 | South Dakota | 5 | 0.00% |
| 25 | Connecticut | 1,289 | 0.82% | 50 | Vermont | 2 | 0.00% |
| | | | | | District of Columbia | 1,975 | 1.26% |

Source: U.S. Department of Health and Human Services, National Center for Health Statistics
Unpublished data (November 22, 1991)

# Births to Black Teenage Mothers as a Percent of Black Live Births in 1989

## National Rate = 22.17% of Black Live Births*

| RANK | STATE | PERCENT | | RANK | STATE | PERCENT |
|---|---|---|---|---|---|---|
| 1 | Mississippi | 28.76 | | 26 | Minnesota | 21.62 |
| 2 | Wisconsin | 28.71 | | 27 | New Jersey | 20.82 |
| 3 | Arkansas | 28.24 | | 28 | Virginia | 19.97 |
| 4 | Kentucky | 26.67 | | 29 | Arizona | 19.02 |
| 5 | Alabama | 26.29 | | 30 | Maryland | 18.87 |
| 6 | Illinois | 26.16 | | 31 | Connecticut | 18.40 |
| 7 | Iowa | 25.63 | | 32 | Colorado | 18.33 |
| 8 | Indiana | 25.59 | | 33 | Rhode Island | 17.25 |
| 9 | Michigan | 25.39 | | 34 | Oregon | 17.11 |
| 10 | Missouri | 25.36 | | 35 | California | 16.26 |
| 11 | Delaware | 25.22 | | 36 | New York | 15.30 |
| 12 | Tennessee | 24.75 | | 37 | Washington | 14.62 |
| 13 | Ohio | 24.69 | | 38 | New Mexico | 14.36 |
| 14 | North Carolina | 24.57 | | 39 | Massachusetts | 14.23 |
| 15 | West Virginia | 24.46 | | 40 | Utah | 9.41 |
| 16 | Nebraska | 24.13 | | 41 | Wyoming | 9.09 |
| 17 | Louisiana | 23.99 | | 42 | Alaska | 9.08 |
| 18 | Florida | 23.70 | | 43 | Maine | 8.87 |
| 19 | South Carolina | 23.61 | | 44 | New Hampshire | 7.61 |
| 20 | Georgia | 23.52 | | 45 | Montana | 7.14 |
| 21 | Oklahoma | 23.32 | | 46 | Idaho | 6.45 |
| 22 | Texas | 22.97 | | 47 | North Dakota | 6.25 |
| 23 | Pennsylvania | 22.81 | | 48 | Hawaii | 5.66 |
| 24 | Kansas | 22.52 | | 49 | Vermont | 5.00 |
| 25 | Nevada | 22.31 | | 50 | South Dakota | 3.85 |
| | | | | | District of Columbia | 21.31 |

Source: U.S. Department of Health and Human Services, National Center for Health Statistics
   Unpublished data (November 22, 1991)
*Calculated by the editors.

# Births to Women 35 to 49 Years Old in 1989

## National Total = 339,504 Live Births

| RANK | STATE | BIRTHS | % | RANK | STATE | BIRTHS | % |
|------|-------|--------|---|------|-------|--------|---|
| 1 | California | 58,405 | 17.20% | 26 | Alabama | 3,654 | 1.08% |
| 2 | New York | 32,308 | 9.52% | 27 | South Carolina | 3,455 | 1.02% |
| 3 | Texas | 21,743 | 6.40% | 28 | Kentucky | 3,039 | 0.90% |
| 4 | Illinois | 16,315 | 4.81% | 29 | Utah | 2,947 | 0.87% |
| 5 | Florida | 16,043 | 4.73% | 30 | Kansas | 2,819 | 0.83% |
| 6 | Pennsylvania | 14,429 | 4.25% | 31 | Iowa | 2,693 | 0.79% |
| 7 | New Jersey | 13,161 | 3.88% | 32 | Oklahoma | 2,684 | 0.79% |
| 8 | Ohio | 11,613 | 3.42% | 33 | Mississippi | 2,207 | 0.65% |
| 9 | Michigan | 10,872 | 3.20% | 34 | New Mexico | 2,174 | 0.64% |
| 10 | Massachusetts | 10,419 | 3.07% | 35 | Hawaii | 2,160 | 0.64% |
| 11 | Virginia | 8,712 | 2.57% | 36 | Arkansas | 1,786 | 0.53% |
| 12 | Maryland | 7,605 | 2.24% | 36 | Nebraska | 1,786 | 0.53% |
| 13 | Georgia | 7,284 | 2.15% | 38 | Nevada | 1,532 | 0.45% |
| 14 | Washington | 7,010 | 2.06% | 39 | West Virginia | 1,316 | 0.39% |
| 15 | North Carolina | 6,478 | 1.91% | 40 | Maine | 1,286 | 0.38% |
| 16 | Minnesota | 5,980 | 1.76% | 41 | Idaho | 1,280 | 0.38% |
| 17 | Wisconsin | 5,640 | 1.66% | 42 | Rhode Island | 1,226 | 0.36% |
| 18 | Connecticut | 5,428 | 1.60% | 43 | Alaska | 1,211 | 0.36% |
| 19 | Missouri | 5,329 | 1.57% | 44 | New Hampshire | 1,160 | 0.34% |
| 20 | Arizona | 5,262 | 1.55% | 45 | Montana | 951 | 0.28% |
| 21 | Colorado | 5,248 | 1.55% | 46 | Vermont | 840 | 0.25% |
| 22 | Indiana | 5,115 | 1.51% | 47 | South Dakota | 824 | 0.24% |
| 23 | Louisiana | 4,563 | 1.34% | 48 | Delaware | 784 | 0.23% |
| 24 | Tennessee | 4,337 | 1.28% | 49 | North Dakota | 748 | 0.22% |
| 25 | Oregon | 3,891 | 1.15% | 50 | Wyoming | 514 | 0.15% |
| | | | | | District of Columbia | 1,238 | 0.36% |

*Source: U.S. Department of Health and Human Services, National Center for Health Statistics*
   *Unpublished data (November 22, 1991)*

# Births to Women 35 to 49 Years Old as a Percent of Live Births in 1989

## National Rate = 8.40% of Live Births*

| RANK | STATE | PERCENT | RANK | STATE | PERCENT |
|---|---|---|---|---|---|
| 1 | Massachusetts | 11.38 | 26 | Nevada | 7.81 |
| 2 | Hawaii | 11.15 | 27 | Wyoming | 7.45 |
| 3 | New York | 11.09 | 28 | South Dakota | 7.43 |
| 4 | Connecticut | 10.97 | 29 | Nebraska | 7.38 |
| 5 | New Jersey | 10.80 | 30 | Maine | 7.36 |
| 6 | Alaska | 10.38 | 31 | Michigan | 7.32 |
| 7 | California | 10.25 | 32 | Delaware | 7.31 |
| 8 | Colorado | 9.96 | 33 | Kansas | 7.28 |
| 9 | Vermont | 9.89 | 34 | Ohio | 7.08 |
| 10 | Maryland | 9.72 | 35 | Texas | 7.07 |
| 11 | Oregon | 9.43 | 36 | Iowa | 6.90 |
| 12 | Washington | 9.30 | 37 | Missouri | 6.84 |
| 13 | Virginia | 9.00 | 38 | Georgia | 6.61 |
| 14 | Minnesota | 8.86 | 39 | New Hampshire | 6.51 |
| 15 | Illinois | 8.57 | 40 | North Carolina | 6.34 |
| 16 | Pennsylvania | 8.55 | 41 | Louisiana | 6.27 |
| 17 | Florida | 8.31 | 42 | Indiana | 6.13 |
| 18 | Rhode Island | 8.30 | 43 | South Carolina | 6.03 |
| 19 | Utah | 8.29 | 44 | West Virginia | 5.94 |
| 20 | Montana | 8.14 | 45 | Tennessee | 5.93 |
| 21 | Idaho | 8.06 | 46 | Alabama | 5.84 |
| 22 | New Mexico | 7.95 | 47 | Kentucky | 5.69 |
| 23 | Arizona | 7.83 | 48 | Oklahoma | 5.66 |
| 23 | Wisconsin | 7.83 | 49 | Mississippi | 5.13 |
| 25 | North Dakota | 7.82 | 50 | Arkansas | 4.97 |
|  |  |  |  | District of Columbia | 10.50 |

Source: U.S. Department of Health and Human Services, National Center for Health Statistics
Unpublished data (November 22, 1991)
*Calculated by the editors.

# Births to White Women 35 to 49 Years Old in 1989

## National Total = 279,442 Live Births

| RANK | STATE | BIRTHS | % | RANK | STATE | BIRTHS | % |
|------|-------|--------|---|------|-------|--------|---|
| 1 | California | 46,317 | 16.57% | 25 | Utah | 2,798 | 1.00% |
| 2 | New York | 24,941 | 8.93% | 27 | Louisiana | 2,783 | 1.00% |
| 3 | Texas | 18,794 | 6.73% | 28 | Iowa | 2,611 | 0.93% |
| 4 | Illinois | 13,279 | 4.75% | 29 | Kansas | 2,601 | 0.93% |
| 5 | Florida | 12,892 | 4.61% | 30 | Alabama | 2,394 | 0.86% |
| 6 | Pennsylvania | 12,738 | 4.56% | 31 | South Carolina | 2,295 | 0.82% |
| 7 | New Jersey | 10,962 | 3.92% | 32 | Oklahoma | 2,215 | 0.79% |
| 8 | Ohio | 10,232 | 3.66% | 33 | New Mexico | 1,736 | 0.62% |
| 9 | Massachusetts | 9,346 | 3.34% | 34 | Nebraska | 1,692 | 0.61% |
| 10 | Michigan | 8,999 | 3.22% | 35 | New Hampshire | 1,503 | 0.54% |
| 11 | Virginia | 7,079 | 2.53% | 36 | Arkansas | 1,389 | 0.50% |
| 12 | Washington | 6,196 | 2.22% | 37 | Nevada | 1,320 | 0.47% |
| 13 | Maryland | 5,718 | 2.05% | 38 | Maine | 1,269 | 0.45% |
| 14 | Minnesota | 5,531 | 1.98% | 39 | West Virginia | 1,267 | 0.45% |
| 15 | Wisconsin | 5,111 | 1.83% | 40 | Idaho | 1,248 | 0.45% |
| 16 | Georgia | 5,047 | 1.81% | 41 | Mississippi | 1,184 | 0.42% |
| 17 | Colorado | 4,913 | 1.76% | 42 | Rhode Island | 1,109 | 0.40% |
| 18 | Connecticut | 4,892 | 1.75% | 43 | Alaska | 910 | 0.33% |
| 19 | North Carolina | 4,868 | 1.74% | 44 | Montana | 877 | 0.31% |
| 20 | Indiana | 4,663 | 1.67% | 45 | Vermont | 833 | 0.30% |
| 21 | Missouri | 4,654 | 1.67% | 46 | Hawaii | 731 | 0.26% |
| 22 | Arizona | 4,518 | 1.62% | 47 | South Dakota | 704 | 0.25% |
| 23 | Oregon | 3,638 | 1.30% | 48 | North Dakota | 698 | 0.25% |
| 24 | Tennessee | 3,438 | 1.23% | 49 | Delaware | 661 | 0.24% |
| 25 | Kentucky | 2,798 | 1.00% | 50 | Wyoming | 494 | 0.18% |
| | | | | | District of Columbia | 556 | 0.20% |

Source: U.S. Department of Health and Human Services, National Center for Health Statistics
Unpublished data (November 22, 1991)

# Births to White Women 35 to 49 Years Old as a Percent of White Live Births in 1989

## National Rate = 8.92% of White Live Births*

| RANK | STATE | PERCENT | RANK | STATE | PERCENT |
|------|-------|---------|------|-------|---------|
| 1 | Hawaii | 16.33 | 26 | Nevada | 8.09 |
| 2 | Alaska | 12.20 | 27 | Arizona | 8.04 |
| 3 | Massachusetts | 11.97 | 28 | New Mexico | 7.87 |
| 4 | New Jersey | 11.96 | 29 | Michigan | 7.86 |
| 5 | Connecticut | 11.86 | 30 | South Dakota | 7.82 |
| 6 | New York | 11.77 | 31 | Nebraska | 7.71 |
| 7 | Maryland | 11.39 | 32 | Kansas | 7.70 |
| 8 | Colorado | 10.35 | 33 | Wyoming | 7.66 |
| 9 | California | 10.33 | 34 | Ohio | 7.57 |
| 10 | Virginia | 10.17 | 35 | Maine | 7.43 |
| 11 | Vermont | 9.93 | 36 | Georgia | 7.37 |
| 12 | Oregon | 9.70 | 36 | Missouri | 7.37 |
| 13 | Washington | 9.63 | 36 | Texas | 7.37 |
| 14 | Illinois | 9.52 | 39 | North Carolina | 7.11 |
| 15 | Pennsylvania | 9.20 | 40 | Iowa | 7.05 |
| 16 | Minnesota | 9.12 | 41 | Louisiana | 6.75 |
| 17 | Florida | 9.00 | 42 | South Carolina | 6.71 |
| 18 | Montana | 8.88 | 43 | Indiana | 6.40 |
| 19 | Rhode Island | 8.65 | 44 | Tennessee | 6.30 |
| 20 | New Hampshire | 8.62 | 45 | Oklahoma | 6.22 |
| 21 | Utah | 8.42 | 46 | West Virginia | 6.00 |
| 22 | North Dakota | 8.41 | 47 | Alabama | 5.97 |
| 23 | Delaware | 8.31 | 48 | Kentucky | 5.88 |
| 24 | Wisconsin | 8.24 | 49 | Mississippi | 5.39 |
| 25 | Idaho | 8.23 | 50 | Arkansas | 5.19 |

District of Columbia          32.61

Source: U.S. Department of Health and Human Services, National Center for Health Statistics
   Unpublished data (November 22, 1991)
*Calculated by the editors.

# Births to Black Women 35 to 49 Years Old in 1989

## National Total = 38,282 Live Births

| RANK | STATE | BIRTHS | % | RANK | STATE | BIRTHS | % |
|---|---|---|---|---|---|---|---|
| 1 | New York | 5,712 | 14.92% | 26 | Kentucky | 203 | 0.53% |
| 2 | California | 3,077 | 8.04% | 27 | Washington | 164 | 0.43% |
| 3 | Florida | 2,824 | 7.38% | 28 | Colorado | 148 | 0.39% |
| 4 | Illinois | 2,236 | 5.84% | 29 | Kansas | 125 | 0.33% |
| 5 | Georgia | 2,066 | 5.40% | 30 | Arizona | 111 | 0.29% |
| 6 | Texas | 2,014 | 5.26% | 31 | Minnesota | 99 | 0.26% |
| 7 | Louisiana | 1,640 | 4.28% | 32 | Delaware | 98 | 0.26% |
| 8 | Michigan | 1,602 | 4.18% | 33 | Nevada | 92 | 0.24% |
| 9 | New Jersey | 1,521 | 3.97% | 34 | Rhode Island | 65 | 0.17% |
| 10 | Maryland | 1,482 | 3.87% | 35 | Oregon | 47 | 0.12% |
| 11 | North Carolina | 1,452 | 3.79% | 36 | Nebraska | 42 | 0.11% |
| 12 | Pennsylvania | 1,323 | 3.46% | 37 | Iowa | 40 | 0.10% |
| 13 | Virginia | 1,231 | 3.22% | 38 | West Virginia | 39 | 0.10% |
| 14 | Alabama | 1,198 | 3.13% | 39 | Alaska | 29 | 0.08% |
| 15 | Ohio | 1,181 | 3.09% | 40 | New Mexico | 27 | 0.07% |
| 16 | South Carolina | 1,108 | 2.89% | 41 | Hawaii | 22 | 0.06% |
| 17 | Mississippi | 986 | 2.58% | 42 | Utah | 19 | 0.05% |
| 18 | Tennessee | 823 | 2.15% | 43 | New Hampshire | 11 | 0.03% |
| 19 | Massachusetts | 644 | 1.68% | 44 | Maine | 7 | 0.02% |
| 20 | Missouri | 558 | 1.46% | 45 | Wyoming | 5 | 0.01% |
| 21 | Connecticut | 390 | 1.02% | 46 | South Dakota | 2 | 0.01% |
| 22 | Arkansas | 373 | 0.97% | 46 | Vermont | 2 | 0.01% |
| 23 | Indiana | 363 | 0.95% | 48 | Idaho | 1 | 0.00% |
| 24 | Wisconsin | 268 | 0.70% | 48 | Montana | 1 | 0.00% |
| 25 | Oklahoma | 215 | 0.56% | 48 | North Dakota | 1 | 0.00% |
| | | | | | District of Columbia | 595 | 1.55% |

Source: U.S. Department of Health and Human Services, National Center for Health Statistics
Unpublished data (November 22, 1991)

# Births to Black Women 35 to 49 Years Old as a Percent of Black Live Births in 1989

## National Rate = 5.40% of Black Live Births*

| RANK | STATE | PERCENT | RANK | STATE | PERCENT |
|---|---|---|---|---|---|
| 1 | New York | 8.62 | 26 | Nevada | 4.52 |
| 2 | Massachusetts | 6.77 | 27 | Texas | 4.46 |
| 3 | Florida | 6.06 | 28 | Ohio | 4.40 |
| 4 | New Jersey | 6.04 | 29 | Arkansas | 4.34 |
| 5 | New Hampshire | 5.98 | 30 | West Virginia | 4.20 |
| 6 | Maryland | 5.96 | 31 | Missouri | 4.18 |
| 7 | Maine | 5.65 | 32 | Alaska | 4.11 |
| 8 | Connecticut | 5.57 | 32 | Washington | 4.11 |
| 9 | Alabama | 5.48 | 34 | Oregon | 3.90 |
| 10 | Louisiana | 5.47 | 35 | Oklahoma | 3.89 |
| 11 | California | 5.43 | 36 | Delaware | 3.79 |
| 12 | Michigan | 5.19 | 36 | Kentucky | 3.79 |
| 13 | Georgia | 5.16 | 38 | Indiana | 3.77 |
| 14 | Utah | 5.11 | 39 | Wisconsin | 3.71 |
| 14 | Virginia | 5.11 | 40 | New Mexico | 3.69 |
| 16 | Rhode Island | 5.10 | 41 | Arizona | 3.58 |
| 17 | Wyoming | 5.05 | 42 | Kansas | 3.35 |
| 18 | Vermont | 5.00 | 42 | Minnesota | 3.35 |
| 19 | Illinois | 4.96 | 44 | Iowa | 3.17 |
| 20 | South Carolina | 4.92 | 45 | Nebraska | 2.72 |
| 21 | Pennsylvania | 4.84 | 46 | Hawaii | 2.35 |
| 22 | Mississippi | 4.80 | 47 | South Dakota | 1.54 |
| 23 | North Carolina | 4.73 | 48 | Montana | 1.43 |
| 24 | Tennessee | 4.61 | 49 | Idaho | 1.08 |
| 25 | Colorado | 4.55 | 50 | North Dakota | 0.89 |
| | | | | District of Columbia | 6.42 |

Source: U.S. Department of Health and Human Services, National Center for Health Statistics
   Unpublished data (November 22, 1991)
*Calculated by the editors.

# Births by Cesarean in 1989

## National Total = 826,955 Cesarean Births*

| RANK | STATE | BIRTHS | % | RANK | STATE | BIRTHS | % |
|---|---|---|---|---|---|---|---|
| 1 | California | 128,737 | 15.57% | 26 | Colorado | 9,227 | 1.12% |
| 2 | New York | 67,861 | 8.21% | 27 | Kansas | 9,063 | 1.10% |
| 3 | Texas | 52,597 | 6.36% | 28 | Connecticut | 8,706 | 1.05% |
| 4 | Florida | 49,090 | 5.94% | 29 | Oregon | 8,096 | 0.98% |
| 5 | Illinois | 42,369 | 5.12% | 30 | Iowa | 7,615 | 0.92% |
| 6 | Ohio | 39,542 | 4.78% | 31 | Utah | 6,278 | 0.76% |
| 7 | Pennsylvania | 37,762 | 4.57% | 32 | West Virginia | 5,392 | 0.65% |
| 8 | Michigan | 33,651 | 4.07% | 33 | New Mexico | 5,068 | 0.61% |
| 9 | New Jersey | 30,705 | 3.71% | 34 | Hawaii | 4,042 | 0.49% |
| 10 | Georgia | 25,262 | 3.05% | 35 | New Hampshire | 3,948 | 0.48% |
| 11 | North Carolina | 23,617 | 2.86% | 36 | Maine | 3,402 | 0.41% |
| 12 | Massachusetts | 20,708 | 2.50% | 37 | Idaho | 3,072 | 0.37% |
| 13 | Missouri | 17,915 | 2.17% | 38 | Delaware | 2,513 | 0.30% |
| 14 | Virginia | 17,609 | 2.13% | 39 | Rhode Island | 2,431 | 0.29% |
| 15 | Tennessee | 17,489 | 2.11% | 40 | Montana | 2,355 | 0.28% |
| 16 | Indiana | 17,368 | 2.10% | 41 | South Dakota | 1,909 | 0.23% |
| 17 | Alabama | 15,937 | 1.93% | 42 | North Dakota | 1,841 | 0.22% |
| 18 | Washington | 13,523 | 1.64% | 43 | Alaska | 1,762 | 0.21% |
| 19 | South Carolina | 12,948 | 1.57% | 44 | Vermont | 1,575 | 0.19% |
| 20 | Wisconsin | 12,723 | 1.54% | 45 | Wyoming | 1,286 | 0.16% |
| 21 | Kentucky | 12,645 | 1.53% | – | Louisiana** | N/A | N/A |
| 22 | Arizona | 12,364 | 1.50% | – | Maryland** | N/A | N/A |
| 23 | Minnesota | 12,023 | 1.45% | – | Nebraska** | N/A | N/A |
| 24 | Mississippi | 10,986 | 1.33% | – | Nevada** | N/A | N/A |
| 25 | Arkansas | 9,457 | 1.14% | – | Oklahoma** | N/A | N/A |
| | | | | | District of Columbia | 2,486 | 0.30% |

Source: U.S. Department of Health and Human Services, National Center for Health Statistics
     Unpublished data (May 8, 1992)
*Total reflects births in 45 states shown.
**Not available.

# Rate of Live Births by Cesarean in 1989

## National Rate = 22.8% of Live Births*

| RANK | STATE | RATE | RANK | STATE | RATE |
|------|-------|------|------|-------|------|
| 1 | Arkansas | 27.0 | 26 | Hawaii | 20.9 |
| 2 | Mississippi | 25.9 | 26 | Indiana | 20.9 |
| 3 | New Jersey | 25.7 | 28 | Montana | 20.2 |
| 4 | Alabama | 25.6 | 29 | Rhode Island | 20.1 |
| 4 | Florida | 25.6 | 29 | Washington | 20.1 |
| 6 | West Virginia | 25.2 | 31 | Iowa | 20.0 |
| 7 | Texas | 25.0 | 32 | Idaho | 19.6 |
| 8 | Kentucky | 24.8 | 32 | Maine | 19.6 |
| 9 | Virginia | 24.5 | 32 | Oregon | 19.6 |
| 10 | Tennessee | 24.3 | 35 | North Dakota | 19.5 |
| 11 | Ohio | 24.2 | 36 | Wyoming | 18.9 |
| 12 | Delaware | 24.0 | 37 | New Mexico | 18.7 |
| 12 | Kansas | 24.0 | 37 | South Dakota | 18.7 |
| 14 | New York | 23.6 | 37 | Vermont | 18.7 |
| 15 | North Carolina | 23.3 | 40 | Minnesota | 18.6 |
| 16 | Missouri | 23.1 | 41 | Arizona | 18.5 |
| 17 | Georgia | 23.0 | 42 | Utah | 17.7 |
| 18 | Massachusetts | 22.9 | 42 | Wisconsin | 17.7 |
| 18 | Michigan | 22.9 | 44 | Colorado | 17.6 |
| 20 | Illinois | 22.7 | 45 | Alaska | 15.2 |
| 20 | South Carolina | 22.7 | – | Louisiana** | N/A |
| 22 | California | 22.6 | – | Maryland** | N/A |
| 23 | Pennsylvania | 22.5 | – | Nebraska** | N/A |
| 24 | New Hampshire | 22.2 | – | Nevada** | N/A |
| 25 | Connecticut | 21.2 | – | Oklahoma** | N/A |

| | |
|---|---|
| District of Columbia | 27.1 |

Source: U.S. Department of Health and Human Services, National Center for Health Statistics

    Unpublished data (May 8, 1992)

*Total reflects births in 45 states shown.

**Not available.

## Births by Vaginal Delivery in 1989

## National Total = 2,793,463 Births by Vaginal Delivery*

| RANK | STATE | BIRTHS | % | RANK | STATE | BIRTHS | % |
|------|-------|--------|---|------|-------|--------|---|
| 1 | California | 439,651 | 15.74% | 26 | Connecticut | 32,300 | 1.16% |
| 2 | New York | 219,331 | 7.85% | 27 | Mississippi | 31,487 | 1.13% |
| 3 | Texas | 157,567 | 5.64% | 28 | Iowa | 30,508 | 1.09% |
| 4 | Illinois | 144,158 | 5.16% | 29 | Utah | 29,145 | 1.04% |
| 5 | Florida | 142,350 | 5.10% | 30 | Kansas | 28,678 | 1.03% |
| 6 | Pennsylvania | 130,187 | 4.66% | 31 | Arkansas | 25,607 | 0.92% |
| 7 | Ohio | 123,625 | 4.43% | 32 | New Mexico | 22,004 | 0.79% |
| 8 | Michigan | 113,048 | 4.05% | 33 | West Virginia | 16,008 | 0.57% |
| 9 | New Jersey | 88,912 | 3.18% | 34 | Hawaii | 15,316 | 0.55% |
| 10 | Georgia | 84,717 | 3.03% | 35 | Maine | 13,956 | 0.50% |
| 11 | North Carolina | 77,751 | 2.78% | 36 | New Hampshire | 13,816 | 0.49% |
| 12 | Massachusetts | 69,763 | 2.50% | 37 | Idaho | 12,602 | 0.45% |
| 13 | Indiana | 65,737 | 2.35% | 38 | Alaska | 9,817 | 0.35% |
| 14 | Missouri | 59,648 | 2.14% | 39 | Rhode Island | 9,674 | 0.35% |
| 15 | Wisconsin | 59,177 | 2.12% | 40 | Montana | 9,279 | 0.33% |
| 16 | Tennessee | 54,463 | 1.95% | 41 | South Dakota | 8,315 | 0.30% |
| 17 | Arizona | 54,437 | 1.95% | 42 | Delaware | 7,954 | 0.28% |
| 18 | Virginia | 54,320 | 1.94% | 43 | North Dakota | 7,615 | 0.27% |
| 19 | Washington | 53,909 | 1.93% | 44 | Vermont | 6,859 | 0.25% |
| 20 | Minnesota | 52,727 | 1.89% | 45 | Wyoming | 5,529 | 0.20% |
| 21 | Alabama | 46,314 | 1.66% | – | Louisiana** | N/A | N/A |
| 22 | South Carolina | 44,042 | 1.58% | – | Maryland** | N/A | N/A |
| 23 | Colorado | 43,069 | 1.54% | – | Nebraska** | N/A | N/A |
| 24 | Kentucky | 38,282 | 1.37% | – | Nevada** | N/A | N/A |
| 25 | Oregon | 33,107 | 1.19% | – | Oklahoma** | N/A | N/A |
| | | | | | District of Columbia | 6,702 | 0.24% |

Source: U.S. Department of Health and Human Services, National Center for Health Statistics
     Unpublished data (May 8, 1992)
*Total reflects births in 45 states shown.
**Not available.

# Percent of Live Births by Vaginal Delivery in 1989

## National Rate = 73.5% of Live Births*

| RANK | STATE | PERCENT | RANK | STATE | PERCENT |
|------|-------|---------|------|-------|---------|
| 1 | Alaska | 84.2 | 25 | North Carolina | 76.1 |
| 2 | Wisconsin | 82.2 | 27 | Illinois | 75.7 |
| 3 | Utah | 81.9 | 28 | Ohio | 75.4 |
| 4 | Colorado | 81.7 | 29 | New York | 75.3 |
| 5 | Arizona | 81.0 | 30 | South Dakota | 75.0 |
| 6 | Vermont | 80.8 | 31 | Tennessee | 74.4 |
| 7 | New Mexico | 80.4 | 32 | Delaware | 74.1 |
| 8 | Oregon | 80.2 | 33 | Alabama | 74.0 |
| 9 | Wyoming | 80.1 | 33 | Kansas | 74.0 |
| 10 | Maine | 79.9 | 35 | Florida | 73.7 |
| 11 | North Dakota | 79.6 | 36 | Mississippi | 73.1 |
| 12 | Montana | 79.5 | 37 | New Jersey | 73.0 |
| 13 | Idaho | 79.3 | 38 | West Virginia | 72.2 |
| 14 | Hawaii | 79.1 | 39 | Kentucky | 71.7 |
| 15 | Indiana | 78.8 | 40 | Washington | 71.5 |
| 16 | Iowa | 78.2 | 41 | Arkansas | 71.3 |
| 17 | Minnesota | 78.1 | 42 | Rhode Island | 65.5 |
| 18 | New Hampshire | 77.6 | 43 | Connecticut | 65.3 |
| 19 | California | 77.1 | 44 | Virginia | 56.1 |
| 19 | Pennsylvania | 77.1 | 45 | Texas | 51.2 |
| 21 | Georgia | 76.8 | – | Louisiana** | N/A |
| 21 | South Carolina | 76.8 | – | Maryland** | N/A |
| 23 | Missouri | 76.6 | – | Nebraska** | N/A |
| 24 | Massachusetts | 76.2 | – | Nevada** | N/A |
| 25 | Michigan | 76.1 | – | Oklahoma** | N/A |

District of Columbia     56.8

Source: U.S. Department of Health and Human Services, National Center for Health Statistics
     Unpublished data (May 8, 1992)

*Calculated by the editors.  Total reflects births in 45 states shown.

**Not available.

# Births by Vaginal Delivery after a Previous Cesarean Delivery in 1989

## National Total = 71,019 Births by Vaginal Delivery after a Previous Cesarean Delivery*

| RANK | STATE | BIRTHS | % | RANK | STATE | BIRTHS | % |
|------|-------|--------|---|------|-------|--------|---|
| 1 | California | 8,673 | 12.21% | 26 | South Carolina | 836 | 1.18% |
| 2 | New York | 7,298 | 10.28% | 27 | Iowa | 792 | 1.12% |
| 3 | Florida | 3,912 | 5.51% | 28 | Kentucky | 696 | 0.98% |
| 4 | Illinois | 3,855 | 5.43% | 29 | Kansas | 670 | 0.94% |
| 5 | Pennsylvania | 3,710 | 5.22% | 30 | Mississippi | 635 | 0.89% |
| 6 | Texas | 3,486 | 4.91% | 31 | New Mexico | 567 | 0.80% |
| 7 | Michigan | 3,096 | 4.36% | 32 | Arkansas | 541 | 0.76% |
| 8 | Ohio | 2,998 | 4.22% | 33 | New Hampshire | 460 | 0.65% |
| 9 | Massachusetts | 2,102 | 2.96% | 34 | Idaho | 399 | 0.56% |
| 10 | New Jersey | 2,015 | 2.84% | 35 | Hawaii | 398 | 0.56% |
| 11 | Washington | 1,933 | 2.72% | 36 | Alaska | 369 | 0.52% |
| 12 | Wisconsin | 1,822 | 2.57% | 37 | Maine | 343 | 0.48% |
| 13 | Minnesota | 1,771 | 2.49% | 38 | Rhode Island | 312 | 0.44% |
| 14 | Georgia | 1,740 | 2.45% | 39 | Montana | 282 | 0.40% |
| 15 | Missouri | 1,613 | 2.27% | 40 | Vermont | 249 | 0.35% |
| 16 | North Carolina | 1,552 | 2.19% | 41 | North Dakota | 243 | 0.34% |
| 17 | Arizona | 1,537 | 2.16% | 42 | West Virginia | 227 | 0.32% |
| 18 | Colorado | 1,462 | 2.06% | 43 | South Dakota | 215 | 0.30% |
| 19 | Virginia | 1,347 | 1.90% | 44 | Wyoming | 167 | 0.24% |
| 20 | Oregon | 1,303 | 1.83% | 45 | Delaware | 126 | 0.18% |
| 21 | Tennessee | 1,173 | 1.65% | – | Louisiana** | N/A | N/A |
| 22 | Indiana | 1,162 | 1.64% | – | Maryland** | N/A | N/A |
| 23 | Connecticut | 981 | 1.38% | – | Nebraska** | N/A | N/A |
| 24 | Utah | 937 | 1.32% | – | Nevada** | N/A | N/A |
| 25 | Alabama | 865 | 1.22% | – | Oklahoma** | N/A | N/A |
| | | | | | District of Columbia | 149 | 0.21% |

Source: U.S. Department of Health and Human Services, National Center for Health Statistics
    Unpublished data (May 8, 1992)

*Total reflects births in 45 states shown.

**Not available.

# Rate of Vaginal Births after a Previous Cesarean in 1989

## National Rate = 18.9% of Live Births*

| RANK | STATE | RATE | RANK | STATE | RATE |
|---|---|---|---|---|---|
| 1 | Alaska | 36.9 | 26 | Illinois | 19.3 |
| 2 | Colorado | 32.5 | 27 | Virginia | 18.8 |
| 3 | Oregon | 30.3 | 28 | Florida | 18.6 |
| 4 | Vermont | 30.0 | 28 | Michigan | 18.6 |
| 5 | Washington | 28.0 | 30 | North Carolina | 16.9 |
| 6 | Utah | 27.6 | 31 | Tennessee | 16.8 |
| 7 | Minnesota | 27.3 | 32 | Ohio | 16.3 |
| 8 | Wisconsin | 25.8 | 33 | Georgia | 16.2 |
| 9 | Arizona | 25.7 | 34 | South Carolina | 15.5 |
| 10 | Wyoming | 25.5 | 35 | California | 15.4 |
| 11 | Idaho | 24.6 | 35 | New Jersey | 15.4 |
| 12 | New Hampshire | 24.2 | 37 | Texas | 15.0 |
| 12 | New Mexico | 24.2 | 38 | Kansas | 14.8 |
| 14 | Rhode Island | 24.1 | 39 | Indiana | 14.7 |
| 15 | Connecticut | 23.5 | 40 | Alabama | 14.1 |
| 16 | North Dakota | 23.3 | 41 | Arkansas | 13.6 |
| 17 | Hawaii | 22.7 | 42 | Kentucky | 13.5 |
| 17 | Montana | 22.7 | 43 | Mississippi | 13.0 |
| 19 | New York | 22.5 | 44 | Delaware | 12.9 |
| 20 | South Dakota | 22.1 | 45 | West Virginia | 10.1 |
| 21 | Maine | 21.9 | – | Louisiana** | N/A |
| 22 | Massachusetts | 21.6 | – | Maryland** | N/A |
| 23 | Iowa | 20.6 | – | Nebraska** | N/A |
| 24 | Pennsylvania | 20.5 | – | Nevada** | N/A |
| 25 | Missouri | 20.0 | – | Oklahoma** | N/A |
|  |  |  |  | District of Columbia | 14.4 |

Source: U.S. Department of Health and Human Services, National Center for Health Statistics
Unpublished data (May 8, 1992)

*Number of vaginal births after previous cesarean delivery per 100 live births to women with a previous cesarean delivery. Total reflects percentage for 45 states shown.

**Not available.

42

# Reported Legal Abortions in 1988

## National Total = 1,371,285 Reported Legal Abortions*

| RANK | STATE | ABORTIONS | % | RANK | STATE | ABORTIONS | % |
|---|---|---|---|---|---|---|---|
| 1 | California | 334,887 | 24.42% | 26 | Indiana | 13,003 | 0.95% |
| 2 | New York | 142,862 | 10.42% | 27 | Colorado | 12,425 | 0.91% |
| 3 | Texas | 81,474 | 5.94% | 28 | Kentucky | 11,631 | 0.85% |
| 4 | Florida | 65,153 | 4.75% | 29 | Oklahoma | 11,073 | 0.81% |
| 5 | Pennsylvania | 50,786 | 3.70% | 30 | Rhode Island | 7,615 | 0.56% |
| 6 | Illinois | 50,478 | 3.68% | 31 | Kansas | 7,534 | 0.55% |
| 7 | Michigan | 46,747 | 3.41% | 32 | Nevada | 6,936 | 0.51% |
| 8 | Massachusetts | 38,841 | 2.83% | 33 | Iowa | 6,405 | 0.47% |
| 9 | North Carolina | 37,629 | 2.74% | 34 | Hawaii | 6,040 | 0.44% |
| 10 | New Jersey | 35,987 | 2.62% | 35 | Nebraska | 6,006 | 0.44% |
| 11 | Georgia | 35,213 | 2.57% | 36 | Delaware | 5,458 | 0.40% |
| 12 | Ohio | 34,543 | 2.52% | 37 | Arkansas | 5,439 | 0.40% |
| 13 | Virginia | 34,029 | 2.48% | 38 | Mississippi | 5,170 | 0.38% |
| 14 | Washington | 29,802 | 2.17% | 39 | New Mexico | 5,126 | 0.37% |
| 15 | Maryland | 23,707 | 1.73% | 40 | Utah | 4,732 | 0.35% |
| 16 | Tennessee | 21,589 | 1.57% | 41 | Maine | 4,723 | 0.34% |
| 17 | Connecticut | 20,219 | 1.47% | 42 | New Hampshire | 4,156 | 0.30% |
| 18 | Wisconsin | 17,986 | 1.31% | 43 | West Virginia | 3,467 | 0.25% |
| 19 | Minnesota | 17,975 | 1.31% | 44 | Vermont | 3,309 | 0.24% |
| 20 | Missouri | 17,382 | 1.27% | 45 | Montana | 2,866 | 0.21% |
| 21 | Arizona | 15,922 | 1.16% | 46 | North Dakota | 2,221 | 0.16% |
| 22 | Louisiana | 15,367 | 1.12% | 47 | Idaho | 1,650 | 0.12% |
| 23 | Alabama | 14,746 | 1.08% | 48 | Alaska | 1,463 | 0.11% |
| 24 | South Carolina | 14,133 | 1.03% | 49 | South Dakota | 898 | 0.07% |
| 25 | Oregon | 13,309 | 0.97% | 50 | Wyoming | 351 | 0.03% |
| | | | | | District of Columbia | 20,822 | 1.52% |

Source: U.S. Department of Health and Human Services, Centers for Disease Control
"Special Focus on Reproductive Health Surveillance" (Morbidity and Mortality Weekly Report, Vol. 40, No. SS-2, July 1991)
*By state of occurrence.

# Reported Legal Abortions per 1,000 Live Births in 1988

## National Ratio = 352 Reported Legal Abortions per 1,000 Live Births*

| RANK | STATE | RATIO | | RANK | STATE | RATIO |
|------|-------|-------|---|------|-------|-------|
| 1 | California | 628 | | 26 | South Carolina | 257 |
| 2 | Rhode Island | 537 | | 27 | Wisconsin | 254 |
| 3 | Delaware | 525 | | 28 | Nebraska | 251 |
| 4 | New York | 519 | | 29 | Montana | 245 |
| 5 | Massachusetts | 441 | | 30 | Alabama | 243 |
| 6 | Connecticut | 421 | | 30 | Arizona | 243 |
| 7 | Washington | 411 | | 32 | New Hampshire | 239 |
| 8 | Vermont | 408 | | 33 | Colorado | 233 |
| 9 | North Carolina | 386 | | 34 | Kentucky | 228 |
| 10 | Nevada | 377 | | 34 | Missouri | 228 |
| 11 | Virginia | 367 | | 36 | North Dakota | 220 |
| 12 | Florida | 356 | | 37 | Ohio | 215 |
| 13 | Georgia | 335 | | 38 | Louisiana | 208 |
| 13 | Michigan | 335 | | 39 | Kansas | 195 |
| 15 | Oregon | 334 | | 40 | New Mexico | 190 |
| 16 | Hawaii | 319 | | 41 | Iowa | 168 |
| 17 | Maryland | 310 | | 42 | Indiana | 160 |
| 18 | Pennsylvania | 307 | | 43 | West Virginia | 159 |
| 19 | New Jersey | 306 | | 44 | Arkansas | 155 |
| 20 | Tennessee | 305 | | 45 | Alaska | 132 |
| 21 | Maine | 275 | | 46 | Utah | 131 |
| 22 | Illinois | 273 | | 47 | Mississippi | 123 |
| 23 | Minnesota | 269 | | 48 | Idaho | 105 |
| 23 | Texas | 269 | | 49 | South Dakota | 80 |
| 25 | Oklahoma | 262 | | 50 | Wyoming | 49 |

District of Columbia*          N/R

Source: U.S. Department of Health and Human Services, Centers for Disease Control
    "Special Focus on Reproductive Health Surveillance" (Morbidity and Mortality Weekly Report, Vol. 40, No. SS-2, July 1991)
*By state of occurrence. District of Columbia's ratio was not listed but was noted as being greater than 1,000 abortions per 1,000 live births.

# Reported Legal Abortions per 1,000 Women Ages 15–44 in 1988

## National Rate = 24 Reported Legal Abortions per 1,000 Women Ages 15–44*

| RANK | STATE | RATE |
|---|---|---|
| 1 | California | 49 |
| 2 | Delaware | 36 |
| 3 | New York | 34 |
| 4 | Rhode Island | 33 |
| 5 | Connecticut | 28 |
| 5 | Nevada | 28 |
| 7 | Washington | 27 |
| 8 | Hawaii | 26 |
| 8 | Massachusetts | 26 |
| 8 | Vermont | 26 |
| 11 | North Carolina | 25 |
| 12 | Virginia | 24 |
| 13 | Florida | 23 |
| 13 | Georgia | 23 |
| 15 | Michigan | 21 |
| 15 | Oregon | 21 |
| 17 | Arizona | 20 |
| 17 | Maryland | 20 |
| 17 | Tennessee | 20 |
| 17 | Texas | 20 |
| 21 | New Jersey | 19 |
| 21 | Pennsylvania | 19 |
| 23 | Illinois | 18 |
| 23 | Maine | 18 |
| 25 | Minnesota | 17 |

| RANK | STATE | RATE |
|---|---|---|
| 25 | Nebraska | 17 |
| 25 | South Carolina | 17 |
| 28 | Alabama | 16 |
| 28 | Colorado | 16 |
| 28 | Montana | 16 |
| 28 | Wisconsin | 16 |
| 32 | Louisiana | 15 |
| 32 | New Hampshire | 15 |
| 32 | New Mexico | 15 |
| 32 | North Dakota | 15 |
| 32 | Oklahoma | 15 |
| 37 | Missouri | 14 |
| 37 | Ohio | 14 |
| 39 | Kansas | 13 |
| 39 | Kentucky | 13 |
| 39 | Utah | 13 |
| 42 | Alaska | 11 |
| 43 | Arkansas | 10 |
| 43 | Indiana | 10 |
| 43 | Iowa | 10 |
| 46 | Mississippi | 9 |
| 47 | Idaho | 8 |
| 47 | West Virginia | 8 |
| 49 | South Dakota | 5 |
| 50 | Wyoming | 3 |

| | District of Columbia* | N/R |
|---|---|---|

Source: U.S. Department of Health and Human Services, Centers for Disease Control
    "Special Focus on Reproductive Health Surveillance" (Morbidity and Mortality Weekly Report, Vol. 40, No. SS-2, July 1991)
*By state of occurrence. District of Columbia's rate was not listed but was noted as being greater than 100 abortions per 1,000 women ages 15 to 44.

# Percentage of Reported Legal Abortions Obtained by Out–Of–State Residents in 1988
## (Selected States Only)
## National Rate = 8.6% of Reported Legal Abortions Obtained by Out–Of–State Residents*

| RANK | STATE | PERCENT | RANK | STATE | PERCENT |
|---|---|---|---|---|---|
| 1 | North Dakota | 44.1 | 26 | South Carolina | 5.5 |
| 2 | Vermont | 29.1 | 27 | Indiana | 4.6 |
| 3 | Montana | 25.0 | 27 | Texas | 4.6 |
| 4 | Nebraska | 21.0 | 29 | Connecticut | 4.3 |
| 5 | Tennessee | 17.8 | 30 | Kansas | 4.2 |
| 6 | Mississippi | 15.2 | 30 | New Mexico | 4.2 |
| 7 | Utah | 14.5 | 32 | Kentucky | 3.2 |
| 8 | South Dakota | 13.1 | 32 | New Jersey | 3.2 |
| 9 | Wyoming | 12.1 | 34 | Illinois | 2.7 |
| 10 | Nevada | 11.9 | 35 | Arkansas | 2.0 |
| 11 | Missouri | 11.3 | 36 | Maine | 1.9 |
| 12 | Minnesota | 10.2 | 37 | Maryland | 1.2 |
| 13 | Oregon | 9.2 | 38 | Hawaii | 0.6 |
| 14 | Georgia | 8.9 | – | Alabama** | N/A |
| 15 | Arizona | 8.3 | – | Alaska** | N/A |
| 16 | Idaho | 7.8 | – | California** | N/A |
| 17 | North Carolina | 7.7 | – | Delaware** | N/A |
| 18 | Colorado | 7.4 | – | Florida** | N/A |
| 19 | Wisconsin | 7.1 | – | Iowa** | N/A |
| 20 | Ohio | 7.0 | – | Louisiana** | N/A |
| 21 | Massachusetts | 6.8 | – | Michigan** | N/A |
| 22 | New York | 5.9 | – | New Hampshire** | N/A |
| 22 | Pennsylvania | 5.9 | – | Oklahoma** | N/A |
| 22 | Virginia | 5.9 | – | Rhode Island** | N/A |
| 25 | Washington | 5.8 | – | West Virginia** | N/A |

District of Columbia     50.4

*Source: U.S. Department of Health and Human Services, Centers for Disease Control*

    *"Special Focus on Reproductive Health Surveillance" (Morbidity and Mortality Weekly Report, Vol. 40, No. SS-2, July 1991)*

*\*By state of occurrence.*

*\*\*Not reported.*

# Reported Legal Abortions Obtained by Teenagers in 1988
## (Selected States Only)
### Selected States Total = 180,667 Reported Legal Abortions Obtained by Teenagers*

| RANK | STATE | ABORTIONS | % | RANK | STATE | ABORTIONS | % |
|------|-------|-----------|---|------|-------|-----------|---|
| 1 | New York | 31,202 | 17.27% | 26 | Maine | 1,489 | 0.82% |
| 2 | Texas | 16,962 | 9.39% | 27 | Nevada | 1,478 | 0.82% |
| 3 | Pennsylvania | 14,106 | 7.81% | 28 | Hawaii | 1,326 | 0.73% |
| 4 | North Carolina | 11,154 | 6.17% | 29 | New Mexico | 1,263 | 0.70% |
| 5 | Massachusetts | 10,013 | 5.54% | 30 | Utah | 1,189 | 0.66% |
| 6 | Georgia | 9,217 | 5.10% | 31 | Vermont | 908 | 0.50% |
| 7 | Virginia | 8,739 | 4.84% | 32 | Montana | 851 | 0.47% |
| 8 | Washington | 7,260 | 4.02% | 33 | North Dakota | 666 | 0.37% |
| 9 | Tennessee | 6,148 | 3.40% | 34 | Idaho | 422 | 0.23% |
| 10 | Maryland | 5,857 | 3.24% | 35 | South Dakota | 252 | 0.14% |
| 11 | Connecticut | 5,342 | 2.96% | 36 | Wyoming | 111 | 0.06% |
| 12 | Wisconsin | 4,640 | 2.57% | – | Alabama** | N/A | N/A |
| 13 | Minnesota | 4,625 | 2.56% | – | Alaska** | N/A | N/A |
| 14 | Missouri | 4,216 | 2.33% | – | California** | N/A | N/A |
| 15 | South Carolina | 4,017 | 2.22% | – | Delaware** | N/A | N/A |
| 16 | Louisiana | 3,764 | 2.08% | – | Florida** | N/A | N/A |
| 17 | Kentucky | 3,723 | 2.06% | – | Illinois** | N/A | N/A |
| 18 | Oregon | 3,655 | 2.02% | – | Indiana** | N/A | N/A |
| 19 | Arizona | 3,580 | 1.98% | – | Iowa** | N/A | N/A |
| 20 | Colorado | 3,182 | 1.76% | – | Michigan** | N/A | N/A |
| 21 | Kansas | 2,474 | 1.37% | – | New Hampshire** | N/A | N/A |
| 22 | Rhode Island | 1,781 | 0.99% | – | New Jersey** | N/A | N/A |
| 23 | Nebraska | 1,759 | 0.97% | – | Ohio** | N/A | N/A |
| 24 | Arkansas | 1,752 | 0.97% | – | Oklahoma** | N/A | N/A |
| 25 | Mississippi | 1,544 | 0.85% | – | West Virginia** | N/A | N/A |

Source: U.S. Department of Health and Human Services, Centers for Disease Control

    *"Special Focus on Reproductive Health Surveillance"* (Morbidity and Mortality Weekly Report, Vol. 40, No. SS-2, July 1991)

*By state of occurrence. Total is for listed states only.

**Not available.

# Percent of Reported Legal Abortions Obtained by Teenagers in 1988
## (Selected States Only)
## Selected States Percent = 24.99% of Reported Legal Abortions Are Obtained by Teenagers*

| RANK | STATE | PERCENT | RANK | STATE | PERCENT |
|------|-------|---------|------|-------|---------|
| 1 | Kansas | 32.84 | 26 | Maryland | 24.71 |
| 2 | Arkansas | 32.21 | 27 | New Mexico | 24.64 |
| 3 | Kentucky | 32.01 | 28 | Louisiana | 24.49 |
| 4 | Wyoming | 31.62 | 29 | Washington | 24.36 |
| 5 | Maine | 31.53 | 30 | Missouri | 24.25 |
| 6 | North Dakota | 29.99 | 31 | Rhode Island | 23.39 |
| 7 | Mississippi | 29.86 | 32 | Arizona | 22.48 |
| 8 | Montana | 29.69 | 33 | Hawaii | 21.95 |
| 9 | North Carolina | 29.64 | 34 | New York | 21.84 |
| 10 | Nebraska | 29.29 | 35 | Nevada | 21.31 |
| 11 | Tennessee | 28.48 | 36 | Texas | 20.82 |
| 12 | South Carolina | 28.42 | – | Alabama** | N/A |
| 13 | South Dakota | 28.06 | – | Alaska** | N/A |
| 14 | Pennsylvania | 27.78 | – | California** | N/A |
| 15 | Oregon | 27.46 | – | Delaware** | N/A |
| 16 | Vermont | 27.44 | – | Florida** | N/A |
| 17 | Connecticut | 26.42 | – | Illinois** | N/A |
| 18 | Georgia | 26.17 | – | Indiana** | N/A |
| 19 | Wisconsin | 25.80 | – | Iowa** | N/A |
| 20 | Massachusetts | 25.78 | – | Michigan** | N/A |
| 21 | Minnesota | 25.73 | – | New Hampshire** | N/A |
| 22 | Virginia | 25.68 | – | New Jersey** | N/A |
| 23 | Colorado | 25.61 | – | Ohio** | N/A |
| 24 | Idaho | 25.58 | – | Oklahoma** | N/A |
| 25 | Utah | 25.13 | – | West Virginia** | N/A |

Source: U.S. Department of Health and Human Services, Centers for Disease Control
"Special Focus on Reproductive Health Surveillance" (Morbidity and Mortality Weekly Report, Vol. 40, No. SS–2, July 1991)
*Rates calculated by the editors. By state of occurrence. Percent is for listed states only.
**Not available.

# Reported Legal Abortions Obtained by Teenagers 17 Years and Younger in 1988
## (Selected States Only)
### Selected States Total = 76,327 Reported Legal Abortions*

| RANK | STATE | ABORTIONS | % | RANK | STATE | ABORTIONS | % |
|---|---|---|---|---|---|---|---|
| 1 | New York | 13,279 | 17.40% | 26 | Nevada | 589 | 0.77% |
| 2 | Texas | 6,441 | 8.44% | 27 | New Mexico | 583 | 0.76% |
| 3 | Pennsylvania | 5,888 | 7.71% | 28 | Hawaii | 552 | 0.72% |
| 4 | North Carolina | 5,156 | 6.76% | 29 | Rhode Island | 503 | 0.66% |
| 5 | Georgia | 4,296 | 5.63% | 30 | Utah | 456 | 0.60% |
| 6 | Virginia | 3,791 | 4.97% | 31 | Montana | 412 | 0.54% |
| 7 | Massachusetts | 3,731 | 4.89% | 32 | Vermont | 367 | 0.48% |
| 8 | Washington | 3,021 | 3.96% | 33 | North Dakota | 183 | 0.24% |
| 9 | Maryland | 2,669 | 3.50% | 34 | Idaho | 149 | 0.20% |
| 10 | Tennessee | 2,630 | 3.45% | 35 | South Dakota | 113 | 0.15% |
| 11 | Connecticut | 2,463 | 3.23% | 36 | Wyoming | 56 | 0.07% |
| 12 | Wisconsin | 1,961 | 2.57% | – | Alabama** | N/A | N/A |
| 13 | South Carolina | 1,857 | 2.43% | – | Alaska** | N/A | N/A |
| 14 | Minnesota | 1,834 | 2.40% | – | California** | N/A | N/A |
| 15 | Kentucky | 1,809 | 2.37% | – | Delaware** | N/A | N/A |
| 16 | Missouri | 1,584 | 2.08% | – | Florida** | N/A | N/A |
| 17 | Oregon | 1,551 | 2.03% | – | Illinois** | N/A | N/A |
| 18 | Louisiana | 1,470 | 1.93% | – | Indiana** | N/A | N/A |
| 19 | Colorado | 1,403 | 1.84% | – | Iowa** | N/A | N/A |
| 20 | Arizona | 1,311 | 1.72% | – | Michigan** | N/A | N/A |
| 21 | Kansas | 1,200 | 1.57% | – | New Hampshire** | N/A | N/A |
| 22 | Mississippi | 772 | 1.01% | – | New Jersey** | N/A | N/A |
| 23 | Arkansas | 770 | 1.01% | – | Ohio** | N/A | N/A |
| 24 | Maine | 750 | 0.98% | – | Oklahoma** | N/A | N/A |
| 25 | Nebraska | 727 | 0.95% | – | West Virginia** | N/A | N/A |

Source: U.S. Department of Health and Human Services, Centers for Disease Control
    "Special Focus on Reproductive Health Surveillance" (Morbidity and Mortality Weekly Report, Vol. 40, No. SS-2, July 1991)
*Totals calculated by the editors. By state of occurrence. Total is for listed states only.
**Not available.

## Percent of Reported Legal Abortions Obtained by Teenagers 17 Years and Younger in 1988
### (Selected States Only)
### Selected State Rate = 10.26% of Reported Legal Abortions*

| RANK | STATE | PERCENT | RANK | STATE | PERCENT |
|---|---|---|---|---|---|
| 1 | Wyoming | 15.95 | 26 | Massachusetts | 9.61 |
| 2 | Kansas | 15.93 | 27 | Louisiana | 9.57 |
| 3 | Maine | 15.88 | 28 | New York | 9.29 |
| 4 | Kentucky | 15.55 | 29 | Hawaii | 9.14 |
| 5 | Mississippi | 14.93 | 30 | Missouri | 9.11 |
| 6 | Montana | 14.38 | 31 | Idaho | 9.03 |
| 7 | Arkansas | 14.16 | 32 | Nevada | 8.49 |
| 8 | North Carolina | 13.70 | 33 | North Dakota | 8.24 |
| 9 | South Carolina | 13.14 | 34 | Arizona | 8.23 |
| 10 | South Dakota | 12.58 | 35 | Texas | 7.91 |
| 11 | Georgia | 12.20 | 36 | Rhode Island | 6.61 |
| 12 | Connecticut | 12.18 | – | Alabama** | N/A |
| 12 | Tennessee | 12.18 | – | Alaska** | N/A |
| 14 | Nebraska | 12.10 | – | California** | N/A |
| 15 | Oregon | 11.65 | – | Delaware** | N/A |
| 16 | Pennsylvania | 11.59 | – | Florida** | N/A |
| 17 | New Mexico | 11.37 | – | Illinois** | N/A |
| 18 | Colorado | 11.29 | – | Indiana** | N/A |
| 19 | Maryland | 11.26 | – | Iowa** | N/A |
| 20 | Virginia | 11.14 | – | Michigan** | N/A |
| 21 | Vermont | 11.09 | – | New Hampshire** | N/A |
| 22 | Wisconsin | 10.90 | – | New Jersey** | N/A |
| 23 | Minnesota | 10.20 | – | Ohio** | N/A |
| 24 | Washington | 10.14 | – | Oklahoma** | N/A |
| 25 | Utah | 9.64 | – | West Virginia** | N/A |

Source: U.S. Department of Health and Human Services, Centers for Disease Control

"Special Focus on Reproductive Health Surveillance" (Morbidity and Mortality Weekly Report, Vol. 40, No. SS-2, July 1991)

*Rates calculated by the editors. By state of occurrence. Percent is for listed states only.

**Not available.

# Percent of Teenage Abortions Obtained by Teenagers 17 Years and Younger in 1988
## (Selected States Only)
### Selected States Rate = 42.2% of Teenage Abortions*

| RANK | STATE | PERCENT | RANK | STATE | PERCENT |
|------|-------|---------|------|-------|---------|
| 1 | Wyoming | 50.4 | 26 | Nevada | 39.8 |
| 2 | Maine | 50.3 | 27 | Minnesota | 39.7 |
| 3 | Mississippi | 50.0 | 28 | Louisiana | 39.2 |
| 4 | Kansas | 48.5 | 29 | Utah | 38.4 |
| 4 | Kentucky | 48.5 | 30 | Texas | 37.9 |
| 6 | Montana | 48.4 | 31 | Missouri | 37.6 |
| 7 | Georgia | 46.6 | 32 | Massachusetts | 37.3 |
| 8 | Connecticut | 46.2 | 33 | Arizona | 36.6 |
| 8 | North Carolina | 46.2 | 34 | Idaho | 35.3 |
| 8 | South Carolina | 46.2 | 35 | Rhode Island | 28.1 |
| 11 | New Mexico | 46.1 | 36 | North Dakota | 27.6 |
| 12 | Maryland | 45.6 | – | Alabama** | N/A |
| 13 | South Dakota | 44.8 | – | Alaska** | N/A |
| 14 | Colorado | 44.1 | – | California** | N/A |
| 15 | Arkansas | 43.9 | – | Delaware** | N/A |
| 16 | Virginia | 43.3 | – | Florida** | N/A |
| 17 | Tennessee | 42.8 | – | Illinois** | N/A |
| 18 | New York | 42.6 | – | Indiana** | N/A |
| 19 | Oregon | 42.5 | – | Iowa** | N/A |
| 20 | Wisconsin | 42.2 | – | Michigan** | N/A |
| 21 | Pennsylvania | 41.8 | – | New Hampshire** | N/A |
| 22 | Hawaii | 41.7 | – | New Jersey** | N/A |
| 22 | Washington | 41.7 | – | Ohio** | N/A |
| 24 | Nebraska | 41.3 | – | Oklahoma** | N/A |
| 25 | Vermont | 40.4 | – | West Virginia** | N/A |

Source: U.S. Department of Health and Human Services, Centers for Disease Control

*"Special Focus on Reproductive Health Surveillance"* (Morbidity and Mortality Weekly Report, Vol. 40, No. SS-2, July 1991)

*Rates calculated by the editors. By state of occurrence. Percent is for listed states only.

**Not available.

# Reported Legal Abortions Performed at 12 Weeks or Less of Gestation in 1988
## (Selected States Only)
## Selected States Total = 590,769 Abortions Performed at 12 Weeks or Less of Gestation*

| RANK | STATE | ABORTIONS | % | RANK | STATE | ABORTIONS | % |
|---|---|---|---|---|---|---|---|
| 1 | New York | 119,633 | 20.25% | 26 | New Mexico | 4,474 | 0.76% |
| 2 | Texas | 70,424 | 11.92% | 27 | Utah | 4,287 | 0.73% |
| 3 | Virginia | 32,490 | 5.50% | 28 | Maine | 4,035 | 0.68% |
| 4 | North Carolina | 31,686 | 5.36% | 29 | Vermont | 3,178 | 0.54% |
| 5 | New Jersey | 29,408 | 4.98% | 30 | Montana | 2,655 | 0.45% |
| 6 | Georgia | 28,197 | 4.77% | 31 | North Dakota | 2,072 | 0.35% |
| 7 | Washington | 26,891 | 4.55% | 32 | Idaho | 1,592 | 0.27% |
| 8 | Maryland | 21,293 | 3.60% | 33 | South Dakota | 894 | 0.15% |
| 9 | Tennessee | 19,459 | 3.29% | 34 | Wyoming | 347 | 0.06% |
| 10 | Connecticut | 18,252 | 3.09% | – | Alabama** | N/A | N/A |
| 11 | Minnesota | 15,673 | 2.65% | – | Alaska** | N/A | N/A |
| 12 | Missouri | 15,011 | 2.54% | – | California** | N/A | N/A |
| 13 | Wisconsin | 14,624 | 2.48% | – | Delaware** | N/A | N/A |
| 14 | Arizona | 14,064 | 2.38% | – | Florida** | N/A | N/A |
| 15 | South Carolina | 14,054 | 2.38% | – | Illinois** | N/A | N/A |
| 16 | Louisiana | 13,142 | 2.22% | – | Indiana** | N/A | N/A |
| 17 | Oregon | 11,831 | 2.00% | – | Iowa** | N/A | N/A |
| 18 | Colorado | 10,866 | 1.84% | – | Massachusetts** | N/A | N/A |
| 19 | Kentucky | 8,570 | 1.45% | – | Michigan** | N/A | N/A |
| 20 | Rhode Island | 7,036 | 1.19% | – | Nebraska** | N/A | N/A |
| 21 | Nevada | 6,387 | 1.08% | – | New Hampshire** | N/A | N/A |
| 22 | Kansas | 6,152 | 1.04% | – | Ohio** | N/A | N/A |
| 23 | Hawaii | 5,319 | 0.90% | – | Oklahoma** | N/A | N/A |
| 24 | Arkansas | 5,010 | 0.85% | – | Pennsylvania** | N/A | N/A |
| 25 | Mississippi | 4,539 | 0.77% | – | West Virginia** | N/A | N/A |
| | | | | | District of Columbia | 17,224 | 2.92% |

Source: U.S. Department of Health and Human Services, Centers for Disease Control

   "Special Focus on Reproductive Health Surveillance" (Morbidity and Mortality Weekly Report, Vol. 40, No. SS-2, July 1991)

*By state of occurrence. Total is for listed states only.

**Not available.

# Percent of Reported Legal Abortions Performed at 12 Weeks or Less of Gestation in 1988
## (Selected States Only)
### Selected States Rate = 86.5% of Reported Legal Abortions*

| RANK | STATE | PERCENT | RANK | STATE | PERCENT |
|---|---|---|---|---|---|
| 1 | South Dakota | 99.6 | 26 | Missouri | 86.3 |
| 2 | South Carolina | 99.4 | 27 | Louisiana | 85.5 |
| 3 | Wyoming | 98.9 | 28 | Maine | 85.4 |
| 4 | Idaho | 96.4 | 29 | North Carolina | 84.2 |
| 5 | Vermont | 96.0 | 30 | New York | 83.7 |
| 6 | Virginia | 95.6 | 31 | New Jersey | 81.8 |
| 7 | North Dakota | 93.3 | 32 | Kansas | 81.7 |
| 8 | Montana | 92.6 | 33 | Georgia | 80.1 |
| 9 | Rhode Island | 92.5 | 34 | Kentucky | 73.6 |
| 10 | Arkansas | 92.1 | – | Alabama** | N/A |
| 10 | Nevada | 92.1 | – | Alaska** | N/A |
| 12 | Utah | 90.6 | – | California** | N/A |
| 13 | Connecticut | 90.2 | – | Delaware** | N/A |
| 13 | Washington | 90.2 | – | Florida** | N/A |
| 15 | Tennessee | 90.1 | – | Illinois** | N/A |
| 16 | Maryland | 89.8 | – | Indiana** | N/A |
| 17 | Oregon | 88.9 | – | Iowa* | N/A |
| 18 | Arizona | 88.4 | – | Massachusetts** | N/A |
| 19 | Hawaii | 88.1 | – | Michigan** | N/A |
| 20 | Mississippi | 87.8 | – | Nebraska** | N/A |
| 21 | Colorado | 87.5 | – | New Hampshire** | N/A |
| 21 | Wisconsin | 87.5 | – | Ohio** | N/A |
| 23 | New Mexico | 87.3 | – | Oklahoma** | N/A |
| 24 | Minnesota | 87.2 | – | Pennsylvania** | N/A |
| 25 | Texas | 86.4 | – | West Virginia** | N/A |

District of Columbia     82.6

Source: U.S. Department of Health and Human Services, Centers for Disease Control
    "Special Focus on Reproductive Health Surveillance" (Morbidity and Mortality Weekly Report, Vol. 40, No. SS-2, July 1991)
*Rates calculated by the editors. By state of occurrence. Total is for listed states only.
**Not available.

# Reported Legal Abortions Performed At or After 21 Weeks of Gestation in 1988
## (Selected States Only)
## Selected States Total = 7,457 Reported Legal Abortions*

| RANK | STATE | ABORTIONS | % | RANK | STATE | ABORTIONS | % |
|------|-------|-----------|---|------|-------|-----------|---|
| 1 | New York | 2,534 | 33.98% | 26 | Arkansas | 6 | 0.08% |
| 2 | Texas | 1,391 | 18.65% | 27 | Vermont | 5 | 0.07% |
| 3 | Georgia | 674 | 9.04% | 28 | Idaho | 1 | 0.01% |
| 4 | Washington | 396 | 5.31% | 29 | Maine | 0 | 0.00% |
| 5 | Kentucky | 393 | 5.27% | 29 | Montana | 0 | 0.00% |
| 6 | Kansas | 308 | 4.13% | 29 | North Dakota | 0 | 0.00% |
| 7 | New Jersey | 277 | 3.71% | 29 | South Dakota | 0 | 0.00% |
| 8 | Oregon | 211 | 2.83% | 29 | Utah | 0 | 0.00% |
| 9 | Wisconsin | 173 | 2.32% | 29 | Wyoming | 0 | 0.00% |
| 10 | Louisiana | 172 | 2.31% | – | Alabama** | N/A | N/A |
| 11 | Minnesota | 162 | 2.17% | – | Alaska** | N/A | N/A |
| 12 | Virginia | 138 | 1.85% | – | California** | N/A | N/A |
| 13 | North Carolina | 115 | 1.54% | – | Delaware** | N/A | N/A |
| 14 | Colorado | 110 | 1.48% | – | Florida** | N/A | N/A |
| 15 | Missouri | 75 | 1.01% | – | Illinois** | N/A | N/A |
| 16 | Tennessee | 57 | 0.76% | – | Indiana** | N/A | N/A |
| 17 | Arizona | 55 | 0.74% | – | Iowa** | N/A | N/A |
| 18 | Maryland | 49 | 0.66% | – | Massachusetts** | N/A | N/A |
| 19 | Hawaii | 31 | 0.42% | – | Michigan** | N/A | N/A |
| 20 | South Carolina | 21 | 0.28% | – | Nebraska** | N/A | N/A |
| 21 | New Mexico | 15 | 0.20% | – | New Hampshire** | N/A | N/A |
| 22 | Nevada | 12 | 0.16% | – | Ohio** | N/A | N/A |
| 23 | Connecticut | 11 | 0.15% | – | Oklahoma** | N/A | N/A |
| 24 | Mississippi | 10 | 0.13% | – | Pennsylvania** | N/A | N/A |
| 25 | Rhode Island | 8 | 0.11% | – | West Virginia** | N/A | N/A |
| | | | | | District of Columbia | 47 | 0.63% |

Source: U.S. Department of Health and Human Services, Centers for Disease Control

*Special Focus on Reproductive Health Surveillance" (Morbidity and Mortality Weekly Report, Vol. 40, No. SS-2, July 1991)

*By state of occurrence. Total is for listed states only.

**Not available.

# Percent of Reported Legal Abortions Performed At or After 21 Weeks of Gestation in 1988
## (Selected States Only)
## Selected States Rate = 1.1% of Reported Legal Abortions*

| RANK | STATE | PERCENT | RANK | STATE | PERCENT |
|---|---|---|---|---|---|
| 1 | Kansas | 4.1 | 24 | Idaho | 0.1 |
| 2 | Kentucky | 3.4 | 24 | Rhode Island | 0.1 |
| 3 | Georgia | 1.9 | 24 | South Carolina | 0.1 |
| 4 | New York | 1.8 | 29 | Maine | 0.0 |
| 5 | Texas | 1.7 | 29 | Montana | 0.0 |
| 6 | Oregon | 1.6 | 29 | North Dakota | 0.0 |
| 7 | Washington | 1.3 | 29 | South Dakota | 0.0 |
| 8 | Louisiana | 1.1 | 29 | Utah | 0.0 |
| 9 | Wisconsin | 1.0 | 29 | Wyoming | 0.0 |
| 10 | Colorado | 0.9 | – | Alabama** | N/A |
| 10 | Minnesota | 0.9 | – | Alaska** | N/A |
| 12 | New Jersey | 0.8 | – | California** | N/A |
| 13 | Hawaii | 0.5 | – | Delaware** | N/A |
| 14 | Missouri | 0.4 | – | Florida** | N/A |
| 14 | Virginia | 0.4 | – | Illinois** | N/A |
| 16 | Arizona | 0.3 | – | Indiana** | N/A |
| 16 | New Mexico | 0.3 | – | Iowa** | N/A |
| 16 | North Carolina | 0.3 | – | Massachusetts** | N/A |
| 16 | Tennessee | 0.3 | – | Michigan** | N/A |
| 20 | Maryland | 0.2 | – | Nebraska** | N/A |
| 20 | Mississippi | 0.2 | – | New Hampshire** | N/A |
| 20 | Nevada | 0.2 | – | Ohio** | N/A |
| 20 | Vermont | 0.2 | – | Oklahoma** | N/A |
| 24 | Arkansas | 0.1 | – | Pennsylvania** | N/A |
| 24 | Connecticut | 0.1 | – | West Virginia** | N/A |

District of Columbia                    0.2

Source: U.S. Department of Health and Human Services, Centers for Disease Control
   *Special Focus on Reproductive Health Surveillance"* (Morbidity and Mortality Weekly Report, Vol. 40, No. SS-2, July 1991)
*Rates calculated by the editors. By state of occurrence. Percent is for listed states only.
**Not available.

# II. DEATHS

# II. DEATHS (continued)

# II. DEATHS (continued)

# Deaths in 1991

## National Total = 2,165,000 Deaths*

| RANK | STATE | DEATHS | % | RANK | STATE | DEATHS | % |
|---|---|---|---|---|---|---|---|
| 1 | California | 218,735 | 10.10% | 26 | Arizona | 29,329 | 1.35% |
| 2 | New York | 166,795 | 7.70% | 27 | Connecticut | 27,745 | 1.28% |
| 3 | Florida | 135,280 | 6.25% | 28 | Iowa | 25,906 | 1.20% |
| 4 | Texas | 128,926 | 5.96% | 29 | Mississippi | 25,625 | 1.18% |
| 5 | Pennsylvania | 123,536 | 5.71% | 30 | Oregon | 25,205 | 1.16% |
| 6 | Illinois | 104,389 | 4.82% | 31 | Arkansas | 24,230 | 1.12% |
| 7 | Ohio | 99,104 | 4.58% | 32 | Kansas | 22,511 | 1.04% |
| 8 | Michigan | 79,972 | 3.69% | 33 | Colorado | 22,334 | 1.03% |
| 9 | New Jersey | 69,983 | 3.23% | 34 | West Virginia | 19,801 | 0.91% |
| 10 | North Carolina | 58,909 | 2.72% | 35 | Nebraska | 14,665 | 0.68% |
| 11 | Missouri | 53,461 | 2.47% | 36 | New Mexico | 11,116 | 0.51% |
| 12 | Georgia | 52,708 | 2.43% | 37 | Maine | 10,952 | 0.51% |
| 13 | Indiana | 51,780 | 2.39% | 38 | Rhode Island | 9,294 | 0.43% |
| 14 | Massachusetts | 51,366 | 2.37% | 39 | Nevada | 9,243 | 0.43% |
| 15 | Virginia | 49,151 | 2.27% | 40 | Utah | 9,199 | 0.42% |
| 16 | Tennessee | 45,351 | 2.09% | 41 | New Hampshire | 8,513 | 0.39% |
| 17 | Wisconsin | 43,749 | 2.02% | 42 | Idaho | 7,789 | 0.36% |
| 18 | Louisiana | 38,290 | 1.77% | 43 | Montana | 7,071 | 0.33% |
| 19 | Alabama | 38,027 | 1.76% | 44 | Hawaii | 6,715 | 0.31% |
| 20 | Maryland | 37,982 | 1.75% | 45 | South Dakota | 6,594 | 0.30% |
| 21 | Washington | 37,682 | 1.74% | 46 | Delaware | 5,880 | 0.27% |
| 22 | Kentucky | 35,281 | 1.63% | 47 | North Dakota | 5,648 | 0.26% |
| 23 | Minnesota | 35,270 | 1.63% | 48 | Vermont | 4,541 | 0.21% |
| 24 | Oklahoma | 30,349 | 1.40% | 49 | Wyoming | 3,167 | 0.15% |
| 25 | South Carolina | 29,983 | 1.38% | 50 | Alaska | 2,145 | 0.10% |
| | | | | | District of Columbia | 6,961 | 0.32% |

Source: U.S. Department of Health and Human Services, National Center for Health Statistics
   "Monthly Vital Statistics Report" (Vol. 40, No. 13, September 30, 1992)
*Data are provisional estimates by state of residence.

# Death Rate in 1991

## National Rate = 8.5 Deaths per 1,000 Population*

| RANK | STATE | RATE | | RANK | STATE | RATE |
|------|-------|------|---|------|-------|------|
| 1 | West Virginia | 10.9 | | 24 | North Dakota | 8.7 |
| 2 | Missouri | 10.3 | | 27 | Massachusetts | 8.6 |
| 3 | Pennsylvania | 10.2 | | 27 | Michigan | 8.6 |
| 4 | Florida | 10.1 | | 27 | Oregon | 8.6 |
| 5 | Arkansas | 10.0 | | 30 | Connecticut | 8.5 |
| 6 | Mississippi | 9.8 | | 31 | Delaware | 8.4 |
| 7 | Kentucky | 9.5 | | 32 | South Carolina | 8.3 |
| 7 | Oklahoma | 9.5 | | 33 | Arizona | 7.9 |
| 9 | Alabama | 9.2 | | 33 | Georgia | 7.9 |
| 9 | New York | 9.2 | | 33 | Maryland | 7.9 |
| 9 | Rhode Island | 9.2 | | 33 | Minnesota | 7.9 |
| 9 | South Dakota | 9.2 | | 37 | Virginia | 7.8 |
| 13 | Indiana | 9.1 | | 38 | Vermont | 7.7 |
| 13 | Iowa | 9.1 | | 39 | Washington | 7.6 |
| 15 | Nebraska | 9.0 | | 40 | Idaho | 7.5 |
| 15 | New Jersey | 9.0 | | 40 | Nevada | 7.5 |
| 15 | Ohio | 9.0 | | 42 | New Hampshire | 7.4 |
| 15 | Tennessee | 9.0 | | 42 | Texas | 7.4 |
| 19 | Illinois | 8.9 | | 44 | California | 7.2 |
| 19 | Wisconsin | 8.9 | | 45 | New Mexico | 7.1 |
| 21 | Kansas | 8.8 | | 46 | Wyoming | 6.8 |
| 21 | Louisiana | 8.8 | | 47 | Colorado | 6.7 |
| 21 | Montana | 8.8 | | 48 | Hawaii | 5.9 |
| 24 | Maine | 8.7 | | 49 | Utah | 5.3 |
| 24 | North Carolina | 8.7 | | 50 | Alaska | 4.0 |

District of Columbia     11.9

Source: U.S. Department of Health and Human Services, National Center for Health Statistics
   "Monthly Vital Statistics Report" (Vol. 40, No. 13, September 30, 1992)
*Data are provisional estimates by state of residence.

# Deaths in 1990

## National Total = 2,162,000 Deaths*

| RANK | STATE | DEATHS | % | | RANK | STATE | DEATHS | % |
|---|---|---|---|---|---|---|---|---|
| 1 | California | 214,692 | 9.93% | | 26 | Arizona | 28,653 | 1.33% |
| 2 | New York | 168,004 | 7.77% | | 27 | Iowa | 28,220 | 1.31% |
| 3 | Florida | 134,499 | 6.22% | | 28 | Connecticut | 26,935 | 1.25% |
| 4 | Texas | 126,756 | 5.86% | | 29 | Oregon | 25,725 | 1.19% |
| 5 | Pennsylvania | 122,928 | 5.69% | | 30 | Mississippi | 25,254 | 1.17% |
| 6 | Illinois | 103,478 | 4.79% | | 31 | Arkansas | 24,922 | 1.15% |
| 7 | Ohio | 99,049 | 4.58% | | 32 | Kansas | 22,348 | 1.03% |
| 8 | Michigan | 78,979 | 3.65% | | 33 | Colorado | 21,545 | 1.00% |
| 9 | New Jersey | 70,446 | 3.26% | | 34 | West Virginia | 19,502 | 0.90% |
| 10 | North Carolina | 57,532 | 2.66% | | 35 | Nebraska | 14,785 | 0.68% |
| 11 | Massachusetts | 55,092 | 2.55% | | 36 | Maine | 11,160 | 0.52% |
| 12 | Georgia | 52,617 | 2.43% | | 37 | New Mexico | 10,934 | 0.51% |
| 13 | Missouri | 51,558 | 2.38% | | 38 | Rhode Island | 9,380 | 0.43% |
| 14 | Indiana | 49,940 | 2.31% | | 39 | Utah | 9,325 | 0.43% |
| 15 | Virginia | 48,374 | 2.24% | | 40 | Nevada | 8,890 | 0.41% |
| 16 | Tennessee | 45,228 | 2.09% | | 41 | New Hampshire | 8,447 | 0.39% |
| 17 | Wisconsin | 42,744 | 1.98% | | 42 | Idaho | 7,603 | 0.35% |
| 18 | Alabama | 41,289 | 1.91% | | 43 | Montana | 6,964 | 0.32% |
| 19 | Maryland | 39,132 | 1.81% | | 44 | Hawaii | 6,741 | 0.31% |
| 20 | Louisiana | 36,832 | 1.70% | | 45 | South Dakota | 6,394 | 0.30% |
| 21 | Washington | 36,525 | 1.69% | | 46 | Delaware | 5,803 | 0.27% |
| 22 | Kentucky | 35,544 | 1.64% | | 47 | North Dakota | 5,657 | 0.26% |
| 23 | Minnesota | 34,802 | 1.61% | | 48 | Vermont | 4,601 | 0.21% |
| 24 | Oklahoma | 30,314 | 1.40% | | 49 | Wyoming | 3,248 | 0.15% |
| 25 | South Carolina | 29,891 | 1.38% | | 50 | Alaska | 2,198 | 0.10% |
| | | | | | | District of Columbia | 7,518 | 0.35% |

Source: U.S. Department of Health and Human Services, National Center for Health Statistics
"Monthly Vital Statistics Report" (Vol. 40, No. 13, September 30, 1992)
*Data are provisional estimates by state of residence.

# Death Rate in 1990

## National Rate = 8.6 Deaths per 1,000 Population*

| RANK | STATE | RATE | | RANK | STATE | RATE |
|---|---|---|---|---|---|---|
| 1 | West Virginia | 10.6 | | 25 | North Carolina | 8.6 |
| 2 | Arkansas | 10.3 | | 25 | North Dakota | 8.6 |
| 2 | Florida | 10.3 | | 28 | Delaware | 8.5 |
| 4 | Pennsylvania | 10.2 | | 28 | Michigan | 8.5 |
| 5 | Alabama | 10.0 | | 30 | Louisiana | 8.4 |
| 6 | Iowa | 9.9 | | 30 | South Carolina | 8.4 |
| 6 | Missouri | 9.9 | | 32 | Connecticut | 8.3 |
| 8 | Mississippi | 9.6 | | 33 | Maryland | 8.2 |
| 9 | Kentucky | 9.5 | | 34 | Georgia | 8.0 |
| 10 | Oklahoma | 9.4 | | 34 | Vermont | 8.0 |
| 11 | Massachusetts | 9.3 | | 36 | Arizona | 7.9 |
| 11 | New York | 9.3 | | 36 | Minnesota | 7.9 |
| 11 | Rhode Island | 9.3 | | 38 | Virginia | 7.8 |
| 14 | Nebraska | 9.1 | | 39 | Nevada | 7.6 |
| 14 | New Jersey | 9.1 | | 40 | New Hampshire | 7.5 |
| 14 | Tennessee | 9.1 | | 40 | Washington | 7.5 |
| 17 | Maine | 9.0 | | 42 | Idaho | 7.4 |
| 17 | Ohio | 9.0 | | 42 | Texas | 7.4 |
| 19 | Indiana | 8.9 | | 44 | California | 7.2 |
| 19 | Oregon | 8.9 | | 45 | New Mexico | 7.1 |
| 19 | South Dakota | 8.9 | | 46 | Wyoming | 6.9 |
| 22 | Illinois | 8.8 | | 47 | Colorado | 6.5 |
| 22 | Kansas | 8.8 | | 48 | Hawaii | 6.0 |
| 24 | Wisconsin | 8.7 | | 49 | Utah | 5.4 |
| 25 | Montana | 8.6 | | 50 | Alaska | 4.2 |
| | | | | | District of Columbia | 12.6 |

Source: U.S. Department of Health and Human Services, National Center for Health Statistics
    *"Monthly Vital Statistics Report" (Vol. 40, No. 13, September 30, 1992)*
*Data are provisional estimates by state of residence.*

# Deaths in 1980

## National Total = 1,990,000 Deaths*

| RANK | STATE | DEATHS | % | RANK | STATE | DEATHS | % |
|---|---|---|---|---|---|---|---|
| 1 | California | 187,000 | 9.40% | 25 | Iowa | 27,000 | 1.36% |
| 2 | New York | 173,000 | 8.69% | 27 | South Carolina | 25,000 | 1.26% |
| 3 | Pennsylvania | 124,000 | 6.23% | 28 | Mississippi | 24,000 | 1.21% |
| 4 | Texas | 108,000 | 5.43% | 29 | Arkansas | 23,000 | 1.16% |
| 5 | Florida | 105,000 | 5.28% | 30 | Kansas | 22,000 | 1.11% |
| 6 | Illinois | 103,000 | 5.18% | 30 | Oregon | 22,000 | 1.11% |
| 7 | Ohio | 98,000 | 4.92% | 32 | Arizona | 21,000 | 1.06% |
| 8 | Michigan | 75,000 | 3.77% | 33 | Colorado | 19,000 | 0.95% |
| 9 | New Jersey | 69,000 | 3.47% | 33 | West Virginia | 19,000 | 0.95% |
| 10 | Massachusetts | 55,000 | 2.76% | 35 | Nebraska | 14,000 | 0.70% |
| 11 | Missouri | 50,000 | 2.51% | 36 | Maine | 11,000 | 0.55% |
| 12 | North Carolina | 48,000 | 2.41% | 37 | New Mexico | 9,000 | 0.45% |
| 13 | Indiana | 47,000 | 2.36% | 37 | Rhode Island | 9,000 | 0.45% |
| 14 | Georgia | 44,000 | 2.21% | 39 | New Hampshire | 8,000 | 0.40% |
| 15 | Virginia | 43,000 | 2.16% | 39 | Utah | 8,000 | 0.40% |
| 16 | Tennessee | 41,000 | 2.06% | 41 | Idaho | 7,000 | 0.35% |
| 16 | Wisconsin | 41,000 | 2.06% | 41 | Montana | 7,000 | 0.35% |
| 18 | Alabama | 36,000 | 1.81% | 41 | South Dakota | 7,000 | 0.35% |
| 18 | Louisiana | 36,000 | 1.81% | 44 | Nevada | 6,000 | 0.30% |
| 20 | Kentucky | 34,000 | 1.71% | 44 | North Dakota | 6,000 | 0.30% |
| 20 | Maryland | 34,000 | 1.71% | 46 | Delaware | 5,000 | 0.25% |
| 22 | Minnesota | 33,000 | 1.66% | 46 | Hawaii | 5,000 | 0.25% |
| 23 | Washington | 32,000 | 1.61% | 46 | Vermont | 5,000 | 0.25% |
| 24 | Oklahoma | 28,000 | 1.41% | 49 | Wyoming | 3,000 | 0.15% |
| 25 | Connecticut | 27,000 | 1.36% | 50 | Alaska | 2,000 | 0.10% |
| | | | | | District of Columbia | 7,000 | 0.35% |

Source: U.S. Department of Health and Human Services, Centers for Disease Control, National Center for Health Statistics
"Vital Statistics of the United States 1980" and "Monthly Vital Statistics Report"
*By state of residence.

60

# Death Rate in 1980

## National Rate = 8.8 Deaths per 1,000 Population*

| RANK | STATE | RATE |
|------|-------|------|
| 1 | Florida | 10.7 |
| 2 | Pennsylvania | 10.4 |
| 3 | Missouri | 10.1 |
| 4 | Arkansas | 9.9 |
| 4 | West Virginia | 9.9 |
| 6 | New York | 9.8 |
| 6 | Rhode Island | 9.8 |
| 8 | Maine | 9.6 |
| 8 | Massachusetts | 9.6 |
| 10 | South Dakota | 9.5 |
| 11 | Mississippi | 9.4 |
| 11 | New Jersey | 9.4 |
| 13 | Iowa | 9.3 |
| 13 | Kansas | 9.3 |
| 13 | Oklahoma | 9.3 |
| 16 | Kentucky | 9.2 |
| 16 | Nebraska | 9.2 |
| 18 | Alabama | 9.1 |
| 18 | Ohio | 9.1 |
| 20 | Illinois | 9.0 |
| 20 | Vermont | 9.0 |
| 22 | Tennessee | 8.9 |
| 23 | Connecticut | 8.8 |
| 24 | Wisconsin | 8.7 |
| 25 | Indiana | 8.6 |

| RANK | STATE | RATE |
|------|-------|------|
| 25 | North Dakota | 8.6 |
| 27 | Delaware | 8.5 |
| 27 | Louisiana | 8.5 |
| 27 | Montana | 8.5 |
| 30 | New Hampshire | 8.3 |
| 30 | Oregon | 8.3 |
| 32 | Minnesota | 8.2 |
| 32 | North Carolina | 8.2 |
| 34 | Georgia | 8.1 |
| 34 | Maryland | 8.1 |
| 34 | Michigan | 8.1 |
| 34 | South Carolina | 8.1 |
| 38 | Virginia | 8.0 |
| 39 | Arizona | 7.9 |
| 39 | California | 7.9 |
| 41 | Washington | 7.7 |
| 42 | Texas | 7.6 |
| 43 | Nevada | 7.4 |
| 44 | Idaho | 7.2 |
| 45 | New Mexico | 7.0 |
| 46 | Wyoming | 6.9 |
| 47 | Colorado | 6.6 |
| 48 | Utah | 5.6 |
| 49 | Hawaii | 5.2 |
| 50 | Alaska | 4.3 |

| | | |
|---|---|---|
| | District of Columbia | 11.1 |

Source: U.S. Department of Health and Human Services, Centers for Disease Control, National Center for Health Statistics
    "Vital Statistics of the United States 1980" and "Monthly Vital Statistics Report"
*By state of residence.

# Infant Deaths in 1992

## National Total = 36,100 Infant Deaths*

| RANK | STATE | INFANT DEATHS | % | RANK | STATE | INFANT DEATHS | % |
|------|-------|---------------|---|------|-------|---------------|---|
| 1 | Texas | 2,498 | 6.92% | 26 | Colorado | 424 | 1.17% |
| 2 | Illinois | 2,075 | 5.75% | 27 | Arkansas | 354 | 0.98% |
| 3 | Florida | 1,661 | 4.60% | 28 | Kansas | 334 | 0.93% |
| 4 | Pennsylvania | 1,534 | 4.25% | 29 | Oregon | 325 | 0.90% |
| 5 | Ohio | 1,513 | 4.19% | 30 | Iowa | 289 | 0.80% |
| 6 | Michigan | 1,495 | 4.14% | 31 | New Mexico | 258 | 0.71% |
| 7 | Georgia | 1,217 | 3.37% | 32 | Utah | 228 | 0.63% |
| 8 | North Carolina | 1,077 | 2.98% | 33 | West Virginia | 206 | 0.57% |
| 9 | New Jersey | 1,016 | 2.81% | 34 | Nebraska | 184 | 0.51% |
| 10 | Virginia | 905 | 2.51% | 35 | Nevada | 167 | 0.46% |
| 11 | Missouri | 775 | 2.15% | 36 | Hawaii | 144 | 0.40% |
| 12 | Louisiana | 761 | 2.11% | 37 | Delaware | 137 | 0.38% |
| 13 | Indiana | 744 | 2.06% | 38 | Idaho | 134 | 0.37% |
| 14 | Tennessee | 739 | 2.05% | 39 | Maine | 107 | 0.30% |
| 15 | Alabama | 676 | 1.87% | 40 | Rhode Island | 104 | 0.29% |
| 16 | Maryland | 668 | 1.85% | 41 | Alaska | 103 | 0.29% |
| 17 | South Carolina | 594 | 1.65% | 42 | South Dakota | 99 | 0.27% |
| 18 | Massachusetts | 590 | 1.63% | 43 | New Hampshire | 96 | 0.27% |
| 19 | Wisconsin | 589 | 1.63% | 44 | Montana | 85 | 0.24% |
| 20 | Arizona | 584 | 1.62% | 45 | North Dakota | 83 | 0.23% |
| 21 | Washington | 580 | 1.61% | 46 | Wyoming | 57 | 0.16% |
| 22 | Minnesota | 501 | 1.39% | 47 | Vermont | 47 | 0.13% |
| 23 | Mississippi | 476 | 1.32% | – | California** | N/A | N/A |
| 24 | Kentucky | 459 | 1.27% | – | Connecticut** | N/A | N/A |
| 25 | Oklahoma | 457 | 1.27% | – | New York** | N/A | N/A |
| | | | | | District of Columbia | 204 | 0.57% |

Source: U.S. Department of Health and Human Services, National Center for Health Statistics
"Monthly Vital Statistics Report" (Vol. 41, No. 2, June 26, 1992)

*For 12 month period ending February 1992. Provisional data. Deaths under 1 year old. Total includes states not shown separately.

** Not available.

# Infant Mortality Rate in 1992

## National Rate = 8.9 Infant Deaths per 1,000 Live Births*

| RANK | STATE | RATE | RANK | STATE | RATE |
|------|-------|------|------|-------|------|
| 1 | Delaware | 12.4 | 26 | Florida | 8.6 |
| 2 | Georgia | 11.0 | 27 | Wyoming | 8.5 |
| 2 | Mississippi | 11.0 | 28 | Kentucky | 8.3 |
| 4 | Illinois | 10.7 | 28 | Maryland | 8.3 |
| 5 | Alabama | 10.6 | 30 | Wisconsin | 8.2 |
| 6 | North Carolina | 10.4 | 31 | Idaho | 7.9 |
| 7 | South Carolina | 10.3 | 31 | Iowa | 7.9 |
| 8 | Louisiana | 10.2 | 33 | Colorado | 7.8 |
| 9 | Arkansas | 10.1 | 33 | Washington | 7.8 |
| 9 | Tennessee | 10.1 | 35 | Nebraska | 7.7 |
| 11 | Missouri | 10.0 | 35 | Texas | 7.7 |
| 12 | Michigan | 9.8 | 37 | Oregon | 7.6 |
| 13 | Oklahoma | 9.7 | 38 | Minnesota | 7.4 |
| 14 | Ohio | 9.5 | 39 | Montana | 7.3 |
| 15 | Virginia | 9.3 | 40 | Hawaii | 7.2 |
| 15 | West Virginia | 9.3 | 40 | Nevada | 7.2 |
| 17 | Pennsylvania | 9.2 | 42 | Rhode Island | 7.1 |
| 18 | Alaska | 9.1 | 43 | Massachusetts | 6.7 |
| 18 | New Mexico | 9.1 | 44 | Maine | 6.3 |
| 18 | North Dakota | 9.1 | 44 | Utah | 6.3 |
| 21 | South Dakota | 9.0 | 46 | Vermont | 6.1 |
| 22 | Arizona | 8.8 | 47 | New Hampshire | 6.0 |
| 22 | Indiana | 8.8 | – | California** | N/A |
| 22 | New Jersey | 8.8 | – | Connecticut** | N/A |
| 25 | Kansas | 8.7 | – | New York** | N/A |

District of Columbia                        21.0

Source: U.S. Department of Health and Human Services, National Center for Health Statistics
   "Monthly Vital Statistics Report" (Vol. 41, No. 2, June 26, 1992)
*State rates are for 12 month period ending February 1992. Provisional data. Deaths under 1 year old. National rate reflects 12 month period ending January 1992.
** Not available.

63

# Infant Deaths in 1991

## National Total = 36,500 Infant Deaths*

| RANK | STATE | DEATHS | % | RANK | STATE | DEATHS | % |
|---|---|---|---|---|---|---|---|
| 1 | California | 4,748 | 13.01% | 26 | Oklahoma | 467 | 1.28% |
| 2 | New York | 2,734 | 7.49% | 27 | Kentucky | 452 | 1.24% |
| 3 | Texas | 2,510 | 6.88% | 28 | Colorado | 446 | 1.22% |
| 4 | Illinois | 2,006 | 5.50% | 29 | Arkansas | 361 | 0.99% |
| 5 | Florida | 1,722 | 4.72% | 30 | Connecticut | 355 | 0.97% |
| 6 | Pennsylvania | 1,587 | 4.35% | 31 | Kansas | 352 | 0.96% |
| 7 | Michigan | 1,521 | 4.17% | 32 | Oregon | 326 | 0.89% |
| 8 | Ohio | 1,500 | 4.11% | 33 | Iowa | 279 | 0.76% |
| 9 | Georgia | 1,364 | 3.74% | 34 | New Mexico | 239 | 0.65% |
| 10 | North Carolina | 1,123 | 3.08% | 35 | Utah | 210 | 0.58% |
| 11 | New Jersey | 1,013 | 2.78% | 36 | West Virginia | 199 | 0.55% |
| 12 | Virginia | 938 | 2.57% | 37 | Nebraska | 177 | 0.48% |
| 13 | Missouri | 799 | 2.19% | 38 | Nevada | 162 | 0.44% |
| 14 | Indiana | 794 | 2.18% | 39 | Idaho | 150 | 0.41% |
| 15 | Louisiana | 716 | 1.96% | 40 | Delaware | 142 | 0.39% |
| 16 | Tennessee | 709 | 1.94% | 41 | Hawaii | 131 | 0.36% |
| 17 | Maryland | 684 | 1.87% | 42 | Rhode Island | 114 | 0.31% |
| 18 | Alabama | 675 | 1.85% | 43 | Maine | 105 | 0.29% |
| 19 | South Carolina | 617 | 1.69% | 43 | New Hampshire | 105 | 0.29% |
| 20 | Massachusetts | 591 | 1.62% | 45 | Alaska | 101 | 0.28% |
| 21 | Arizona | 588 | 1.61% | 46 | South Dakota | 99 | 0.27% |
| 22 | Wisconsin | 584 | 1.60% | 47 | Montana | 88 | 0.24% |
| 23 | Washington | 564 | 1.55% | 48 | North Dakota | 82 | 0.22% |
| 24 | Minnesota | 491 | 1.35% | 49 | Wyoming | 49 | 0.13% |
| 25 | Mississippi | 490 | 1.34% | 50 | Vermont | 47 | 0.13% |
| | | | | | District of Columbia | 199 | 0.55% |

Source: U.S. Department of Health and Human Services, National Center for Health Statistics
"Monthly Vital Statistics Report" (Vol. 40, No. 13, September 30, 1992)
*Data are provisional estimates by state of residence. Infant deaths are those occurring under 1 year.

# Infant Mortality Rate in 1991

## National Rate = 8.9 Infant Deaths per 1,000 Live Births*

| RANK | STATE | RATE | RANK | STATE | RATE |
|---|---|---|---|---|---|
| 1 | Delaware | 12.7 | 25 | Idaho | 8.7 |
| 2 | Georgia | 12.4 | 27 | New Jersey | 8.6 |
| 3 | Mississippi | 11.3 | 28 | New Mexico | 8.5 |
| 4 | Alabama | 11.2 | 29 | Colorado | 8.3 |
| 5 | North Carolina | 11.0 | 30 | Kentucky | 8.2 |
| 6 | South Carolina | 10.7 | 31 | Maryland | 8.1 |
| 7 | Arkansas | 10.4 | 31 | Wisconsin | 8.1 |
| 8 | Illinois | 10.3 | 33 | California | 7.8 |
| 9 | Missouri | 10.2 | 33 | Rhode Island | 7.8 |
| 10 | Michigan | 9.9 | 35 | Iowa | 7.7 |
| 10 | Oklahoma | 9.9 | 35 | Texas | 7.7 |
| 12 | Tennessee | 9.7 | 37 | Montana | 7.6 |
| 12 | Virginia | 9.7 | 37 | Oregon | 7.6 |
| 14 | Louisiana | 9.6 | 39 | Connecticut | 7.4 |
| 15 | Ohio | 9.5 | 39 | Nebraska | 7.4 |
| 16 | Indiana | 9.4 | 39 | Washington | 7.4 |
| 16 | Kansas | 9.4 | 42 | Minnesota | 7.3 |
| 16 | New York | 9.4 | 43 | Wyoming | 7.2 |
| 16 | Pennsylvania | 9.4 | 44 | Nevada | 7.1 |
| 20 | Alaska | 9.0 | 45 | Massachusetts | 6.8 |
| 20 | North Dakota | 9.0 | 46 | Hawaii | 6.5 |
| 20 | South Dakota | 9.0 | 46 | New Hampshire | 6.5 |
| 20 | West Virginia | 9.0 | 48 | Maine | 6.3 |
| 24 | Florida | 8.9 | 49 | Vermont | 6.1 |
| 25 | Arizona | 8.7 | 50 | Utah | 6.0 |

District of Columbia                    20.0

*Source: U.S. Department of Health and Human Services, National Center for Health Statistics*

*"Monthly Vital Statistics Report" (Vol. 40, No. 13, September 30, 1992)*

*\*Data are provisional estimates by state of residence. Infant deaths are those occurring under 1 year.*

# Births to Deaths Ratio in 1991

## National Ratio = 1.90 Births for Every Death in 1991 *

| RANK | STATE | RATIO | RANK | STATE | RATIO |
|------|-------|-------|------|-------|-------|
| 1 | Alaska | 5.24 | 26 | Mississippi | 1.70 |
| 2 | Utah | 3.81 | 26 | Oregon | 1.70 |
| 3 | Hawaii | 2.98 | 26 | Vermont | 1.70 |
| 4 | California | 2.77 | 29 | Massachusetts | 1.68 |
| 5 | New Mexico | 2.53 | 29 | New Jersey | 1.68 |
| 5 | Texas | 2.53 | 31 | South Dakota | 1.67 |
| 7 | Nevada | 2.49 | 32 | Kansas | 1.66 |
| 8 | Colorado | 2.42 | 33 | Indiana | 1.64 |
| 9 | Arizona | 2.31 | 33 | Wisconsin | 1.64 |
| 10 | Maryland | 2.22 | 35 | Montana | 1.63 |
| 11 | Idaho | 2.21 | 35 | Nebraska | 1.63 |
| 12 | Wyoming | 2.15 | 37 | North Dakota | 1.61 |
| 13 | Georgia | 2.09 | 37 | Tennessee | 1.61 |
| 14 | Washington | 2.01 | 39 | Ohio | 1.60 |
| 15 | Virginia | 1.97 | 40 | Alabama | 1.59 |
| 16 | Louisiana | 1.95 | 41 | Rhode Island | 1.57 |
| 17 | South Carolina | 1.93 | 42 | Kentucky | 1.56 |
| 18 | Michigan | 1.92 | 42 | Oklahoma | 1.56 |
| 19 | Delaware | 1.90 | 44 | Maine | 1.51 |
| 19 | Minnesota | 1.90 | 45 | Missouri | 1.46 |
| 21 | New Hampshire | 1.89 | 46 | Florida | 1.44 |
| 22 | Illinois | 1.86 | 47 | Arkansas | 1.43 |
| 23 | New York | 1.75 | 48 | Iowa | 1.39 |
| 24 | Connecticut | 1.74 | 49 | Pennsylvania | 1.36 |
| 24 | North Carolina | 1.74 | 50 | West Virginia | 1.12 |
| | | | | District of Columbia | 1.43 |

Source: U.S. Department of Health and Human Services, National Center for Health Statistics
    "Monthly Vital Statistics Report" (Vol. 40, No. 13, September 30, 1992)
*Calculated by the editors.  Data are provisional estimates by state of residence.

# Infant Deaths in 1990

## National Total = 38,100 Infant Deaths*

| RANK | STATE | DEATHS | % | RANK | STATE | DEATHS | % |
|---|---|---|---|---|---|---|---|
| 1 | California | 4,722 | 12.39% | 26 | Kentucky | 495 | 1.30% |
| 2 | New York | 2,975 | 7.81% | 27 | Oklahoma | 463 | 1.22% |
| 3 | Texas | 2,552 | 6.70% | 28 | Colorado | 443 | 1.16% |
| 4 | Illinois | 2,132 | 5.60% | 29 | Connecticut | 413 | 1.08% |
| 5 | Florida | 1,930 | 5.07% | 30 | Arkansas | 362 | 0.95% |
| 6 | Michigan | 1,672 | 4.39% | 31 | Iowa | 341 | 0.90% |
| 7 | Pennsylvania | 1,646 | 4.32% | 32 | Oregon | 331 | 0.87% |
| 8 | Ohio | 1,558 | 4.09% | 33 | Kansas | 310 | 0.81% |
| 9 | Georgia | 1,246 | 3.27% | 34 | Utah | 264 | 0.69% |
| 10 | North Carolina | 1,156 | 3.03% | 35 | New Mexico | 252 | 0.66% |
| 11 | New Jersey | 1,117 | 2.93% | 36 | West Virginia | 211 | 0.55% |
| 12 | Virginia | 1,020 | 2.68% | 37 | Nebraska | 188 | 0.49% |
| 13 | Indiana | 843 | 2.21% | 38 | Nevada | 181 | 0.48% |
| 14 | Maryland | 771 | 2.02% | 39 | Idaho | 149 | 0.39% |
| 15 | Louisiana | 761 | 2.00% | 40 | Hawaii | 148 | 0.39% |
| 16 | Tennessee | 759 | 1.99% | 41 | New Hampshire | 120 | 0.31% |
| 17 | Massachusetts | 713 | 1.87% | 42 | Alaska | 118 | 0.31% |
| 18 | Missouri | 702 | 1.84% | 43 | Maine | 114 | 0.30% |
| 19 | South Carolina | 680 | 1.78% | 44 | Montana | 112 | 0.29% |
| 20 | Alabama | 654 | 1.72% | 45 | South Dakota | 107 | 0.28% |
| 21 | Washington | 616 | 1.62% | 46 | Delaware | 106 | 0.28% |
| 22 | Arizona | 610 | 1.60% | 47 | Rhode Island | 104 | 0.27% |
| 23 | Wisconsin | 606 | 1.59% | 48 | North Dakota | 72 | 0.19% |
| 24 | Mississippi | 536 | 1.41% | 49 | Wyoming | 56 | 0.15% |
| 25 | Minnesota | 502 | 1.32% | 50 | Vermont | 53 | 0.14% |
| | | | | | District of Columbia | 203 | 0.53% |

Source: U.S. Department of Health and Human Services, National Center for Health Statistics
"Monthly Vital Statistics Report" (Vol. 40, No. 13, September 30, 1992)
*Data are provisional estimates by state of residence. Infant deaths are those occurring under 1 year.

# Infant Mortality Rate in 1990

## National Rate = 9.1 Infant Deaths per 1,000 Live Births*

| RANK | STATE | RATE | | RANK | STATE | RATE |
|------|-------|------|---|------|-------|------|
| 1 | Mississippi | 12.2 | | 26 | Arizona | 8.9 |
| 2 | South Carolina | 11.5 | | 27 | New Mexico | 8.8 |
| 3 | Georgia | 11.0 | | 28 | Iowa | 8.7 |
| 3 | North Carolina | 11.0 | | 29 | Kentucky | 8.6 |
| 5 | Illinois | 10.9 | | 29 | Missouri | 8.6 |
| 6 | Louisiana | 10.6 | | 31 | Nevada | 8.5 |
| 7 | Michigan | 10.5 | | 32 | Colorado | 8.4 |
| 8 | Tennessee | 10.4 | | 33 | Wisconsin | 8.3 |
| 9 | Virginia | 10.2 | | 34 | Wyoming | 8.0 |
| 10 | Alaska | 10.1 | | 35 | Connecticut | 7.9 |
| 11 | Arkansas | 10.0 | | 35 | Washington | 7.9 |
| 12 | Indiana | 9.9 | | 37 | Nebraska | 7.8 |
| 12 | New York | 9.9 | | 37 | Texas | 7.8 |
| 14 | Oklahoma | 9.8 | | 39 | Kansas | 7.7 |
| 14 | South Dakota | 9.8 | | 40 | California | 7.6 |
| 16 | Florida | 9.7 | | 40 | Massachusetts | 7.6 |
| 17 | Alabama | 9.6 | | 40 | North Dakota | 7.6 |
| 17 | Pennsylvania | 9.6 | | 43 | Oregon | 7.5 |
| 19 | Montana | 9.5 | | 44 | Hawaii | 7.3 |
| 19 | Ohio | 9.5 | | 44 | Minnesota | 7.3 |
| 19 | West Virginia | 9.5 | | 44 | Utah | 7.3 |
| 22 | Delaware | 9.4 | | 47 | New Hampshire | 7.0 |
| 23 | Maryland | 9.2 | | 47 | Rhode Island | 7.0 |
| 24 | Idaho | 9.0 | | 49 | Maine | 6.7 |
| 24 | New Jersey | 9.0 | | 50 | Vermont | 6.4 |

District of Columbia     18.6

Source: U.S. Department of Health and Human Services, National Center for Health Statistics
   "Monthly Vital Statistics Report" (Vol. 40, No. 13, September 30, 1992)
*Data are provisional estimates by state of residence. Infant deaths are those occurring under 1 year.

# Infant Mortality Rate in 1980

## National Rate = 12.6 Infant Deaths per 1,000 Live Births*

| RANK | STATE | RATE | RANK | STATE | RATE |
|---|---|---|---|---|---|
| 1 | Mississippi | 17.0 | 25 | Texas | 12.2 |
| 2 | South Carolina | 15.6 | 27 | North Dakota | 12.1 |
| 3 | Alabama | 15.1 | 28 | Indiana | 11.9 |
| 4 | Illinois | 14.8 | 29 | Iowa | 11.8 |
| 5 | Florida | 14.6 | 29 | Washington | 11.8 |
| 6 | Georgia | 14.5 | 29 | West Virginia | 11.8 |
| 6 | North Carolina | 14.5 | 32 | Nebraska | 11.5 |
| 8 | Louisiana | 14.3 | 32 | New Mexico | 11.5 |
| 9 | Maryland | 14.0 | 34 | Connecticut | 11.2 |
| 10 | Delaware | 13.9 | 35 | California | 11.1 |
| 11 | Virginia | 13.6 | 36 | Rhode Island | 11.0 |
| 12 | Tennessee | 13.5 | 37 | South Dakota | 10.9 |
| 13 | Pennsylvania | 13.2 | 38 | Idaho | 10.7 |
| 14 | Kentucky | 12.9 | 38 | Nevada | 10.7 |
| 15 | Michigan | 12.8 | 38 | Vermont | 10.7 |
| 15 | Ohio | 12.8 | 41 | Massachusetts | 10.5 |
| 17 | Arkansas | 12.7 | 42 | Kansas | 10.4 |
| 17 | Oklahoma | 12.7 | 42 | Utah | 10.4 |
| 19 | New Jersey | 12.5 | 44 | Hawaii | 10.3 |
| 19 | New York | 12.5 | 44 | Wisconsin | 10.3 |
| 21 | Arizona | 12.4 | 46 | Colorado | 10.1 |
| 21 | Missouri | 12.4 | 47 | Minnesota | 10.0 |
| 21 | Montana | 12.4 | 48 | New Hampshire | 9.9 |
| 24 | Alaska | 12.3 | 49 | Wyoming | 9.8 |
| 25 | Oregon | 12.2 | 50 | Maine | 9.2 |

District of Columbia     25.0

Source: U.S. Department of Health and Human Services, Centers for Disease Control, National Center for Health Statistics
  "Vital Statistics of the United States, 1980" (Vol. I–Natality, issued 1984) and unpublished data
*Deaths of infants under 1 year old, exclusive of fetal deaths. By state of residence.

# White Infant Deaths in 1989

## National Total = 25,794 White Infant Deaths*

| RANK | STATE | DEATHS | % | RANK | STATE | DEATHS | % |
|---|---|---|---|---|---|---|---|
| 1 | California | 3,571 | 13.84% | 26 | Oregon | 329 | 1.28% |
| 2 | Texas | 2,043 | 7.92% | 27 | South Carolina | 312 | 1.21% |
| 3 | New York | 1,831 | 7.10% | 28 | Connecticut | 298 | 1.16% |
| 4 | Illinois | 1,282 | 4.97% | 29 | Oklahoma | 294 | 1.14% |
| 5 | Ohio | 1,148 | 4.45% | 30 | Iowa | 291 | 1.13% |
| 6 | Florida | 1,144 | 4.44% | 31 | Kansas | 280 | 1.09% |
| 7 | Pennsylvania | 1,111 | 4.31% | 32 | Utah | 255 | 0.99% |
| 8 | Michigan | 950 | 3.68% | 33 | Arkansas | 227 | 0.88% |
| 9 | Indiana | 674 | 2.61% | 34 | West Virginia | 198 | 0.77% |
| 10 | New Jersey | 651 | 2.52% | 35 | Mississippi | 190 | 0.74% |
| 11 | Georgia | 624 | 2.42% | 36 | New Mexico | 173 | 0.67% |
| 12 | North Carolina | 591 | 2.29% | 37 | Nebraska | 156 | 0.60% |
| 13 | Washington | 573 | 2.22% | 38 | Idaho | 144 | 0.56% |
| 14 | Massachusetts | 549 | 2.13% | 39 | New Hampshire | 141 | 0.55% |
| 15 | Missouri | 541 | 2.10% | 40 | Rhode Island | 128 | 0.50% |
| 16 | Virginia | 519 | 2.01% | 41 | Maine | 124 | 0.48% |
| 17 | Wisconsin | 514 | 1.99% | 42 | Nevada | 121 | 0.47% |
| 18 | Arizona | 495 | 1.92% | 43 | Montana | 98 | 0.38% |
| 19 | Tennessee | 459 | 1.78% | 44 | Delaware | 76 | 0.29% |
| 20 | Maryland | 416 | 1.61% | 45 | South Dakota | 64 | 0.25% |
| 21 | Colorado | 405 | 1.57% | 46 | Wyoming | 63 | 0.24% |
| 22 | Kentucky | 399 | 1.55% | 47 | North Dakota | 62 | 0.24% |
| 23 | Minnesota | 386 | 1.50% | 48 | Vermont | 59 | 0.23% |
| 24 | Alabama | 375 | 1.45% | 49 | Alaska | 54 | 0.21% |
| 25 | Louisiana | 352 | 1.36% | 50 | Hawaii | 28 | 0.11% |
| | | | | | District of Columbia | 26 | 0.10% |

Source: U.S. Department of Health and Human Services, National Center for Health Statistics
"Monthly Vital Statistics Report" (Vol. 40, No. 8(S)2, January 7, 1992)
*Deaths of infants under 1 year old, exclusive of fetal deaths. Based on race of the mother.

# White Infant Mortality Rate in 1989

## National Rate = 8.24 White Infant Deaths per 1,000 Live White Births*

| RANK | STATE | RATE | RANK | STATE | RATE |
|------|-------|------|------|-------|------|
| 1 | Rhode Island | 9.98 | 26 | Kansas | 8.29 |
| 2 | Montana | 9.93 | 26 | Maryland | 8.29 |
| 3 | Wyoming | 9.77 | 26 | Wisconsin | 8.29 |
| 4 | Delaware | 9.55 | 29 | Oklahoma | 8.26 |
| 5 | Idaho | 9.50 | 30 | New Hampshire | 8.09 |
| 6 | West Virginia | 9.38 | 31 | Pennsylvania | 8.03 |
| 7 | Alabama | 9.35 | 32 | Texas | 8.01 |
| 8 | Indiana | 9.26 | 33 | Florida | 7.98 |
| 9 | Illinois | 9.19 | 34 | California | 7.96 |
| 10 | South Carolina | 9.12 | 35 | Iowa | 7.86 |
| 11 | Georgia | 9.11 | 36 | New Mexico | 7.84 |
| 12 | Washington | 8.91 | 37 | Utah | 7.67 |
| 13 | Arizona | 8.81 | 38 | North Dakota | 7.47 |
| 14 | Oregon | 8.77 | 39 | Virginia | 7.45 |
| 15 | Mississippi | 8.65 | 40 | Nevada | 7.42 |
| 16 | New York | 8.64 | 41 | Maine | 7.26 |
| 17 | North Carolina | 8.63 | 42 | Alaska | 7.24 |
| 18 | Missouri | 8.56 | 43 | Connecticut | 7.22 |
| 19 | Colorado | 8.53 | 44 | Nebraska | 7.11 |
| 19 | Louisiana | 8.53 | 44 | South Dakota | 7.11 |
| 21 | Ohio | 8.49 | 46 | New Jersey | 7.10 |
| 22 | Arkansas | 8.47 | 47 | Massachusetts | 7.03 |
| 23 | Tennessee | 8.42 | 47 | Vermont | 7.03 |
| 24 | Kentucky | 8.38 | 49 | Minnesota | 6.37 |
| 25 | Michigan | 8.30 | 50 | Hawaii | 6.25 |

District of Columbia     15.25

Source: U.S. Department of Health and Human Services, National Center for Health Statistics
   "Monthly Vital Statistics Report" (Vol. 40, No. 8(S)2, January 7, 1992)
*Rates calculated by the editors. Based on race of the mother. Deaths of infants under 1 year old, exclusive of fetal deaths.

# Black Infant Deaths in 1989

## National Total = 12,527 Black Infant Deaths*

| RANK | STATE | DEATHS | % | RANK | STATE | DEATHS | % |
|---|---|---|---|---|---|---|---|
| 1 | New York | 1,205 | 9.62% | 26 | Oklahoma | 70 | 0.56% |
| 2 | California | 932 | 7.44% | 27 | Washington | 63 | 0.50% |
| 3 | Illinois | 931 | 7.43% | 28 | Arizona | 55 | 0.44% |
| 4 | Florida | 742 | 5.92% | 28 | Minnesota | 55 | 0.44% |
| 5 | Texas | 728 | 5.81% | 30 | Kansas | 52 | 0.42% |
| 6 | Georgia | 725 | 5.79% | 31 | Delaware | 50 | 0.40% |
| 7 | Michigan | 673 | 5.37% | 32 | Colorado | 45 | 0.36% |
| 8 | Pennsylvania | 579 | 4.62% | 33 | Nevada | 35 | 0.28% |
| 9 | North Carolina | 537 | 4.29% | 34 | Nebraska | 26 | 0.21% |
| 10 | Louisiana | 477 | 3.81% | 35 | Iowa | 23 | 0.18% |
| 11 | Ohio | 471 | 3.76% | 36 | Oregon | 22 | 0.18% |
| 12 | New Jersey | 464 | 3.70% | 37 | Rhode Island | 20 | 0.16% |
| 13 | Virginia | 436 | 3.48% | 38 | New Mexico | 11 | 0.09% |
| 14 | South Carolina | 419 | 3.34% | 38 | West Virginia | 11 | 0.09% |
| 15 | Maryland | 381 | 3.04% | 40 | Hawaii | 8 | 0.06% |
| 16 | Alabama | 377 | 3.01% | 41 | Utah | 6 | 0.05% |
| 17 | Tennessee | 327 | 2.61% | 42 | Alaska | 5 | 0.04% |
| 18 | Mississippi | 304 | 2.43% | 43 | Idaho | 1 | 0.01% |
| 19 | Missouri | 223 | 1.78% | 43 | New Hampshire | 1 | 0.01% |
| 20 | Indiana | 178 | 1.42% | 43 | North Dakota | 1 | 0.01% |
| 21 | Massachusetts | 138 | 1.10% | 43 | South Dakota | 1 | 0.01% |
| 22 | Arkansas | 137 | 1.09% | 47 | Maine | 0 | 0.00% |
| 23 | Connecticut | 130 | 1.04% | 47 | Montana | 0 | 0.00% |
| 24 | Wisconsin | 116 | 0.93% | 47 | Vermont | 0 | 0.00% |
| 25 | Kentucky | 92 | 0.73% | 47 | Wyoming | 0 | 0.00% |
|  |  |  |  |  | District of Columbia | 244 | 1.95% |

Source: U.S. Department of Health and Human Services, National Center for Health Statistics
    "Monthly Vital Statistics Report" (Vol. 40, No. 8(S)2, January 7, 1992)
*Deaths of infants under 1 year old, exclusive of fetal deaths. Based on race of the mother.

# Black Infant Mortality Rate in 1989

## National Rate = 17.66 Black Infant Deaths per 1,000 Live Black Births*

| RANK | STATE | RATE | RANK | STATE | RATE |
|------|-------|------|------|-------|------|
| 1 | Michigan | 21.81 | 26 | Texas | 16.12 |
| 2 | Pennsylvania | 21.20 | 27 | Wisconsin | 16.08 |
| 3 | Illinois | 20.65 | 28 | Arkansas | 15.95 |
| 4 | Delaware | 19.31 | 29 | Florida | 15.92 |
| 5 | Minnesota | 18.64 | 30 | Louisiana | 15.90 |
| 6 | South Carolina | 18.61 | 31 | Washington | 15.77 |
| 7 | Connecticut | 18.56 | 32 | Rhode Island | 15.69 |
| 8 | Indiana | 18.50 | 33 | Maryland | 15.31 |
| 9 | New Jersey | 18.44 | 34 | New Mexico | 15.05 |
| 10 | Tennessee | 18.30 | 35 | Mississippi | 14.80 |
| 11 | Oregon | 18.27 | 36 | Massachusetts | 14.51 |
| 12 | Iowa | 18.25 | 37 | Kansas | 13.93 |
| 13 | New York | 18.18 | 38 | Colorado | 13.84 |
| 14 | Georgia | 18.09 | 39 | Oklahoma | 12.67 |
| 14 | Virginia | 18.09 | 40 | West Virginia | 11.85 |
| 16 | Arizona | 17.76 | 41 | Idaho | 10.75 |
| 17 | Ohio | 17.55 | 42 | North Dakota | 8.93 |
| 18 | North Carolina | 17.49 | 43 | Hawaii | 8.55 |
| 19 | Alabama | 17.25 | 44 | South Dakota | 7.69 |
| 20 | Nevada | 17.20 | 45 | Alaska | 7.09 |
| 21 | Kentucky | 17.16 | 46 | New Hampshire | 5.43 |
| 22 | Nebraska | 16.82 | 47 | Maine | 0.00 |
| 23 | Missouri | 16.69 | 47 | Montana | 0.00 |
| 24 | California | 16.46 | 47 | Vermont | 0.00 |
| 25 | Utah | 16.13 | 47 | Wyoming | 0.00 |

District of Columbia     26.32

Source: U.S. Department of Health and Human Services, National Center for Health Statistics
"Monthly Vital Statistics Report" (Vol. 40, No. 8(S)2, January 7, 1992)
*Rates calculated by the editors. Based on race of the mother. Deaths of infants under 1 year old, exclusive of fetal deaths.

# White Infant Mortality Rate in 1980

## National Rate = 11.0 White Infant Deaths per 1,000 Live Births*

| RANK | STATE | RATE | | RANK | STATE | RATE |
|------|-------|------|---|------|-------|------|
| 1 | Oregon | 12.2 | | 25 | New York | 10.8 |
| 2 | North Carolina | 12.1 | | 25 | South Carolina | 10.8 |
| 2 | Oklahoma | 12.1 | | 28 | Idaho | 10.7 |
| 4 | Kentucky | 12.0 | | 28 | Nebraska | 10.7 |
| 5 | Pennsylvania | 11.9 | | 28 | Vermont | 10.7 |
| 5 | Tennessee | 11.9 | | 31 | California | 10.6 |
| 5 | Virginia | 11.9 | | 31 | Michigan | 10.6 |
| 8 | Arizona | 11.8 | | 33 | Indiana | 10.5 |
| 8 | Florida | 11.8 | | 33 | Louisiana | 10.5 |
| 8 | Montana | 11.8 | | 33 | Utah | 10.5 |
| 11 | Illinois | 11.7 | | 36 | Arkansas | 10.3 |
| 11 | North Dakota | 11.7 | | 36 | New Jersey | 10.3 |
| 13 | Alabama | 11.6 | | 38 | Connecticut | 10.2 |
| 13 | Hawaii | 11.6 | | 39 | Massachusetts | 10.1 |
| 13 | Maryland | 11.6 | | 40 | Nevada | 10.0 |
| 16 | Iowa | 11.5 | | 41 | New Hampshire | 9.9 |
| 16 | Washington | 11.5 | | 42 | Colorado | 9.8 |
| 18 | West Virginia | 11.4 | | 42 | Delaware | 9.8 |
| 19 | New Mexico | 11.3 | | 44 | Wisconsin | 9.7 |
| 20 | Ohio | 11.2 | | 45 | Minnesota | 9.6 |
| 20 | Texas | 11.2 | | 46 | Kansas | 9.5 |
| 22 | Mississippi | 11.1 | | 47 | Alaska | 9.4 |
| 22 | Missouri | 11.1 | | 47 | Maine | 9.4 |
| 24 | Rhode Island | 10.9 | | 49 | Wyoming | 9.3 |
| 25 | Georgia | 10.8 | | 50 | South Dakota | 9.0 |

| | | |
|---|---|---|
| District of Columbia | | 17.8 |

Source: U.S. Department of Health and Human Services, Centers for Disease Control, National Center for Health Statistics,
   "Vital Statistics of the United States, 1980" (Vol. I–Natality, issued 1984) and unpublished data
*Deaths of infants under 1 year old, exclusive of fetal deaths. By state of residence.

# Black Infant Mortality Rate in 1980

## National Rate = 21.4 Black Infant Deaths per 1,000 Live Births*

| RANK | STATE | RATE | RANK | STATE | RATE |
|------|-------|------|------|-------|------|
| 1 | Delaware | 27.9 | 24 | Nevada | 20.6 |
| 2 | North Dakota** | 27.5 | 27 | Maryland | 20.4 |
| 3 | Utah** | 27.3 | 28 | Arkansas | 20.0 |
| 4 | Iowa | 27.2 | 28 | Minnesota | 20.0 |
| 5 | Illinois | 26.3 | 28 | New York | 20.0 |
| 6 | Wyoming** | 25.9 | 28 | North Carolina | 20.0 |
| 7 | Nebraska | 25.2 | 32 | Virginia | 19.8 |
| 8 | Michigan | 24.2 | 33 | Alaska** | 19.5 |
| 9 | Mississippi | 23.7 | 34 | Tennessee | 19.3 |
| 10 | Indiana | 23.4 | 35 | Colorado | 19.1 |
| 11 | New Mexico** | 23.1 | 35 | Connecticut | 19.1 |
| 11 | Pennsylvania | 23.1 | 37 | Texas | 18.8 |
| 13 | Ohio | 23.0 | 38 | Wisconsin | 18.5 |
| 14 | South Carolina | 22.9 | 39 | Arizona | 18.4 |
| 15 | Florida | 22.8 | 40 | California | 18.0 |
| 16 | New Hampshire** | 22.5 | 41 | Rhode Island** | 17.4 |
| 17 | Kentucky | 22.0 | 42 | Massachusetts | 16.8 |
| 18 | New Jersey | 21.9 | 43 | Washington | 16.4 |
| 19 | Oklahoma | 21.8 | 44 | Oregon** | 15.9 |
| 20 | Alabama | 21.6 | 45 | Hawaii** | 11.8 |
| 21 | West Virginia | 21.5 | 46 | Idaho | 0.0 |
| 22 | Georgia | 21.0 | 46 | Maine | 0.0 |
| 23 | Missouri | 20.7 | 46 | Montana | 0.0 |
| 24 | Kansas | 20.6 | 46 | South Dakota | 0.0 |
| 24 | Louisiana | 20.6 | 46 | Vermont | 0.0 |
| | | | | District of Columbia | 26.7 |

Source: U.S. Department of Health and Human Services, Centers for Disease Control, National Center for Health Statistics
   "Vital Statistics of the United States, 1980" (Vol. I–Natality, issued 1984) and unpublished data
*Deaths of infants under 1 year old, exclusive of fetal deaths. By state of residence.
**Based on a frequency of less than 20 infant deaths.

# Neonatal Deaths in 1989

## National Total = 25,168 Neonatal Deaths*

| RANK | STATE | DEATHS | % | RANK | STATE | DEATHS | % |
|------|-------|--------|---|------|-------|--------|---|
| 1 | California | 2,961 | 11.76% | 26 | Kentucky | 283 | 1.12% |
| 2 | New York | 2,090 | 8.30% | 27 | Minnesota | 278 | 1.10% |
| 3 | Texas | 1,730 | 6.87% | 28 | Colorado | 272 | 1.08% |
| 4 | Illinois | 1,428 | 5.67% | 29 | Oklahoma | 234 | 0.93% |
| 5 | Florida | 1,253 | 4.98% | 30 | Arkansas | 216 | 0.86% |
| 6 | Pennsylvania | 1,183 | 4.70% | 31 | Iowa | 214 | 0.85% |
| 7 | Michigan | 1,071 | 4.26% | 32 | Oregon | 208 | 0.83% |
| 8 | Ohio | 1,033 | 4.10% | 33 | Kansas | 183 | 0.73% |
| 9 | Georgia | 887 | 3.52% | 34 | Utah | 158 | 0.63% |
| 10 | North Carolina | 775 | 3.08% | 35 | New Mexico | 146 | 0.58% |
| 11 | New Jersey | 751 | 2.98% | 36 | West Virginia | 139 | 0.55% |
| 12 | Virginia | 687 | 2.73% | 37 | Rhode Island | 115 | 0.46% |
| 13 | Indiana | 540 | 2.15% | 38 | Nebraska | 108 | 0.43% |
| 14 | Louisiana | 529 | 2.10% | 39 | Idaho | 100 | 0.40% |
| 15 | Maryland | 509 | 2.02% | 40 | Delaware | 92 | 0.37% |
| 16 | Alabama | 502 | 1.99% | 41 | Maine | 89 | 0.35% |
| 17 | Tennessee | 500 | 1.99% | 41 | New Hampshire | 89 | 0.35% |
| 18 | Massachusetts | 484 | 1.92% | 43 | Hawaii | 82 | 0.33% |
| 19 | South Carolina | 467 | 1.86% | 44 | Nevada | 76 | 0.30% |
| 20 | Missouri | 462 | 1.84% | 45 | Montana | 65 | 0.26% |
| 21 | Wisconsin | 391 | 1.55% | 46 | South Dakota | 51 | 0.20% |
| 22 | Washington | 381 | 1.51% | 47 | Alaska | 50 | 0.20% |
| 23 | Arizona | 371 | 1.47% | 48 | North Dakota | 45 | 0.18% |
| 24 | Connecticut | 315 | 1.25% | 49 | Vermont | 41 | 0.16% |
| 25 | Mississippi | 310 | 1.23% | 50 | Wyoming | 36 | 0.14% |
| | | | | | District of Columbia | 188 | 0.75% |

*Source: U.S. Department of Health and Human Services, National Center for Health Statistics*
 *"Monthly Vital Statistics Report" (Vol. 40, No. 8(S)2, January 7, 1992)*
*Deaths of infants under 28 days, exclusive of fetal deaths.

# Neonatal Death Rate in 1989

## National Rate = 6.23 Neonatal Deaths per 1,000 Live Births*

| RANK | STATE | RATE | | RANK | STATE | RATE |
|------|-------|------|---|------|-------|------|
| 1 | Delaware | 8.57 | | 26 | Montana | 5.57 |
| 2 | South Carolina | 8.15 | | 27 | Arizona | 5.52 |
| 3 | Georgia | 8.04 | | 28 | Iowa | 5.48 |
| 4 | Alabama | 8.02 | | 29 | Wisconsin | 5.43 |
| 5 | Rhode Island | 7.79 | | 30 | New Mexico | 5.34 |
| 6 | North Carolina | 7.59 | | 31 | Kentucky | 5.30 |
| 7 | Illinois | 7.50 | | 32 | Massachusetts | 5.29 |
| 8 | Louisiana | 7.27 | | 33 | Wyoming | 5.22 |
| 9 | Michigan | 7.21 | | 34 | California | 5.19 |
| 10 | Mississippi | 7.20 | | 35 | Colorado | 5.16 |
| 11 | New York | 7.17 | | 36 | Maine | 5.10 |
| 12 | Virginia | 7.10 | | 37 | Washington | 5.06 |
| 13 | Pennsylvania | 7.01 | | 38 | Oregon | 5.04 |
| 14 | Tennessee | 6.83 | | 39 | New Hampshire | 5.00 |
| 15 | Maryland | 6.50 | | 40 | Oklahoma | 4.94 |
| 16 | Florida | 6.49 | | 41 | Vermont | 4.83 |
| 17 | Indiana | 6.47 | | 42 | Kansas | 4.72 |
| 18 | Connecticut | 6.37 | | 43 | North Dakota | 4.70 |
| 19 | Idaho | 6.30 | | 44 | South Dakota | 4.60 |
| 19 | Ohio | 6.30 | | 45 | Nebraska | 4.46 |
| 21 | West Virginia | 6.27 | | 46 | Utah | 4.44 |
| 22 | New Jersey | 6.16 | | 47 | Alaska | 4.29 |
| 23 | Arkansas | 6.01 | | 48 | Hawaii | 4.23 |
| 24 | Missouri | 5.93 | | 49 | Minnesota | 4.12 |
| 25 | Texas | 5.62 | | 50 | Nevada | 3.88 |
| | | | | | District of Columbia | 15.95 |

Source: U.S. Department of Health and Human Services, National Center for Health Statistics
"Monthly Vital Statistics Report" (Vol. 40, No. 8(S)2, January 7, 1992)
*Rates calculated by the editors. Deaths of infants under 28 days, exclusive of fetal deaths.

# White Neonatal Deaths in 1989

## National Total = 16,428 White Neonatal Deaths*

| RANK | STATE | DEATHS | % | RANK | STATE | DEATHS | % |
|---|---|---|---|---|---|---|---|
| 1 | California | 2,201 | 13.40% | 26 | Connecticut | 220 | 1.34% |
| 2 | New York | 1,257 | 7.65% | 27 | South Carolina | 200 | 1.22% |
| 3 | Texas | 1,237 | 7.53% | 28 | Oregon | 194 | 1.18% |
| 4 | Illinois | 834 | 5.08% | 29 | Iowa | 191 | 1.16% |
| 5 | Pennsylvania | 792 | 4.82% | 30 | Oklahoma | 181 | 1.10% |
| 6 | Ohio | 739 | 4.50% | 31 | Kansas | 153 | 0.93% |
| 7 | Florida | 738 | 4.49% | 32 | Utah | 142 | 0.86% |
| 8 | Michigan | 608 | 3.70% | 33 | Arkansas | 139 | 0.85% |
| 9 | New Jersey | 454 | 2.76% | 34 | West Virginia | 134 | 0.82% |
| 10 | Indiana | 425 | 2.59% | 35 | Mississippi | 133 | 0.81% |
| 11 | Georgia | 393 | 2.39% | 36 | New Mexico | 113 | 0.69% |
| 12 | North Carolina | 379 | 2.31% | 37 | Rhode Island | 100 | 0.61% |
| 13 | Massachusetts | 376 | 2.29% | 38 | Idaho | 93 | 0.57% |
| 14 | Virginia | 370 | 2.25% | 39 | New Hampshire | 89 | 0.54% |
| 15 | Missouri | 339 | 2.06% | 40 | Nebraska | 87 | 0.53% |
| 16 | Washington | 326 | 1.98% | 41 | Maine | 85 | 0.52% |
| 17 | Wisconsin | 317 | 1.93% | 42 | Nevada | 59 | 0.36% |
| 18 | Arizona | 308 | 1.87% | 43 | Delaware | 58 | 0.35% |
| 19 | Tennessee | 279 | 1.70% | 44 | Montana | 52 | 0.32% |
| 20 | Alabama | 257 | 1.56% | 45 | Vermont | 41 | 0.25% |
| 21 | Maryland | 253 | 1.54% | 46 | North Dakota | 37 | 0.23% |
| 22 | Minnesota | 235 | 1.43% | 47 | South Dakota | 34 | 0.21% |
| 23 | Colorado | 233 | 1.42% | 47 | Wyoming | 34 | 0.21% |
| 24 | Kentucky | 229 | 1.39% | 49 | Alaska | 26 | 0.16% |
| 25 | Louisiana | 228 | 1.39% | 50 | Hawaii | 12 | 0.07% |
| | | | | | District of Columbia | 14 | 0.09% |

Source: U.S. Department of Health and Human Services, National Center for Health Statistics

   "Monthly Vital Statistics Report" (Vol. 40, No. 8(S)2, January 7, 1992)

*Deaths of infants under 28 days, exclusive of fetal deaths. Based on race of the mother.

# White Neonatal Death Rate in 1989

## National Rate = 5.25 Neonatal Deaths per 1,000 Live White Births*

| RANK | STATE | RATE | RANK | STATE | RATE |
|---|---|---|---|---|---|
| 1 | Rhode Island | 7.80 | 26 | Florida | 5.15 |
| 2 | Delaware | 7.29 | 27 | New Mexico | 5.12 |
| 3 | Alabama | 6.40 | 27 | Tennessee | 5.12 |
| 4 | West Virginia | 6.35 | 29 | New Hampshire | 5.11 |
| 5 | Idaho | 6.14 | 29 | Wisconsin | 5.11 |
| 6 | Mississippi | 6.05 | 31 | Oklahoma | 5.09 |
| 7 | Illinois | 5.98 | 32 | Washington | 5.07 |
| 8 | New York | 5.93 | 33 | Maryland | 5.04 |
| 9 | South Carolina | 5.85 | 34 | Maine | 4.98 |
| 10 | Indiana | 5.84 | 35 | New Jersey | 4.95 |
| 11 | Georgia | 5.74 | 36 | California | 4.91 |
| 12 | Pennsylvania | 5.72 | 36 | Colorado | 4.91 |
| 13 | North Carolina | 5.54 | 38 | Vermont | 4.89 |
| 14 | Louisiana | 5.53 | 39 | Texas | 4.85 |
| 15 | Arizona | 5.48 | 40 | Massachusetts | 4.82 |
| 16 | Ohio | 5.47 | 41 | Kentucky | 4.81 |
| 17 | Missouri | 5.37 | 42 | Kansas | 4.53 |
| 18 | Connecticut | 5.33 | 43 | North Dakota | 4.46 |
| 19 | Michigan | 5.31 | 44 | Utah | 4.27 |
| 19 | Virginia | 5.31 | 45 | Nebraska | 3.97 |
| 21 | Montana | 5.27 | 46 | Minnesota | 3.88 |
| 21 | Wyoming | 5.27 | 47 | South Dakota | 3.78 |
| 23 | Arkansas | 5.19 | 48 | Nevada | 3.62 |
| 24 | Oregon | 5.17 | 49 | Alaska | 3.49 |
| 25 | Iowa | 5.16 | 50 | Hawaii | 2.68 |

District of Columbia     8.21

Source: U.S. Department of Health and Human Services, National Center for Health Statistics
     "Monthly Vital Statistics Report" (Vol. 40, No. 8(S)2, January 7, 1992)
*Rates calculated by the editors. Deaths of infants under 28 days, exclusive of fetal deaths. Based on race of the mother.

# Black Neonatal Deaths in 1989

## National Total = 8,021 Black Neonatal Deaths*

| RANK | STATE | DEATHS | % | RANK | STATE | DEATHS | % |
|---|---|---|---|---|---|---|---|
| 1 | New York | 803 | 10.01% | 26 | Washington | 37 | 0.46% |
| 2 | Illinois | 577 | 7.19% | 27 | Oklahoma | 35 | 0.44% |
| 3 | California | 538 | 6.71% | 28 | Delaware | 33 | 0.41% |
| 4 | Florida | 507 | 6.32% | 28 | Minnesota | 33 | 0.41% |
| 5 | Georgia | 488 | 6.08% | 30 | Colorado | 32 | 0.40% |
| 6 | Texas | 464 | 5.78% | 31 | Arizona | 28 | 0.35% |
| 7 | Michigan | 453 | 5.65% | 32 | Kansas | 25 | 0.31% |
| 8 | North Carolina | 380 | 4.74% | 33 | Iowa | 17 | 0.21% |
| 9 | Pennsylvania | 375 | 4.68% | 34 | Nebraska | 16 | 0.20% |
| 10 | Virginia | 307 | 3.83% | 35 | Nevada | 15 | 0.19% |
| 11 | Louisiana | 298 | 3.72% | 36 | Rhode Island | 13 | 0.16% |
| 12 | Ohio | 291 | 3.63% | 37 | Oregon | 10 | 0.12% |
| 13 | New Jersey | 281 | 3.50% | 38 | New Mexico | 6 | 0.07% |
| 14 | South Carolina | 266 | 3.32% | 39 | Utah | 5 | 0.06% |
| 15 | Maryland | 249 | 3.10% | 39 | West Virginia | 5 | 0.06% |
| 16 | Alabama | 243 | 3.03% | 41 | Hawaii | 4 | 0.05% |
| 17 | Tennessee | 220 | 2.74% | 42 | Alaska | 3 | 0.04% |
| 18 | Mississippi | 176 | 2.19% | 43 | Idaho | 1 | 0.01% |
| 19 | Missouri | 120 | 1.50% | 44 | Maine | 0 | 0.00% |
| 20 | Indiana | 114 | 1.42% | 44 | Montana | 0 | 0.00% |
| 21 | Massachusetts | 100 | 1.25% | 44 | New Hampshire | 0 | 0.00% |
| 22 | Connecticut | 90 | 1.12% | 44 | North Dakota | 0 | 0.00% |
| 23 | Arkansas | 75 | 0.94% | 44 | South Dakota | 0 | 0.00% |
| 24 | Wisconsin | 61 | 0.76% | 44 | Vermont | 0 | 0.00% |
| 25 | Kentucky | 53 | 0.66% | 44 | Wyoming | 0 | 0.00% |
|  |  |  |  |  | District of Columbia | 174 | 2.17% |

Source: U.S. Department of Health and Human Services, National Center for Health Statistics
"Monthly Vital Statistics Report" (Vol. 40, No. 8(S)2, January 7, 1992)
*Deaths of infants under 28 days, exclusive of fetal deaths. Based on race of the mother.

# Black Neonatal Death Rate in 1989

## National Rate = 11.31 Black Neonatal Deaths per 1,000 Live Black Births*

| RANK | STATE | RATE | RANK | STATE | RATE |
|---|---|---|---|---|---|
| 1 | Michigan | 14.68 | 26 | Louisiana | 9.93 |
| 2 | Pennsylvania | 13.73 | 27 | Kentucky | 9.88 |
| 3 | Iowa | 13.49 | 28 | Colorado | 9.84 |
| 4 | Utah | 13.44 | 29 | California | 9.50 |
| 5 | Connecticut | 12.85 | 30 | Washington | 9.26 |
| 6 | Illinois | 12.80 | 31 | Arizona | 9.04 |
| 7 | Delaware | 12.75 | 32 | Missouri | 8.98 |
| 8 | Virginia | 12.74 | 33 | Arkansas | 8.73 |
| 9 | North Carolina | 12.38 | 34 | Mississippi | 8.57 |
| 10 | Tennessee | 12.31 | 35 | Wisconsin | 8.45 |
| 11 | Georgia | 12.18 | 36 | Oregon | 8.31 |
| 12 | New York | 12.11 | 37 | New Mexico | 8.21 |
| 13 | Indiana | 11.85 | 38 | Nevada | 7.37 |
| 14 | South Carolina | 11.81 | 39 | Kansas | 6.70 |
| 15 | Minnesota | 11.18 | 40 | Oklahoma | 6.34 |
| 16 | New Jersey | 11.17 | 41 | West Virginia | 5.39 |
| 17 | Alabama | 11.12 | 42 | Hawaii | 4.27 |
| 18 | Florida | 10.88 | 43 | Alaska | 4.26 |
| 19 | Ohio | 10.84 | 44 | Maine | 0.00 |
| 20 | Idaho | 10.75 | 44 | Montana | 0.00 |
| 21 | Massachusetts | 10.51 | 44 | New Hampshire | 0.00 |
| 22 | Nebraska | 10.35 | 44 | North Dakota | 0.00 |
| 23 | Texas | 10.27 | 44 | South Dakota | 0.00 |
| 24 | Rhode Island | 10.20 | 44 | Vermont | 0.00 |
| 25 | Maryland | 10.01 | 44 | Wyoming | 0.00 |

District of Columbia          18.77

Source:  U.S. Department of Health and Human Services, National Center for Health Statistics

    "Monthly Vital Statistics Report" (Vol. 40, No. 8(S)2, January 7, 1992)

*Rates calculated by the editors.  Deaths of infants under 28 days, exclusive of fetal deaths.  Based on race of the mother.

# Deaths by AIDS in 1991

## National Total = 13,882 Deaths by AIDS*

| RANK | STATE | DEATHS | % | RANK | STATE | DEATHS | % |
|------|-------|--------|---|------|-------|--------|---|
| 1 | California | 2,865 | 20.64% | 26 | Nevada | 91 | 0.66% |
| 2 | Florida | 1,846 | 13.30% | 27 | Oklahoma | 81 | 0.58% |
| 3 | New York | 1,656 | 11.93% | 28 | Hawaii | 78 | 0.56% |
| 4 | Texas | 957 | 6.89% | 29 | Wisconsin | 76 | 0.55% |
| 5 | New Jersey | 737 | 5.31% | 30 | Kentucky | 63 | 0.45% |
| 6 | Illinois | 560 | 4.03% | 31 | Mississippi | 55 | 0.40% |
| 7 | Georgia | 444 | 3.20% | 32 | Arkansas | 53 | 0.38% |
| 8 | Pennsylvania | 412 | 2.97% | 33 | New Mexico | 49 | 0.35% |
| 9 | Maryland | 364 | 2.62% | 34 | Kansas | 47 | 0.34% |
| 10 | Massachusetts | 301 | 2.17% | 35 | Iowa | 42 | 0.30% |
| 11 | Louisiana | 272 | 1.96% | 36 | Delaware | 34 | 0.24% |
| 12 | Washington | 250 | 1.80% | 37 | Utah | 34 | 0.24% |
| 13 | Ohio | 245 | 1.76% | 38 | Rhode Island | 31 | 0.22% |
| 14 | Michigan | 221 | 1.59% | 39 | Arizona | 25 | 0.18% |
| 15 | Virginia | 202 | 1.46% | 40 | West Virginia | 22 | 0.16% |
| 16 | North Carolina | 196 | 1.41% | 41 | Nebraska | 21 | 0.15% |
| 17 | Missouri | 192 | 1.38% | 42 | New Hampshire | 15 | 0.11% |
| 18 | Colorado | 188 | 1.35% | 43 | Maine | 14 | 0.10% |
| 19 | Oregon | 149 | 1.07% | 44 | Montana | 11 | 0.08% |
| 20 | Tennessee | 141 | 1.02% | 45 | Idaho | 10 | 0.07% |
| 21 | Connecticut | 122 | 0.88% | 46 | Vermont | 9 | 0.06% |
| 22 | Alabama | 118 | 0.85% | 47 | Wyoming | 6 | 0.04% |
| 22 | Minnesota | 110 | 0.79% | 48 | Alaska | 4 | 0.03% |
| 24 | Indiana | 104 | 0.75% | 49 | South Dakota | 3 | 0.02% |
| 25 | South Carolina | 100 | 0.72% | 50 | North Dakota | 0 | 0.00% |

| | | | |
|---|---|---|---|
| | District of Columbia | 256 | 1.84% |

Source: U.S. Department of Health and Human Services, Centers for Disease Control
"Health, United States, 1991"

*As of September 30, 1991. Numbers reflect reporting delays and differ from figures released earlier. AIDS is Acquired Immunodeficiency Syndrome.

# Deaths by AIDS in 1990

## National Total = 25,747 Deaths by AIDS*

| RANK | STATE | DEATHS | % | RANK | STATE | DEATHS | % |
|---|---|---|---|---|---|---|---|
| 1 | California | 5,149 | 20.00% | 26 | Minnesota | 161 | 0.63% |
| 2 | New York | 4,902 | 19.04% | 27 | Mississippi | 125 | 0.49% |
| 3 | Florida | 2,565 | 9.96% | 28 | Kentucky | 116 | 0.45% |
| 4 | Texas | 2,092 | 8.13% | 29 | Nevada | 115 | 0.45% |
| 5 | New Jersey | 1,244 | 4.83% | 30 | Oklahoma | 112 | 0.44% |
| 6 | Illinois | 873 | 3.39% | 31 | Wisconsin | 110 | 0.43% |
| 7 | Pennsylvania | 815 | 3.17% | 32 | Hawaii | 106 | 0.41% |
| 8 | Georgia | 806 | 3.13% | 33 | Kansas | 78 | 0.30% |
| 9 | Maryland | 600 | 2.33% | 34 | Arkansas | 69 | 0.27% |
| 10 | Massachusetts | 567 | 2.20% | 35 | Delaware | 68 | 0.26% |
| 11 | Ohio | 418 | 1.62% | 36 | Rhode Island | 67 | 0.26% |
| 12 | Louisiana | 388 | 1.51% | 37 | Utah | 62 | 0.24% |
| 13 | Virginia | 384 | 1.49% | 38 | New Mexico | 56 | 0.22% |
| 14 | Michigan | 363 | 1.41% | 39 | West Virginia | 46 | 0.18% |
| 15 | Washington | 353 | 1.37% | 40 | Maine | 41 | 0.16% |
| 16 | Missouri | 301 | 1.17% | 41 | Iowa | 34 | 0.13% |
| 17 | North Carolina | 295 | 1.15% | 42 | Nebraska | 32 | 0.12% |
| 18 | Connecticut | 269 | 1.04% | 43 | New Hampshire | 26 | 0.10% |
| 19 | Colorado | 263 | 1.02% | 44 | Idaho | 20 | 0.08% |
| 20 | South Carolina | 231 | 0.90% | 45 | Vermont | 13 | 0.05% |
| 21 | Tennessee | 202 | 0.78% | 46 | Montana | 8 | 0.03% |
| 22 | Oregon | 201 | 0.78% | 47 | Alaska | 7 | 0.03% |
| 22 | Indiana | 185 | 0.72% | 48 | Wyoming | 4 | 0.02% |
| 24 | Arizona | 171 | 0.66% | 49 | South Dakota | 2 | 0.01% |
| 25 | Alabama | 167 | 0.65% | 50 | North Dakota | 1 | 0.00% |
| | | | | | District of Columbia | 464 | 1.80% |

Source: U.S. Department of Health and Human Services, Centers for Disease Control
    "Health, United States, 1991"

*As of September 30, 1991. Numbers are for the entire year of 1990, reflect reporting delays and differ from figures released earlier. AIDS is Acquired Immunodeficiency Syndrome.

# Death Rate by AIDS in 1990

## National Rate = 10.35 Deaths by AIDS per 100,000 Population in 1990*

| RANK | STATE | RATE | RANK | STATE | RATE |
|------|-------|------|------|-------|------|
| 1 | New York | 27.25 | 26 | Tennessee | 4.14 |
| 2 | Florida | 19.83 | 27 | Alabama | 4.13 |
| 3 | California | 17.30 | 28 | Michigan | 3.91 |
| 4 | New Jersey | 16.09 | 29 | Ohio | 3.85 |
| 5 | Maryland | 12.55 | 30 | New Mexico | 3.70 |
| 6 | Georgia | 12.44 | 31 | Minnesota | 3.68 |
| 7 | Texas | 12.32 | 32 | Utah | 3.60 |
| 8 | Delaware | 10.21 | 33 | Oklahoma | 3.56 |
| 9 | Nevada | 9.57 | 34 | Indiana | 3.34 |
| 10 | Hawaii | 9.56 | 34 | Maine | 3.34 |
| 11 | Massachusetts | 9.42 | 36 | Kansas | 3.15 |
| 12 | Louisiana | 9.19 | 36 | Kentucky | 3.15 |
| 13 | Connecticut | 8.18 | 38 | Arkansas | 2.94 |
| 14 | Colorado | 7.98 | 39 | West Virginia | 2.56 |
| 15 | Illinois | 7.64 | 40 | New Hampshire | 2.34 |
| 16 | Washington | 7.25 | 41 | Vermont | 2.31 |
| 17 | Oregon | 7.07 | 42 | Wisconsin | 2.25 |
| 18 | Pennsylvania | 6.86 | 43 | Nebraska | 2.03 |
| 19 | Rhode Island | 6.68 | 44 | Idaho | 1.99 |
| 20 | South Carolina | 6.63 | 45 | Alaska | 1.27 |
| 21 | Virginia | 6.21 | 46 | Iowa | 1.22 |
| 22 | Missouri | 5.88 | 47 | Montana | 1.00 |
| 23 | Mississippi | 4.86 | 48 | Wyoming | 0.88 |
| 24 | Arizona | 4.67 | 49 | South Dakota | 0.29 |
| 25 | North Carolina | 4.45 | 50 | North Dakota | 0.16 |
|  |  |  |  | District of Columbia | 76.45 |

Source: U.S. Department of Health and Human Services, Centers for Disease Control
    "Health, United States, 1991"
*Calculated by the editors using 1990 Census resident population figures. As of September 30, 1991. Numbers are for the entire year of 1990, reflect reporting delays and differ from figures released earlier. AIDS is Acquired Immunodeficiency Syndrome.

# Deaths by AIDS through 1991

## National Total = 122,203 Deaths by AIDS*

| RANK | STATE | DEATHS | % | RANK | STATE | DEATHS | % |
|---|---|---|---|---|---|---|---|
| 1 | New York | 27,412 | 22.43% | 26 | Minnesota | 634 | 0.52% |
| 2 | California | 24,644 | 20.17% | 27 | Oklahoma | 554 | 0.45% |
| 3 | Florida | 11,621 | 9.51% | 28 | Nevada | 488 | 0.40% |
| 4 | Texas | 8,907 | 7.29% | 29 | Mississippi | 487 | 0.40% |
| 5 | New Jersey | 7,662 | 6.27% | 30 | Hawaii | 478 | 0.39% |
| 6 | Illinois | 3,812 | 3.12% | 31 | Wisconsin | 459 | 0.38% |
| 7 | Pennsylvania | 3,564 | 2.92% | 32 | Kentucky | 450 | 0.37% |
| 8 | Georgia | 3,217 | 2.63% | 33 | Arkansas | 344 | 0.28% |
| 9 | Massachusetts | 2,522 | 2.06% | 34 | Kansas | 343 | 0.28% |
| 10 | Maryland | 2,461 | 2.01% | 35 | Rhode Island | 282 | 0.23% |
| 11 | Louisiana | 1,817 | 1.49% | 36 | New Mexico | 257 | 0.21% |
| 12 | Ohio | 1,718 | 1.41% | 37 | Utah | 249 | 0.20% |
| 13 | Virginia | 1,665 | 1.36% | 38 | Delaware | 239 | 0.20% |
| 14 | Washington | 1,580 | 1.29% | 39 | Iowa | 178 | 0.15% |
| 15 | Michigan | 1,523 | 1.25% | 40 | West Virginia | 147 | 0.12% |
| 16 | Connecticut | 1,340 | 1.10% | 41 | Nebraska | 145 | 0.12% |
| 17 | North Carolina | 1,302 | 1.07% | 42 | Maine | 136 | 0.11% |
| 18 | Missouri | 1,285 | 1.05% | 43 | New Hampshire | 128 | 0.10% |
| 19 | Colorado | 1,205 | 0.99% | 44 | Idaho | 61 | 0.05% |
| 20 | Arizona | 820 | 0.67% | 45 | Vermont | 52 | 0.04% |
| 21 | Tennessee | 804 | 0.66% | 46 | Alaska | 49 | 0.04% |
| 22 | Oregon | 778 | 0.64% | 47 | Montana | 44 | 0.04% |
| 22 | South Carolina | 778 | 0.64% | 48 | Wyoming | 27 | 0.02% |
| 24 | Indiana | 735 | 0.60% | 49 | North Dakota | 18 | 0.01% |
| 25 | Alabama | 698 | 0.57% | 50 | South Dakota | 14 | 0.01% |
| | | | | | District of Columbia | 2,070 | 1.69% |

Source: U.S. Department of Health and Human Services, Centers for Disease Control
   "Health, United States, 1991"

*Cumulative deaths as of September 30, 1991. Numbers reflect reporting delays and differ from figures released earlier. AIDS is Acquired Immunodeficiency Syndrome.

# Estimated Deaths by Cancer in 1992

## National Estimated Total = 520,000 Deaths by Cancer*

| RANK | STATE | DEATHS | % | RANK | STATE | DEATHS | % |
|---|---|---|---|---|---|---|---|
| 1 | California | 52,000 | 10.00% | 26 | Oklahoma | 6,800 | 1.31% |
| 2 | New York | 40,000 | 7.69% | 26 | South Carolina | 6,800 | 1.31% |
| 3 | Florida | 35,000 | 6.73% | 28 | Oregon | 6,300 | 1.21% |
| 4 | Pennsylvania | 30,200 | 5.81% | 29 | Iowa | 6,200 | 1.19% |
| 5 | Texas | 28,000 | 5.38% | 30 | Arkansas | 5,900 | 1.13% |
| 6 | Illinois | 24,300 | 4.67% | 31 | Mississippi | 5,700 | 1.10% |
| 7 | Ohio | 24,100 | 4.63% | 32 | Kansas | 5,100 | 0.98% |
| 8 | Michigan | 18,700 | 3.60% | 33 | Colorado | 4,900 | 0.94% |
| 9 | New Jersey | 18,200 | 3.50% | 34 | West Virginia | 4,700 | 0.90% |
| 10 | North Carolina | 14,000 | 2.69% | 35 | Nebraska | 3,300 | 0.63% |
| 11 | Massachusetts | 13,600 | 2.62% | 36 | Maine | 3,000 | 0.58% |
| 12 | Georgia | 12,200 | 2.35% | 37 | Rhode Island | 2,500 | 0.48% |
| 12 | Indiana | 12,200 | 2.35% | 38 | Nevada | 2,400 | 0.46% |
| 12 | Virginia | 12,200 | 2.35% | 38 | New Hampshire | 2,400 | 0.46% |
| 15 | Missouri | 11,500 | 2.21% | 38 | New Mexico | 2,400 | 0.46% |
| 16 | Tennessee | 10,900 | 2.10% | 41 | Utah | 1,900 | 0.37% |
| 17 | Wisconsin | 10,200 | 1.96% | 42 | Hawaii | 1,700 | 0.33% |
| 18 | Maryland | 9,900 | 1.90% | 42 | Idaho | 1,700 | 0.33% |
| 19 | Alabama | 9,300 | 1.79% | 42 | Montana | 1,700 | 0.33% |
| 20 | Washington | 9,100 | 1.75% | 45 | Delaware | 1,600 | 0.31% |
| 21 | Louisiana | 9,000 | 1.73% | 46 | South Dakota | 1,500 | 0.29% |
| 22 | Minnesota | 8,500 | 1.63% | 47 | North Dakota | 1,300 | 0.25% |
| 23 | Kentucky | 8,300 | 1.60% | 48 | Vermont | 1,100 | 0.21% |
| 24 | Arizona | 7,400 | 1.42% | 49 | Wyoming | 800 | 0.15% |
| 25 | Connecticut | 7,300 | 1.40% | 50 | Alaska | 500 | 0.10% |
| | | | | | District of Columbia | 1,700 | 0.33% |

Source: American Cancer Society

*"Cancer Facts & Figures – 1992"* (Copyright 1992, Reprinted with permission from the American Cancer Society)

*These estimates are based on cancer mortality data from 1982 through 1988.*

# Estimated Death Rate by Cancer in 1992

## National Estimated Rate = 206.20 Deaths by Cancer per 100,000 Population*

| RANK | STATE | RATE | RANK | STATE | RATE |
|------|-------|------|------|-------|------|
| 1 | Florida | 263.61 | 26 | Montana | 210.40 |
| 2 | West Virginia | 260.97 | 27 | North Carolina | 207.81 |
| 3 | Pennsylvania | 252.49 | 27 | Nebraska | 207.16 |
| 4 | Rhode Island | 249.00 | 29 | Wisconsin | 205.85 |
| 5 | Arkansas | 248.74 | 29 | North Dakota | 204.72 |
| 6 | Maine | 242.91 | 31 | Kansas | 204.41 |
| 7 | Delaware | 235.29 | 31 | Maryland | 203.70 |
| 8 | New Jersey | 234.54 | 33 | Michigan | 199.62 |
| 9 | Alabama | 227.44 | 33 | Arizona | 197.33 |
| 10 | Massachusetts | 226.82 | 35 | Virginia | 194.08 |
| 11 | Kentucky | 223.54 | 36 | Vermont | 194.00 |
| 12 | Missouri | 222.95 | 37 | Minnesota | 191.79 |
| 12 | Connecticut | 221.82 | 37 | South Carolina | 191.01 |
| 14 | Iowa | 221.82 | 39 | Nevada | 186.92 |
| 14 | New York | 221.51 | 40 | Georgia | 184.21 |
| 14 | Ohio | 220.31 | 40 | Washington | 181.35 |
| 14 | Tennessee | 220.07 | 42 | Wyoming | 173.91 |
| 18 | Mississippi | 219.91 | 42 | California | 171.17 |
| 19 | Indiana | 217.47 | 42 | Idaho | 163.62 |
| 20 | New Hampshire | 217.19 | 45 | Texas | 161.39 |
| 20 | Oregon | 215.61 | 45 | New Mexico | 155.04 |
| 20 | Oklahoma | 214.17 | 47 | Hawaii | 149.78 |
| 20 | South Dakota | 213.37 | 48 | Colorado | 145.10 |
| 24 | Louisiana | 211.67 | 49 | Utah | 107.34 |
| 25 | Illinois | 210.52 | 50 | Alaska | 87.72 |
| | | | | District of Columbia | 284.28 |

Source: American Cancer Society

"Cancer Facts & Figures - 1992" (Copyright 1992, Reprinted with permission from the American Cancer Society)

*Calculated by the editors using 1991 Census resident population figures. These estimates are based on cancer mortality data from 1982 through 1988.

# Estimated Deaths by Female Breast Cancer in 1992

## National Estimated Total = 46,000 Deaths by Female Breast Cancer*

| RANK | STATE | DEATHS | % | RANK | STATE | DEATHS | % |
|---|---|---|---|---|---|---|---|
| 1 | California | 4,500 | 9.78% | 25 | Iowa | 600 | 1.30% |
| 2 | New York | 4,000 | 8.70% | 27 | Oklahoma | 550 | 1.20% |
| 3 | Florida | 2,900 | 6.30% | 27 | Oregon | 550 | 1.20% |
| 4 | Pennsylvania | 2,800 | 6.09% | 27 | South Carolina | 550 | 1.20% |
| 5 | Illinois | 2,200 | 4.78% | 30 | Colorado | 475 | 1.03% |
| 5 | Ohio | 2,200 | 4.78% | 31 | Kansas | 450 | 0.98% |
| 5 | Texas | 2,200 | 4.78% | 32 | Arkansas | 425 | 0.92% |
| 8 | Michigan | 1,700 | 3.70% | 32 | Mississippi | 425 | 0.92% |
| 8 | New Jersey | 1,700 | 3.70% | 34 | West Virginia | 350 | 0.76% |
| 10 | Massachusetts | 1,400 | 3.04% | 35 | Nebraska | 300 | 0.65% |
| 11 | North Carolina | 1,300 | 2.83% | 36 | Rhode Island | 250 | 0.54% |
| 12 | Georgia | 1,100 | 2.39% | 37 | Maine | 225 | 0.49% |
| 12 | Indiana | 1,100 | 2.39% | 37 | New Hampshire | 225 | 0.49% |
| 12 | Virginia | 1,100 | 2.39% | 37 | New Mexico | 225 | 0.49% |
| 15 | Missouri | 1,000 | 2.17% | 40 | Nevada | 200 | 0.43% |
| 16 | Maryland | 900 | 1.96% | 40 | Utah | 200 | 0.43% |
| 16 | Tennessee | 900 | 1.96% | 42 | Delaware | 175 | 0.38% |
| 16 | Wisconsin | 900 | 1.96% | 43 | South Dakota | 150 | 0.33% |
| 19 | Minnesota | 800 | 1.74% | 44 | Hawaii | 125 | 0.27% |
| 19 | Washington | 800 | 1.74% | 44 | Idaho | 125 | 0.27% |
| 21 | Alabama | 700 | 1.52% | 44 | Montana | 125 | 0.27% |
| 21 | Connecticut | 700 | 1.52% | 44 | Vermont | 125 | 0.27% |
| 23 | Kentucky | 650 | 1.41% | 48 | North Dakota | 100 | 0.22% |
| 23 | Louisiana | 650 | 1.41% | 49 | Wyoming | 75 | 0.16% |
| 25 | Arizona | 600 | 1.30% | 50 | Alaska | 50 | 0.11% |
| | | | | | District of Columbia | 150 | 0.33% |

Source: American Cancer Society

*"Cancer Facts & Figures - 1992"* (Copyright 1992, Reprinted with permission from the American Cancer Society)

*These estimates are based on cancer mortality data from 1982 through 1988.*

# Estimated Death Rate by Female Breast Cancer in 1992

## National Estimated Rate = 36.09 Deaths by Female Breast Cancer per 100,000 Female Population*

| RANK | STATE | RATE | RANK | STATE | RATE |
|------|-------|------|------|-------|------|
| 1 | Delaware | 50.99 | 26 | Tennessee | 35.60 |
| 2 | Rhode Island | 47.90 | 27 | Michigan | 35.55 |
| 3 | Pennsylvania | 45.25 | 28 | Arkansas | 34.90 |
| 4 | Massachusetts | 44.76 | 29 | Virginia | 34.88 |
| 5 | Vermont | 43.51 | 30 | Kentucky | 34.21 |
| 6 | Florida | 43.44 | 31 | Oklahoma | 34.06 |
| 7 | New York | 42.71 | 32 | Nevada | 33.90 |
| 8 | New Jersey | 42.56 | 33 | Alabama | 33.26 |
| 9 | South Dakota | 42.43 | 34 | Wyoming | 33.10 |
| 10 | Iowa | 41.90 | 35 | Georgia | 33.00 |
| 11 | Connecticut | 41.32 | 36 | Washington | 32.61 |
| 12 | New Hampshire | 39.77 | 37 | Arizona | 32.35 |
| 13 | Ohio | 39.14 | 38 | Mississippi | 31.66 |
| 14 | Indiana | 38.52 | 39 | North Dakota | 31.19 |
| 15 | North Carolina | 38.07 | 40 | Montana | 30.99 |
| 16 | Oregon | 38.06 | 41 | South Carolina | 30.59 |
| 17 | Missouri | 37.70 | 42 | California | 30.28 |
| 18 | West Virginia | 37.56 | 43 | Louisiana | 29.70 |
| 19 | Illinois | 37.43 | 44 | New Mexico | 29.23 |
| 20 | Nebraska | 37.09 | 45 | Colorado | 28.56 |
| 21 | Maryland | 36.54 | 46 | Texas | 25.52 |
| 22 | Wisconsin | 36.02 | 47 | Idaho | 24.71 |
| 23 | Minnesota | 35.88 | 48 | Utah | 23.07 |
| 24 | Maine | 35.71 | 49 | Hawaii | 22.96 |
| 25 | Kansas | 35.63 | 50 | Alaska | 19.22 |
| | | | | District of Columbia | 46.31 |

Source: American Cancer Society

"Cancer Facts & Figures – 1992" (Copyright 1992, Reprinted with permission from the American Cancer Society)

*Calculated by the editors using 1990 Census resident population figures. These estimates are based on cancer mortality data from 1982 through 1988.

# Estimated Deaths by Colon and Rectum Cancer in 1992

## National Total = 58,300 Deaths by Colon and Rectum Cancer*

| RANK | STATE | DEATHS | % | RANK | STATE | DEATHS | % |
|---|---|---|---|---|---|---|---|
| 1 | California | 5,500 | 9.43% | 26 | Arizona | 750 | 1.29% |
| 2 | New York | 5,100 | 8.75% | 27 | Oklahoma | 700 | 1.20% |
| 3 | Florida | 4,000 | 6.86% | 27 | South Carolina | 700 | 1.20% |
| 4 | Pennsylvania | 3,700 | 6.35% | 29 | Kansas | 650 | 1.11% |
| 5 | Illinois | 3,000 | 5.15% | 29 | Oregon | 650 | 1.11% |
| 6 | Ohio | 2,800 | 4.80% | 31 | Arkansas | 600 | 1.03% |
| 7 | Texas | 2,600 | 4.46% | 31 | Mississippi | 600 | 1.03% |
| 8 | New Jersey | 2,300 | 3.95% | 33 | Colorado | 550 | 0.94% |
| 9 | Michigan | 2,000 | 3.43% | 33 | West Virginia | 550 | 0.94% |
| 10 | Massachusetts | 1,700 | 2.92% | 35 | Nebraska | 375 | 0.64% |
| 11 | North Carolina | 1,500 | 2.57% | 36 | Maine | 350 | 0.60% |
| 12 | Indiana | 1,300 | 2.23% | 37 | New Hampshire | 300 | 0.51% |
| 12 | Virginia | 1,300 | 2.23% | 37 | Rhode Island | 300 | 0.51% |
| 14 | Georgia | 1,200 | 2.06% | 39 | New Mexico | 275 | 0.47% |
| 14 | Missouri | 1,200 | 2.06% | 40 | Hawaii | 225 | 0.39% |
| 14 | Tennessee | 1,200 | 2.06% | 40 | Nevada | 225 | 0.39% |
| 14 | Wisconsin | 1,200 | 2.06% | 42 | Idaho | 200 | 0.34% |
| 18 | Maryland | 1,100 | 1.89% | 42 | Montana | 200 | 0.34% |
| 19 | Minnesota | 1,000 | 1.72% | 42 | Utah | 200 | 0.34% |
| 20 | Connecticut | 900 | 1.54% | 45 | Delaware | 175 | 0.30% |
| 20 | Kentucky | 900 | 1.54% | 45 | South Dakota | 175 | 0.30% |
| 20 | Louisiana | 900 | 1.54% | 47 | North Dakota | 150 | 0.26% |
| 20 | Washington | 900 | 1.54% | 48 | Vermont | 125 | 0.21% |
| 24 | Alabama | 850 | 1.46% | 49 | Wyoming | 75 | 0.13% |
| 25 | Iowa | 800 | 1.37% | 50 | Alaska | 50 | 0.09% |
|  |  |  |  |  | District of Columbia | 200 | 0.34% |

Source: American Cancer Society

"Cancer Facts & Figures – 1992" (Copyright 1992, Reprinted with permission from the American Cancer Society)

*These estimates are based on cancer mortality data from 1982 through 1988.

# Estimated Death Rate by Colon and Rectum Cancer in 1992

## National Estimated Rate = 23.12 Deaths by Colon and Rectum Cancer per 100,000 Population*

| RANK | STATE | RATE | RANK | STATE | RATE |
|------|-------|------|------|-------|------|
| 1 | Pennsylvania | 30.93 | 26 | Mississippi | 23.15 |
| 2 | West Virginia | 30.54 | 27 | Maryland | 22.63 |
| 3 | Florida | 30.13 | 28 | Minnesota | 22.56 |
| 4 | Rhode Island | 29.88 | 29 | North Carolina | 22.27 |
| 5 | New Jersey | 29.64 | 30 | Oregon | 22.25 |
| 6 | Iowa | 28.62 | 31 | Oklahoma | 22.05 |
| 7 | Massachusetts | 28.35 | 31 | Vermont | 22.05 |
| 8 | Maine | 28.34 | 33 | Michigan | 21.35 |
| 9 | New York | 28.24 | 34 | Louisiana | 21.17 |
| 10 | Connecticut | 27.35 | 35 | Alabama | 20.79 |
| 11 | New Hampshire | 27.15 | 36 | Virginia | 20.68 |
| 12 | Kansas | 26.05 | 37 | Arizona | 20.00 |
| 13 | Illinois | 25.99 | 38 | Hawaii | 19.82 |
| 14 | Delaware | 25.74 | 39 | South Carolina | 19.66 |
| 15 | Ohio | 25.60 | 40 | Idaho | 19.25 |
| 16 | Arkansas | 25.30 | 41 | Georgia | 18.12 |
| 17 | South Dakota | 24.89 | 42 | California | 18.10 |
| 18 | Montana | 24.75 | 43 | Washington | 17.94 |
| 19 | Kentucky | 24.24 | 44 | New Mexico | 17.76 |
| 20 | Tennessee | 24.23 | 45 | Nevada | 17.52 |
| 21 | Wisconsin | 24.22 | 46 | Wyoming | 16.30 |
| 22 | North Dakota | 23.62 | 47 | Colorado | 16.29 |
| 23 | Nebraska | 23.54 | 48 | Texas | 14.99 |
| 24 | Missouri | 23.26 | 49 | Utah | 11.30 |
| 25 | Indiana | 23.17 | 50 | Alaska | 8.77 |

District of Columbia     33.44

*Source: American Cancer Society*

    *"Cancer Facts & Figures - 1992" (Copyright 1992, Reprinted with permission from the American Cancer Society)*

*\*Calculated by the editors using 1991 Census resident population figures. These estimates are based on cancer mortality data from 1982 through 1988.*

# Estimated Deaths by Leukemia in 1992

## National Estimated Total = 18,200 Deaths by Leukemia*

| RANK | STATE | DEATHS | % | RANK | STATE | DEATHS | % |
|---|---|---|---|---|---|---|---|
| 1 | California | 2,000 | 10.99% | 24 | South Carolina | 250 | 1.37% |
| 2 | New York | 1,300 | 7.14% | 27 | Arkansas | 225 | 1.24% |
| 3 | Florida | 1,100 | 6.04% | 27 | Connecticut | 225 | 1.24% |
| 3 | Pennsylvania | 1,100 | 6.04% | 27 | Iowa | 225 | 1.24% |
| 3 | Texas | 1,100 | 6.04% | 27 | Kansas | 225 | 1.24% |
| 6 | Ohio | 850 | 4.67% | 27 | Kentucky | 225 | 1.24% |
| 7 | Illinois | 800 | 4.40% | 32 | Mississippi | 200 | 1.10% |
| 8 | Michigan | 700 | 3.85% | 33 | Colorado | 175 | 0.96% |
| 9 | New Jersey | 600 | 3.30% | 34 | West Virginia | 150 | 0.82% |
| 10 | Massachusetts | 450 | 2.47% | 35 | Nebraska | 125 | 0.69% |
| 10 | North Carolina | 450 | 2.47% | 36 | Maine | 100 | 0.55% |
| 12 | Indiana | 425 | 2.34% | 36 | New Mexico | 100 | 0.55% |
| 13 | Georgia | 400 | 2.20% | 38 | Utah | 80 | 0.44% |
| 13 | Missouri | 400 | 2.20% | 39 | Nevada | 75 | 0.41% |
| 15 | Tennessee | 375 | 2.06% | 39 | Rhode Island | 75 | 0.41% |
| 15 | Virginia | 375 | 2.06% | 41 | Idaho | 70 | 0.38% |
| 15 | Wisconsin | 375 | 2.06% | 41 | North Dakota | 70 | 0.38% |
| 18 | Minnesota | 350 | 1.92% | 43 | New Hampshire | 60 | 0.33% |
| 19 | Maryland | 325 | 1.79% | 43 | South Dakota | 60 | 0.33% |
| 19 | Washington | 325 | 1.79% | 45 | Delaware | 50 | 0.27% |
| 21 | Alabama | 300 | 1.65% | 45 | Hawaii | 50 | 0.27% |
| 22 | Arizona | 275 | 1.51% | 45 | Montana | 50 | 0.27% |
| 22 | Louisiana | 275 | 1.51% | 45 | Vermont | 50 | 0.27% |
| 24 | Oklahoma | 250 | 1.37% | 45 | Wyoming | 50 | 0.27% |
| 24 | Oregon | 250 | 1.37% | 50 | Alaska | 25 | 0.14% |
| | | | | | District of Columbia | 60 | 0.33% |

Source: American Cancer Society

"Cancer Facts & Figures – 1992" (Copyright 1992, Reprinted with permission from the American Cancer Society)

*These estimates are based on cancer mortality data from 1982 through 1988.

# Estimated Death Rate by Leukemia in 1992

## National Estimated Rate = 7.22 Deaths by Leukemia per 100,000 Population*

| RANK | STATE | RATE | RANK | STATE | RATE |
|------|-------|------|------|-------|------|
| 1 | North Dakota | 11.02 | 26 | Delaware | 7.35 |
| 2 | Wyoming | 10.87 | 27 | Alabama | 7.34 |
| 3 | Arkansas | 9.49 | 28 | Arizona | 7.33 |
| 4 | Pennsylvania | 9.20 | 29 | New York | 7.20 |
| 5 | Kansas | 9.02 | 30 | South Carolina | 7.02 |
| 6 | Vermont | 8.82 | 31 | Illinois | 6.93 |
| 7 | Oregon | 8.56 | 32 | Connecticut | 6.84 |
| 8 | South Dakota | 8.53 | 33 | Idaho | 6.74 |
| 9 | West Virginia | 8.33 | 34 | Maryland | 6.69 |
| 10 | Florida | 8.29 | 35 | North Carolina | 6.68 |
| 11 | Maine | 8.10 | 36 | California | 6.58 |
| 12 | Iowa | 8.05 | 37 | Washington | 6.48 |
| 13 | Minnesota | 7.90 | 38 | Louisiana | 6.47 |
| 14 | Oklahoma | 7.87 | 39 | New Mexico | 6.46 |
| 15 | Nebraska | 7.85 | 40 | Texas | 6.34 |
| 16 | Ohio | 7.77 | 41 | Montana | 6.19 |
| 17 | Missouri | 7.75 | 42 | Kentucky | 6.06 |
| 18 | New Jersey | 7.73 | 43 | Georgia | 6.04 |
| 19 | Mississippi | 7.72 | 44 | Virginia | 5.97 |
| 20 | Indiana | 7.58 | 45 | Nevada | 5.84 |
| 21 | Tennessee | 7.57 | 46 | New Hampshire | 5.43 |
| 21 | Wisconsin | 7.57 | 47 | Colorado | 5.18 |
| 23 | Massachusetts | 7.51 | 48 | Utah | 4.52 |
| 24 | Michigan | 7.47 | 49 | Hawaii | 4.41 |
| 24 | Rhode Island | 7.47 | 50 | Alaska | 4.39 |
| | | | | District of Columbia | 10.03 |

Source: American Cancer Society

"Cancer Facts & Figures – 1992" (Copyright 1992, Reprinted with permission from the American Cancer Society)

*Calculated by the editors using 1991 Census resident population figures. These estimates are based on cancer mortality data from 1982 through 1988.

# Estimated Deaths by Lung Cancer in 1992

## National Estimated Total = 146,000 Deaths by Lung Cancer*

| RANK | STATE | DEATHS | % | RANK | STATE | DEATHS | % |
|------|-------|--------|---|------|-------|--------|---|
| 1 | California | 14,200 | 9.73% | 25 | Minnesota | 2,000 | 1.37% |
| 2 | Florida | 10,500 | 7.19% | 25 | South Carolina | 2,000 | 1.37% |
| 3 | New York | 10,000 | 6.85% | 28 | Connecticut | 1,900 | 1.30% |
| 4 | Pennsylvania | 8,200 | 5.62% | 29 | Oregon | 1,800 | 1.23% |
| 5 | Texas | 7,800 | 5.34% | 30 | Iowa | 1,700 | 1.16% |
| 6 | Ohio | 6,900 | 4.73% | 30 | Mississippi | 1,700 | 1.16% |
| 7 | Illinois | 6,700 | 4.59% | 32 | West Virginia | 1,500 | 1.03% |
| 8 | Michigan | 5,200 | 3.56% | 33 | Kansas | 1,400 | 0.96% |
| 9 | New Jersey | 4,800 | 3.29% | 34 | Colorado | 1,200 | 0.82% |
| 10 | North Carolina | 4,200 | 2.88% | 35 | Nebraska | 900 | 0.62% |
| 11 | Indiana | 3,700 | 2.53% | 36 | Nevada | 850 | 0.58% |
| 12 | Georgia | 3,600 | 2.47% | 37 | Maine | 800 | 0.55% |
| 12 | Massachusetts | 3,600 | 2.47% | 38 | Rhode Island | 650 | 0.45% |
| 12 | Virginia | 3,600 | 2.47% | 39 | New Hampshire | 600 | 0.41% |
| 15 | Missouri | 3,500 | 2.40% | 40 | New Mexico | 550 | 0.38% |
| 15 | Tennessee | 3,500 | 2.40% | 41 | Hawaii | 450 | 0.31% |
| 17 | Kentucky | 2,900 | 1.99% | 41 | Montana | 450 | 0.31% |
| 17 | Maryland | 2,900 | 1.99% | 43 | Delaware | 425 | 0.29% |
| 19 | Alabama | 2,800 | 1.92% | 43 | Idaho | 425 | 0.29% |
| 20 | Louisiana | 2,700 | 1.85% | 45 | South Dakota | 375 | 0.26% |
| 21 | Washington | 2,600 | 1.78% | 46 | North Dakota | 325 | 0.22% |
| 22 | Wisconsin | 2,400 | 1.64% | 47 | Utah | 300 | 0.21% |
| 23 | Arizona | 2,200 | 1.51% | 47 | Vermont | 300 | 0.21% |
| 24 | Oklahoma | 2,100 | 1.44% | 49 | Alaska | 200 | 0.14% |
| 25 | Arkansas | 2,000 | 1.37% | 50 | Wyoming | 175 | 0.12% |
|  |  |  |  |  | District of Columbia | 425 | 0.29% |

Source: American Cancer Society

*"Cancer Facts & Figures - 1992"* (Copyright 1992, Reprinted with permission from the American Cancer Society)

*These estimates are based on cancer mortality data from 1982 through 1988.

# Estimated Death Rate by Lung Cancer in 1992

## National Estimated Rate = 57.90 Deaths by Lung Cancer per 100,000 Population*

| RANK | STATE | RATE | RANK | STATE | RATE |
|---|---|---|---|---|---|
| 1 | Arkansas | 84.32 | 26 | Connecticut | 57.73 |
| 2 | West Virginia | 83.29 | 27 | Virginia | 57.27 |
| 3 | Florida | 79.08 | 28 | Nebraska | 56.50 |
| 4 | Kentucky | 78.10 | 29 | South Carolina | 56.18 |
| 5 | Tennessee | 70.66 | 30 | Kansas | 56.11 |
| 6 | Pennsylvania | 68.56 | 31 | Montana | 55.69 |
| 7 | Alabama | 68.48 | 32 | Michigan | 55.51 |
| 8 | Missouri | 67.86 | 33 | New York | 55.38 |
| 9 | Nevada | 66.20 | 34 | Georgia | 54.36 |
| 10 | Oklahoma | 66.14 | 35 | New Hampshire | 54.30 |
| 11 | Indiana | 65.95 | 36 | South Dakota | 53.34 |
| 12 | Mississippi | 65.59 | 37 | Vermont | 52.91 |
| 13 | Maine | 64.78 | 38 | Washington | 51.81 |
| 14 | Rhode Island | 64.74 | 39 | North Dakota | 51.18 |
| 15 | Louisiana | 63.50 | 40 | Wisconsin | 48.44 |
| 16 | Ohio | 63.08 | 41 | California | 46.74 |
| 17 | Delaware | 62.50 | 42 | Minnesota | 45.13 |
| 18 | North Carolina | 62.34 | 43 | Texas | 44.96 |
| 19 | New Jersey | 61.86 | 44 | Idaho | 40.90 |
| 20 | Oregon | 61.60 | 45 | Hawaii | 39.65 |
| 21 | Iowa | 60.82 | 46 | Wyoming | 38.04 |
| 22 | Massachusetts | 60.04 | 47 | Colorado | 35.53 |
| 23 | Maryland | 59.67 | 47 | New Mexico | 35.53 |
| 24 | Arizona | 58.67 | 49 | Alaska | 35.09 |
| 25 | Illinois | 58.04 | 50 | Utah | 16.95 |
| | | | | District of Columbia | 71.07 |

Source: American Cancer Society
"Cancer Facts & Figures – 1992" (Copyright 1992, Reprinted with permission from the American Cancer Society)
*Calculated by the editors using 1991 Census resident population figures. These estimates are based on cancer mortality data from 1982 through 1988.

# Estimated Deaths by Oral Cancer in 1992

## National Estimated Total = 7,950 Deaths by Oral Cancer*

| RANK | STATE | DEATHS | % | RANK | STATE | DEATHS | % |
|------|-------|--------|-----|------|-------|--------|-----|
| 1 | California | 800 | 10.06% | 24 | Minnesota | 100 | 1.26% |
| 2 | New York | 700 | 8.81% | 24 | Oregon | 100 | 1.26% |
| 3 | Florida | 650 | 8.18% | 24 | Washington | 100 | 1.26% |
| 4 | Texas | 425 | 5.35% | 29 | Mississippi | 90 | 1.13% |
| 5 | Pennsylvania | 350 | 4.40% | 30 | Colorado | 80 | 1.01% |
| 6 | Illinois | 325 | 4.09% | 31 | Arizona | 75 | 0.94% |
| 6 | Ohio | 325 | 4.09% | 32 | Arkansas | 70 | 0.88% |
| 8 | Michigan | 300 | 3.77% | 32 | Kansas | 70 | 0.88% |
| 9 | New Jersey | 275 | 3.46% | 34 | Rhode Island | 60 | 0.75% |
| 10 | Georgia | 250 | 3.14% | 34 | West Virginia | 60 | 0.75% |
| 10 | Massachusetts | 250 | 3.14% | 36 | Maine | 50 | 0.63% |
| 12 | North Carolina | 225 | 2.83% | 37 | New Hampshire | 40 | 0.50% |
| 13 | Alabama | 175 | 2.20% | 38 | Delaware | 30 | 0.38% |
| 13 | Virginia | 175 | 2.20% | 38 | Hawaii | 30 | 0.38% |
| 15 | Indiana | 150 | 1.89% | 38 | Idaho | 30 | 0.38% |
| 15 | Louisiana | 150 | 1.89% | 38 | Montana | 30 | 0.38% |
| 15 | Maryland | 150 | 1.89% | 38 | Nebraska | 30 | 0.38% |
| 15 | South Carolina | 150 | 1.89% | 38 | Nevada | 30 | 0.38% |
| 15 | Tennessee | 150 | 1.89% | 38 | New Mexico | 30 | 0.38% |
| 15 | Wisconsin | 150 | 1.89% | 45 | North Dakota | 25 | 0.31% |
| 21 | Connecticut | 125 | 1.57% | 46 | South Dakota | 20 | 0.25% |
| 21 | Missouri | 125 | 1.57% | 46 | Utah | 20 | 0.25% |
| 21 | Oklahoma | 125 | 1.57% | 48 | Alaska | 10 | 0.13% |
| 24 | Iowa | 100 | 1.26% | 48 | Vermont | 10 | 0.13% |
| 24 | Kentucky | 100 | 1.26% | 48 | Wyoming | 10 | 0.13% |
| | | | | | District of Columbia | 50 | 0.63% |

*Source: American Cancer Society*

*"Cancer Facts & Figures - 1992" (Copyright 1992, Reprinted with permission from the American Cancer Society)*

*\*These estimates are based on cancer mortality data from 1982 through 1988.*

# Estimated Death Rate by Oral Cancer in 1992

## National Estimated Rate = 3.15 Deaths by Oral Cancer per 100,000 Population*

| RANK | STATE | RATE | RANK | STATE | RATE |
|------|-------|------|------|-------|------|
| 1 | Rhode Island | 5.98 | 26 | Ohio | 2.97 |
| 2 | Florida | 4.90 | 27 | Arkansas | 2.95 |
| 3 | Delaware | 4.41 | 28 | Pennsylvania | 2.93 |
| 4 | Alabama | 4.28 | 29 | Idaho | 2.89 |
| 5 | South Carolina | 4.21 | 30 | South Dakota | 2.84 |
| 6 | Massachusetts | 4.17 | 31 | Illinois | 2.82 |
| 7 | Maine | 4.05 | 32 | Kansas | 2.81 |
| 8 | North Dakota | 3.94 | 33 | Virginia | 2.78 |
| 8 | Oklahoma | 3.94 | 34 | Kentucky | 2.69 |
| 10 | New York | 3.88 | 35 | Indiana | 2.67 |
| 11 | Connecticut | 3.80 | 36 | Hawaii | 2.64 |
| 12 | Georgia | 3.77 | 37 | California | 2.63 |
| 13 | Montana | 3.71 | 38 | Texas | 2.45 |
| 14 | New Hampshire | 3.62 | 39 | Missouri | 2.42 |
| 15 | Iowa | 3.58 | 40 | Colorado | 2.37 |
| 16 | New Jersey | 3.54 | 41 | Nevada | 2.34 |
| 17 | Louisiana | 3.53 | 42 | Minnesota | 2.26 |
| 18 | Mississippi | 3.47 | 43 | Wyoming | 2.17 |
| 19 | Oregon | 3.42 | 44 | Arizona | 2.00 |
| 20 | North Carolina | 3.34 | 45 | Washington | 1.99 |
| 21 | West Virginia | 3.33 | 46 | New Mexico | 1.94 |
| 22 | Michigan | 3.20 | 47 | Nebraska | 1.88 |
| 23 | Maryland | 3.09 | 48 | Vermont | 1.76 |
| 24 | Tennessee | 3.03 | 49 | Alaska | 1.75 |
| 24 | Wisconsin | 3.03 | 50 | Utah | 1.13 |
| | | | | District of Columbia | 8.36 |

*Source: American Cancer Society*

*"Cancer Facts & Figures – 1992" (Copyright 1992, Reprinted with permission from the American Cancer Society)*

*\*Calculated by the editors using 1991 Census resident population figures. These estimates are based on cancer mortality data from 1982 through 1988.*

# Estimated Deaths by Pancreas Cancer in 1992

## National Estimated Total = 25,000 Deaths by Pancreas Cancer*

| RANK | STATE | DEATHS | % | RANK | STATE | DEATHS | % |
|------|-------|--------|---|------|-------|--------|---|
| 1 | California | 2,700 | 10.80% | 25 | South Carolina | 325 | 1.30% |
| 2 | New York | 2,000 | 8.00% | 27 | Arkansas | 300 | 1.20% |
| 3 | Florida | 1,700 | 6.80% | 27 | Iowa | 300 | 1.20% |
| 4 | Pennsylvania | 1,300 | 5.20% | 27 | Mississippi | 300 | 1.20% |
| 4 | Texas | 1,300 | 5.20% | 27 | Oklahoma | 300 | 1.20% |
| 6 | Illinois | 1,200 | 4.80% | 27 | Oregon | 300 | 1.20% |
| 7 | Ohio | 1,100 | 4.40% | 32 | Colorado | 250 | 1.00% |
| 8 | Michigan | 900 | 3.60% | 32 | Kansas | 250 | 1.00% |
| 9 | New Jersey | 850 | 3.40% | 34 | West Virginia | 200 | 0.80% |
| 10 | North Carolina | 700 | 2.80% | 35 | Nebraska | 150 | 0.60% |
| 11 | Massachusetts | 650 | 2.60% | 36 | Maine | 125 | 0.50% |
| 12 | Georgia | 550 | 2.20% | 36 | Nevada | 125 | 0.50% |
| 12 | Indiana | 550 | 2.20% | 36 | New Mexico | 125 | 0.50% |
| 12 | Missouri | 550 | 2.20% | 39 | Idaho | 100 | 0.40% |
| 12 | Virginia | 550 | 2.20% | 39 | New Hampshire | 100 | 0.40% |
| 16 | Maryland | 500 | 2.00% | 39 | Rhode Island | 100 | 0.40% |
| 16 | Minnesota | 500 | 2.00% | 39 | Utah | 100 | 0.40% |
| 16 | Tennessee | 500 | 2.00% | 43 | Hawaii | 90 | 0.36% |
| 19 | Louisiana | 475 | 1.90% | 44 | Montana | 80 | 0.32% |
| 19 | Wisconsin | 475 | 1.90% | 45 | North Dakota | 70 | 0.28% |
| 21 | Alabama | 450 | 1.80% | 45 | South Dakota | 70 | 0.28% |
| 22 | Washington | 425 | 1.70% | 47 | Delaware | 60 | 0.24% |
| 23 | Connecticut | 400 | 1.60% | 48 | Vermont | 50 | 0.20% |
| 24 | Kentucky | 350 | 1.40% | 49 | Alaska | 30 | 0.12% |
| 25 | Arizona | 325 | 1.30% | 49 | Wyoming | 30 | 0.12% |
| | | | | | District of Columbia | 70 | 0.28% |

Source: American Cancer Society

"Cancer Facts & Figures – 1992" (Copyright 1992, Reprinted with permission from the American Cancer Society)

*These estimates are based on cancer mortality data from 1982 through 1988.

# Estimated Death Rate by Pancreas Cancer in 1992

## National Estimated Rate = 9.91 Deaths by Pancreas Cancer per 100,000 Population*

| RANK | STATE | RATE | | RANK | STATE | RATE |
|---|---|---|---|---|---|---|
| 1 | Florida | 12.80 | | 26 | Montana | 9.90 |
| 2 | Arkansas | 12.65 | | 27 | Indiana | 9.80 |
| 3 | Connecticut | 12.15 | | 28 | Nevada | 9.74 |
| 4 | Mississippi | 11.57 | | 29 | Idaho | 9.62 |
| 5 | Minnesota | 11.28 | | 30 | Michigan | 9.61 |
| 6 | Louisiana | 11.17 | | 31 | Wisconsin | 9.59 |
| 7 | West Virginia | 11.10 | | 32 | Oklahoma | 9.45 |
| 8 | New York | 11.08 | | 33 | Kentucky | 9.43 |
| 9 | North Dakota | 11.02 | | 34 | Nebraska | 9.42 |
| 10 | Alabama | 11.01 | | 35 | South Carolina | 9.13 |
| 11 | New Jersey | 10.95 | | 36 | New Hampshire | 9.05 |
| 12 | Pennsylvania | 10.87 | | 37 | California | 8.89 |
| 13 | Massachusetts | 10.84 | | 38 | Delaware | 8.82 |
| 14 | Iowa | 10.73 | | 38 | Vermont | 8.82 |
| 15 | Missouri | 10.66 | | 40 | Virginia | 8.75 |
| 16 | Illinois | 10.40 | | 41 | Arizona | 8.67 |
| 17 | North Carolina | 10.39 | | 42 | Washington | 8.47 |
| 18 | Maryland | 10.29 | | 43 | Georgia | 8.30 |
| 19 | Oregon | 10.27 | | 44 | New Mexico | 8.07 |
| 20 | Maine | 10.12 | | 45 | Hawaii | 7.93 |
| 21 | Tennessee | 10.09 | | 46 | Texas | 7.49 |
| 22 | Ohio | 10.06 | | 47 | Colorado | 7.40 |
| 23 | Kansas | 10.02 | | 48 | Wyoming | 6.52 |
| 24 | Rhode Island | 9.96 | | 49 | Utah | 5.65 |
| 24 | South Dakota | 9.96 | | 50 | Alaska | 5.26 |

District of Columbia          11.71

Source: American Cancer Society

   "Cancer Facts & Figures – 1992" (Copyright 1992, Reprinted with permission from the American Cancer Society)

*Calculated by the editors using 1991 Census resident population figures. These estimates are based on cancer mortality data from 1982 through 1988.

# Estimated Deaths by Prostate Cancer in 1992

## National Estimated Total = 34,000 Deaths by Prostate Cancer*

| RANK | STATE | DEATHS | % | RANK | STATE | DEATHS | % |
|------|-------|--------|------|------|-------|--------|------|
| 1 | California | 3,400 | 10.00% | 26 | Kentucky | 450 | 1.32% |
| 2 | Florida | 2,600 | 7.65% | 26 | Oregon | 450 | 1.32% |
| 3 | New York | 2,500 | 7.35% | 28 | Connecticut | 400 | 1.18% |
| 4 | Pennsylvania | 2,000 | 5.88% | 28 | Oklahoma | 400 | 1.18% |
| 5 | Texas | 1,600 | 4.71% | 30 | Arkansas | 375 | 1.10% |
| 6 | Illinois | 1,500 | 4.41% | 30 | Mississippi | 375 | 1.10% |
| 6 | Ohio | 1,500 | 4.41% | 32 | Colorado | 350 | 1.03% |
| 8 | Michigan | 1,300 | 3.82% | 32 | Kansas | 350 | 1.03% |
| 9 | New Jersey | 1,000 | 2.94% | 34 | West Virginia | 300 | 0.88% |
| 9 | North Carolina | 1,000 | 2.94% | 35 | Nebraska | 225 | 0.66% |
| 11 | Georgia | 850 | 2.50% | 36 | Maine | 175 | 0.51% |
| 11 | Virginia | 850 | 2.50% | 36 | New Hampshire | 175 | 0.51% |
| 13 | Massachusetts | 800 | 2.35% | 36 | New Mexico | 175 | 0.51% |
| 14 | Indiana | 750 | 2.21% | 36 | Utah | 175 | 0.51% |
| 14 | Wisconsin | 750 | 2.21% | 40 | Idaho | 150 | 0.44% |
| 16 | Missouri | 700 | 2.06% | 40 | Rhode Island | 150 | 0.44% |
| 16 | Washington | 700 | 2.06% | 42 | Montana | 125 | 0.37% |
| 18 | Minnesota | 650 | 1.91% | 42 | Nevada | 125 | 0.37% |
| 18 | Tennessee | 650 | 1.91% | 42 | North Dakota | 125 | 0.37% |
| 20 | Alabama | 600 | 1.76% | 42 | South Dakota | 125 | 0.37% |
| 20 | Maryland | 600 | 1.76% | 46 | Delaware | 100 | 0.29% |
| 22 | Louisiana | 550 | 1.62% | 46 | Hawaii | 100 | 0.29% |
| 23 | Arizona | 500 | 1.47% | 46 | Vermont | 100 | 0.29% |
| 24 | Iowa | 475 | 1.40% | 49 | Wyoming | 50 | 0.15% |
| 24 | South Carolina | 475 | 1.40% | 50 | Alaska | 25 | 0.07% |
|  |  |  |  |  | District of Columbia | 150 | 0.44% |

*Source: American Cancer Society*

*"Cancer Facts & Figures - 1992" (Copyright 1992, Reprinted with permission from the American Cancer Society)*

*These estimates are based on cancer mortality data from 1982 through 1988.*

# Estimated Death Rate by Prostate Cancer in 1992

## National Estimated Rate = 28.04 Deaths by Prostate Cancer per 100,000 Male Population*

| RANK | STATE | RATE | RANK | STATE | RATE |
|------|-------|------|------|-------|------|
| 1 | Florida | 41.52 | 26 | Ohio | 28.70 |
| 2 | North Dakota | 39.28 | 27 | Missouri | 28.41 |
| 3 | South Dakota | 36.50 | 28 | South Carolina | 28.13 |
| 4 | Vermont | 36.30 | 29 | Virginia | 28.02 |
| 5 | Iowa | 35.32 | 30 | Indiana | 27.90 |
| 6 | Pennsylvania | 35.12 | 31 | Massachusetts | 27.69 |
| 7 | West Virginia | 34.82 | 32 | Tennessee | 27.67 |
| 8 | Arkansas | 33.10 | 33 | Arizona | 27.61 |
| 9 | Oregon | 32.21 | 34 | Louisiana | 27.08 |
| 10 | New Hampshire | 32.20 | 35 | Georgia | 27.03 |
| 11 | Montana | 31.58 | 36 | Illinois | 27.02 |
| 12 | Wisconsin | 31.34 | 37 | New Jersey | 26.77 |
| 13 | Rhode Island | 31.15 | 38 | Oklahoma | 26.13 |
| 14 | North Carolina | 31.11 | 39 | Maryland | 25.88 |
| 15 | Alabama | 30.99 | 40 | Kentucky | 25.21 |
| 16 | Delaware | 30.96 | 41 | Connecticut | 25.11 |
| 17 | Mississippi | 30.47 | 42 | New Mexico | 23.48 |
| 18 | Minnesota | 30.30 | 43 | California | 22.82 |
| 19 | Idaho | 29.94 | 44 | Wyoming | 22.03 |
| 20 | Maine | 29.27 | 45 | Colorado | 21.46 |
| 21 | Nebraska | 29.24 | 46 | Utah | 20.45 |
| 22 | Washington | 29.00 | 47 | Nevada | 20.43 |
| 23 | New York | 28.98 | 48 | Texas | 19.13 |
| 24 | Kansas | 28.82 | 49 | Hawaii | 17.73 |
| 25 | Michigan | 28.81 | 50 | Alaska | 8.62 |

District of Columbia       53.01

Source: American Cancer Society

    "Cancer Facts & Figures - 1992" (Copyright 1992, Reprinted with permission from the American Cancer Society)

*Calculated by the editors using 1990 Census resident population figures. These estimates are based on cancer mortality data from 1982 through 1988.

# Estimated Deaths by Skin Melanoma in 1992

## National Estimated Total = 6,700 Deaths by Skin Melanoma*

| RANK | STATE | DEATHS | % | RANK | STATE | DEATHS | % |
|---|---|---|---|---|---|---|---|
| 1 | California | 800 | 11.94% | 25 | Connecticut | 90 | 1.34% |
| 2 | New York | 500 | 7.46% | 25 | Iowa | 90 | 1.34% |
| 3 | Florida | 475 | 7.09% | 25 | Oregon | 90 | 1.34% |
| 4 | Pennsylvania | 375 | 5.60% | 25 | South Carolina | 90 | 1.34% |
| 5 | Texas | 350 | 5.22% | 30 | Louisiana | 80 | 1.19% |
| 6 | Illinois | 250 | 3.73% | 31 | Arkansas | 70 | 1.04% |
| 6 | New Jersey | 250 | 3.73% | 31 | Kansas | 70 | 1.04% |
| 6 | Ohio | 250 | 3.73% | 33 | Mississippi | 60 | 0.90% |
| 9 | North Carolina | 225 | 3.36% | 33 | Nebraska | 60 | 0.90% |
| 10 | Massachusetts | 200 | 2.99% | 33 | West Virginia | 60 | 0.90% |
| 11 | Georgia | 175 | 2.61% | 36 | Maine | 40 | 0.60% |
| 11 | Michigan | 175 | 2.61% | 36 | New Mexico | 40 | 0.60% |
| 13 | Indiana | 150 | 2.24% | 36 | Utah | 40 | 0.60% |
| 13 | Virginia | 150 | 2.24% | 39 | Idaho | 30 | 0.45% |
| 15 | Maryland | 125 | 1.87% | 39 | Nevada | 30 | 0.45% |
| 15 | Missouri | 125 | 1.87% | 41 | Delaware | 25 | 0.37% |
| 15 | Tennessee | 125 | 1.87% | 41 | Montana | 25 | 0.37% |
| 15 | Washington | 125 | 1.87% | 41 | New Hampshire | 25 | 0.37% |
| 15 | Wisconsin | 125 | 1.87% | 41 | Rhode Island | 25 | 0.37% |
| 20 | Alabama | 100 | 1.49% | 45 | Hawaii | 20 | 0.30% |
| 20 | Arizona | 100 | 1.49% | 45 | North Dakota | 20 | 0.30% |
| 20 | Kentucky | 100 | 1.49% | 45 | South Dakota | 20 | 0.30% |
| 20 | Minnesota | 100 | 1.49% | 45 | Vermont | 20 | 0.30% |
| 20 | Oklahoma | 100 | 1.49% | 49 | Alaska | 10 | 0.15% |
| 25 | Colorado | 90 | 1.34% | 49 | Wyoming | 10 | 0.15% |
| | | | | | District of Columbia | 20 | 0.30% |

Source: American Cancer Society

"Cancer Facts & Figures – 1992" (Copyright 1992, Reprinted with permission from the American Cancer Society)

*These estimates are based on cancer mortality data from 1982 through 1988.

# Estimated Death Rate by Skin Melanoma in 1992

## National Estimated Rate = 2.66 Deaths by Skin Melanoma per 100,000 Population*

| RANK | STATE | RATE | | RANK | STATE | RATE |
|------|-------|------|---|------|-------|------|
| 1 | Nebraska | 3.77 | | 26 | Georgia | 2.64 |
| 2 | Delaware | 3.68 | | 27 | California | 2.63 |
| 3 | Florida | 3.58 | | 28 | New Mexico | 2.58 |
| 4 | Vermont | 3.53 | | 29 | Maryland | 2.57 |
| 5 | Massachusetts | 3.34 | | 30 | South Carolina | 2.53 |
| 5 | North Carolina | 3.34 | | 31 | Tennessee | 2.52 |
| 7 | West Virginia | 3.33 | | 31 | Wisconsin | 2.52 |
| 8 | Maine | 3.24 | | 33 | Rhode Island | 2.49 |
| 9 | Iowa | 3.22 | | 33 | Washington | 2.49 |
| 9 | New Jersey | 3.22 | | 35 | Alabama | 2.45 |
| 11 | North Dakota | 3.15 | | 36 | Missouri | 2.42 |
| 11 | Oklahoma | 3.15 | | 37 | Virginia | 2.39 |
| 13 | Pennsylvania | 3.14 | | 38 | Nevada | 2.34 |
| 14 | Montana | 3.09 | | 39 | Mississippi | 2.31 |
| 15 | Oregon | 3.08 | | 40 | Ohio | 2.29 |
| 16 | Arkansas | 2.95 | | 41 | Minnesota | 2.26 |
| 17 | Idaho | 2.89 | | 41 | New Hampshire | 2.26 |
| 18 | South Dakota | 2.84 | | 41 | Utah | 2.26 |
| 19 | Kansas | 2.81 | | 44 | Illinois | 2.17 |
| 20 | New York | 2.77 | | 44 | Wyoming | 2.17 |
| 21 | Connecticut | 2.73 | | 46 | Texas | 2.02 |
| 22 | Kentucky | 2.69 | | 47 | Louisiana | 1.88 |
| 23 | Arizona | 2.67 | | 48 | Michigan | 1.87 |
| 23 | Colorado | 2.67 | | 49 | Hawaii | 1.76 |
| 23 | Indiana | 2.67 | | 50 | Alaska | 1.75 |
| | | | | | District of Columbia | 3.34 |

Source: American Cancer Society

"Cancer Facts & Figures - 1992" (Copyright 1992, Reprinted with permission from the American Cancer Society)

*Calculated by the editors using 1991 Census resident population figures. These estimates are based on cancer mortality data from 1982 through 1988.

# Estimated Deaths by Cancer of the Uterus in 1992

## National Estimated Total = 10,000 Deaths by Cancer of the Uterus*

| RANK | STATE | DEATHS | % | RANK | STATE | DEATHS | % |
|---|---|---|---|---|---|---|---|
| 1 | California | 1,000 | 10.00% | 24 | Oregon | 125 | 1.25% |
| 2 | New York | 850 | 8.50% | 24 | South Carolina | 125 | 1.25% |
| 3 | Florida | 600 | 6.00% | 28 | Arkansas | 100 | 1.00% |
| 3 | Pennsylvania | 600 | 6.00% | 28 | Connecticut | 100 | 1.00% |
| 5 | Illinois | 500 | 5.00% | 28 | Iowa | 100 | 1.00% |
| 5 | Ohio | 500 | 5.00% | 28 | Kansas | 100 | 1.00% |
| 5 | Texas | 500 | 5.00% | 28 | Washington | 100 | 1.00% |
| 8 | Michigan | 400 | 4.00% | 28 | West Virginia | 100 | 1.00% |
| 9 | New Jersey | 375 | 3.75% | 34 | Colorado | 75 | 0.75% |
| 10 | North Carolina | 275 | 2.75% | 35 | Maine | 60 | 0.60% |
| 11 | Massachusetts | 250 | 2.50% | 36 | Idaho | 50 | 0.50% |
| 12 | Georgia | 225 | 2.25% | 36 | Nebraska | 50 | 0.50% |
| 12 | Indiana | 225 | 2.25% | 36 | New Hampshire | 50 | 0.50% |
| 12 | Tennessee | 225 | 2.25% | 36 | New Mexico | 50 | 0.50% |
| 12 | Virginia | 225 | 2.25% | 36 | Rhode Island | 50 | 0.50% |
| 16 | Alabama | 200 | 2.00% | 36 | Utah | 50 | 0.50% |
| 16 | Louisiana | 200 | 2.00% | 42 | Nevada | 40 | 0.40% |
| 16 | Missouri | 200 | 2.00% | 43 | Delaware | 30 | 0.30% |
| 19 | Kentucky | 175 | 1.75% | 43 | Hawaii | 30 | 0.30% |
| 19 | Oklahoma | 175 | 1.75% | 43 | Montana | 30 | 0.30% |
| 19 | Wisconsin | 175 | 1.75% | 46 | North Dakota | 25 | 0.25% |
| 22 | Maryland | 150 | 1.50% | 46 | South Dakota | 25 | 0.25% |
| 22 | Minnesota | 150 | 1.50% | 48 | Vermont | 20 | 0.20% |
| 24 | Arizona | 125 | 1.25% | 48 | Wyoming | 20 | 0.20% |
| 24 | Mississippi | 125 | 1.25% | 50 | Alaska | 10 | 0.10% |
| | | | | | District of Columbia | 60 | 0.60% |

Source: American Cancer Society

"Cancer Facts & Figures – 1992" (Copyright 1992, Reprinted with permission from the American Cancer Society)

*These estimates are based on cancer mortality data from 1982 through 1988.

# Estimated Death Rate by Cancer of the Uterus in 1992

## National Rate = 7.84 Deaths by Cancer of the Uterus per 100,000 Female Population*

| RANK | STATE | RATE | RANK | STATE | RATE |
|------|-------|------|------|-------|------|
| 1 | Oklahoma | 10.84 | 26 | Indiana | 7.88 |
| 2 | West Virginia | 10.73 | 27 | North Dakota | 7.80 |
| 3 | Idaho | 9.89 | 28 | Missouri | 7.54 |
| 4 | Pennsylvania | 9.70 | 29 | Montana | 7.44 |
| 5 | Rhode Island | 9.58 | 30 | Virginia | 7.14 |
| 6 | Maine | 9.52 | 31 | South Dakota | 7.07 |
| 7 | Alabama | 9.50 | 32 | Wisconsin | 7.00 |
| 8 | New Jersey | 9.39 | 33 | Iowa | 6.98 |
| 9 | Mississippi | 9.31 | 34 | Vermont | 6.96 |
| 10 | Kentucky | 9.21 | 35 | South Carolina | 6.95 |
| 11 | Louisiana | 9.14 | 36 | Nevada | 6.78 |
| 12 | New York | 9.08 | 37 | Georgia | 6.75 |
| 13 | Florida | 8.99 | 38 | Arizona | 6.74 |
| 14 | Ohio | 8.90 | 39 | California | 6.73 |
| 14 | Tennessee | 8.90 | 39 | Minnesota | 6.73 |
| 16 | New Hampshire | 8.84 | 41 | New Mexico | 6.50 |
| 17 | Wyoming | 8.83 | 42 | Nebraska | 6.18 |
| 18 | Delaware | 8.74 | 43 | Maryland | 6.09 |
| 19 | Oregon | 8.65 | 44 | Connecticut | 5.90 |
| 20 | Illinois | 8.51 | 45 | Texas | 5.80 |
| 21 | Michigan | 8.36 | 46 | Utah | 5.77 |
| 22 | Arkansas | 8.21 | 47 | Hawaii | 5.51 |
| 23 | North Carolina | 8.05 | 48 | Colorado | 4.51 |
| 24 | Massachusetts | 7.99 | 49 | Washington | 4.08 |
| 25 | Kansas | 7.92 | 50 | Alaska | 3.84 |
| | | | | District of Columbia | 18.52 |

Source: American Cancer Society

*"Cancer Facts & Figures – 1992"* (Copyright 1992, Reprinted with permission from the American Cancer Society)

*Calculated by the editors using 1990 Census resident population figures. These estimates are based on cancer mortality data from 1982 through 1988.*

# Deaths by Atherosclerosis in 1988

## National Total = 22,086 Deaths by Atherosclerosis*

| RANK | STATE | DEATHS | % | RANK | STATE | DEATHS | % |
|------|-------|--------|------|------|-------|--------|------|
| 1 | California | 2,353 | 10.65% | 26 | Colorado | 357 | 1.62% |
| 2 | New York | 1,562 | 7.07% | 27 | Kansas | 337 | 1.53% |
| 3 | Florida | 1,210 | 5.48% | 28 | Arizona | 317 | 1.44% |
| 4 | Michigan | 1,188 | 5.38% | 29 | Maryland | 295 | 1.34% |
| 5 | Texas | 1,163 | 5.27% | 30 | Nebraska | 258 | 1.17% |
| 6 | Illinois | 1,052 | 4.76% | 31 | Connecticut | 256 | 1.16% |
| 7 | Pennsylvania | 1,043 | 4.72% | 32 | Arkansas | 208 | 0.94% |
| 8 | Ohio | 1,017 | 4.60% | 32 | West Virginia | 208 | 0.94% |
| 9 | Indiana | 674 | 3.05% | 34 | Mississippi | 196 | 0.89% |
| 10 | Massachusetts | 631 | 2.86% | 35 | South Carolina | 179 | 0.81% |
| 11 | New Jersey | 619 | 2.80% | 36 | Maine | 173 | 0.78% |
| 12 | Iowa | 500 | 2.26% | 37 | New Hampshire | 107 | 0.48% |
| 13 | Washington | 473 | 2.14% | 38 | New Mexico | 106 | 0.48% |
| 14 | Missouri | 440 | 1.99% | 39 | North Dakota | 98 | 0.44% |
| 15 | Tennessee | 429 | 1.94% | 40 | Rhode Island | 93 | 0.42% |
| 16 | Minnesota | 423 | 1.92% | 41 | Montana | 88 | 0.40% |
| 16 | Wisconsin | 423 | 1.92% | 42 | Idaho | 83 | 0.38% |
| 18 | North Carolina | 416 | 1.88% | 43 | Utah | 74 | 0.34% |
| 19 | Virginia | 412 | 1.87% | 44 | South Dakota | 69 | 0.31% |
| 20 | Georgia | 394 | 1.78% | 45 | Nevada | 67 | 0.30% |
| 21 | Oklahoma | 389 | 1.76% | 46 | Vermont | 49 | 0.22% |
| 22 | Oregon | 388 | 1.76% | 47 | Delaware | 38 | 0.17% |
| 23 | Alabama | 382 | 1.73% | 47 | Hawaii | 38 | 0.17% |
| 24 | Kentucky | 379 | 1.72% | 49 | Wyoming | 29 | 0.13% |
| 25 | Louisiana | 375 | 1.70% | 50 | Alaska | 5 | 0.02% |
| | | | | | District of Columbia | 23 | 0.10% |

Source: U.S. Department of Health and Human Services, Centers for Disease Control, National Center for Health Statistics
"Vital Statistics of the United States, 1988" (Vol II, Part B, issued 1990)
*By state of residence.  Atherosclerosis is a form of hardening of the arteries.

# Death Rate by Atherosclerosis in 1988

## National Rate = 8.99 Deaths per 100,000 Population*

| RANK | STATE | RATE | RANK | STATE | RATE |
|------|-------|------|------|-------|------|
| 1 | Iowa | 17.64 | 26 | Tennessee | 8.76 |
| 2 | Nebraska | 16.10 | 27 | New York | 8.72 |
| 3 | North Dakota | 14.69 | 28 | Wisconsin | 8.71 |
| 4 | Maine | 14.36 | 29 | Pennsylvania | 8.69 |
| 5 | Oregon | 14.02 | 30 | Arkansas | 8.68 |
| 6 | Kansas | 13.51 | 31 | Missouri | 8.56 |
| 7 | Michigan | 12.86 | 32 | Louisiana | 8.51 |
| 8 | Indiana | 12.13 | 33 | California | 8.31 |
| 9 | Oklahoma | 12.00 | 34 | Idaho | 8.28 |
| 10 | West Virginia | 11.09 | 35 | New Jersey | 8.02 |
| 11 | Montana | 10.93 | 36 | Connecticut | 7.92 |
| 12 | Colorado | 10.81 | 37 | Mississippi | 7.48 |
| 13 | Massachusetts | 10.71 | 38 | New Mexico | 7.03 |
| 14 | Washington | 10.18 | 39 | Texas | 6.91 |
| 15 | Kentucky | 10.17 | 40 | Virginia | 6.85 |
| 16 | New Hampshire | 9.86 | 41 | North Carolina | 6.41 |
| 17 | Minnesota | 9.82 | 42 | Maryland | 6.38 |
| 18 | Florida | 9.81 | 43 | Nevada | 6.36 |
| 19 | South Dakota | 9.68 | 44 | Georgia | 6.21 |
| 20 | Ohio | 9.37 | 45 | Wyoming | 6.05 |
| 21 | Rhode Island | 9.37 | 46 | Delaware | 5.76 |
| 22 | Alabama | 9.31 | 47 | South Carolina | 5.16 |
| 23 | Arizona | 9.09 | 48 | Utah | 4.38 |
| 24 | Illinois | 9.06 | 49 | Hawaii | 3.46 |
| 25 | Vermont | 8.80 | 50 | Alaska | 0.95 |
| | | | | District of Columbia | 3.73 |

Source: U.S. Department of Health and Human Services, Centers for Disease Control, National Center for Health Statistics
   "Vital Statistics of the United States, 1988" (Vol. II, Part B, issued 1990)
*By state of residence. Atherosclerosis is a form of hardening of the arteries. Rates calculated by the editors.

# Deaths by Cerebrovascular Diseases in 1989

## National Total = 145,551 Deaths by Cerebrovascular Diseases*

| RANK | STATE | DEATHS | % | RANK | STATE | DEATHS | % |
|------|-------|--------|-----|------|-------|--------|-----|
| 1 | California | 15,755 | 10.82% | 26 | Iowa | 2,142 | 1.47% |
| 2 | New York | 9,145 | 6.28% | 27 | Arkansas | 2,035 | 1.40% |
| 3 | Florida | 8,410 | 5.78% | 28 | Oregon | 2,025 | 1.39% |
| 4 | Texas | 8,380 | 5.76% | 29 | Mississippi | 1,893 | 1.30% |
| 5 | Pennsylvania | 7,729 | 5.31% | 30 | Connecticut | 1,789 | 1.23% |
| 6 | Illinois | 6,865 | 4.72% | 31 | Arizona | 1,641 | 1.13% |
| 7 | Ohio | 6,277 | 4.31% | 32 | Kansas | 1,622 | 1.11% |
| 8 | Michigan | 5,198 | 3.57% | 33 | Colorado | 1,322 | 0.91% |
| 9 | North Carolina | 4,613 | 3.17% | 34 | West Virginia | 1,178 | 0.81% |
| 10 | New Jersey | 4,111 | 2.82% | 35 | Nebraska | 1,157 | 0.79% |
| 11 | Indiana | 3,798 | 2.61% | 36 | Maine | 726 | 0.50% |
| 12 | Georgia | 3,755 | 2.58% | 37 | Utah | 638 | 0.44% |
| 13 | Tennessee | 3,550 | 2.44% | 38 | Rhode Island | 606 | 0.42% |
| 14 | Missouri | 3,460 | 2.38% | 39 | Idaho | 577 | 0.40% |
| 15 | Massachusetts | 3,430 | 2.36% | 40 | New Hampshire | 566 | 0.39% |
| 16 | Virginia | 3,319 | 2.28% | 41 | New Mexico | 563 | 0.39% |
| 17 | Wisconsin | 3,242 | 2.23% | 42 | South Dakota | 511 | 0.35% |
| 18 | Alabama | 2,869 | 1.97% | 43 | Hawaii | 491 | 0.34% |
| 19 | Minnesota | 2,846 | 1.96% | 44 | Nevada | 450 | 0.31% |
| 20 | Washington | 2,686 | 1.85% | 45 | Montana | 431 | 0.30% |
| 21 | Kentucky | 2,513 | 1.73% | 46 | North Dakota | 403 | 0.28% |
| 22 | Louisiana | 2,472 | 1.70% | 47 | Delaware | 323 | 0.22% |
| 23 | South Carolina | 2,462 | 1.69% | 48 | Vermont | 298 | 0.20% |
| 24 | Maryland | 2,284 | 1.57% | 49 | Wyoming | 170 | 0.12% |
| 25 | Oklahoma | 2,282 | 1.57% | 50 | Alaska | 97 | 0.07% |
|  |  |  |  |  | District of Columbia | 446 | 0.31% |

Source: U.S. Department of Health and Human Services, Centers for Disease Control, National Center for Health Statistics
"Monthly Vital Statistics Report" (Vol. 40, No. 8(S)2, January 7, 1992)
*By state of residence.  Cerebrovascular disease includes stroke and other disorders of the blood vessels of the brain.

# Death Rate by Cerebrovascular Disease in 1989

## National Rate = 58.6 Deaths per 100,000 Population*

| RANK | STATE | RATE | RANK | STATE | RATE |
|------|-------|------|------|-------|------|
| 1 | Arkansas | 84.6 | 26 | Massachusetts | 58.0 |
| 2 | Iowa | 75.4 | 27 | Ohio | 57.6 |
| 3 | Mississippi | 72.2 | 28 | Idaho | 56.9 |
| 4 | Tennessee | 71.9 | 29 | Louisiana | 56.4 |
| 5 | Nebraska | 71.8 | 29 | Washington | 56.4 |
| 5 | Oregon | 71.8 | 31 | Michigan | 56.1 |
| 7 | South Dakota | 71.5 | 32 | Connecticut | 55.2 |
| 8 | Oklahoma | 70.8 | 33 | Virginia | 54.4 |
| 9 | North Carolina | 70.2 | 34 | California | 54.2 |
| 10 | South Carolina | 70.1 | 35 | Montana | 53.5 |
| 11 | Alabama | 69.7 | 36 | New Jersey | 53.1 |
| 12 | Indiana | 67.9 | 37 | Vermont | 52.6 |
| 13 | Kentucky | 67.4 | 38 | New Hampshire | 51.1 |
| 14 | Missouri | 67.1 | 39 | New York | 50.9 |
| 15 | Wisconsin | 66.6 | 40 | Texas | 49.3 |
| 16 | Florida | 66.4 | 41 | Maryland | 48.7 |
| 17 | Minnesota | 65.4 | 42 | Delaware | 48.0 |
| 18 | Kansas | 64.5 | 43 | Arizona | 46.1 |
| 19 | Pennsylvania | 64.2 | 44 | Hawaii | 44.2 |
| 20 | West Virginia | 63.4 | 45 | Nevada | 40.5 |
| 21 | North Dakota | 61.1 | 46 | Colorado | 39.9 |
| 22 | Rhode Island | 60.7 | 47 | Utah | 37.4 |
| 23 | Maine | 59.4 | 48 | New Mexico | 36.8 |
| 24 | Illinois | 58.9 | 49 | Wyoming | 35.8 |
| 25 | Georgia | 58.3 | 50 | Alaska | 18.4 |
| | | | | District of Columbia | 73.8 |

Source: U.S. Department of Health and Human Services, Centers for Disease Control, National Center for Health Statistics,
"Monthly Vital Statistics Report" (Vol. 40, No. 8(S)2, January 7, 1992)

*By state of residence. Cerebrovascular disease includes stroke and other disorders of the blood vessels of the brain.

# Deaths by Chronic Liver Disease and Cirrhosis in 1988

## National Total = 26,409 Deaths by Chronic Liver Diseases and Cirrhosis*

| RANK | STATE | DEATHS | % | RANK | STATE | DEATHS | % |
|---|---|---|---|---|---|---|---|
| 1 | California | 4,154 | 15.73% | 26 | Minnesota | 295 | 1.12% |
| 2 | New York | 2,549 | 9.65% | 27 | Oklahoma | 288 | 1.09% |
| 3 | Florida | 1,683 | 6.37% | 28 | Oregon | 287 | 1.09% |
| 4 | Texas | 1,417 | 5.37% | 29 | Colorado | 275 | 1.04% |
| 5 | Illinois | 1,255 | 4.75% | 30 | Mississippi | 211 | 0.80% |
| 6 | Pennsylvania | 1,235 | 4.68% | 31 | New Mexico | 193 | 0.73% |
| 7 | Michigan | 1,079 | 4.09% | 32 | Iowa | 192 | 0.73% |
| 8 | New Jersey | 1,043 | 3.95% | 33 | Nevada | 180 | 0.68% |
| 9 | Ohio | 965 | 3.65% | 34 | Kansas | 178 | 0.67% |
| 10 | Massachusetts | 728 | 2.76% | 35 | Arkansas | 168 | 0.64% |
| 11 | North Carolina | 702 | 2.66% | 36 | West Virginia | 165 | 0.62% |
| 12 | Georgia | 585 | 2.22% | 37 | Rhode Island | 130 | 0.49% |
| 13 | Virginia | 544 | 2.06% | 38 | Maine | 127 | 0.48% |
| 14 | Indiana | 461 | 1.75% | 39 | New Hampshire | 120 | 0.45% |
| 15 | Maryland | 455 | 1.72% | 40 | Nebraska | 102 | 0.39% |
| 15 | Washington | 455 | 1.72% | 41 | Montana | 87 | 0.33% |
| 17 | Arizona | 450 | 1.70% | 42 | Utah | 81 | 0.31% |
| 18 | Tennessee | 410 | 1.55% | 43 | Hawaii | 79 | 0.30% |
| 19 | Alabama | 404 | 1.53% | 44 | Idaho | 65 | 0.25% |
| 20 | Wisconsin | 394 | 1.49% | 45 | Delaware | 64 | 0.24% |
| 21 | Missouri | 373 | 1.41% | 46 | Vermont | 61 | 0.23% |
| 22 | Connecticut | 330 | 1.25% | 47 | North Dakota | 58 | 0.22% |
| 23 | Louisiana | 328 | 1.24% | 48 | South Dakota | 52 | 0.20% |
| 24 | Kentucky | 326 | 1.23% | 49 | Alaska | 45 | 0.17% |
| 24 | South Carolina | 326 | 1.23% | 50 | Wyoming | 41 | 0.16% |
| | | | | | District of Columbia | 214 | 0.81% |

Source: U.S. Department of Health and Human Services, Centers for Disease Control, National Center for Health Statistics,
     "Vital Statistics of the United States, 1988" (Vol II, Part B, issued 1990)
*By state of residence.

# Death Rate by Chronic Liver Disease and Cirrhosis in 1988

## National Rate = 10.74 Deaths per 100,000 Population*

| RANK | STATE | RATE | RANK | STATE | RATE |
|------|-------|------|------|-------|------|
| 1 | Nevada | 17.08 | 26 | Virginia | 9.04 |
| 2 | California | 14.67 | 27 | Ohio | 8.89 |
| 3 | New York | 14.23 | 28 | Oklahoma | 8.88 |
| 4 | Florida | 13.64 | 29 | West Virginia | 8.80 |
| 5 | New Jersey | 13.51 | 30 | Kentucky | 8.75 |
| 6 | Rhode Island | 13.09 | 31 | North Dakota | 8.70 |
| 7 | Arizona | 12.90 | 32 | Alaska | 8.59 |
| 8 | New Mexico | 12.81 | 33 | Wyoming | 8.56 |
| 9 | Massachusetts | 12.36 | 34 | Texas | 8.41 |
| 10 | Michigan | 11.68 | 35 | Tennessee | 8.38 |
| 11 | New Hampshire | 11.06 | 36 | Colorado | 8.33 |
| 12 | Vermont | 10.95 | 37 | Indiana | 8.30 |
| 13 | North Carolina | 10.82 | 38 | Wisconsin | 8.12 |
| 14 | Montana | 10.81 | 39 | Mississippi | 8.05 |
| 15 | Illinois | 10.81 | 40 | Louisiana | 7.44 |
| 16 | Maine | 10.54 | 41 | South Dakota | 7.29 |
| 17 | Oregon | 10.37 | 42 | Missouri | 7.26 |
| 18 | Pennsylvania | 10.29 | 43 | Hawaii | 7.19 |
| 19 | Connecticut | 10.21 | 44 | Kansas | 7.13 |
| 20 | Alabama | 9.85 | 45 | Arkansas | 7.01 |
| 21 | Maryland | 9.84 | 46 | Minnesota | 6.85 |
| 22 | Washington | 9.79 | 47 | Iowa | 6.77 |
| 23 | Delaware | 9.70 | 48 | Idaho | 6.48 |
| 24 | South Carolina | 9.39 | 49 | Nebraska | 6.37 |
| 25 | Georgia | 9.22 | 50 | Utah | 4.79 |
| | | | | District of Columbia | 34.68 |

Source: U.S. Department of Health and Human Services, Centers for Disease Control, National Center for Health Statistics,
"Vital Statistics of the United States, 1988" (Vol. II, Part B, issued 1990)
*By state of residence. Rates calculated by the editors.

# Deaths by Chronic Obstructive Pulmonary Diseases in 1988

## National Total = 82,853 Deaths by Chronic Pulmonary Diseases*

| RANK | STATE | DEATHS | % | RANK | STATE | DEATHS | % |
|------|-------|--------|---|------|-------|--------|---|
| 1 | California | 9,684 | 11.69% | 26 | Iowa | 1,205 | 1.45% |
| 2 | New York | 5,549 | 6.70% | 27 | Oregon | 1,195 | 1.44% |
| 3 | Florida | 5,317 | 6.42% | 28 | Louisiana | 1,140 | 1.38% |
| 4 | Pennsylvania | 4,325 | 5.22% | 29 | Kansas | 1,008 | 1.22% |
| 5 | Texas | 4,092 | 4.94% | 30 | South Carolina | 950 | 1.15% |
| 6 | Ohio | 4,070 | 4.91% | 31 | Connecticut | 946 | 1.14% |
| 7 | Illinois | 3,529 | 4.26% | 32 | West Virginia | 903 | 1.09% |
| 8 | Michigan | 2,902 | 3.50% | 33 | Arkansas | 866 | 1.05% |
| 9 | New Jersey | 2,261 | 2.73% | 34 | Mississippi | 804 | 0.97% |
| 10 | North Carolina | 2,098 | 2.53% | 35 | Nebraska | 583 | 0.70% |
| 11 | Missouri | 2,081 | 2.51% | 36 | Nevada | 557 | 0.67% |
| 12 | Indiana | 2,078 | 2.51% | 37 | Maine | 555 | 0.67% |
| 13 | Massachusetts | 2,024 | 2.44% | 38 | New Mexico | 471 | 0.57% |
| 14 | Washington | 1,846 | 2.23% | 39 | Idaho | 403 | 0.49% |
| 15 | Georgia | 1,842 | 2.22% | 40 | Montana | 383 | 0.46% |
| 16 | Tennessee | 1,742 | 2.10% | 41 | Utah | 374 | 0.45% |
| 17 | Virginia | 1,641 | 1.98% | 42 | New Hampshire | 364 | 0.44% |
| 18 | Wisconsin | 1,589 | 1.92% | 43 | Rhode Island | 341 | 0.41% |
| 19 | Kentucky | 1,530 | 1.85% | 44 | Vermont | 252 | 0.30% |
| 20 | Arizona | 1,461 | 1.76% | 45 | South Dakota | 240 | 0.29% |
| 21 | Alabama | 1,439 | 1.74% | 46 | North Dakota | 203 | 0.25% |
| 22 | Maryland | 1,407 | 1.70% | 47 | Delaware | 199 | 0.24% |
| 23 | Minnesota | 1,297 | 1.57% | 48 | Wyoming | 197 | 0.24% |
| 24 | Colorado | 1,296 | 1.56% | 49 | Hawaii | 192 | 0.23% |
| 25 | Oklahoma | 1,206 | 1.46% | 50 | Alaska | 71 | 0.09% |
| | | | | | District of Columbia | 145 | 0.18% |

Source: U.S. Department of Health and Human Services, Centers for Disease Control, National Center for Health Statistics,
"Vital Statistics of the United States, 1988" (Vol. II, Part B, issued 1990)
*By state of residence. Includes allied conditions.

# Death Rate by Chronic Obstructive Pulmonary Diseases in 1988

## National Rate = 33.71 Deaths per 100,000 Population*

| RANK | STATE | RATE | RANK | STATE | RATE |
|------|-------|------|------|-------|------|
| 1 | Nevada | 52.85 | 26 | Rhode Island | 34.34 |
| 2 | West Virginia | 48.13 | 27 | California | 34.20 |
| 3 | Montana | 47.58 | 28 | South Dakota | 33.66 |
| 4 | Maine | 46.06 | 29 | New Hampshire | 33.55 |
| 5 | Vermont | 45.24 | 30 | Wisconsin | 32.73 |
| 6 | Oregon | 43.19 | 31 | North Carolina | 32.33 |
| 7 | Florida | 43.10 | 32 | Michigan | 31.41 |
| 8 | Iowa | 42.52 | 33 | New Mexico | 31.25 |
| 9 | Arizona | 41.87 | 34 | New York | 30.98 |
| 10 | Wyoming | 41.13 | 35 | Mississippi | 30.69 |
| 11 | Kentucky | 41.05 | 36 | Maryland | 30.44 |
| 12 | Missouri | 40.48 | 37 | North Dakota | 30.43 |
| 13 | Kansas | 40.40 | 38 | Illinois | 30.39 |
| 14 | Idaho | 40.18 | 39 | Delaware | 30.15 |
| 15 | Washington | 39.72 | 40 | Minnesota | 30.11 |
| 16 | Colorado | 39.26 | 41 | New Jersey | 29.28 |
| 17 | Ohio | 37.49 | 42 | Connecticut | 29.26 |
| 18 | Indiana | 37.40 | 43 | Georgia | 29.04 |
| 19 | Oklahoma | 37.20 | 44 | South Carolina | 27.38 |
| 20 | Nebraska | 36.39 | 45 | Virginia | 27.28 |
| 21 | Arkansas | 36.16 | 46 | Louisiana | 25.86 |
| 22 | Pennsylvania | 36.04 | 47 | Texas | 24.30 |
| 23 | Tennessee | 35.59 | 48 | Utah | 22.13 |
| 24 | Alabama | 35.08 | 49 | Hawaii | 17.49 |
| 25 | Massachusetts | 34.37 | 50 | Alaska | 13.55 |

District of Columbia          23.50

Source: U.S. Department of Health and Human Services, Centers for Disease Control, National Center for Health Statistics,
     "Vital Statistics of the United States, 1988" (Vol. II, Part B, issued 1990)
*By state of residence. Includes allied conditions. Rates calculated by the editors.

# Deaths by Diabetes Mellitus in 1988

## National Total = 40,368 Deaths by Diabetes Mellitus*

| RANK | STATE | DEATHS | % | RANK | STATE | DEATHS | % |
|---|---|---|---|---|---|---|---|
| 1 | California | 3,405 | 8.43% | 26 | Oklahoma | 539 | 1.34% |
| 2 | New York | 3,249 | 8.05% | 27 | Connecticut | 530 | 1.31% |
| 3 | Pennsylvania | 2,624 | 6.50% | 28 | Mississippi | 498 | 1.23% |
| 4 | Florida | 2,139 | 5.30% | 29 | Iowa | 458 | 1.13% |
| 5 | Ohio | 2,135 | 5.29% | 30 | Oregon | 443 | 1.10% |
| 6 | Texas | 2,058 | 5.10% | 31 | Arkansas | 419 | 1.04% |
| 7 | Illinois | 1,835 | 4.55% | 32 | Kansas | 409 | 1.01% |
| 8 | New Jersey | 1,532 | 3.80% | 33 | West Virginia | 390 | 0.97% |
| 9 | Michigan | 1,520 | 3.77% | 34 | Colorado | 371 | 0.92% |
| 10 | North Carolina | 1,326 | 3.28% | 35 | Rhode Island | 284 | 0.70% |
| 11 | Indiana | 1,222 | 3.03% | 36 | Maine | 276 | 0.68% |
| 12 | Massachusetts | 922 | 2.28% | 37 | New Mexico | 258 | 0.64% |
| 13 | Georgia | 912 | 2.26% | 38 | Nebraska | 249 | 0.62% |
| 14 | Louisiana | 863 | 2.14% | 39 | Utah | 221 | 0.55% |
| 15 | Kentucky | 847 | 2.10% | 40 | New Hampshire | 178 | 0.44% |
| 16 | Missouri | 824 | 2.04% | 41 | Idaho | 163 | 0.40% |
| 17 | Alabama | 792 | 1.96% | 42 | Montana | 153 | 0.38% |
| 18 | Wisconsin | 788 | 1.95% | 43 | Delaware | 147 | 0.36% |
| 19 | Maryland | 773 | 1.91% | 43 | Hawaii | 147 | 0.36% |
| 20 | Virginia | 753 | 1.87% | 45 | Nevada | 123 | 0.30% |
| 21 | Tennessee | 739 | 1.83% | 46 | North Dakota | 115 | 0.28% |
| 22 | Washington | 655 | 1.62% | 47 | South Dakota | 95 | 0.24% |
| 23 | Minnesota | 557 | 1.38% | 48 | Vermont | 93 | 0.23% |
| 24 | South Carolina | 550 | 1.36% | 49 | Wyoming | 70 | 0.17% |
| 25 | Arizona | 543 | 1.35% | 50 | Alaska | 40 | 0.10% |
| | | | | | District of Columbia | 136 | 0.34% |

Source: U.S. Department of Health and Human Services, Centers for Disease Control, National Center for Health Statistics,
"Vital Statistics of the United States, 1988" (Vol II, Part B, issued 1990)
*By state of residence.

# Death Rate by Diabetes Mellitus in 1988

## National Rate = 16.42 Deaths per 100,000 Population*

| RANK | STATE | RATE | RANK | STATE | RATE |
|------|-------|------|------|-------|------|
| 1 | Rhode Island | 28.60 | 26 | Kansas | 16.39 |
| 2 | Maine | 22.90 | 27 | Idaho | 16.25 |
| 3 | Kentucky | 22.73 | 28 | Wisconsin | 16.23 |
| 4 | Delaware | 22.27 | 29 | Iowa | 16.16 |
| 5 | Indiana | 21.99 | 30 | Missouri | 16.03 |
| 6 | Pennsylvania | 21.86 | 31 | Oregon | 16.01 |
| 7 | West Virginia | 20.79 | 32 | South Carolina | 15.85 |
| 8 | North Carolina | 20.43 | 33 | Illinois | 15.80 |
| 9 | New Jersey | 19.84 | 34 | Massachusetts | 15.66 |
| 10 | Ohio | 19.67 | 35 | Arizona | 15.56 |
| 11 | Louisiana | 19.58 | 36 | Nebraska | 15.54 |
| 12 | Alabama | 19.31 | 37 | Tennessee | 15.10 |
| 13 | Mississippi | 19.01 | 38 | Wyoming | 14.61 |
| 14 | Montana | 19.01 | 39 | Georgia | 14.38 |
| 15 | New York | 18.14 | 40 | Washington | 14.09 |
| 16 | Arkansas | 17.49 | 41 | Hawaii | 13.39 |
| 17 | Florida | 17.34 | 42 | South Dakota | 13.32 |
| 18 | North Dakota | 17.24 | 43 | Utah | 13.08 |
| 19 | New Mexico | 17.12 | 44 | Minnesota | 12.93 |
| 20 | Maryland | 16.72 | 45 | Virginia | 12.52 |
| 21 | Vermont | 16.70 | 46 | Texas | 12.22 |
| 22 | Oklahoma | 16.63 | 47 | California | 12.03 |
| 23 | Michigan | 16.45 | 48 | Nevada | 11.67 |
| 24 | New Hampshire | 16.41 | 49 | Colorado | 11.24 |
| 25 | Connecticut | 16.39 | 50 | Alaska | 7.63 |

District of Columbia     22.04

*Source: U.S. Department of Health and Human Services, Centers for Disease Control, National Center for Health Statistics,*
    *"Vital Statistics of the United States, 1988" (Vol. II, Part B, issued 1990)*
*By state of residence. Rates calculated by the editors.*

# Deaths by Diseases of the Heart in 1989

## National Total = 733,867 Deaths by Diseases of the Heart*

| RANK | STATE | DEATHS | % | RANK | STATE | DEATHS | % |
|---|---|---|---|---|---|---|---|
| 1 | California | 69,610 | 9.49% | 26 | Iowa | 9,681 | 1.32% |
| 2 | New York | 64,823 | 8.83% | 27 | Mississippi | 9,627 | 1.31% |
| 3 | Florida | 46,304 | 6.31% | 28 | South Carolina | 9,556 | 1.30% |
| 4 | Pennsylvania | 45,086 | 6.14% | 29 | Arizona | 8,768 | 1.19% |
| 5 | Texas | 40,287 | 5.49% | 30 | Arkansas | 8,341 | 1.14% |
| 6 | Illinois | 36,709 | 5.00% | 31 | Kansas | 7,734 | 1.05% |
| 7 | Ohio | 35,357 | 4.82% | 32 | Oregon | 7,588 | 1.03% |
| 8 | Michigan | 28,098 | 3.83% | 33 | West Virginia | 7,332 | 1.00% |
| 9 | New Jersey | 24,317 | 3.31% | 34 | Colorado | 6,102 | 0.83% |
| 10 | North Carolina | 18,980 | 2.59% | 35 | Nebraska | 5,128 | 0.70% |
| 11 | Massachusetts | 17,836 | 2.43% | 36 | Maine | 3,814 | 0.52% |
| 12 | Missouri | 17,704 | 2.41% | 37 | Rhode Island | 3,417 | 0.47% |
| 13 | Indiana | 17,112 | 2.33% | 38 | New Mexico | 3,014 | 0.41% |
| 14 | Georgia | 16,754 | 2.28% | 39 | New Hampshire | 2,818 | 0.38% |
| 15 | Virginia | 15,778 | 2.15% | 40 | Nevada | 2,729 | 0.37% |
| 16 | Tennessee | 15,467 | 2.11% | 41 | Utah | 2,728 | 0.37% |
| 17 | Wisconsin | 14,888 | 2.03% | 42 | South Dakota | 2,401 | 0.33% |
| 18 | Alabama | 13,182 | 1.80% | 43 | Idaho | 2,315 | 0.32% |
| 19 | Louisiana | 12,754 | 1.74% | 44 | Montana | 2,041 | 0.28% |
| 20 | Kentucky | 12,253 | 1.67% | 45 | Hawaii | 1,994 | 0.27% |
| 21 | Maryland | 12,108 | 1.65% | 46 | Delaware | 1,961 | 0.27% |
| 22 | Washington | 11,199 | 1.53% | 47 | North Dakota | 1,874 | 0.26% |
| 23 | Minnesota | 10,879 | 1.48% | 48 | Vermont | 1,475 | 0.20% |
| 24 | Oklahoma | 10,698 | 1.46% | 49 | Wyoming | 968 | 0.13% |
| 25 | Connecticut | 9,829 | 1.34% | 50 | Alaska | 476 | 0.06% |
| | | | | | District of Columbia | 1,973 | 0.27% |

Source: U.S. Department of Health and Human Services, Centers for Disease Control, National Center for Health Statistics,
     "Monthly Vital Statistics Report" (Vol. 40, No. 8(S)2, January 7, 1992)
*By state of residence.

# Death Rate by Diseases of the Heart in 1989

## National Rate = 295.6 Deaths per 100,000 Population*

| RANK | STATE | RATE | RANK | STATE | RATE |
|------|-------|------|------|-------|------|
| 1 | West Virginia | 394.8 | 26 | Delaware | 291.4 |
| 2 | Pennsylvania | 374.5 | 27 | Louisiana | 291.1 |
| 3 | Mississippi | 367.3 | 28 | North Carolina | 288.8 |
| 4 | Florida | 365.4 | 29 | North Dakota | 283.9 |
| 5 | New York | 361.1 | 30 | South Carolina | 272.1 |
| 6 | Arkansas | 346.7 | 31 | Oregon | 269.1 |
| 7 | Missouri | 343.2 | 32 | Georgia | 260.3 |
| 8 | Rhode Island | 342.4 | 33 | Vermont | 260.1 |
| 9 | Iowa | 340.9 | 34 | Virginia | 258.7 |
| 10 | South Dakota | 335.8 | 35 | Maryland | 257.9 |
| 11 | Oklahoma | 331.8 | 36 | New Hampshire | 254.6 |
| 12 | Kentucky | 328.8 | 37 | Montana | 253.2 |
| 13 | Ohio | 324.2 | 38 | Minnesota | 249.9 |
| 14 | Alabama | 320.1 | 39 | Arizona | 246.6 |
| 15 | Nebraska | 318.3 | 40 | Nevada | 245.6 |
| 16 | Illinois | 314.9 | 41 | California | 239.5 |
| 17 | New Jersey | 314.3 | 42 | Texas | 237.1 |
| 18 | Tennessee | 313.1 | 43 | Washington | 235.2 |
| 19 | Maine | 312.1 | 44 | Idaho | 228.3 |
| 20 | Kansas | 307.8 | 45 | Wyoming | 203.8 |
| 21 | Indiana | 306.0 | 46 | New Mexico | 197.3 |
| 22 | Wisconsin | 305.9 | 47 | Colorado | 184.0 |
| 23 | Connecticut | 303.5 | 48 | Hawaii | 179.3 |
| 24 | Michigan | 303.0 | 49 | Utah | 159.8 |
| 25 | Massachusetts | 301.6 | 50 | Alaska | 90.3 |
| | | | | District of Columbia | 326.7 |

Source: U.S. Department of Health and Human Services, Centers for Disease Control, National Center for Health Statistics,
    "Monthly Vital Statistics Report" (Vol. 40, No. 8(S)2, January 7, 1992)
*By state of residence.

# Deaths by Malignant Neoplasms in 1989

## National Total = 496,152 Deaths by Malignant Neoplasms*

| RANK | STATE | DEATHS | % | RANK | STATE | DEATHS | % |
|---|---|---|---|---|---|---|---|
| 1 | California | 48,165 | 9.71% | 26 | South Carolina | 6,495 | 1.31% |
| 2 | New York | 38,093 | 7.68% | 27 | Arizona | 6,458 | 1.30% |
| 3 | Florida | 32,580 | 6.57% | 28 | Iowa | 6,187 | 1.25% |
| 4 | Pennsylvania | 29,211 | 5.89% | 29 | Oregon | 5,821 | 1.17% |
| 5 | Texas | 27,414 | 5.53% | 30 | Arkansas | 5,526 | 1.11% |
| 6 | Illinois | 23,929 | 4.82% | 31 | Mississippi | 5,269 | 1.06% |
| 7 | Ohio | 23,218 | 4.68% | 32 | Kansas | 5,011 | 1.01% |
| 8 | Michigan | 18,337 | 3.70% | 33 | Colorado | 4,705 | 0.95% |
| 9 | New Jersey | 17,990 | 3.63% | 34 | West Virginia | 4,380 | 0.88% |
| 10 | Massachusetts | 13,630 | 2.75% | 35 | Nebraska | 3,308 | 0.67% |
| 11 | North Carolina | 12,976 | 2.62% | 36 | Maine | 2,815 | 0.57% |
| 12 | Missouri | 11,623 | 2.34% | 37 | Rhode Island | 2,449 | 0.49% |
| 13 | Indiana | 11,361 | 2.29% | 38 | New Mexico | 2,249 | 0.45% |
| 14 | Virginia | 11,262 | 2.27% | 39 | New Hampshire | 2,168 | 0.44% |
| 15 | Georgia | 11,150 | 2.25% | 40 | Nevada | 2,080 | 0.42% |
| 16 | Tennessee | 10,151 | 2.05% | 41 | Utah | 1,858 | 0.37% |
| 17 | Wisconsin | 9,815 | 1.98% | 42 | Idaho | 1,672 | 0.34% |
| 18 | Maryland | 9,498 | 1.91% | 43 | Montana | 1,578 | 0.32% |
| 19 | Washington | 8,718 | 1.76% | 44 | Hawaii | 1,574 | 0.32% |
| 20 | Alabama | 8,608 | 1.73% | 45 | South Dakota | 1,444 | 0.29% |
| 21 | Louisiana | 8,508 | 1.71% | 46 | Delaware | 1,429 | 0.29% |
| 22 | Kentucky | 8,257 | 1.66% | 47 | North Dakota | 1,357 | 0.27% |
| 23 | Minnesota | 8,018 | 1.62% | 48 | Vermont | 1,094 | 0.22% |
| 24 | Connecticut | 7,135 | 1.44% | 49 | Wyoming | 754 | 0.15% |
| 25 | Oklahoma | 6,681 | 1.35% | 50 | Alaska | 440 | 0.09% |
|  |  |  |  |  | District of Columbia | 1,703 | 0.34% |

Source: U.S. Department of Health and Human Services, Centers for Disease Control, National Center for Health Statistics,
   "Monthly Vital Statistics Report" (Vol. 40, No. 8(S)2, January 7, 1992)
*By state of residence.  Neoplasms are abnormal tissue, tumors.  Includes many cancers.

# Death Rate by Malignant Neoplasms in 1989

## National Rate = 199.9 Deaths per 100,000 Population*

| RANK | STATE | RATE | RANK | STATE | RATE |
|------|-------|------|------|-------|------|
| 1 | Florida | 257.1 | 26 | Wisconsin | 201.7 |
| 2 | Rhode Island | 245.4 | 27 | Mississippi | 201.0 |
| 3 | Pennsylvania | 242.6 | 28 | Kansas | 199.4 |
| 4 | West Virginia | 235.9 | 29 | Michigan | 197.7 |
| 5 | New Jersey | 232.5 | 30 | North Carolina | 197.5 |
| 6 | Massachusetts | 230.5 | 31 | Montana | 195.8 |
| 7 | Maine | 230.4 | 31 | New Hampshire | 195.8 |
| 8 | Arkansas | 229.7 | 33 | Louisiana | 194.2 |
| 9 | Missouri | 225.3 | 34 | Vermont | 192.9 |
| 10 | Kentucky | 221.5 | 35 | Nevada | 187.2 |
| 11 | Connecticut | 220.3 | 36 | South Carolina | 184.9 |
| 12 | Iowa | 217.9 | 37 | Virginia | 184.7 |
| 13 | Ohio | 212.9 | 38 | Minnesota | 184.2 |
| 14 | Delaware | 212.3 | 39 | Washington | 183.1 |
| 15 | New York | 212.2 | 40 | Arizona | 181.6 |
| 16 | Alabama | 209.0 | 41 | Georgia | 173.2 |
| 17 | Oklahoma | 207.2 | 42 | California | 165.7 |
| 18 | Oregon | 206.4 | 43 | Idaho | 164.9 |
| 19 | North Dakota | 205.6 | 44 | Texas | 161.3 |
| 20 | Tennessee | 205.5 | 45 | Wyoming | 158.7 |
| 21 | Illinois | 205.3 | 46 | New Mexico | 147.2 |
| 21 | Nebraska | 205.3 | 47 | Colorado | 141.8 |
| 23 | Indiana | 203.1 | 48 | Hawaii | 141.5 |
| 24 | Maryland | 202.3 | 49 | Utah | 108.8 |
| 25 | South Dakota | 202.0 | 50 | Alaska | 83.5 |

District of Columbia          282.0

Source: U.S. Department of Health and Human Services, Centers for Disease Control, National Center for Health Statistics,
   "Monthly Vital Statistics Report" (Vol. 40, No. 8(S)2, January 7, 1992)
*By state of residence. Neoplasms are abnormal tissue, tumors. Includes many cancers.

# Deaths by Pneumonia and Influenza in 1988

## National Total = 77,662 Deaths by Pneumonia and Influenza*

| RANK | STATE | DEATHS | % | RANK | STATE | DEATHS | % |
|------|-------|--------|---|------|-------|--------|---|
| 1 | California | 9,344 | 12.03% | 26 | Louisiana | 1,021 | 1.31% |
| 2 | New York | 6,932 | 8.93% | 27 | Arizona | 998 | 1.29% |
| 3 | Texas | 3,999 | 5.15% | 27 | Arkansas | 998 | 1.29% |
| 4 | Pennsylvania | 3,996 | 5.15% | 29 | Colorado | 984 | 1.27% |
| 5 | Illinois | 3,849 | 4.96% | 30 | Kansas | 950 | 1.22% |
| 6 | Florida | 3,366 | 4.33% | 31 | Oregon | 924 | 1.19% |
| 7 | Ohio | 3,248 | 4.18% | 32 | South Carolina | 745 | 0.96% |
| 8 | Michigan | 2,691 | 3.47% | 33 | Nebraska | 732 | 0.94% |
| 9 | Massachusetts | 2,530 | 3.26% | 34 | Mississippi | 710 | 0.91% |
| 10 | New Jersey | 2,404 | 3.10% | 35 | West Virginia | 689 | 0.89% |
| 11 | Missouri | 1,937 | 2.49% | 36 | Utah | 410 | 0.53% |
| 12 | North Carolina | 1,927 | 2.48% | 37 | New Mexico | 366 | 0.47% |
| 13 | Wisconsin | 1,799 | 2.32% | 38 | Maine | 355 | 0.46% |
| 14 | Virginia | 1,745 | 2.25% | 39 | Idaho | 343 | 0.44% |
| 15 | Georgia | 1,653 | 2.13% | 40 | South Dakota | 308 | 0.40% |
| 16 | Tennessee | 1,626 | 2.09% | 41 | New Hampshire | 306 | 0.39% |
| 17 | Indiana | 1,601 | 2.06% | 42 | Nevada | 263 | 0.34% |
| 18 | Minnesota | 1,536 | 1.98% | 43 | Rhode Island | 259 | 0.33% |
| 19 | Kentucky | 1,338 | 1.72% | 44 | Montana | 249 | 0.32% |
| 20 | Washington | 1,316 | 1.69% | 45 | North Dakota | 210 | 0.27% |
| 21 | Maryland | 1,291 | 1.66% | 46 | Hawaii | 197 | 0.25% |
| 22 | Iowa | 1,259 | 1.62% | 47 | Vermont | 186 | 0.24% |
| 23 | Alabama | 1,181 | 1.52% | 48 | Delaware | 151 | 0.19% |
| 24 | Oklahoma | 1,167 | 1.50% | 49 | Wyoming | 149 | 0.19% |
| 25 | Connecticut | 1,102 | 1.42% | 50 | Alaska | 46 | 0.06% |
|  |  |  |  |  | District of Columbia | 276 | 0.36% |

Source: U.S. Department of Health and Human Services, Centers for Disease Control, National Center for Health Statistics,
*"Vital Statistics of the United States, 1988"* (Vol II, Part B, issued 1990)
*By state of residence.

# Death Rate by Pneumonia and Influenza in 1988

## National Rate = 31.59 Deaths per 100,000 Population*

| RANK | STATE | RATE | RANK | STATE | RATE |
|------|-------|------|------|-------|------|
| 1 | Nebraska | 45.69 | 26 | Ohio | 29.92 |
| 2 | Iowa | 44.42 | 27 | Colorado | 29.81 |
| 3 | South Dakota | 43.20 | 28 | North Carolina | 29.70 |
| 4 | Massachusetts | 42.96 | 29 | Maine | 29.46 |
| 5 | Arkansas | 41.67 | 30 | Michigan | 29.12 |
| 6 | New York | 38.71 | 31 | Virginia | 29.01 |
| 7 | Kansas | 38.08 | 32 | Indiana | 28.82 |
| 8 | Missouri | 37.68 | 33 | Alabama | 28.79 |
| 9 | Wisconsin | 37.05 | 34 | Arizona | 28.60 |
| 10 | West Virginia | 36.73 | 35 | Washington | 28.31 |
| 11 | Oklahoma | 36.00 | 36 | New Hampshire | 28.20 |
| 12 | Kentucky | 35.90 | 37 | Maryland | 27.93 |
| 13 | Minnesota | 35.66 | 38 | Florida | 27.29 |
| 14 | Idaho | 34.20 | 39 | Mississippi | 27.10 |
| 15 | Connecticut | 34.09 | 40 | Rhode Island | 26.08 |
| 16 | Oregon | 33.39 | 41 | Georgia | 26.06 |
| 17 | Vermont | 33.39 | 42 | Nevada | 24.95 |
| 18 | Pennsylvania | 33.30 | 43 | New Mexico | 24.29 |
| 19 | Tennessee | 33.22 | 44 | Utah | 24.26 |
| 20 | Illinois | 33.14 | 45 | Texas | 23.75 |
| 21 | California | 33.00 | 46 | Louisiana | 23.16 |
| 22 | North Dakota | 31.48 | 47 | Delaware | 22.88 |
| 23 | New Jersey | 31.14 | 48 | South Carolina | 21.47 |
| 24 | Wyoming | 31.11 | 49 | Hawaii | 17.94 |
| 25 | Montana | 30.93 | 50 | Alaska | 8.78 |

District of Columbia      44.73

Source: U.S. Department of Health and Human Services, Centers for Disease Control, National Center for Health Statistics,
    "Vital Statistics of the United States, 1988" (Vol. II, Part B, issued 1990)
*By state of residence.  Rates calculated by the editors.

# Deaths by Complications of Pregnancy and Childbirth in 1988

## National Total = 330 Deaths by Complications of Pregnancy and Childbirth*

| RANK | STATE | DEATHS | % | RANK | STATE | DEATHS | % |
|---|---|---|---|---|---|---|---|
| 1 | California | 50 | 15.15% | 24 | Minnesota | 4 | 1.21% |
| 2 | New York | 35 | 10.61% | 24 | Missouri | 4 | 1.21% |
| 3 | Texas | 24 | 7.27% | 24 | South Carolina | 4 | 1.21% |
| 4 | Illinois | 14 | 4.24% | 29 | Arizona | 3 | 0.91% |
| 5 | Florida | 12 | 3.64% | 29 | Maine | 3 | 0.91% |
| 5 | North Carolina | 12 | 3.64% | 29 | Massachusetts | 3 | 0.91% |
| 7 | Michigan | 11 | 3.33% | 32 | Connecticut | 2 | 0.61% |
| 8 | Louisiana | 10 | 3.03% | 32 | Hawaii | 2 | 0.61% |
| 8 | New Jersey | 10 | 3.03% | 32 | Nebraska | 2 | 0.61% |
| 8 | Virginia | 10 | 3.03% | 32 | New Mexico | 2 | 0.61% |
| 11 | Georgia | 9 | 2.73% | 32 | Oregon | 2 | 0.61% |
| 11 | Tennessee | 9 | 2.73% | 32 | Utah | 2 | 0.61% |
| 13 | Alabama | 8 | 2.42% | 38 | Delaware | 1 | 0.30% |
| 13 | Pennsylvania | 8 | 2.42% | 38 | Idaho | 1 | 0.30% |
| 15 | Indiana | 7 | 2.12% | 38 | Montana | 1 | 0.30% |
| 15 | Mississippi | 7 | 2.12% | 38 | Nevada | 1 | 0.30% |
| 15 | Ohio | 7 | 2.12% | 38 | New Hampshire | 1 | 0.30% |
| 18 | Arkansas | 6 | 1.82% | 38 | Rhode Island | 1 | 0.30% |
| 18 | Oklahoma | 6 | 1.82% | 38 | South Dakota | 1 | 0.30% |
| 18 | Wisconsin | 6 | 1.82% | 38 | Vermont | 1 | 0.30% |
| 21 | Colorado | 5 | 1.52% | 38 | Washington | 1 | 0.30% |
| 21 | Iowa | 5 | 1.52% | 38 | West Virginia | 1 | 0.30% |
| 21 | Kentucky | 5 | 1.52% | 38 | Wyoming | 1 | 0.30% |
| 24 | Kansas | 4 | 1.21% | 49 | Alaska | 0 | 0.00% |
| 24 | Maryland | 4 | 1.21% | 49 | North Dakota | 0 | 0.00% |
| | | | | | District of Columbia | 2 | 0.61% |

Source: U.S. Department of Health and Human Services, Centers for Disease Control, National Center for Health Statistics,
   "Vital Statistics of the United States, 1988" (Vol II, Part B, issued 1990)
*By state of residence.

# Death Rate by Complications of Pregnancy and Childbirth in 1988

## National Rate = .134 Deaths per 100,000 Population*

| RANK | STATE | RATE | RANK | STATE | RATE |
|------|-------|------|------|-------|------|
| 1 | Mississippi | 0.267 | 26 | Nebraska | 0.125 |
| 2 | Arkansas | 0.251 | 27 | Montana | 0.124 |
| 3 | Maine | 0.249 | 28 | Wisconsin | 0.124 |
| 4 | Louisiana | 0.227 | 29 | Illinois | 0.121 |
| 5 | Wyoming | 0.209 | 30 | Michigan | 0.119 |
| 6 | New York | 0.195 | 31 | Utah | 0.118 |
| 7 | Alabama | 0.195 | 32 | South Carolina | 0.115 |
| 8 | Oklahoma | 0.185 | 33 | Rhode Island | 0.101 |
| 9 | North Carolina | 0.185 | 34 | Idaho | 0.100 |
| 10 | Tennessee | 0.184 | 35 | Florida | 0.097 |
| 11 | Hawaii | 0.182 | 36 | Nevada | 0.095 |
| 12 | Vermont | 0.180 | 37 | Minnesota | 0.093 |
| 13 | California | 0.177 | 38 | New Hampshire | 0.092 |
| 14 | Iowa | 0.176 | 39 | Maryland | 0.087 |
| 15 | Virginia | 0.166 | 40 | Arizona | 0.086 |
| 16 | Kansas | 0.160 | 41 | Missouri | 0.078 |
| 17 | Delaware | 0.152 | 42 | Oregon | 0.072 |
| 18 | Colorado | 0.151 | 43 | Pennsylvania | 0.067 |
| 19 | Texas | 0.143 | 44 | Ohio | 0.064 |
| 20 | Georgia | 0.142 | 45 | Connecticut | 0.062 |
| 21 | South Dakota | 0.140 | 46 | West Virginia | 0.053 |
| 22 | Kentucky | 0.134 | 47 | Massachusetts | 0.051 |
| 23 | New Mexico | 0.133 | 48 | Washington | 0.022 |
| 24 | New Jersey | 0.130 | 49 | Alaska | 0.000 |
| 25 | Indiana | 0.126 | 49 | North Dakota | 0.000 |
|  |  |  |  | District of Columbia | 0.324 |

Source: U.S. Department of Health and Human Services, Centers for Disease Control, National Center for Health Statistics,
     "Vital Statistics of the United States, 1988" (Vol. II, Part B, issued 1990)
*By state of residence. Rates calculated by the editors.

# Deaths by Suicide in 1989

## National Total = 30,232 Deaths by Suicide*

| RANK | STATE | SUICIDES | % | RANK | STATE | SUICIDES | % |
|---|---|---|---|---|---|---|---|
| 1 | California | 3,704 | 12.25% | 26 | Oregon | 470 | 1.55% |
| 2 | Texas | 2,126 | 7.03% | 27 | South Carolina | 424 | 1.40% |
| 3 | Florida | 2,076 | 6.87% | 28 | Oklahoma | 416 | 1.38% |
| 4 | New York | 1,519 | 5.02% | 29 | Iowa | 315 | 1.04% |
| 5 | Pennsylvania | 1,451 | 4.80% | 30 | Mississippi | 314 | 1.04% |
| 6 | Ohio | 1,235 | 4.09% | 31 | Connecticut | 303 | 1.00% |
| 7 | Illinois | 1,171 | 3.87% | 32 | New Mexico | 298 | 0.99% |
| 8 | Michigan | 1,045 | 3.46% | 33 | Kansas | 285 | 0.94% |
| 9 | North Carolina | 871 | 2.88% | 34 | Nevada | 257 | 0.85% |
| 10 | Georgia | 855 | 2.83% | 35 | Arkansas | 246 | 0.81% |
| 11 | Virginia | 814 | 2.69% | 36 | West Virginia | 231 | 0.76% |
| 12 | Indiana | 678 | 2.24% | 37 | Utah | 211 | 0.70% |
| 13 | Arizona | 671 | 2.22% | 38 | Nebraska | 174 | 0.58% |
| 14 | Missouri | 665 | 2.20% | 39 | Maine | 170 | 0.56% |
| 15 | Tennessee | 652 | 2.16% | 40 | Montana | 161 | 0.53% |
| 16 | Washington | 648 | 2.14% | 41 | Idaho | 160 | 0.53% |
| 17 | Wisconsin | 597 | 1.97% | 42 | New Hampshire | 126 | 0.42% |
| 18 | Colorado | 549 | 1.82% | 43 | Hawaii | 109 | 0.36% |
| 19 | Louisiana | 542 | 1.79% | 44 | Rhode Island | 100 | 0.33% |
| 20 | Maryland | 525 | 1.74% | 45 | Delaware | 95 | 0.31% |
| 21 | Minnesota | 515 | 1.70% | 46 | Vermont | 94 | 0.31% |
| 22 | Alabama | 506 | 1.67% | 47 | South Dakota | 90 | 0.30% |
| 23 | New Jersey | 503 | 1.66% | 48 | Alaska | 89 | 0.29% |
| 24 | Massachusetts | 491 | 1.62% | 49 | Wyoming | 82 | 0.27% |
| 25 | Kentucky | 482 | 1.59% | 50 | North Dakota | 70 | 0.23% |
| | | | | | District of Columbia | 51 | 0.17% |

Source: U.S. Department of Health and Human Services, Centers for Disease Control, National Center for Health Statistics,
"Monthly Vital Statistics Report" (Vol. 40, No. 8(S)2, January 7, 1992)
*By state of residence.

# Death Rate by Suicide in 1989

## National Rate = 12.2 Deaths by Suicide per 100,000 Population*

| RANK | STATE | RATE | RANK | STATE | RATE |
|------|-------|------|------|-------|------|
| 1 | Nevada | 23.1 | 25 | Utah | 12.4 |
| 2 | Montana | 20.0 | 25 | West Virginia | 12.4 |
| 3 | New Mexico | 19.5 | 28 | Alabama | 12.3 |
| 4 | Arizona | 18.9 | 28 | Wisconsin | 12.3 |
| 5 | Wyoming | 17.3 | 30 | Indiana | 12.1 |
| 6 | Alaska | 16.9 | 30 | Pennsylvania | 12.1 |
| 7 | Oregon | 16.7 | 30 | South Carolina | 12.1 |
| 8 | Colorado | 16.6 | 33 | Mississippi | 12.0 |
| 8 | Vermont | 16.6 | 34 | Minnesota | 11.8 |
| 10 | Florida | 16.4 | 35 | New Hampshire | 11.4 |
| 11 | Idaho | 15.8 | 36 | Kansas | 11.3 |
| 12 | Delaware | 14.1 | 36 | Michigan | 11.3 |
| 13 | Maine | 13.9 | 36 | Ohio | 11.3 |
| 14 | Washington | 13.6 | 39 | Maryland | 11.2 |
| 15 | Georgia | 13.3 | 40 | Iowa | 11.1 |
| 15 | North Carolina | 13.3 | 41 | Nebraska | 10.8 |
| 15 | Virginia | 13.3 | 42 | North Dakota | 10.6 |
| 18 | Tennessee | 13.2 | 43 | Arkansas | 10.2 |
| 19 | Kentucky | 12.9 | 44 | Illinois | 10.0 |
| 19 | Missouri | 12.9 | 44 | Rhode Island | 10.0 |
| 19 | Oklahoma | 12.9 | 46 | Hawaii | 9.8 |
| 22 | California | 12.7 | 47 | Connecticut | 9.4 |
| 23 | South Dakota | 12.6 | 48 | New York | 8.5 |
| 24 | Texas | 12.5 | 49 | Massachusetts | 8.3 |
| 25 | Louisiana | 12.4 | 50 | New Jersey | 6.5 |
| | | | | District of Columbia | 8.4 |

Source: U.S. Department of Health and Human Services, Centers for Disease Control, National Center for Health Statistics,
"Monthly Vital Statistics Report" (Vol. 40, No. 8(S)2, January 7, 1992)
*By state of residence.

125

# Deaths by Syphilis in 1988

## National Total = 85 Deaths by Syphilis*

| RANK | STATE | DEATHS | % | RANK | STATE | DEATHS | % |
|------|-------|--------|------|------|-------|--------|------|
| 1 | Florida | 11 | 12.94% | 19 | Washington | 1 | 1.18% |
| 2 | California | 10 | 11.76% | 27 | Alabama | 0 | 0.00% |
| 3 | New York | 9 | 10.59% | 27 | Alaska | 0 | 0.00% |
| 4 | Texas | 8 | 9.41% | 27 | Arkansas | 0 | 0.00% |
| 5 | North Carolina | 4 | 4.71% | 27 | Delaware | 0 | 0.00% |
| 6 | Indiana | 3 | 3.53% | 27 | Hawaii | 0 | 0.00% |
| 6 | Louisiana | 3 | 3.53% | 27 | Idaho | 0 | 0.00% |
| 6 | Missouri | 3 | 3.53% | 27 | Kansas | 0 | 0.00% |
| 6 | Ohio | 3 | 3.53% | 27 | Kentucky | 0 | 0.00% |
| 6 | Pennsylvania | 3 | 3.53% | 27 | Maine | 0 | 0.00% |
| 6 | Virginia | 3 | 3.53% | 27 | Minnesota | 0 | 0.00% |
| 12 | Arizona | 2 | 2.35% | 27 | Mississippi | 0 | 0.00% |
| 12 | Colorado | 2 | 2.35% | 27 | Montana | 0 | 0.00% |
| 12 | Connecticut | 2 | 2.35% | 27 | Nebraska | 0 | 0.00% |
| 12 | Georgia | 2 | 2.35% | 27 | Nevada | 0 | 0.00% |
| 12 | Massachusetts | 2 | 2.35% | 27 | New Hampshire | 0 | 0.00% |
| 12 | Michigan | 2 | 2.35% | 27 | New Mexico | 0 | 0.00% |
| 12 | Tennessee | 2 | 2.35% | 27 | North Dakota | 0 | 0.00% |
| 19 | Illinois | 1 | 1.18% | 27 | South Carolina | 0 | 0.00% |
| 19 | Iowa | 1 | 1.18% | 27 | South Dakota | 0 | 0.00% |
| 19 | Maryland | 1 | 1.18% | 27 | Utah | 0 | 0.00% |
| 19 | New Jersey | 1 | 1.18% | 27 | Vermont | 0 | 0.00% |
| 19 | Oklahoma | 1 | 1.18% | 27 | West Virginia | 0 | 0.00% |
| 19 | Oregon | 1 | 1.18% | 27 | Wisconsin | 0 | 0.00% |
| 19 | Rhode Island | 1 | 1.18% | 27 | Wyoming | 0 | 0.00% |
| | | | | | District of Columbia | 3 | 3.53% |

Source: U.S. Department of Health and Human Services, Centers for Disease Control, National Center for Health Statistics,
"Vital Statistics of the United States, 1988" (Vol II, Part B, issued 1990)
*By state of residence.

# Death Rate by Syphilis in 1988

## National Rate = .035 Deaths per 100,000 Population*

| RANK | STATE | RATE | RANK | STATE | RATE |
|------|-------|------|------|-------|------|
| 1 | Rhode Island | 0.101 | 26 | Illinois | 0.009 |
| 2 | Florida | 0.089 | 27 | Alabama | 0.000 |
| 3 | Louisiana | 0.068 | 27 | Alaska | 0.000 |
| 4 | Connecticut | 0.062 | 27 | Arkansas | 0.000 |
| 5 | North Carolina | 0.062 | 27 | Delaware | 0.000 |
| 6 | Colorado | 0.061 | 27 | Hawaii | 0.000 |
| 7 | Missouri | 0.058 | 27 | Idaho | 0.000 |
| 8 | Arizona | 0.057 | 27 | Kansas | 0.000 |
| 9 | Indiana | 0.054 | 27 | Kentucky | 0.000 |
| 10 | New York | 0.050 | 27 | Maine | 0.000 |
| 11 | Virginia | 0.050 | 27 | Minnesota | 0.000 |
| 12 | Texas | 0.048 | 27 | Mississippi | 0.000 |
| 13 | Tennessee | 0.041 | 27 | Montana | 0.000 |
| 14 | Oregon | 0.036 | 27 | Nebraska | 0.000 |
| 15 | California | 0.035 | 27 | Nevada | 0.000 |
| 16 | Iowa | 0.035 | 27 | New Hampshire | 0.000 |
| 17 | Massachusetts | 0.034 | 27 | New Mexico | 0.000 |
| 18 | Georgia | 0.032 | 27 | North Dakota | 0.000 |
| 19 | Oklahoma | 0.031 | 27 | South Carolina | 0.000 |
| 20 | Ohio | 0.028 | 27 | South Dakota | 0.000 |
| 21 | Pennsylvania | 0.025 | 27 | Utah | 0.000 |
| 22 | Michigan | 0.022 | 27 | Vermont | 0.000 |
| 23 | Maryland | 0.022 | 27 | West Virginia | 0.000 |
| 24 | Washington | 0.022 | 27 | Wisconsin | 0.000 |
| 25 | New Jersey | 0.013 | 27 | Wyoming | 0.000 |
| | | | | District of Columbia | 0.486 |

Source: U.S. Department of Health and Human Services, Centers for Disease Control, National Center for Health Statistics,
   "Vital Statistics of the United States, 1988" (Vol. II, Part B, issued 1990)
*By state of residence. Rates calculated by the editors.

# Deaths by Tuberculosis in 1988

## National Total = 1,921 Deaths by Tuberculosis*

| RANK | STATE | DEATHS | % | RANK | STATE | DEATHS | % |
|---|---|---|---|---|---|---|---|
| 1 | New York | 290 | 15.10% | 26 | Indiana | 22 | 1.15% |
| 2 | California | 232 | 12.08% | 26 | Washington | 22 | 1.15% |
| 3 | Florida | 145 | 7.55% | 28 | Wisconsin | 17 | 0.88% |
| 4 | Texas | 127 | 6.61% | 29 | Hawaii | 16 | 0.83% |
| 5 | Illinois | 78 | 4.06% | 30 | Oregon | 14 | 0.73% |
| 6 | North Carolina | 73 | 3.80% | 31 | Colorado | 13 | 0.68% |
| 7 | Pennsylvania | 71 | 3.70% | 31 | Connecticut | 13 | 0.68% |
| 8 | New Jersey | 70 | 3.64% | 31 | Iowa | 13 | 0.68% |
| 9 | Georgia | 69 | 3.59% | 34 | Nevada | 10 | 0.52% |
| 10 | Tennessee | 60 | 3.12% | 35 | Minnesota | 7 | 0.36% |
| 11 | Louisiana | 48 | 2.50% | 35 | New Mexico | 7 | 0.36% |
| 12 | Ohio | 47 | 2.45% | 37 | Kansas | 6 | 0.31% |
| 13 | Missouri | 43 | 2.24% | 38 | Delaware | 5 | 0.26% |
| 14 | Michigan | 42 | 2.19% | 38 | Maine | 5 | 0.26% |
| 15 | Alabama | 41 | 2.13% | 40 | Utah | 4 | 0.21% |
| 16 | Virginia | 37 | 1.93% | 41 | South Dakota | 3 | 0.16% |
| 17 | Kentucky | 36 | 1.87% | 42 | Alaska | 2 | 0.10% |
| 18 | Mississippi | 30 | 1.56% | 42 | Montana | 2 | 0.10% |
| 19 | Maryland | 29 | 1.51% | 42 | Nebraska | 2 | 0.10% |
| 20 | Arkansas | 28 | 1.46% | 42 | Rhode Island | 2 | 0.10% |
| 20 | Oklahoma | 28 | 1.46% | 46 | Idaho | 1 | 0.05% |
| 22 | Massachusetts | 26 | 1.35% | 46 | North Dakota | 1 | 0.05% |
| 23 | Arizona | 24 | 1.25% | 46 | Vermont | 1 | 0.05% |
| 24 | South Carolina | 23 | 1.20% | 49 | New Hampshire | 0 | 0.00% |
| 24 | West Virginia | 23 | 1.20% | 49 | Wyoming | 0 | 0.00% |
| | | | | | District of Columbia | 13 | 0.68% |

Source: U.S. Department of Health and Human Services, Centers for Disease Control, National Center for Health Statistics,
    "Vital Statistics of the United States, 1988" (Vol II, Part B, issued 1990)
*By state of residence.

# Death Rate by Tuberculosis in 1988

## National Rate = .78 Deaths per 100,000 Population*

| RANK | STATE | RATE | RANK | STATE | RATE |
|------|-------|------|------|-------|------|
| 1 | New York | 1.62 | 26 | Oregon | 0.51 |
| 2 | Hawaii | 1.46 | 27 | Washington | 0.47 |
| 3 | West Virginia | 1.23 | 28 | New Mexico | 0.46 |
| 4 | Tennessee | 1.23 | 29 | Iowa | 0.46 |
| 5 | Florida | 1.18 | 30 | Michigan | 0.45 |
| 6 | Arkansas | 1.17 | 31 | Massachusetts | 0.44 |
| 7 | Mississippi | 1.15 | 32 | Ohio | 0.43 |
| 8 | North Carolina | 1.12 | 33 | South Dakota | 0.42 |
| 9 | Louisiana | 1.09 | 34 | Maine | 0.41 |
| 10 | Georgia | 1.09 | 35 | Connecticut | 0.40 |
| 11 | Alabama | 1.00 | 36 | Indiana | 0.40 |
| 12 | Kentucky | 0.97 | 37 | Colorado | 0.39 |
| 13 | Nevada | 0.95 | 38 | Alaska | 0.38 |
| 14 | New Jersey | 0.91 | 39 | Wisconsin | 0.35 |
| 15 | Oklahoma | 0.86 | 40 | Montana | 0.25 |
| 16 | Missouri | 0.84 | 41 | Kansas | 0.24 |
| 17 | California | 0.82 | 42 | Utah | 0.24 |
| 18 | Delaware | 0.76 | 43 | Rhode Island | 0.20 |
| 19 | Texas | 0.75 | 44 | Vermont | 0.18 |
| 20 | Arizona | 0.69 | 45 | Minnesota | 0.16 |
| 21 | Illinois | 0.67 | 46 | North Dakota | 0.15 |
| 22 | South Carolina | 0.66 | 47 | Nebraska | 0.12 |
| 23 | Maryland | 0.63 | 48 | Idaho | 0.10 |
| 24 | Virginia | 0.62 | 49 | New Hampshire | 0.00 |
| 25 | Pennsylvania | 0.59 | 49 | Wyoming | 0.00 |

District of Columbia     2.11

Source: U.S. Department of Health and Human Services, Centers for Disease Control, National Center for Health Statistics,
   "Vital Statistics of the United States, 1988" (Vol. II, Part B, issued 1990) (Rates calculated by editors.)
*By state of residence. Rates calculated by the editors.

# III. FACILITIES

# III. FACILITIES (continued)

# Hospitals in 1990

## National Total = 6,649 Hospitals*

| RANK | STATE | HOSPITALS | % | RANK | STATE | HOSPITALS | % |
|---|---|---|---|---|---|---|---|
| 1 | California | 548 | 8.24% | 26 | Washington | 110 | 1.65% |
| 2 | Texas | 537 | 8.08% | 27 | Nebraska | 102 | 1.53% |
| 3 | New York | 305 | 4.59% | 28 | Arkansas | 96 | 1.44% |
| 4 | Pennsylvania | 302 | 4.54% | 29 | Arizona | 91 | 1.37% |
| 5 | Florida | 288 | 4.33% | 30 | South Carolina | 89 | 1.34% |
| 6 | Illinois | 247 | 3.71% | 31 | Colorado | 86 | 1.29% |
| 7 | Ohio | 224 | 3.37% | 32 | Maryland | 82 | 1.23% |
| 8 | Michigan | 205 | 3.08% | 33 | Oregon | 77 | 1.16% |
| 9 | Georgia | 203 | 3.05% | 34 | West Virginia | 68 | 1.02% |
| 10 | Louisiana | 173 | 2.60% | 35 | South Dakota | 66 | 0.99% |
| 11 | Minnesota | 167 | 2.51% | 36 | Connecticut | 63 | 0.95% |
| 12 | Kansas | 160 | 2.41% | 37 | Montana | 62 | 0.93% |
| 12 | Missouri | 160 | 2.41% | 38 | New Mexico | 60 | 0.90% |
| 14 | Massachusetts | 157 | 2.36% | 39 | North Dakota | 57 | 0.86% |
| 15 | Tennessee | 156 | 2.35% | 40 | Utah | 52 | 0.78% |
| 16 | North Carolina | 155 | 2.33% | 41 | Idaho | 50 | 0.75% |
| 17 | Wisconsin | 148 | 2.23% | 42 | Maine | 44 | 0.66% |
| 18 | Alabama | 138 | 2.08% | 43 | New Hampshire | 40 | 0.60% |
| 19 | Oklahoma | 137 | 2.06% | 44 | Wyoming | 32 | 0.48% |
| 20 | Indiana | 135 | 2.03% | 45 | Nevada | 31 | 0.47% |
| 20 | Virginia | 135 | 2.03% | 46 | Alaska | 27 | 0.41% |
| 22 | Iowa | 134 | 2.02% | 47 | Hawaii | 26 | 0.39% |
| 23 | Kentucky | 123 | 1.85% | 48 | Rhode Island | 19 | 0.29% |
| 24 | New Jersey | 119 | 1.79% | 49 | Vermont | 18 | 0.27% |
| 25 | Mississippi | 115 | 1.73% | 50 | Delaware | 13 | 0.20% |
| | | | | | District of Columbia | 17 | 0.26% |

Source: American Hospital Association

"Hospital Statistics: A Comprehensive Summary of U.S. Hospitals 1991-1992" (Copyright, reprinted with permission)

*Federal and nonfederal hospitals.

# Federal Hospitals in 1990

## National Total = 337 Federal Hospitals

| RANK | STATE | HOSPITALS | % | RANK | STATE | HOSPITALS | % |
|---|---|---|---|---|---|---|---|
| 1 | California | 29 | 8.61% | 24 | Montana | 5 | 1.48% |
| 2 | Texas | 21 | 6.23% | 24 | Nebraska | 5 | 1.48% |
| 3 | Arizona | 16 | 4.75% | 24 | North Dakota | 5 | 1.48% |
| 4 | New York | 15 | 4.45% | 24 | Ohio | 5 | 1.48% |
| 5 | Florida | 13 | 3.86% | 24 | Tennessee | 5 | 1.48% |
| 6 | New Mexico | 12 | 3.56% | 31 | Arkansas | 4 | 1.19% |
| 7 | Oklahoma | 11 | 3.26% | 31 | Indiana | 4 | 1.19% |
| 7 | Pennsylvania | 11 | 3.26% | 31 | Kentucky | 4 | 1.19% |
| 9 | South Dakota | 10 | 2.97% | 31 | Minnesota | 4 | 1.19% |
| 10 | Georgia | 9 | 2.67% | 31 | Nevada | 4 | 1.19% |
| 10 | Illinois | 9 | 2.67% | 31 | New Jersey | 4 | 1.19% |
| 10 | North Carolina | 9 | 2.67% | 31 | West Virginia | 4 | 1.19% |
| 13 | Alabama | 8 | 2.37% | 38 | Connecticut | 3 | 0.89% |
| 13 | Alaska | 8 | 2.37% | 38 | Iowa | 3 | 0.89% |
| 13 | Maryland | 8 | 2.37% | 38 | Wisconsin | 3 | 0.89% |
| 13 | Virginia | 8 | 2.37% | 38 | Wyoming | 3 | 0.89% |
| 13 | Washington | 8 | 2.37% | 42 | Delaware | 2 | 0.59% |
| 18 | Kansas | 7 | 2.08% | 42 | Idaho | 2 | 0.59% |
| 18 | Michigan | 7 | 2.08% | 42 | Maine | 2 | 0.59% |
| 18 | Missouri | 7 | 2.08% | 42 | Oregon | 2 | 0.59% |
| 18 | South Carolina | 7 | 2.08% | 42 | Rhode Island | 2 | 0.59% |
| 22 | Colorado | 6 | 1.78% | 42 | Utah | 2 | 0.59% |
| 22 | Louisiana | 6 | 1.78% | 48 | Hawaii | 1 | 0.30% |
| 24 | Massachusetts | 5 | 1.48% | 48 | New Hampshire | 1 | 0.30% |
| 24 | Mississippi | 5 | 1.48% | 48 | Vermont | 1 | 0.30% |
| | | | | | District of Columbia | 2 | 0.59% |

Source: American Hospital Association
"Hospital Statistics: A Comprehensive Summary of U.S. Hospitals 1991–1992" (Copyright, reprinted with permission)

# Nonfederal Hospitals in 1990

## National Total = 6,312 Nonfederal Hospitals

| RANK | STATE | HOSPITALS | % | RANK | STATE | HOSPITALS | % |
|---|---|---|---|---|---|---|---|
| 1 | California | 519 | 8.22% | 26 | Washington | 102 | 1.62% |
| 2 | Texas | 516 | 8.17% | 27 | Nebraska | 97 | 1.54% |
| 3 | Pennsylvania | 291 | 4.61% | 28 | Arkansas | 92 | 1.46% |
| 4 | New York | 290 | 4.59% | 29 | South Carolina | 82 | 1.30% |
| 5 | Florida | 275 | 4.36% | 30 | Colorado | 80 | 1.27% |
| 6 | Illinois | 238 | 3.77% | 31 | Arizona | 75 | 1.19% |
| 7 | Ohio | 219 | 3.47% | 31 | Oregon | 75 | 1.19% |
| 8 | Michigan | 198 | 3.14% | 33 | Maryland | 74 | 1.17% |
| 9 | Georgia | 194 | 3.07% | 34 | West Virginia | 64 | 1.01% |
| 10 | Louisiana | 167 | 2.65% | 35 | Connecticut | 60 | 0.95% |
| 11 | Minnesota | 163 | 2.58% | 36 | Montana | 57 | 0.90% |
| 12 | Kansas | 153 | 2.42% | 37 | South Dakota | 56 | 0.89% |
| 12 | Missouri | 153 | 2.42% | 38 | North Dakota | 52 | 0.82% |
| 14 | Massachusetts | 152 | 2.41% | 39 | Utah | 50 | 0.79% |
| 15 | Tennessee | 151 | 2.39% | 40 | Idaho | 48 | 0.76% |
| 16 | North Carolina | 146 | 2.31% | 40 | New Mexico | 48 | 0.76% |
| 17 | Wisconsin | 145 | 2.30% | 42 | Maine | 42 | 0.67% |
| 18 | Indiana | 131 | 2.08% | 43 | New Hampshire | 39 | 0.62% |
| 18 | Iowa | 131 | 2.08% | 44 | Wyoming | 29 | 0.46% |
| 20 | Alabama | 130 | 2.06% | 45 | Nevada | 27 | 0.43% |
| 21 | Virginia | 127 | 2.01% | 46 | Hawaii | 25 | 0.40% |
| 22 | Oklahoma | 126 | 2.00% | 47 | Alaska | 19 | 0.30% |
| 23 | Kentucky | 119 | 1.89% | 48 | Rhode Island | 17 | 0.27% |
| 24 | New Jersey | 115 | 1.82% | 48 | Vermont | 17 | 0.27% |
| 25 | Mississippi | 110 | 1.74% | 50 | Delaware | 11 | 0.17% |
| | | | | | District of Columbia | 15 | 0.24% |

Source: American Hospital Association

"Hospital Statistics: A Comprehensive Summary of U.S. Hospitals 1991-1992" (Copyright, reprinted with permission)

# Psychiatric Hospitals in 1990

## National Total = 774 Psychiatric Hospitals*

| RANK | STATE | HOSPITALS | % | RANK | STATE | HOSPITALS | % |
|---|---|---|---|---|---|---|---|
| 1 | Texas | 75 | 9.69% | 23 | New Jersey | 11 | 1.42% |
| 2 | California | 64 | 8.27% | 23 | New Mexico | 11 | 1.42% |
| 3 | New York | 47 | 6.07% | 28 | Colorado | 10 | 1.29% |
| 4 | Pennsylvania | 45 | 5.81% | 28 | New Hampshire | 10 | 1.29% |
| 5 | Florida | 44 | 5.68% | 28 | South Carolina | 10 | 1.29% |
| 6 | Georgia | 27 | 3.49% | 31 | Iowa | 8 | 1.03% |
| 7 | Louisiana | 26 | 3.36% | 31 | Utah | 8 | 1.03% |
| 7 | Ohio | 26 | 3.36% | 31 | Washington | 8 | 1.03% |
| 9 | Illinois | 24 | 3.10% | 34 | Arkansas | 6 | 0.78% |
| 9 | Massachusetts | 24 | 3.10% | 34 | Mississippi | 6 | 0.78% |
| 9 | Virginia | 24 | 3.10% | 34 | Nevada | 6 | 0.78% |
| 12 | Michigan | 21 | 2.71% | 37 | Idaho | 5 | 0.65% |
| 12 | North Carolina | 21 | 2.71% | 37 | Oregon | 5 | 0.65% |
| 14 | Connecticut | 17 | 2.20% | 37 | West Virginia | 5 | 0.65% |
| 14 | Indiana | 17 | 2.20% | 40 | Nebraska | 4 | 0.52% |
| 14 | Wisconsin | 17 | 2.20% | 41 | Alaska | 3 | 0.39% |
| 17 | Maryland | 16 | 2.07% | 41 | Delaware | 3 | 0.39% |
| 18 | Missouri | 15 | 1.94% | 41 | Maine | 3 | 0.39% |
| 19 | Arizona | 14 | 1.81% | 41 | Rhode Island | 3 | 0.39% |
| 19 | Tennessee | 14 | 1.81% | 41 | Wyoming | 3 | 0.39% |
| 21 | Kansas | 13 | 1.68% | 46 | North Dakota | 2 | 0.26% |
| 21 | Oklahoma | 13 | 1.68% | 46 | Vermont | 2 | 0.26% |
| 23 | Alabama | 11 | 1.42% | 48 | Hawaii | 1 | 0.13% |
| 23 | Kentucky | 11 | 1.42% | 48 | Montana | 1 | 0.13% |
| 23 | Minnesota | 11 | 1.42% | 48 | South Dakota | 1 | 0.13% |
| | | | | | District of Columbia | 2 | 0.26% |

Source: American Hospital Association
   "Hospital Statistics: A Comprehensive Summary of U.S. Hospitals 1991-1992" (Copyright, reprinted with permission)
*Federal and nonfederal psychiatric hospitals.

# Community Hospitals in 1990

## National Total = 5,384 Community Hospitals*

| RANK | STATE | HOSPITALS | % | RANK | STATE | HOSPITALS | % |
|---|---|---|---|---|---|---|---|
| 1 | California | 445 | 8.27% | 26 | Washington | 91 | 1.69% |
| 2 | Texas | 428 | 7.95% | 27 | Nebraska | 90 | 1.67% |
| 3 | Pennsylvania | 238 | 4.42% | 28 | Arkansas | 86 | 1.60% |
| 4 | New York | 235 | 4.36% | 29 | Oregon | 70 | 1.30% |
| 5 | Florida | 224 | 4.16% | 30 | Colorado | 69 | 1.28% |
| 6 | Illinois | 210 | 3.90% | 30 | South Carolina | 69 | 1.28% |
| 7 | Ohio | 190 | 3.53% | 32 | Arizona | 61 | 1.13% |
| 8 | Michigan | 176 | 3.27% | 33 | West Virginia | 59 | 1.10% |
| 9 | Georgia | 163 | 3.03% | 34 | Montana | 55 | 1.02% |
| 10 | Minnesota | 152 | 2.82% | 35 | South Dakota | 53 | 0.98% |
| 11 | Louisiana | 140 | 2.60% | 36 | Maryland | 52 | 0.97% |
| 12 | Kansas | 138 | 2.56% | 37 | North Dakota | 50 | 0.93% |
| 13 | Missouri | 135 | 2.51% | 38 | Idaho | 43 | 0.80% |
| 14 | Tennessee | 134 | 2.49% | 39 | Utah | 42 | 0.78% |
| 15 | Wisconsin | 129 | 2.40% | 40 | Maine | 39 | 0.72% |
| 16 | Iowa | 124 | 2.30% | 41 | New Mexico | 37 | 0.69% |
| 17 | Alabama | 120 | 2.23% | 42 | Connecticut | 35 | 0.65% |
| 17 | North Carolina | 120 | 2.23% | 43 | New Hampshire | 27 | 0.50% |
| 19 | Indiana | 113 | 2.10% | 43 | Wyoming | 27 | 0.50% |
| 20 | Oklahoma | 111 | 2.06% | 45 | Nevada | 21 | 0.39% |
| 21 | Kentucky | 107 | 1.99% | 46 | Hawaii | 18 | 0.33% |
| 22 | Mississippi | 103 | 1.91% | 47 | Alaska | 16 | 0.30% |
| 23 | Massachusetts | 101 | 1.88% | 48 | Vermont | 15 | 0.28% |
| 24 | Virginia | 97 | 1.80% | 49 | Rhode Island | 12 | 0.22% |
| 25 | New Jersey | 95 | 1.76% | 50 | Delaware | 8 | 0.15% |
|  |  |  |  |  | District of Columbia | 11 | 0.20% |

Source: American Hospital Association

*"Hospital Statistics: A Comprehensive Summary of U.S. Hospitals 1991-1992"* (Copyright, reprinted with permission)

*Community hospitals are a subset of nonfederal hospitals.

# Community Hospitals per 100,000 Population in 1990

## National Rate = 2.16 Community Hospitals per 100,000 Population*

| RANK | STATE | RATE | | RANK | STATE | RATE |
|---|---|---|---|---|---|---|
| 1 | North Dakota | 7.83 | | 26 | New Mexico | 2.44 |
| 2 | South Dakota | 7.61 | | 26 | Utah | 2.44 |
| 3 | Montana | 6.88 | | 28 | New Hampshire | 2.43 |
| 4 | Wyoming | 5.95 | | 29 | Colorado | 2.09 |
| 5 | Nebraska | 5.70 | | 30 | Indiana | 2.04 |
| 6 | Kansas | 5.57 | | 31 | Pennsylvania | 2.00 |
| 7 | Iowa | 4.47 | | 32 | South Carolina | 1.98 |
| 8 | Idaho | 4.27 | | 33 | Michigan | 1.89 |
| 9 | Mississippi | 4.00 | | 34 | Washington | 1.87 |
| 10 | Arkansas | 3.66 | | 35 | Illinois | 1.84 |
| 11 | Oklahoma | 3.53 | | 36 | North Carolina | 1.81 |
| 12 | Minnesota | 3.47 | | 37 | Nevada | 1.75 |
| 13 | Louisiana | 3.32 | | 37 | Ohio | 1.75 |
| 14 | West Virginia | 3.29 | | 39 | Florida | 1.73 |
| 15 | Maine | 3.18 | | 40 | Massachusetts | 1.68 |
| 16 | Alabama | 2.97 | | 41 | Arizona | 1.66 |
| 17 | Alaska | 2.91 | | 42 | Hawaii | 1.62 |
| 18 | Kentucky | 2.90 | | 43 | Virginia | 1.57 |
| 19 | Tennessee | 2.75 | | 44 | California | 1.50 |
| 20 | Vermont | 2.67 | | 45 | New York | 1.31 |
| 21 | Missouri | 2.64 | | 46 | New Jersey | 1.23 |
| 21 | Wisconsin | 2.64 | | 47 | Delaware | 1.20 |
| 23 | Georgia | 2.52 | | 47 | Rhode Island | 1.20 |
| 23 | Texas | 2.52 | | 49 | Maryland | 1.09 |
| 25 | Oregon | 2.46 | | 50 | Connecticut | 1.06 |
| | | | | | District of Columbia | 1.81 |

Source: Morgan Quitno Corporation

*Calculated by the editors using 1990 Census resident population figures and American Hospital Association statistics.

# Community Hospitals per 1,000 Square Miles in 1990

## National Rate = 1.42 Community Hospitals per 1,000 Square Miles*

| RANK | STATE | RATE | | RANK | STATE | RATE |
|------|-------|------|---|------|-------|------|
| 1 | New Jersey | 10.89 | | 26 | Wisconsin | 1.97 |
| 2 | Massachusetts | 9.57 | | 27 | Missouri | 1.94 |
| 3 | Rhode Island | 7.77 | | 28 | Michigan | 1.82 |
| 4 | Connecticut | 6.31 | | 29 | Minnesota | 1.75 |
| 5 | Pennsylvania | 5.17 | | 30 | Kansas | 1.68 |
| 6 | New York | 4.31 | | 31 | Hawaii | 1.65 |
| 7 | Ohio | 4.24 | | 32 | Arkansas | 1.62 |
| 8 | Maryland | 4.19 | | 33 | Oklahoma | 1.59 |
| 9 | Illinois | 3.63 | | 33 | Texas | 1.59 |
| 10 | Florida | 3.41 | | 35 | Vermont | 1.56 |
| 11 | Delaware | 3.21 | | 36 | Washington | 1.28 |
| 12 | Tennessee | 3.18 | | 37 | Nebraska | 1.16 |
| 13 | Indiana | 3.10 | | 38 | Maine | 1.10 |
| 14 | New Hampshire | 2.89 | | 39 | North Dakota | 0.71 |
| 15 | Georgia | 2.74 | | 39 | Oregon | 0.71 |
| 16 | California | 2.72 | | 41 | South Dakota | 0.69 |
| 17 | Louisiana | 2.70 | | 42 | Colorado | 0.66 |
| 18 | Kentucky | 2.65 | | 43 | Arizona | 0.54 |
| 19 | West Virginia | 2.43 | | 44 | Idaho | 0.51 |
| 20 | Alabama | 2.29 | | 45 | Utah | 0.49 |
| 21 | Virginia | 2.27 | | 46 | Montana | 0.37 |
| 22 | North Carolina | 2.23 | | 47 | New Mexico | 0.30 |
| 23 | Iowa | 2.20 | | 48 | Wyoming | 0.28 |
| 24 | South Carolina | 2.16 | | 49 | Nevada | 0.19 |
| 25 | Mississippi | 2.13 | | 50 | Alaska | 0.02 |

District of Columbia        161.76

Source: Morgan Quitno Corporation

*Calculated by the editors using 1990 Census total land area figures and American Hospital Association statistics.

# Nongovernment Not-For-Profit Hospitals in 1990

## National Total = 3,191 Nongovernment Not-For-Profit Hospitals*

| RANK | STATE | HOSPITALS | % | RANK | STATE | HOSPITALS | % |
|---|---|---|---|---|---|---|---|
| 1 | California | 237 | 7.43% | 26 | South Dakota | 45 | 1.41% |
| 2 | Pennsylvania | 225 | 7.05% | 27 | Oregon | 43 | 1.35% |
| 3 | New York | 194 | 6.08% | 28 | Arkansas | 42 | 1.32% |
| 4 | Ohio | 165 | 5.17% | 28 | Montana | 42 | 1.32% |
| 5 | Illinois | 163 | 5.11% | 30 | Alabama | 39 | 1.22% |
| 6 | Michigan | 137 | 4.29% | 30 | Georgia | 39 | 1.22% |
| 7 | Texas | 132 | 4.14% | 30 | Oklahoma | 39 | 1.22% |
| 8 | Wisconsin | 122 | 3.82% | 33 | Colorado | 35 | 1.10% |
| 9 | Florida | 98 | 3.07% | 33 | Maine | 35 | 1.10% |
| 10 | New Jersey | 91 | 2.85% | 35 | Connecticut | 34 | 1.07% |
| 11 | Massachusetts | 89 | 2.79% | 35 | Louisiana | 34 | 1.07% |
| 12 | Minnesota | 86 | 2.70% | 37 | West Virginia | 33 | 1.03% |
| 13 | Missouri | 84 | 2.63% | 38 | Mississippi | 32 | 1.00% |
| 14 | Virginia | 77 | 2.41% | 39 | South Carolina | 29 | 0.91% |
| 15 | North Carolina | 72 | 2.26% | 40 | New Hampshire | 24 | 0.75% |
| 16 | Kentucky | 68 | 2.13% | 40 | Utah | 24 | 0.75% |
| 17 | Kansas | 62 | 1.94% | 42 | New Mexico | 23 | 0.72% |
| 18 | Iowa | 57 | 1.79% | 43 | Vermont | 15 | 0.47% |
| 19 | Indiana | 56 | 1.75% | 44 | Rhode Island | 12 | 0.38% |
| 19 | Tennessee | 56 | 1.75% | 45 | Idaho | 11 | 0.34% |
| 21 | Maryland | 50 | 1.57% | 46 | Hawaii | 10 | 0.31% |
| 22 | North Dakota | 49 | 1.54% | 47 | Wyoming | 9 | 0.28% |
| 22 | Washington | 49 | 1.54% | 48 | Delaware | 8 | 0.25% |
| 24 | Arizona | 46 | 1.44% | 49 | Alaska | 7 | 0.22% |
| 24 | Nebraska | 46 | 1.44% | 50 | Nevada | 6 | 0.19% |
| | | | | | District of Columbia | 10 | 0.31% |

Source: American Hospital Association

*"Hospital Statistics: A Comprehensive Summary of U.S. Hospitals 1991-1992"* (Copyright, reprinted with permission)

*Nongovernment not-for-profit hospitals are a subset of community hospitals.*

# Investor-Owned (For-Profit) Hospitals in 1990

## National Total = 749 Investor-Owned (For-Profit) Hospitals*

| RANK | STATE | HOSPITALS | % | RANK | STATE | HOSPITALS | % |
|---|---|---|---|---|---|---|---|
| 1 | Texas | 138 | 18.42% | 25 | Nevada | 5 | 0.67% |
| 2 | California | 119 | 15.89% | 25 | Washington | 5 | 0.67% |
| 3 | Florida | 93 | 12.42% | 28 | New Mexico | 4 | 0.53% |
| 4 | Tennessee | 46 | 6.14% | 29 | Idaho | 3 | 0.40% |
| 5 | Louisiana | 43 | 5.74% | 29 | New Hampshire | 3 | 0.40% |
| 6 | Georgia | 39 | 5.21% | 31 | Iowa | 2 | 0.27% |
| 7 | Alabama | 32 | 4.27% | 31 | Maryland | 2 | 0.27% |
| 8 | Kentucky | 21 | 2.80% | 31 | Massachusetts | 2 | 0.27% |
| 9 | Arkansas | 15 | 2.00% | 31 | Michigan | 2 | 0.27% |
| 9 | Virginia | 15 | 2.00% | 31 | Wyoming | 2 | 0.27% |
| 9 | West Virginia | 15 | 2.00% | 36 | Alaska | 1 | 0.13% |
| 12 | Mississippi | 14 | 1.87% | 36 | Hawaii | 1 | 0.13% |
| 13 | New York | 13 | 1.74% | 36 | Montana | 1 | 0.13% |
| 13 | North Carolina | 13 | 1.74% | 36 | Nebraska | 1 | 0.13% |
| 13 | Oklahoma | 13 | 1.74% | 36 | New Jersey | 1 | 0.13% |
| 16 | Missouri | 11 | 1.47% | 36 | Ohio | 1 | 0.13% |
| 16 | South Carolina | 11 | 1.47% | 42 | Connecticut | 0 | 0.00% |
| 18 | Illinois | 10 | 1.34% | 42 | Delaware | 0 | 0.00% |
| 19 | Utah | 9 | 1.20% | 42 | Maine | 0 | 0.00% |
| 20 | Arizona | 8 | 1.07% | 42 | Minnesota | 0 | 0.00% |
| 20 | Kansas | 8 | 1.07% | 42 | North Dakota | 0 | 0.00% |
| 20 | Oregon | 8 | 1.07% | 42 | Rhode Island | 0 | 0.00% |
| 23 | Indiana | 7 | 0.93% | 42 | South Dakota | 0 | 0.00% |
| 23 | Pennsylvania | 7 | 0.93% | 42 | Vermont | 0 | 0.00% |
| 25 | Colorado | 5 | 0.67% | 42 | Wisconsin | 0 | 0.00% |
| | | | | | District of Columbia | 0 | 0.00% |

Source: American Hospital Association

*"Hospital Statistics: A Comprehensive Summary of U.S. Hospitals 1991-1992"* (Copyright, reprinted with permission)

*Investor-owned (for-profit) hospitals are a subset of community hospitals.

# State and Local Government-Owned Hospitals in 1990

## National Total = 1,444 State and Local Government-Owned Hospitals*

| RANK | STATE | HOSPITALS | % | RANK | STATE | HOSPITALS | % |
|---|---|---|---|---|---|---|---|
| 1 | Texas | 158 | 10.94% | 26 | Oregon | 19 | 1.32% |
| 2 | California | 89 | 6.16% | 27 | Kentucky | 18 | 1.25% |
| 3 | Georgia | 85 | 5.89% | 28 | Wyoming | 16 | 1.11% |
| 4 | Kansas | 68 | 4.71% | 29 | Montana | 12 | 0.83% |
| 5 | Minnesota | 66 | 4.57% | 30 | West Virginia | 11 | 0.76% |
| 6 | Iowa | 65 | 4.50% | 31 | Massachusetts | 10 | 0.69% |
| 7 | Louisiana | 63 | 4.36% | 31 | Nevada | 10 | 0.69% |
| 8 | Oklahoma | 59 | 4.09% | 31 | New Mexico | 10 | 0.69% |
| 9 | Mississippi | 57 | 3.95% | 34 | Utah | 9 | 0.62% |
| 10 | Indiana | 50 | 3.46% | 35 | Alaska | 8 | 0.55% |
| 11 | Alabama | 49 | 3.39% | 35 | South Dakota | 8 | 0.55% |
| 12 | Nebraska | 43 | 2.98% | 37 | Arizona | 7 | 0.48% |
| 13 | Missouri | 40 | 2.77% | 37 | Hawaii | 7 | 0.48% |
| 14 | Illinois | 37 | 2.56% | 37 | Wisconsin | 7 | 0.48% |
| 14 | Michigan | 37 | 2.56% | 40 | Pennsylvania | 6 | 0.42% |
| 14 | Washington | 37 | 2.56% | 41 | Virginia | 5 | 0.35% |
| 17 | North Carolina | 35 | 2.42% | 42 | Maine | 4 | 0.28% |
| 18 | Florida | 33 | 2.29% | 43 | New Jersey | 3 | 0.21% |
| 19 | Tennessee | 32 | 2.22% | 44 | Connecticut | 1 | 0.07% |
| 20 | Arkansas | 29 | 2.01% | 44 | North Dakota | 1 | 0.07% |
| 20 | Colorado | 29 | 2.01% | 46 | Delaware | 0 | 0.00% |
| 20 | Idaho | 29 | 2.01% | 46 | Maryland | 0 | 0.00% |
| 20 | South Carolina | 29 | 2.01% | 46 | New Hampshire | 0 | 0.00% |
| 24 | New York | 28 | 1.94% | 46 | Rhode Island | 0 | 0.00% |
| 25 | Ohio | 24 | 1.66% | 46 | Vermont | 0 | 0.00% |
| | | | | | District of Columbia | 1 | 0.07% |

Source: American Hospital Association

"Hospital Statistics: A Comprehensive Summary of U.S. Hospitals 1991-1992" (Copyright, reprinted with permission)

*State and local government-owned hospitals are a subset of community hospitals.

# Hospital Beds in 1990

## National Total = 1,213,327 Beds*

| RANK | STATE | BEDS | % | RANK | STATE | BEDS | % |
|---|---|---|---|---|---|---|---|
| 1 | California | 105,381 | 8.69% | 26 | Washington | 15,773 | 1.30% |
| 2 | New York | 104,935 | 8.65% | 27 | Oklahoma | 15,033 | 1.24% |
| 3 | Texas | 79,056 | 6.52% | 28 | South Carolina | 14,550 | 1.20% |
| 4 | Pennsylvania | 68,354 | 5.63% | 29 | Connecticut | 14,533 | 1.20% |
| 5 | Florida | 62,736 | 5.17% | 30 | Colorado | 13,621 | 1.12% |
| 6 | Illinois | 58,056 | 4.78% | 31 | Arizona | 13,432 | 1.11% |
| 7 | Ohio | 52,205 | 4.30% | 32 | Arkansas | 12,867 | 1.06% |
| 8 | Michigan | 41,000 | 3.38% | 33 | Nebraska | 10,561 | 0.87% |
| 9 | New Jersey | 38,143 | 3.14% | 34 | Oregon | 10,322 | 0.85% |
| 10 | Georgia | 34,681 | 2.86% | 35 | West Virginia | 10,175 | 0.84% |
| 11 | Massachusetts | 33,904 | 2.79% | 36 | New Mexico | 6,597 | 0.54% |
| 12 | North Carolina | 30,122 | 2.48% | 37 | Maine | 5,636 | 0.46% |
| 13 | Missouri | 29,575 | 2.44% | 38 | Utah | 5,585 | 0.46% |
| 14 | Tennessee | 29,480 | 2.43% | 39 | South Dakota | 5,428 | 0.45% |
| 15 | Virginia | 29,298 | 2.41% | 40 | North Dakota | 5,298 | 0.44% |
| 16 | Indiana | 26,501 | 2.18% | 41 | Montana | 4,984 | 0.41% |
| 17 | Minnesota | 24,715 | 2.04% | 42 | New Hampshire | 4,953 | 0.41% |
| 18 | Louisiana | 23,890 | 1.97% | 43 | Rhode Island | 4,464 | 0.37% |
| 19 | Wisconsin | 23,756 | 1.96% | 44 | Nevada | 4,118 | 0.34% |
| 20 | Alabama | 23,552 | 1.94% | 45 | Hawaii | 4,093 | 0.34% |
| 21 | Maryland | 20,636 | 1.70% | 46 | Idaho | 3,893 | 0.32% |
| 22 | Kentucky | 18,845 | 1.55% | 47 | Wyoming | 2,925 | 0.24% |
| 23 | Iowa | 17,251 | 1.42% | 48 | Delaware | 2,837 | 0.23% |
| 24 | Mississippi | 17,151 | 1.41% | 49 | Vermont | 2,270 | 0.19% |
| 25 | Kansas | 16,139 | 1.33% | 50 | Alaska | 1,976 | 0.16% |
| | | | | | District of Columbia | 8,041 | 0.66% |

Source: American Hospital Association
"Hospital Statistics: A Comprehensive Summary of U.S. Hospitals 1991-1992" (Copyright, reprinted with permission)
*In federal and nonfederal hospitals.

# Hospital Beds per 100,000 Population in 1990

## National Rate = 488 Beds per 100,000 Population*

| RANK | STATE | RATE | RANK | STATE | RATE |
|------|-------|------|------|-------|------|
| 1 | North Dakota | 829 | 26 | Indiana | 478 |
| 2 | South Dakota | 780 | 26 | Oklahoma | 478 |
| 3 | Nebraska | 669 | 28 | Virginia | 474 |
| 4 | Mississippi | 667 | 29 | Texas | 465 |
| 5 | Kansas | 651 | 30 | Maine | 459 |
| 6 | Wyoming | 645 | 31 | North Carolina | 454 |
| 7 | Montana | 624 | 32 | New Hampshire | 447 |
| 8 | Iowa | 621 | 33 | Rhode Island | 445 |
| 9 | Tennessee | 604 | 34 | Connecticut | 442 |
| 10 | Alabama | 583 | 35 | Michigan | 441 |
| 10 | New York | 583 | 36 | New Mexico | 435 |
| 12 | Missouri | 578 | 37 | Maryland | 432 |
| 13 | Pennsylvania | 575 | 38 | Delaware | 426 |
| 14 | West Virginia | 567 | 39 | South Carolina | 417 |
| 15 | Louisiana | 566 | 40 | Colorado | 413 |
| 16 | Minnesota | 565 | 41 | Vermont | 403 |
| 17 | Massachusetts | 564 | 42 | Idaho | 387 |
| 18 | Arkansas | 547 | 43 | Hawaii | 369 |
| 19 | Georgia | 535 | 44 | Arizona | 366 |
| 20 | Kentucky | 511 | 45 | Oregon | 363 |
| 21 | Illinois | 508 | 46 | Alaska | 359 |
| 22 | New Jersey | 493 | 47 | California | 354 |
| 23 | Wisconsin | 486 | 48 | Nevada | 343 |
| 24 | Florida | 485 | 49 | Utah | 324 |
| 25 | Ohio | 481 | 49 | Washington | 324 |

District of Columbia     1,325

Source: Morgan Quitno Corporation

*Calculated by the editors using 1990 Census resident population figures and American Hospital Association Statistics. Beds in federal and nonfederal hospitals.

# Average Number of Beds per Hospital in 1990

## National Rate = 182 Beds per Hospital*

| RANK | STATE | RATE | RANK | STATE | RATE |
|------|-------|------|------|-------|------|
| 1 | New York | 344 | 26 | West Virginia | 150 |
| 2 | New Jersey | 321 | 27 | Mississippi | 149 |
| 3 | Maryland | 252 | 28 | Arizona | 148 |
| 4 | Illinois | 235 | 28 | Minnesota | 148 |
| 4 | Rhode Island | 235 | 30 | Texas | 147 |
| 6 | Ohio | 233 | 31 | Washington | 143 |
| 7 | Connecticut | 231 | 32 | Louisiana | 138 |
| 8 | Pennsylvania | 226 | 33 | Arkansas | 134 |
| 9 | Delaware | 218 | 33 | Oregon | 134 |
| 9 | Florida | 218 | 35 | Nevada | 133 |
| 11 | Virginia | 217 | 36 | Iowa | 129 |
| 12 | Massachusetts | 216 | 37 | Maine | 128 |
| 13 | Michigan | 200 | 38 | Vermont | 126 |
| 14 | Indiana | 196 | 39 | New Hampshire | 124 |
| 15 | North Carolina | 194 | 40 | New Mexico | 110 |
| 16 | California | 192 | 40 | Oklahoma | 110 |
| 17 | Tennessee | 189 | 42 | Utah | 107 |
| 18 | Missouri | 185 | 43 | Nebraska | 104 |
| 19 | Alabama | 171 | 44 | Kansas | 101 |
| 19 | Georgia | 171 | 45 | North Dakota | 93 |
| 21 | South Carolina | 163 | 46 | Wyoming | 91 |
| 22 | Wisconsin | 161 | 47 | South Dakota | 82 |
| 23 | Colorado | 158 | 48 | Montana | 80 |
| 24 | Hawaii | 157 | 49 | Idaho | 78 |
| 25 | Kentucky | 153 | 50 | Alaska | 73 |

District of Columbia            473

*Source: Morgan Quitno Corporation*

*\*Calculated by the editors using 1990 Census resident population figures and American Hospital Association Statistics.  Beds in federal and nonfederal hospitals.*

# Beds in Federal Hospitals in 1990

## National Total = 98,255 Federal Hospital Beds

| RANK | STATE | BEDS | % | RANK | STATE | BEDS | % |
|---|---|---|---|---|---|---|---|
| 1 | California | 8,679 | 8.83% | 26 | Louisiana | 1,327 | 1.35% |
| 2 | Texas | 8,212 | 8.36% | 27 | Minnesota | 1,323 | 1.35% |
| 3 | New York | 7,226 | 7.35% | 28 | South Carolina | 1,234 | 1.26% |
| 4 | Illinois | 4,659 | 4.74% | 29 | Indiana | 1,205 | 1.23% |
| 5 | Pennsylvania | 4,628 | 4.71% | 30 | Iowa | 1,187 | 1.21% |
| 6 | Florida | 4,368 | 4.45% | 31 | West Virginia | 1,041 | 1.06% |
| 7 | Ohio | 3,520 | 3.58% | 32 | South Dakota | 1,016 | 1.03% |
| 8 | Massachusetts | 3,035 | 3.09% | 33 | Oklahoma | 936 | 0.95% |
| 9 | Georgia | 2,931 | 2.98% | 34 | Oregon | 918 | 0.93% |
| 10 | Virginia | 2,571 | 2.62% | 35 | New Mexico | 850 | 0.87% |
| 11 | North Carolina | 2,557 | 2.60% | 36 | Connecticut | 728 | 0.74% |
| 12 | Maryland | 2,500 | 2.54% | 37 | Nebraska | 726 | 0.74% |
| 13 | Missouri | 2,496 | 2.54% | 38 | Alaska | 508 | 0.52% |
| 14 | Tennessee | 2,492 | 2.54% | 39 | Wyoming | 499 | 0.51% |
| 15 | Alabama | 2,261 | 2.30% | 40 | Hawaii | 483 | 0.49% |
| 16 | Michigan | 2,194 | 2.23% | 41 | Utah | 422 | 0.43% |
| 17 | New Jersey | 2,189 | 2.23% | 42 | Maine | 370 | 0.38% |
| 18 | Arizona | 2,048 | 2.08% | 43 | Delaware | 321 | 0.33% |
| 19 | Washington | 1,903 | 1.94% | 44 | Montana | 307 | 0.31% |
| 20 | Mississippi | 1,705 | 1.74% | 45 | North Dakota | 303 | 0.31% |
| 21 | Wisconsin | 1,673 | 1.70% | 46 | Nevada | 280 | 0.28% |
| 22 | Kansas | 1,649 | 1.68% | 47 | Rhode Island | 271 | 0.28% |
| 23 | Colorado | 1,549 | 1.58% | 48 | New Hampshire | 240 | 0.24% |
| 24 | Kentucky | 1,419 | 1.44% | 49 | Idaho | 202 | 0.21% |
| 25 | Arkansas | 1,379 | 1.40% | 50 | Vermont | 171 | 0.17% |
| | | | | | District of Columbia | 1,544 | 1.57% |

Source: American Hospital Association

"Hospital Statistics: A Comprehensive Summary of U.S. Hospitals 1991-1992" (Copyright, reprinted with permission)

# Beds in Nonfederal Hospitals in 1990

## National Total = 1,115,072 Nonfederal Hospital Beds

| RANK | STATE | BEDS | % | RANK | STATE | BEDS | % |
|------|-------|------|---|------|-------|------|---|
| 1 | New York | 97,709 | 8.76% | 26 | Oklahoma | 14,097 | 1.26% |
| 2 | California | 96,702 | 8.67% | 27 | Washington | 13,870 | 1.24% |
| 3 | Texas | 70,844 | 6.35% | 28 | Connecticut | 13,805 | 1.24% |
| 4 | Pennsylvania | 63,726 | 5.71% | 29 | South Carolina | 13,316 | 1.19% |
| 5 | Florida | 58,368 | 5.23% | 30 | Colorado | 12,072 | 1.08% |
| 6 | Illinois | 53,397 | 4.79% | 31 | Arkansas | 11,488 | 1.03% |
| 7 | Ohio | 48,685 | 4.37% | 32 | Arizona | 11,384 | 1.02% |
| 8 | Michigan | 38,806 | 3.48% | 33 | Nebraska | 9,835 | 0.88% |
| 9 | New Jersey | 35,954 | 3.22% | 34 | Oregon | 9,404 | 0.84% |
| 10 | Georgia | 31,750 | 2.85% | 35 | West Virginia | 9,134 | 0.82% |
| 11 | Massachusetts | 30,869 | 2.77% | 36 | New Mexico | 5,747 | 0.52% |
| 12 | North Carolina | 27,565 | 2.47% | 37 | Maine | 5,266 | 0.47% |
| 13 | Missouri | 27,079 | 2.43% | 38 | Utah | 5,163 | 0.46% |
| 14 | Tennessee | 26,988 | 2.42% | 39 | North Dakota | 4,995 | 0.45% |
| 15 | Virginia | 26,727 | 2.40% | 40 | New Hampshire | 4,713 | 0.42% |
| 16 | Indiana | 25,296 | 2.27% | 41 | Montana | 4,677 | 0.42% |
| 17 | Minnesota | 23,392 | 2.10% | 42 | South Dakota | 4,412 | 0.40% |
| 18 | Louisiana | 22,563 | 2.02% | 43 | Rhode Island | 4,193 | 0.38% |
| 19 | Wisconsin | 22,083 | 1.98% | 44 | Nevada | 3,838 | 0.34% |
| 20 | Alabama | 21,291 | 1.91% | 45 | Idaho | 3,691 | 0.33% |
| 21 | Maryland | 18,136 | 1.63% | 46 | Hawaii | 3,610 | 0.32% |
| 22 | Kentucky | 17,426 | 1.56% | 47 | Delaware | 2,516 | 0.23% |
| 23 | Iowa | 16,064 | 1.44% | 48 | Wyoming | 2,426 | 0.22% |
| 24 | Mississippi | 15,446 | 1.39% | 49 | Vermont | 2,099 | 0.19% |
| 25 | Kansas | 14,490 | 1.30% | 50 | Alaska | 1,468 | 0.13% |
| | | | | | District of Columbia | 6,497 | 0.58% |

Source: American Hospital Association

*"Hospital Statistics: A Comprehensive Summary of U.S. Hospitals 1991-1992"* (Copyright, reprinted with permission)

# Beds in Psychiatric Hospitals in 1990

## National Total = 171,891 Psychiatric Hospital Beds*

| RANK | STATE | BEDS | % | RANK | STATE | BEDS | % |
|---|---|---|---|---|---|---|---|
| 1 | New York | 21,093 | 12.27% | 26 | South Carolina | 1,969 | 1.15% |
| 2 | California | 14,150 | 8.23% | 27 | Colorado | 1,915 | 1.11% |
| 3 | Pennsylvania | 11,597 | 6.75% | 28 | Washington | 1,775 | 1.03% |
| 4 | Texas | 11,247 | 6.54% | 29 | Kentucky | 1,682 | 0.98% |
| 5 | Florida | 7,227 | 4.20% | 30 | Oklahoma | 1,600 | 0.93% |
| 6 | North Carolina | 6,060 | 3.53% | 31 | New Mexico | 1,555 | 0.90% |
| 7 | Illinois | 5,986 | 3.48% | 32 | Arizona | 1,411 | 0.82% |
| 8 | Virginia | 5,976 | 3.48% | 33 | Oregon | 1,331 | 0.77% |
| 9 | Georgia | 5,948 | 3.46% | 34 | New Hampshire | 1,171 | 0.68% |
| 10 | Michigan | 5,664 | 3.30% | 35 | Maine | 771 | 0.45% |
| 11 | Ohio | 5,391 | 3.14% | 36 | Utah | 755 | 0.44% |
| 12 | Massachusetts | 5,224 | 3.04% | 37 | Nebraska | 720 | 0.42% |
| 13 | Minnesota | 4,450 | 2.59% | 38 | West Virginia | 699 | 0.41% |
| 14 | New Jersey | 4,382 | 2.55% | 39 | Arkansas | 645 | 0.38% |
| 15 | Wisconsin | 4,060 | 2.36% | 40 | Wyoming | 622 | 0.36% |
| 16 | Maryland | 3,985 | 2.32% | 41 | North Dakota | 583 | 0.34% |
| 17 | Indiana | 3,834 | 2.23% | 42 | Delaware | 510 | 0.30% |
| 18 | Alabama | 3,355 | 1.95% | 43 | Idaho | 491 | 0.29% |
| 19 | Louisiana | 3,060 | 1.78% | 44 | Nevada | 465 | 0.27% |
| 20 | Tennessee | 2,771 | 1.61% | 45 | Vermont | 383 | 0.22% |
| 21 | Kansas | 2,630 | 1.53% | 46 | Rhode Island | 371 | 0.22% |
| 22 | Connecticut | 2,610 | 1.52% | 47 | Alaska | 274 | 0.16% |
| 23 | Missouri | 2,542 | 1.48% | 48 | Hawaii | 205 | 0.12% |
| 24 | Mississippi | 2,504 | 1.46% | 49 | South Dakota | 60 | 0.03% |
| 25 | Iowa | 2,461 | 1.43% | 50 | Montana | 21 | 0.01% |
| | | | | | District of Columbia | 1,700 | 0.99% |

*Source: American Hospital Association*

*"Hospital Statistics: A Comprehensive Summary of U.S. Hospitals 1991–1992" (Copyright, reprinted with permission)*

*\*Federal and nonfederal psychiatric hospitals.*

# Beds in Community Hospitals in 1990

## National Total = 927,360 Community Hospital Beds*

| RANK | STATE | BEDS | % | RANK | STATE | BEDS | % |
|---|---|---|---|---|---|---|---|
| 1 | California | 80,031 | 8.63% | 26 | Washington | 11,915 | 1.28% |
| 2 | New York | 74,476 | 8.03% | 27 | Kansas | 11,796 | 1.27% |
| 3 | Texas | 59,345 | 6.40% | 28 | South Carolina | 11,208 | 1.21% |
| 4 | Pennsylvania | 52,389 | 5.65% | 29 | Arkansas | 10,843 | 1.17% |
| 5 | Florida | 50,594 | 5.46% | 30 | Colorado | 10,316 | 1.11% |
| 6 | Illinois | 46,065 | 4.97% | 31 | Arizona | 9,973 | 1.08% |
| 7 | Ohio | 43,143 | 4.65% | 32 | Connecticut | 9,627 | 1.04% |
| 8 | Michigan | 33,951 | 3.66% | 33 | Nebraska | 8,611 | 0.93% |
| 9 | New Jersey | 28,846 | 3.11% | 34 | West Virginia | 8,435 | 0.91% |
| 10 | Georgia | 25,500 | 2.75% | 35 | Oregon | 8,073 | 0.87% |
| 11 | Missouri | 24,355 | 2.63% | 36 | Montana | 4,633 | 0.50% |
| 12 | Tennessee | 23,517 | 2.54% | 37 | Maine | 4,495 | 0.48% |
| 13 | North Carolina | 21,934 | 2.37% | 38 | North Dakota | 4,412 | 0.48% |
| 14 | Massachusetts | 21,875 | 2.36% | 39 | Utah | 4,408 | 0.48% |
| 15 | Indiana | 21,866 | 2.36% | 40 | South Dakota | 4,200 | 0.45% |
| 16 | Virginia | 20,005 | 2.16% | 41 | New Mexico | 4,192 | 0.45% |
| 17 | Minnesota | 19,434 | 2.10% | 42 | New Hampshire | 3,470 | 0.37% |
| 18 | Louisiana | 19,085 | 2.06% | 43 | Nevada | 3,373 | 0.36% |
| 19 | Wisconsin | 18,687 | 2.02% | 44 | Idaho | 3,200 | 0.35% |
| 20 | Alabama | 18,638 | 2.01% | 45 | Rhode Island | 3,180 | 0.34% |
| 21 | Kentucky | 15,718 | 1.69% | 46 | Hawaii | 2,887 | 0.31% |
| 22 | Iowa | 14,239 | 1.54% | 47 | Wyoming | 2,143 | 0.23% |
| 23 | Maryland | 13,472 | 1.45% | 48 | Delaware | 2,006 | 0.22% |
| 24 | Mississippi | 12,907 | 1.39% | 49 | Vermont | 1,716 | 0.19% |
| 25 | Oklahoma | 12,425 | 1.34% | 50 | Alaska | 1,194 | 0.13% |
| | | | | | District of Columbia | 4,557 | 0.49% |

Source: American Hospital Association

*"Hospital Statistics: A Comprehensive Summary of U.S. Hospitals 1991–1992"* (Copyright, reprinted with permission)

*Community hospital beds are a subset of nonfederal hospital beds.

# Beds in Community Hospitals per 100,000 Population in 1990

## National Rate = 373 Beds per 100,000 Population*

| RANK | STATE | RATE | RANK | STATE | RATE |
|------|-------|------|------|-------|------|
| 1 | North Dakota | 691 | 26 | New Jersey | 373 |
| 2 | South Dakota | 603 | 27 | Maine | 366 |
| 3 | Montana | 580 | 28 | Michigan | 365 |
| 4 | Nebraska | 546 | 29 | Massachusetts | 364 |
| 5 | Iowa | 513 | 30 | Texas | 349 |
| 6 | Mississippi | 502 | 31 | North Carolina | 331 |
| 7 | Tennessee | 482 | 32 | Virginia | 323 |
| 8 | Kansas | 476 | 33 | South Carolina | 321 |
| 8 | Missouri | 476 | 34 | Idaho | 318 |
| 10 | Wyoming | 472 | 35 | Rhode Island | 317 |
| 11 | West Virginia | 470 | 36 | Colorado | 313 |
| 12 | Alabama | 461 | 36 | New Hampshire | 313 |
| 12 | Arkansas | 461 | 38 | Vermont | 305 |
| 14 | Louisiana | 452 | 39 | Delaware | 301 |
| 15 | Minnesota | 444 | 40 | Connecticut | 293 |
| 16 | Pennsylvania | 441 | 41 | Oregon | 284 |
| 17 | Kentucky | 427 | 42 | Maryland | 282 |
| 18 | New York | 414 | 43 | Nevada | 281 |
| 19 | Illinois | 403 | 44 | New Mexico | 277 |
| 20 | Ohio | 398 | 45 | Arizona | 272 |
| 21 | Oklahoma | 395 | 46 | California | 269 |
| 22 | Georgia | 394 | 47 | Hawaii | 261 |
| 22 | Indiana | 394 | 48 | Utah | 256 |
| 24 | Florida | 391 | 49 | Washington | 245 |
| 25 | Wisconsin | 382 | 50 | Alaska | 217 |
|  |  |  |  | District of Columbia | 751 |

Source: Morgan Quitno Corporation

*Calculated by the editors using 1990 Census resident population figures and American Hospital Association statistics. Community hospitals are a subset of nonfederal hospitals.

# Average Number of Beds per Community Hospital in 1990

## National Rate = 172 Beds per Community Hospital*

| RANK | STATE | RATE | RANK | STATE | RATE |
|---|---|---|---|---|---|
| 1 | New York | 317 | 26 | Kentucky | 147 |
| 2 | New Jersey | 304 | 27 | Wisconsin | 145 |
| 3 | Connecticut | 275 | 28 | West Virginia | 143 |
| 4 | Rhode Island | 265 | 29 | Texas | 139 |
| 5 | Maryland | 259 | 30 | Louisiana | 136 |
| 6 | Delaware | 251 | 31 | Washington | 131 |
| 7 | Ohio | 227 | 32 | New Hampshire | 129 |
| 8 | Florida | 226 | 33 | Minnesota | 128 |
| 9 | Pennsylvania | 220 | 34 | Arkansas | 126 |
| 10 | Illinois | 219 | 35 | Mississippi | 125 |
| 11 | Massachusetts | 217 | 36 | Iowa | 115 |
| 12 | Virginia | 206 | 36 | Maine | 115 |
| 13 | Indiana | 194 | 36 | Oregon | 115 |
| 14 | Michigan | 193 | 39 | Vermont | 114 |
| 15 | North Carolina | 183 | 40 | New Mexico | 113 |
| 16 | California | 180 | 41 | Oklahoma | 112 |
| 16 | Missouri | 180 | 42 | Utah | 105 |
| 18 | Tennessee | 176 | 43 | Nebraska | 96 |
| 19 | Arizona | 163 | 44 | North Dakota | 88 |
| 20 | South Carolina | 162 | 45 | Kansas | 85 |
| 21 | Nevada | 161 | 46 | Montana | 84 |
| 22 | Hawaii | 160 | 47 | South Dakota | 79 |
| 23 | Georgia | 156 | 47 | Wyoming | 79 |
| 24 | Alabama | 155 | 49 | Alaska | 75 |
| 25 | Colorado | 150 | 50 | Idaho | 74 |

District of Columbia     414

Source: Morgan Quitno Corporation

*Calculated by the editors using American Hospital Association statistics. Community hospitals are a subset of nonfederal hospitals.

# Beds in Nongovernment Not–For–Profit Hospitals in 1990

## National Total = 656,755 Beds*

| RANK | STATE | BEDS | % | RANK | STATE | BEDS | % |
|------|-------|------|---|------|-------|------|---|
| 1 | New York | 59,669 | 9.09% | 26 | Alabama | 7,256 | 1.10% |
| 2 | Pennsylvania | 51,284 | 7.81% | 27 | Colorado | 7,129 | 1.09% |
| 3 | California | 50,321 | 7.66% | 28 | Arkansas | 7,022 | 1.07% |
| 4 | Illinois | 40,704 | 6.20% | 29 | Kansas | 6,863 | 1.04% |
| 5 | Ohio | 38,726 | 5.90% | 30 | Oklahoma | 6,687 | 1.02% |
| 6 | Michigan | 29,291 | 4.46% | 31 | West Virginia | 6,400 | 0.97% |
| 7 | New Jersey | 27,874 | 4.24% | 32 | Oregon | 6,223 | 0.95% |
| 8 | Texas | 26,952 | 4.10% | 33 | South Carolina | 5,666 | 0.86% |
| 9 | Florida | 24,886 | 3.79% | 34 | Nebraska | 5,559 | 0.85% |
| 10 | Massachusetts | 19,755 | 3.01% | 35 | Mississippi | 4,734 | 0.72% |
| 11 | Missouri | 19,332 | 2.94% | 36 | North Dakota | 4,360 | 0.66% |
| 12 | Wisconsin | 17,427 | 2.65% | 37 | Maine | 4,182 | 0.64% |
| 13 | Indiana | 14,944 | 2.28% | 38 | Montana | 3,914 | 0.60% |
| 14 | Virginia | 14,811 | 2.26% | 39 | South Dakota | 3,851 | 0.59% |
| 15 | Minnesota | 13,849 | 2.11% | 40 | Rhode Island | 3,180 | 0.48% |
| 16 | North Carolina | 13,527 | 2.06% | 41 | New Hampshire | 3,171 | 0.48% |
| 17 | Tennessee | 13,427 | 2.04% | 42 | Utah | 2,758 | 0.42% |
| 18 | Maryland | 12,914 | 1.97% | 43 | New Mexico | 2,368 | 0.36% |
| 19 | Kentucky | 10,420 | 1.59% | 44 | Hawaii | 2,136 | 0.33% |
| 20 | Iowa | 9,429 | 1.44% | 45 | Delaware | 2,006 | 0.31% |
| 21 | Connecticut | 9,395 | 1.43% | 46 | Vermont | 1,716 | 0.26% |
| 22 | Georgia | 8,625 | 1.31% | 47 | Idaho | 1,242 | 0.19% |
| 23 | Washington | 8,458 | 1.29% | 48 | Nevada | 996 | 0.15% |
| 24 | Louisiana | 7,917 | 1.21% | 49 | Wyoming | 718 | 0.11% |
| 25 | Arizona | 7,899 | 1.20% | 50 | Alaska | 707 | 0.11% |
| | | | | | District of Columbia | 4,075 | 0.62% |

Source: American Hospital Association
   "Hospital Statistics: A Comprehensive Summary of U.S. Hospitals 1991-1992" (Copyright, reprinted with permission)
*Nongovernment not-for-profit hospital beds are a subset of community hospital beds.

# Beds in Investor-Owned (For-Profit) Hospitals in 1990

## National Total = 101,377 Beds*

| RANK | STATE | BEDS | % | RANK | STATE | BEDS | % |
|------|-------|------|---|------|-------|------|---|
| 1 | Texas | 18,699 | 18.45% | 26 | Washington | 587 | 0.58% |
| 2 | Florida | 17,576 | 17.34% | 27 | Oregon | 585 | 0.58% |
| 3 | California | 14,604 | 14.41% | 28 | Maryland | 558 | 0.55% |
| 4 | Tennessee | 4,705 | 4.64% | 29 | Pennsylvania | 553 | 0.55% |
| 5 | Louisiana | 4,667 | 4.60% | 30 | Idaho | 409 | 0.40% |
| 6 | Georgia | 4,593 | 4.53% | 31 | Nebraska | 407 | 0.40% |
| 7 | Alabama | 3,943 | 3.89% | 32 | New Hampshire | 299 | 0.29% |
| 8 | Kentucky | 3,223 | 3.18% | 33 | Massachusetts | 276 | 0.27% |
| 9 | Virginia | 3,006 | 2.97% | 34 | Alaska | 238 | 0.23% |
| 10 | New York | 2,592 | 2.56% | 35 | Iowa | 216 | 0.21% |
| 11 | Missouri | 1,687 | 1.66% | 36 | Wyoming | 172 | 0.17% |
| 12 | South Carolina | 1,631 | 1.61% | 37 | Hawaii | 159 | 0.16% |
| 13 | Mississippi | 1,610 | 1.59% | 38 | New Jersey | 151 | 0.15% |
| 14 | Arkansas | 1,477 | 1.46% | 39 | Michigan | 142 | 0.14% |
| 15 | North Carolina | 1,445 | 1.43% | 40 | Montana | 44 | 0.04% |
| 16 | Nevada | 1,415 | 1.40% | 41 | Ohio | 43 | 0.04% |
| 17 | Oklahoma | 1,347 | 1.33% | 42 | Connecticut | 0 | 0.00% |
| 18 | Kansas | 1,301 | 1.28% | 42 | Delaware | 0 | 0.00% |
| 19 | Arizona | 1,132 | 1.12% | 42 | Maine | 0 | 0.00% |
| 20 | Colorado | 1,120 | 1.10% | 42 | Minnesota | 0 | 0.00% |
| 21 | West Virginia | 1,105 | 1.09% | 42 | North Dakota | 0 | 0.00% |
| 22 | Illinois | 1,051 | 1.04% | 42 | Rhode Island | 0 | 0.00% |
| 23 | Utah | 961 | 0.95% | 42 | South Dakota | 0 | 0.00% |
| 24 | Indiana | 960 | 0.95% | 42 | Vermont | 0 | 0.00% |
| 25 | New Mexico | 688 | 0.68% | 42 | Wisconsin | 0 | 0.00% |
| | | | | | District of Columbia | 0 | 0.00% |

Source: American Hospital Association

"Hospital Statistics: A Comprehensive Summary of U.S. Hospitals 1991-1992" (Copyright, reprinted with permission)

*Investor-owned (for-profit) hospital beds are a subset of community hospital beds.

# Beds in State and Local Government–Owned Hospitals in 1990

## National Total = 169,228 Beds*

| RANK | STATE | BEDS | % | RANK | STATE | BEDS | % |
|------|-------|------|---|------|-------|------|---|
| 1 | California | 15,106 | 8.93% | 26 | Colorado | 2,067 | 1.22% |
| 2 | Texas | 13,694 | 8.09% | 27 | Massachusetts | 1,844 | 1.09% |
| 3 | Georgia | 12,282 | 7.26% | 28 | Idaho | 1,549 | 0.92% |
| 4 | New York | 12,215 | 7.22% | 29 | Oregon | 1,265 | 0.75% |
| 5 | Florida | 8,132 | 4.81% | 30 | Wisconsin | 1,260 | 0.74% |
| 6 | Alabama | 7,439 | 4.40% | 31 | Wyoming | 1,253 | 0.74% |
| 7 | North Carolina | 6,962 | 4.11% | 32 | New Mexico | 1,136 | 0.67% |
| 8 | Mississippi | 6,563 | 3.88% | 33 | Nevada | 962 | 0.57% |
| 9 | Louisiana | 6,501 | 3.84% | 34 | Arizona | 942 | 0.56% |
| 10 | Indiana | 5,962 | 3.52% | 35 | West Virginia | 930 | 0.55% |
| 11 | Minnesota | 5,585 | 3.30% | 36 | New Jersey | 821 | 0.49% |
| 12 | Tennessee | 5,385 | 3.18% | 37 | Utah | 689 | 0.41% |
| 13 | Iowa | 4,594 | 2.71% | 38 | Montana | 675 | 0.40% |
| 14 | Michigan | 4,518 | 2.67% | 39 | Hawaii | 592 | 0.35% |
| 15 | Oklahoma | 4,391 | 2.59% | 40 | Pennsylvania | 552 | 0.33% |
| 16 | Ohio | 4,374 | 2.58% | 41 | South Dakota | 349 | 0.21% |
| 17 | Illinois | 4,310 | 2.55% | 42 | Maine | 313 | 0.18% |
| 18 | South Carolina | 3,911 | 2.31% | 43 | Alaska | 249 | 0.15% |
| 19 | Kansas | 3,632 | 2.15% | 44 | Connecticut | 232 | 0.14% |
| 20 | Missouri | 3,336 | 1.97% | 45 | North Dakota | 52 | 0.03% |
| 21 | Washington | 2,870 | 1.70% | 46 | Delaware | 0 | 0.00% |
| 22 | Nebraska | 2,645 | 1.56% | 46 | Maryland | 0 | 0.00% |
| 23 | Arkansas | 2,344 | 1.39% | 46 | New Hampshire | 0 | 0.00% |
| 24 | Virginia | 2,188 | 1.29% | 46 | Rhode Island | 0 | 0.00% |
| 25 | Kentucky | 2,075 | 1.23% | 46 | Vermont | 0 | 0.00% |
|  |  |  |  |  | District of Columbia | 482 | 0.28% |

Source: American Hospital Association

   "Hospital Statistics: A Comprehensive Summary of U.S. Hospitals 1991-1992" (Copyright, reprinted with permission)

*State and local government-owned hospital beds are a subset of community hospital beds.

# Hospital Admissions in 1990

## National Total = 33,773,574 Admissions*

| RANK | STATE | ADMISSIONS | % | | RANK | STATE | ADMISSIONS | % |
|------|-------|-----------|---|---|------|-------|-----------|---|
| 1 | California | 3,316,969 | 9.82% | | 26 | Mississippi | 434,185 | 1.29% |
| 2 | New York | 2,449,532 | 7.25% | | 27 | Oklahoma | 431,097 | 1.28% |
| 3 | Texas | 2,227,166 | 6.59% | | 28 | Iowa | 404,175 | 1.20% |
| 4 | Pennsylvania | 1,886,477 | 5.59% | | 29 | Colorado | 388,681 | 1.15% |
| 5 | Florida | 1,769,204 | 5.24% | | 30 | Connecticut | 377,463 | 1.12% |
| 6 | Illinois | 1,608,893 | 4.76% | | 31 | Arkansas | 375,428 | 1.11% |
| 7 | Ohio | 1,580,337 | 4.68% | | 32 | Kansas | 335,204 | 0.99% |
| 8 | New Jersey | 1,173,615 | 3.47% | | 33 | Oregon | 321,756 | 0.95% |
| 9 | Michigan | 1,115,998 | 3.30% | | 34 | West Virginia | 298,941 | 0.89% |
| 10 | Georgia | 989,479 | 2.93% | | 35 | Nebraska | 212,324 | 0.63% |
| 11 | Massachusetts | 872,318 | 2.58% | | 36 | New Mexico | 190,546 | 0.56% |
| 12 | North Carolina | 867,970 | 2.57% | | 37 | Utah | 190,235 | 0.56% |
| 13 | Tennessee | 850,816 | 2.52% | | 38 | Maine | 155,909 | 0.46% |
| 14 | Virginia | 798,164 | 2.36% | | 39 | New Hampshire | 138,302 | 0.41% |
| 15 | Missouri | 794,165 | 2.35% | | 40 | Rhode Island | 137,597 | 0.41% |
| 16 | Indiana | 753,940 | 2.23% | | 41 | Nevada | 129,596 | 0.38% |
| 17 | Louisiana | 658,189 | 1.95% | | 42 | Hawaii | 118,199 | 0.35% |
| 18 | Alabama | 639,880 | 1.89% | | 43 | South Dakota | 114,299 | 0.34% |
| 19 | Maryland | 630,293 | 1.87% | | 44 | Montana | 114,026 | 0.34% |
| 20 | Wisconsin | 629,243 | 1.86% | | 45 | North Dakota | 109,302 | 0.32% |
| 21 | Kentucky | 580,166 | 1.72% | | 46 | Idaho | 103,428 | 0.31% |
| 22 | Minnesota | 560,300 | 1.66% | | 47 | Delaware | 92,111 | 0.27% |
| 23 | Washington | 551,655 | 1.63% | | 48 | Vermont | 62,770 | 0.19% |
| 24 | South Carolina | 460,309 | 1.36% | | 49 | Alaska | 59,266 | 0.18% |
| 25 | Arizona | 459,092 | 1.36% | | 50 | Wyoming | 54,821 | 0.16% |
| | | | | | | District of Columbia | 199,743 | 0.59% |

*Source: American Hospital Association*

  *"Hospital Statistics: A Comprehensive Summary of U.S. Hospitals 1991-1992" (Copyright, reprinted with permission)*

*Admissions to federal and nonfederal hospitals.*

# Admissions to Federal Hospitals in 1990

## National Total = 1,759,058 Admissions

| RANK | STATE | ADMISSIONS | % | RANK | STATE | ADMISSIONS | % |
|---|---|---|---|---|---|---|---|
| 1 | California | 183,214 | 10.42% | 26 | Arkansas | 24,228 | 1.38% |
| 2 | Texas | 167,791 | 9.54% | 27 | Kansas | 22,540 | 1.28% |
| 3 | Florida | 91,165 | 5.18% | 28 | New Jersey | 20,260 | 1.15% |
| 4 | New York | 70,974 | 4.03% | 29 | Hawaii | 20,237 | 1.15% |
| 5 | Virginia | 61,980 | 3.52% | 30 | Minnesota | 20,218 | 1.15% |
| 6 | Georgia | 61,420 | 3.49% | 31 | Alaska | 20,107 | 1.14% |
| 7 | Illinois | 60,087 | 3.42% | 32 | South Dakota | 19,193 | 1.09% |
| 8 | North Carolina | 55,192 | 3.14% | 33 | Nebraska | 17,527 | 1.00% |
| 9 | Arizona | 51,691 | 2.94% | 34 | West Virginia | 16,766 | 0.95% |
| 10 | Maryland | 51,489 | 2.93% | 35 | Wisconsin | 16,610 | 0.94% |
| 11 | Washington | 49,035 | 2.79% | 36 | Oregon | 15,291 | 0.87% |
| 12 | Colorado | 43,482 | 2.47% | 37 | Indiana | 14,647 | 0.83% |
| 13 | Pennsylvania | 43,348 | 2.46% | 38 | Iowa | 14,318 | 0.81% |
| 14 | Missouri | 42,370 | 2.41% | 39 | Connecticut | 10,787 | 0.61% |
| 15 | Ohio | 41,129 | 2.34% | 40 | North Dakota | 10,300 | 0.59% |
| 16 | Oklahoma | 38,103 | 2.17% | 41 | Utah | 10,067 | 0.57% |
| 17 | South Carolina | 35,493 | 2.02% | 42 | Nevada | 8,753 | 0.50% |
| 18 | Kentucky | 35,023 | 1.99% | 43 | Montana | 8,492 | 0.48% |
| 19 | Alabama | 34,627 | 1.97% | 44 | Rhode Island | 6,531 | 0.37% |
| 20 | Louisiana | 34,034 | 1.93% | 45 | Wyoming | 5,742 | 0.33% |
| 21 | Tennessee | 33,290 | 1.89% | 46 | Maine | 5,564 | 0.32% |
| 22 | Mississippi | 31,470 | 1.79% | 47 | Idaho | 5,083 | 0.29% |
| 23 | New Mexico | 30,536 | 1.74% | 48 | Delaware | 4,767 | 0.27% |
| 24 | Michigan | 28,062 | 1.60% | 49 | Vermont | 3,332 | 0.19% |
| 25 | Massachusetts | 24,306 | 1.38% | 50 | New Hampshire | 2,751 | 0.16% |
|  |  |  |  |  | District of Columbia | 35,636 | 2.03% |

Source: American Hospital Association

"Hospital Statistics: A Comprehensive Summary of U.S. Hospitals 1991–1992" (Copyright, reprinted with permission)

# Admissions to Nonfederal Hospitals in 1990

## National Total = 32,014,516 Admissions

| RANK | STATE | ADMISSIONS | % | RANK | STATE | ADMISSIONS | % |
|------|-------|-----------|------|------|-------|-----------|------|
| 1 | California | 3,133,755 | 9.79% | 26 | Mississippi | 402,715 | 1.26% |
| 2 | New York | 2,378,558 | 7.43% | 27 | Oklahoma | 392,994 | 1.23% |
| 3 | Texas | 2,059,375 | 6.43% | 28 | Iowa | 389,857 | 1.22% |
| 4 | Pennsylvania | 1,843,129 | 5.76% | 29 | Connecticut | 366,676 | 1.15% |
| 5 | Florida | 1,678,039 | 5.24% | 30 | Arkansas | 351,200 | 1.10% |
| 6 | Illinois | 1,548,806 | 4.84% | 31 | Colorado | 345,199 | 1.08% |
| 7 | Ohio | 1,539,208 | 4.81% | 32 | Kansas | 312,664 | 0.98% |
| 8 | New Jersey | 1,153,355 | 3.60% | 33 | Oregon | 306,465 | 0.96% |
| 9 | Michigan | 1,087,936 | 3.40% | 34 | West Virginia | 282,175 | 0.88% |
| 10 | Georgia | 928,059 | 2.90% | 35 | Nebraska | 194,797 | 0.61% |
| 11 | Massachusetts | 848,012 | 2.65% | 36 | Utah | 180,168 | 0.56% |
| 12 | Tennessee | 817,526 | 2.55% | 37 | New Mexico | 160,010 | 0.50% |
| 13 | North Carolina | 812,778 | 2.54% | 38 | Maine | 150,345 | 0.47% |
| 14 | Missouri | 751,795 | 2.35% | 39 | New Hampshire | 135,551 | 0.42% |
| 15 | Indiana | 739,293 | 2.31% | 40 | Rhode Island | 131,066 | 0.41% |
| 16 | Virginia | 736,184 | 2.30% | 41 | Nevada | 120,843 | 0.38% |
| 17 | Louisiana | 624,155 | 1.95% | 42 | Montana | 105,534 | 0.33% |
| 18 | Wisconsin | 612,633 | 1.91% | 43 | North Dakota | 99,002 | 0.31% |
| 19 | Alabama | 605,253 | 1.89% | 44 | Idaho | 98,345 | 0.31% |
| 20 | Maryland | 578,804 | 1.81% | 45 | Hawaii | 97,962 | 0.31% |
| 21 | Kentucky | 545,143 | 1.70% | 46 | South Dakota | 95,106 | 0.30% |
| 22 | Minnesota | 540,082 | 1.69% | 47 | Delaware | 87,344 | 0.27% |
| 23 | Washington | 502,620 | 1.57% | 48 | Vermont | 59,438 | 0.19% |
| 24 | South Carolina | 424,816 | 1.33% | 49 | Wyoming | 49,079 | 0.15% |
| 25 | Arizona | 407,401 | 1.27% | 50 | Alaska | 39,159 | 0.12% |
| | | | | | District of Columbia | 164,107 | 0.51% |

Source: American Hospital Association
"Hospital Statistics: A Comprehensive Summary of U.S. Hospitals 1991-1992" (Copyright, reprinted with permission)

# Admissions to Psychiatric Hospitals in 1990

## National Total = 779,843 Admissions*

| RANK | STATE | ADMISSIONS | % | RANK | STATE | ADMISSIONS | % |
|---|---|---|---|---|---|---|---|
| 1 | Texas | 72,375 | 9.28% | 26 | New Jersey | 10,125 | 1.30% |
| 2 | California | 56,878 | 7.29% | 27 | Washington | 10,049 | 1.29% |
| 3 | New York | 51,082 | 6.55% | 28 | South Carolina | 9,446 | 1.21% |
| 4 | Pennsylvania | 48,926 | 6.27% | 29 | Connecticut | 8,127 | 1.04% |
| 5 | Georgia | 37,849 | 4.85% | 30 | Kansas | 7,992 | 1.02% |
| 6 | Illinois | 37,634 | 4.83% | 31 | Iowa | 7,688 | 0.99% |
| 7 | Florida | 34,102 | 4.37% | 32 | Mississippi | 6,726 | 0.86% |
| 8 | Ohio | 31,118 | 3.99% | 33 | New Mexico | 6,691 | 0.86% |
| 9 | North Carolina | 30,060 | 3.85% | 34 | West Virginia | 5,436 | 0.70% |
| 10 | Virginia | 27,640 | 3.54% | 35 | Nevada | 4,848 | 0.62% |
| 11 | Massachusetts | 26,624 | 3.41% | 36 | Nebraska | 4,830 | 0.62% |
| 12 | Michigan | 22,410 | 2.87% | 37 | Maine | 4,776 | 0.61% |
| 13 | Wisconsin | 18,683 | 2.40% | 38 | Utah | 4,696 | 0.60% |
| 14 | Tennessee | 17,786 | 2.28% | 39 | Oregon | 4,562 | 0.58% |
| 15 | Louisiana | 17,087 | 2.19% | 40 | Arkansas | 4,381 | 0.56% |
| 16 | Maryland | 15,452 | 1.98% | 41 | Rhode Island | 4,056 | 0.52% |
| 17 | Indiana | 14,063 | 1.80% | 42 | Delaware | 3,254 | 0.42% |
| 18 | Kentucky | 13,170 | 1.69% | 43 | Wyoming | 3,032 | 0.39% |
| 19 | Missouri | 12,903 | 1.65% | 44 | North Dakota | 3,019 | 0.39% |
| 20 | Alabama | 12,475 | 1.60% | 45 | Alaska | 1,958 | 0.25% |
| 21 | Minnesota | 12,423 | 1.59% | 46 | Vermont | 1,733 | 0.22% |
| 22 | Arizona | 10,979 | 1.41% | 47 | Idaho | 1,724 | 0.22% |
| 23 | Oklahoma | 10,875 | 1.39% | 48 | Hawaii | 811 | 0.10% |
| 24 | Colorado | 10,801 | 1.39% | 49 | South Dakota | 620 | 0.08% |
| 25 | New Hampshire | 10,633 | 1.36% | 50 | Montana | 73 | 0.01% |
| | | | | | District of Columbia | 5,162 | 0.66% |

Source: American Hospital Association
   "Hospital Statistics: A Comprehensive Summary of U.S. Hospitals 1991–1992" (Copyright, reprinted with permission)
*Admissions to federal and nonfederal psychiatric hospitals.

# Admissions to Community Hospitals in 1990

## National Total = 31,181,046 Admissions*

| RANK | STATE | ADMISSIONS | % | RANK | STATE | ADMISSIONS | % |
|---|---|---|---|---|---|---|---|
| 1 | California | 3,063,199 | 9.82% | 26 | Mississippi | 395,804 | 1.27% |
| 2 | New York | 2,321,509 | 7.45% | 27 | Iowa | 385,138 | 1.24% |
| 3 | Texas | 1,986,259 | 6.37% | 28 | Oklahoma | 381,928 | 1.22% |
| 4 | Pennsylvania | 1,796,054 | 5.76% | 29 | Connecticut | 355,057 | 1.14% |
| 5 | Florida | 1,638,871 | 5.26% | 30 | Arkansas | 346,819 | 1.11% |
| 6 | Ohio | 1,511,655 | 4.85% | 31 | Colorado | 334,781 | 1.07% |
| 7 | Illinois | 1,499,435 | 4.81% | 32 | Kansas | 304,551 | 0.98% |
| 8 | New Jersey | 1,131,509 | 3.63% | 33 | Oregon | 301,903 | 0.97% |
| 9 | Michigan | 1,069,361 | 3.43% | 34 | West Virginia | 276,739 | 0.89% |
| 10 | Georgia | 888,048 | 2.85% | 35 | Nebraska | 187,977 | 0.60% |
| 11 | Massachusetts | 810,991 | 2.60% | 36 | Utah | 175,472 | 0.56% |
| 12 | Tennessee | 798,172 | 2.56% | 37 | New Mexico | 153,319 | 0.49% |
| 13 | North Carolina | 784,414 | 2.52% | 38 | Maine | 145,569 | 0.47% |
| 14 | Missouri | 737,219 | 2.36% | 39 | Rhode Island | 126,730 | 0.41% |
| 15 | Indiana | 727,241 | 2.33% | 40 | New Hampshire | 124,532 | 0.40% |
| 16 | Virginia | 706,240 | 2.26% | 41 | Nevada | 115,995 | 0.37% |
| 17 | Louisiana | 606,863 | 1.95% | 42 | Montana | 105,405 | 0.34% |
| 18 | Alabama | 597,023 | 1.91% | 43 | Idaho | 96,621 | 0.31% |
| 19 | Wisconsin | 596,654 | 1.91% | 44 | North Dakota | 95,983 | 0.31% |
| 20 | Maryland | 562,280 | 1.80% | 45 | Hawaii | 95,958 | 0.31% |
| 21 | Kentucky | 531,817 | 1.71% | 46 | South Dakota | 94,421 | 0.30% |
| 22 | Minnesota | 529,744 | 1.70% | 47 | Delaware | 84,090 | 0.27% |
| 23 | Washington | 491,518 | 1.58% | 48 | Vermont | 57,705 | 0.19% |
| 24 | South Carolina | 413,045 | 1.32% | 49 | Wyoming | 47,973 | 0.15% |
| 25 | Arizona | 396,422 | 1.27% | 50 | Alaska | 37,201 | 0.12% |
| | | | | | District of Columbia | 157,832 | 0.51% |

Source: American Hospital Association

*"Hospital Statistics: A Comprehensive Summary of U.S. Hospitals 1991-1992"* (Copyright, reprinted with permission)

*Community hospital admissions are a subset of nonfederal hospital admissions.

# Admissions to Nongovernment Not-For-Profit Hospitals in 1990

## National Total = 22,878,443 Admissions*

| RANK | STATE | ADMISSIONS | % | RANK | STATE | ADMISSIONS | % |
|------|-------|-----------|------|------|-------|-----------|------|
| 1 | California | 1,980,635 | 8.66% | 26 | Oregon | 248,317 | 1.09% |
| 2 | New York | 1,903,142 | 8.32% | 27 | Colorado | 242,688 | 1.06% |
| 3 | Pennsylvania | 1,777,967 | 7.77% | 28 | Alabama | 240,682 | 1.05% |
| 4 | Ohio | 1,377,313 | 6.02% | 29 | Arkansas | 231,472 | 1.01% |
| 5 | Illinois | 1,349,604 | 5.90% | 30 | Oklahoma | 220,818 | 0.97% |
| 6 | New Jersey | 1,111,343 | 4.86% | 31 | South Carolina | 216,692 | 0.95% |
| 7 | Texas | 988,368 | 4.32% | 32 | West Virginia | 214,566 | 0.94% |
| 8 | Michigan | 967,620 | 4.23% | 33 | Kansas | 191,328 | 0.84% |
| 9 | Florida | 853,549 | 3.73% | 34 | Mississippi | 163,415 | 0.71% |
| 10 | Massachusetts | 743,211 | 3.25% | 35 | Maine | 134,747 | 0.59% |
| 11 | Missouri | 600,520 | 2.62% | 36 | Nebraska | 133,841 | 0.59% |
| 12 | Wisconsin | 560,107 | 2.45% | 37 | Rhode Island | 126,730 | 0.55% |
| 13 | Maryland | 540,955 | 2.36% | 38 | Utah | 120,460 | 0.53% |
| 14 | Virginia | 519,277 | 2.27% | 39 | New Hampshire | 113,633 | 0.50% |
| 15 | Indiana | 513,314 | 2.24% | 40 | Montana | 98,961 | 0.43% |
| 16 | North Carolina | 487,946 | 2.13% | 41 | North Dakota | 95,164 | 0.42% |
| 17 | Tennessee | 477,683 | 2.09% | 42 | South Dakota | 89,782 | 0.39% |
| 18 | Minnesota | 424,214 | 1.85% | 43 | New Mexico | 86,160 | 0.38% |
| 19 | Washington | 366,137 | 1.60% | 44 | Delaware | 84,090 | 0.37% |
| 20 | Kentucky | 360,314 | 1.57% | 45 | Hawaii | 67,496 | 0.30% |
| 21 | Connecticut | 349,123 | 1.53% | 46 | Vermont | 57,705 | 0.25% |
| 22 | Georgia | 323,629 | 1.41% | 47 | Idaho | 47,060 | 0.21% |
| 23 | Arizona | 323,151 | 1.41% | 48 | Nevada | 37,590 | 0.16% |
| 24 | Iowa | 269,991 | 1.18% | 49 | Alaska | 25,075 | 0.11% |
| 25 | Louisiana | 261,494 | 1.14% | 50 | Wyoming | 15,576 | 0.07% |
| | | | | | District of Columbia | 143,788 | 0.63% |

Source: American Hospital Association
   "Hospital Statistics: A Comprehensive Summary of U.S. Hospitals 1991-1992" (Copyright, reprinted with permission)
*Nongovernment not-for-profit hospital admissions are a subset of community hospital admissions.

# Admissions to Investor-Owned (For-Profit) Hospitals in 1990

## National Total = 3,066,198 Admissions*

| RANK | STATE | ADMISSIONS | % | RANK | STATE | ADMISSIONS | % |
|------|-------|-----------|------|------|-------|-----------|------|
| 1 | Texas | 543,951 | 17.74% | 26 | Maryland | 21,325 | 0.70% |
| 2 | Florida | 508,206 | 16.57% | 27 | Washington | 20,334 | 0.66% |
| 3 | California | 468,047 | 15.26% | 28 | Oregon | 17,246 | 0.56% |
| 4 | Georgia | 148,868 | 4.86% | 29 | Idaho | 14,550 | 0.47% |
| 5 | Tennessee | 140,841 | 4.59% | 30 | New Hampshire | 10,899 | 0.36% |
| 6 | Louisiana | 124,881 | 4.07% | 31 | Nebraska | 10,831 | 0.35% |
| 7 | Alabama | 117,859 | 3.84% | 32 | Hawaii | 7,644 | 0.25% |
| 8 | Kentucky | 106,346 | 3.47% | 33 | Pennsylvania | 7,236 | 0.24% |
| 9 | Virginia | 100,716 | 3.28% | 34 | Alaska | 6,462 | 0.21% |
| 10 | New York | 87,537 | 2.85% | 35 | Massachusetts | 5,607 | 0.18% |
| 11 | South Carolina | 57,673 | 1.88% | 36 | Wyoming | 4,535 | 0.15% |
| 12 | Nevada | 50,114 | 1.63% | 37 | Iowa | 3,750 | 0.12% |
| 13 | Arkansas | 47,656 | 1.55% | 38 | New Jersey | 3,425 | 0.11% |
| 14 | North Carolina | 45,007 | 1.47% | 39 | Ohio | 966 | 0.03% |
| 15 | Missouri | 44,759 | 1.46% | 40 | Michigan | 937 | 0.03% |
| 16 | Kansas | 39,988 | 1.30% | 41 | Montana | 655 | 0.02% |
| 17 | Mississippi | 38,365 | 1.25% | 42 | Connecticut | 0 | 0.00% |
| 18 | Oklahoma | 37,554 | 1.22% | 42 | Delaware | 0 | 0.00% |
| 19 | Arizona | 36,445 | 1.19% | 42 | Maine | 0 | 0.00% |
| 20 | Illinois | 35,686 | 1.16% | 42 | Minnesota | 0 | 0.00% |
| 21 | Colorado | 35,348 | 1.15% | 42 | North Dakota | 0 | 0.00% |
| 22 | Utah | 34,795 | 1.13% | 42 | Rhode Island | 0 | 0.00% |
| 23 | West Virginia | 32,557 | 1.06% | 42 | South Dakota | 0 | 0.00% |
| 24 | New Mexico | 23,516 | 0.77% | 42 | Vermont | 0 | 0.00% |
| 25 | Indiana | 23,081 | 0.75% | 42 | Wisconsin | 0 | 0.00% |
| | | | | | District of Columbia | 0 | 0.00% |

Source: American Hospital Association

*"Hospital Statistics: A Comprehensive Summary of U.S. Hospitals 1991-1992"* (Copyright, reprinted with permission)

*Investor-owned (for-profit) hospital admissions are a subset of community hospital admissions.*

# Admissions to State and Local Government-Owned Hospitals in 1990

## National Total = 5,236,405 Admissions*

| RANK | STATE | ADMISSIONS | % | RANK | STATE | ADMISSIONS | % |
|---|---|---|---|---|---|---|---|
| 1 | California | 614,517 | 11.74% | 26 | Colorado | 56,745 | 1.08% |
| 2 | Texas | 453,940 | 8.67% | 27 | New Mexico | 43,643 | 0.83% |
| 3 | Georgia | 415,551 | 7.94% | 28 | Nebraska | 43,305 | 0.83% |
| 4 | New York | 330,830 | 6.32% | 29 | Arizona | 36,826 | 0.70% |
| 5 | Florida | 277,116 | 5.29% | 30 | Wisconsin | 36,547 | 0.70% |
| 6 | North Carolina | 251,461 | 4.80% | 31 | Oregon | 36,340 | 0.69% |
| 7 | Alabama | 238,482 | 4.55% | 32 | Idaho | 35,011 | 0.67% |
| 8 | Louisiana | 220,488 | 4.21% | 33 | West Virginia | 29,616 | 0.57% |
| 9 | Mississippi | 194,024 | 3.71% | 34 | Nevada | 28,291 | 0.54% |
| 10 | Indiana | 190,846 | 3.64% | 35 | Wyoming | 27,862 | 0.53% |
| 11 | Tennessee | 179,648 | 3.43% | 36 | Hawaii | 20,818 | 0.40% |
| 12 | South Carolina | 138,680 | 2.65% | 37 | Utah | 20,217 | 0.39% |
| 13 | Ohio | 133,376 | 2.55% | 38 | New Jersey | 16,741 | 0.32% |
| 14 | Oklahoma | 123,556 | 2.36% | 39 | Pennsylvania | 10,851 | 0.21% |
| 15 | Illinois | 114,145 | 2.18% | 40 | Maine | 10,822 | 0.21% |
| 16 | Iowa | 111,397 | 2.13% | 41 | Connecticut | 5,934 | 0.11% |
| 17 | Minnesota | 105,530 | 2.02% | 42 | Montana | 5,789 | 0.11% |
| 18 | Washington | 105,047 | 2.01% | 43 | Alaska | 5,664 | 0.11% |
| 19 | Michigan | 100,804 | 1.93% | 44 | South Dakota | 4,639 | 0.09% |
| 20 | Missouri | 91,940 | 1.76% | 45 | North Dakota | 819 | 0.02% |
| 21 | Virginia | 86,247 | 1.65% | 46 | Delaware | 0 | 0.00% |
| 22 | Kansas | 73,235 | 1.40% | 46 | Maryland | 0 | 0.00% |
| 23 | Arkansas | 67,691 | 1.29% | 46 | New Hampshire | 0 | 0.00% |
| 24 | Kentucky | 65,157 | 1.24% | 46 | Rhode Island | 0 | 0.00% |
| 25 | Massachusetts | 62,173 | 1.19% | 46 | Vermont | 0 | 0.00% |
| | | | | | District of Columbia | 14,044 | 0.27% |

*Source: American Hospital Association*

   *"Hospital Statistics: A Comprehensive Summary of U.S. Hospitals 1991-1992" (Copyright, reprinted with permission)*

*State and local government-owned hospital admissions are a subset of community hospital admissions.*

# Average Stay in Community Hospitals in 1990

## National Average = 7.2 Days*

| RANK | STATE | DAYS | | RANK | STATE | DAYS |
|------|-------|------|---|------|-------|------|
| 1 | North Dakota | 10.8 | | 24 | Mississippi | 7.1 |
| 2 | New York | 10.1 | | 27 | Florida | 7.0 |
| 2 | South Dakota | 10.1 | | 27 | South Carolina | 7.0 |
| 4 | Montana | 9.8 | | 27 | Virginia | 7.0 |
| 5 | Nebraska | 9.6 | | 27 | West Virginia | 7.0 |
| 6 | Hawaii | 9.3 | | 31 | Georgia | 6.9 |
| 7 | Minnesota | 8.9 | | 31 | Maryland | 6.9 |
| 8 | Wyoming | 8.8 | | 31 | Oklahoma | 6.9 |
| 9 | Iowa | 8.3 | | 31 | Tennessee | 6.9 |
| 10 | Maine | 8.1 | | 35 | New Hampshire | 6.8 |
| 11 | Kansas | 7.9 | | 36 | Delaware | 6.7 |
| 12 | Pennsylvania | 7.8 | | 36 | Idaho | 6.7 |
| 13 | Connecticut | 7.6 | | 36 | Kentucky | 6.7 |
| 13 | Michigan | 7.6 | | 36 | Ohio | 6.7 |
| 15 | New Jersey | 7.5 | | 40 | Indiana | 6.6 |
| 15 | North Carolina | 7.5 | | 40 | Louisiana | 6.6 |
| 17 | Illinois | 7.4 | | 42 | Nevada | 6.4 |
| 17 | Missouri | 7.4 | | 43 | Texas | 6.2 |
| 17 | Wisconsin | 7.4 | | 44 | California | 6.1 |
| 20 | Massachusetts | 7.3 | | 45 | Alaska | 5.8 |
| 20 | Rhode Island | 7.3 | | 46 | Arizona | 5.7 |
| 20 | Vermont | 7.3 | | 46 | New Mexico | 5.7 |
| 23 | Colorado | 7.2 | | 48 | Oregon | 5.5 |
| 24 | Alabama | 7.1 | | 48 | Washington | 5.5 |
| 24 | Arkansas | 7.1 | | 50 | Utah | 5.4 |
| | | | | | District of Columbia | 7.9 |

*Source: American Hospital Association*

  *"Hospital Statistics: A Comprehensive Summary of U.S. Hospitals 1991–1992" (Copyright, reprinted with permission)*

*\*Community hospitals are a subset of nonfederal hospitals.*

160

# Surgical Operations in Hospitals in 1990

## National Total = 23,091,324 Surgical Operations*

| RANK | STATE | OPERATIONS | % | RANK | STATE | OPERATIONS | % |
|---|---|---|---|---|---|---|---|
| 1 | California | 2,062,025 | 8.93% | 26 | Colorado | 304,852 | 1.32% |
| 2 | New York | 1,646,357 | 7.13% | 27 | Oklahoma | 279,690 | 1.21% |
| 3 | Texas | 1,454,729 | 6.30% | 28 | Arizona | 271,844 | 1.18% |
| 4 | Pennsylvania | 1,420,281 | 6.15% | 29 | Connecticut | 270,179 | 1.17% |
| 5 | Florida | 1,187,758 | 5.14% | 30 | Oregon | 255,765 | 1.11% |
| 6 | Ohio | 1,118,600 | 4.84% | 31 | Arkansas | 225,697 | 0.98% |
| 7 | Illinois | 1,058,198 | 4.58% | 32 | Mississippi | 224,412 | 0.97% |
| 8 | Michigan | 911,809 | 3.95% | 33 | West Virginia | 223,111 | 0.97% |
| 9 | New Jersey | 683,356 | 2.96% | 34 | Kansas | 215,820 | 0.93% |
| 10 | Georgia | 626,828 | 2.71% | 35 | Nebraska | 177,784 | 0.77% |
| 11 | Massachusetts | 624,164 | 2.70% | 36 | Utah | 146,341 | 0.63% |
| 12 | North Carolina | 599,526 | 2.60% | 37 | New Mexico | 132,804 | 0.58% |
| 13 | Missouri | 594,340 | 2.57% | 38 | Rhode Island | 118,830 | 0.51% |
| 14 | Indiana | 587,363 | 2.54% | 39 | Maine | 110,978 | 0.48% |
| 15 | Tennessee | 549,897 | 2.38% | 40 | Nevada | 92,617 | 0.40% |
| 16 | Virginia | 522,145 | 2.26% | 41 | New Hampshire | 86,285 | 0.37% |
| 17 | Maryland | 516,127 | 2.24% | 42 | Delaware | 80,506 | 0.35% |
| 18 | Wisconsin | 474,664 | 2.06% | 43 | Idaho | 75,730 | 0.33% |
| 19 | Washington | 409,206 | 1.77% | 44 | North Dakota | 72,426 | 0.31% |
| 20 | Kentucky | 401,478 | 1.74% | 45 | Hawaii | 71,303 | 0.31% |
| 21 | Louisiana | 397,451 | 1.72% | 46 | South Dakota | 64,390 | 0.28% |
| 22 | Alabama | 394,335 | 1.71% | 47 | Montana | 62,881 | 0.27% |
| 23 | Minnesota | 388,098 | 1.68% | 48 | Vermont | 39,888 | 0.17% |
| 24 | Iowa | 327,565 | 1.42% | 49 | Wyoming | 38,481 | 0.17% |
| 25 | South Carolina | 325,867 | 1.41% | 50 | Alaska | 35,442 | 0.15% |
| | | | | | District of Columbia | 131,101 | 0.57% |

Source: American Hospital Association
"Hospital Statistics: A Comprehensive Summary of U.S. Hospitals 1991-1992" (Copyright, reprinted with permission)
*In federal and nonfederal hospitals.

# Emergency Outpatient Visits to Hospitals in 1990

## National Total = 92,080,647 Visits*

| RANK | STATE | VISITS | % | RANK | STATE | VISITS | % |
|---|---|---|---|---|---|---|---|
| 1 | California | 9,125,587 | 9.91% | 26 | Minnesota | 1,211,253 | 1.32% |
| 2 | New York | 6,991,334 | 7.59% | 27 | Oklahoma | 1,104,605 | 1.20% |
| 3 | Texas | 5,251,840 | 5.70% | 28 | Mississippi | 1,030,334 | 1.12% |
| 4 | Pennsylvania | 5,169,721 | 5.61% | 29 | Colorado | 1,022,152 | 1.11% |
| 5 | Ohio | 4,690,029 | 5.09% | 30 | West Virginia | 990,553 | 1.08% |
| 6 | Florida | 4,673,858 | 5.08% | 31 | Oregon | 965,701 | 1.05% |
| 7 | Illinois | 4,212,719 | 4.58% | 32 | Arkansas | 955,373 | 1.04% |
| 8 | Michigan | 3,386,794 | 3.68% | 33 | Iowa | 943,867 | 1.03% |
| 9 | Georgia | 3,041,183 | 3.30% | 34 | Kansas | 792,239 | 0.86% |
| 10 | Massachusetts | 2,804,197 | 3.05% | 35 | Maine | 621,369 | 0.67% |
| 11 | North Carolina | 2,574,069 | 2.80% | 36 | Utah | 577,111 | 0.63% |
| 12 | New Jersey | 2,471,373 | 2.68% | 37 | Rhode Island | 515,246 | 0.56% |
| 13 | Virginia | 2,295,431 | 2.49% | 38 | New Mexico | 508,164 | 0.55% |
| 14 | Tennessee | 2,266,720 | 2.46% | 39 | New Hampshire | 488,654 | 0.53% |
| 15 | Indiana | 2,062,479 | 2.24% | 40 | Nevada | 415,192 | 0.45% |
| 16 | Missouri | 1,905,011 | 2.07% | 41 | Nebraska | 398,580 | 0.43% |
| 17 | Louisiana | 1,817,352 | 1.97% | 42 | Hawaii | 325,820 | 0.35% |
| 18 | Alabama | 1,719,490 | 1.87% | 43 | Idaho | 299,461 | 0.33% |
| 19 | Washington | 1,710,384 | 1.86% | 44 | Delaware | 269,623 | 0.29% |
| 20 | Kentucky | 1,649,666 | 1.79% | 45 | Montana | 255,859 | 0.28% |
| 21 | Maryland | 1,569,730 | 1.70% | 46 | Alaska | 238,978 | 0.26% |
| 22 | Wisconsin | 1,533,039 | 1.66% | 47 | North Dakota | 207,896 | 0.23% |
| 23 | South Carolina | 1,429,520 | 1.55% | 48 | South Dakota | 207,710 | 0.23% |
| 24 | Arizona | 1,288,766 | 1.40% | 49 | Vermont | 196,133 | 0.21% |
| 25 | Connecticut | 1,270,172 | 1.38% | 50 | Wyoming | 181,704 | 0.20% |
| | | | | | District of Columbia | 446,606 | 0.49% |

Source: American Hospital Association
"Hospital Statistics: A Comprehensive Summary of U.S. Hospitals 1991-1992" (Copyright, reprinted with permission)
*To federal and nonfederal hospitals.

# Medicare or Medicaid Certified Nursing Care Facilities in 1991

## National Total = 15,913 Facilities

| RANK | STATE | FACILITIES | % | RANK | STATE | FACILITIES | % |
|------|-------|-----------|------|------|-------|-----------|------|
| 1 | California | 1,290 | 8.11% | 26 | Connecticut | 240 | 1.51% |
| 2 | Texas | 1,127 | 7.08% | 27 | Nebraska | 237 | 1.49% |
| 3 | Ohio | 988 | 6.21% | 28 | Alabama | 219 | 1.38% |
| 4 | Illinois | 792 | 4.98% | 29 | Maryland | 217 | 1.36% |
| 5 | Pennsylvania | 690 | 4.34% | 30 | Colorado | 204 | 1.28% |
| 6 | New York | 619 | 3.89% | 31 | Oregon | 176 | 1.11% |
| 7 | Indiana | 590 | 3.71% | 32 | Mississippi | 162 | 1.02% |
| 8 | Florida | 554 | 3.48% | 33 | South Carolina | 147 | 0.92% |
| 9 | Massachusetts | 540 | 3.39% | 34 | Maine | 146 | 0.92% |
| 10 | Minnesota | 472 | 2.97% | 35 | Arizona | 132 | 0.83% |
| 11 | Missouri | 469 | 2.95% | 36 | West Virginia | 122 | 0.77% |
| 12 | Iowa | 463 | 2.91% | 37 | South Dakota | 118 | 0.74% |
| 13 | Michigan | 439 | 2.76% | 38 | Rhode Island | 100 | 0.63% |
| 14 | Wisconsin | 418 | 2.63% | 39 | Montana | 99 | 0.62% |
| 15 | Kansas | 415 | 2.61% | 40 | Utah | 90 | 0.57% |
| 16 | Oklahoma | 409 | 2.57% | 41 | North Dakota | 83 | 0.52% |
| 17 | Georgia | 364 | 2.29% | 42 | New Hampshire | 76 | 0.48% |
| 18 | Louisiana | 327 | 2.05% | 43 | New Mexico | 71 | 0.45% |
| 19 | North Carolina | 320 | 2.01% | 44 | Idaho | 70 | 0.44% |
| 20 | New Jersey | 306 | 1.92% | 45 | Vermont | 48 | 0.30% |
| 21 | Tennessee | 300 | 1.89% | 46 | Hawaii | 43 | 0.27% |
| 22 | Washington | 287 | 1.80% | 47 | Delaware | 41 | 0.26% |
| 23 | Kentucky | 282 | 1.77% | 48 | Wyoming | 38 | 0.24% |
| 24 | Virginia | 258 | 1.62% | 49 | Nevada | 36 | 0.23% |
| 25 | Arkansas | 248 | 1.56% | 50 | Alaska | 15 | 0.09% |
| | | | | | District of Columbia | 16 | 0.10% |

Source: U.S. Department of Health and Human Services, Health Care Financing Administration and the U.S. Bureau of the Census unpublished data

*Source: U.S. Department of Health and Human Services, Health Care Financing Administration and the U.S. Bureau of the Census unpublished data*

# Medicare Certified Nursing Care Facilities in 1991

## National Total = 9,453 Medicare Facilities

| RANK | STATE | FACILITIES | % | RANK | STATE | FACILITIES | % |
|---|---|---|---|---|---|---|---|
| 1 | California | 1,125 | 11.90% | 26 | Arizona | 128 | 1.35% |
| 2 | Pennsylvania | 610 | 6.45% | 27 | Oregon | 108 | 1.14% |
| 3 | New York | 581 | 6.15% | 28 | Montana | 90 | 0.95% |
| 4 | Ohio | 552 | 5.84% | 29 | Kansas | 84 | 0.89% |
| 5 | Florida | 490 | 5.18% | 30 | Louisiana | 80 | 0.85% |
| 6 | Illinois | 407 | 4.31% | 31 | Rhode Island | 71 | 0.75% |
| 7 | Texas | 403 | 4.26% | 32 | Idaho | 70 | 0.74% |
| 8 | Minnesota | 381 | 4.03% | 33 | North Dakota | 67 | 0.71% |
| 9 | Massachusetts | 346 | 3.66% | 34 | West Virginia | 60 | 0.63% |
| 10 | Michigan | 319 | 3.37% | 35 | Utah | 59 | 0.62% |
| 11 | Missouri | 279 | 2.95% | 36 | Iowa | 57 | 0.60% |
| 12 | North Carolina | 275 | 2.91% | 37 | Nebraska | 50 | 0.53% |
| 13 | Indiana | 263 | 2.78% | 38 | Arkansas | 47 | 0.50% |
| 14 | New Jersey | 227 | 2.40% | 39 | Mississippi | 44 | 0.47% |
| 15 | Georgia | 216 | 2.28% | 40 | Oklahoma | 37 | 0.39% |
| 16 | Alabama | 208 | 2.20% | 41 | Delaware | 34 | 0.36% |
| 17 | Wisconsin | 205 | 2.17% | 41 | Nevada | 34 | 0.36% |
| 18 | Connecticut | 190 | 2.01% | 43 | South Dakota | 31 | 0.33% |
| 19 | Washington | 181 | 1.91% | 44 | Hawaii | 30 | 0.32% |
| 20 | Maryland | 166 | 1.76% | 45 | Wyoming | 26 | 0.28% |
| 21 | Colorado | 159 | 1.68% | 46 | New Mexico | 24 | 0.25% |
| 22 | Kentucky | 145 | 1.53% | 47 | Maine | 23 | 0.24% |
| 22 | Tennessee | 145 | 1.53% | 48 | Vermont | 21 | 0.22% |
| 24 | Virginia | 139 | 1.47% | 49 | New Hampshire | 18 | 0.19% |
| 25 | South Carolina | 129 | 1.36% | 50 | Alaska | 8 | 0.08% |
| | | | | | District of Columbia | 11 | 0.12% |

Source: U.S. Department of Health and Human Services, Health Care Financing Administration and the U.S. Bureau of the Census
unpublished data

# Medicaid Certified Nursing Care Facilities in 1991

## National Total = 6,460 Medicaid Facilities

| RANK | STATE | FACILITIES | % | RANK | STATE | FACILITIES | % |
|------|-------|-----------|------|------|-------|-----------|------|
| 1 | Texas | 724 | 11.21% | 26 | New Jersey | 79 | 1.22% |
| 2 | Ohio | 436 | 6.75% | 27 | Oregon | 68 | 1.05% |
| 3 | Iowa | 406 | 6.28% | 28 | Florida | 64 | 0.99% |
| 4 | Illinois | 385 | 5.96% | 29 | West Virginia | 62 | 0.96% |
| 5 | Oklahoma | 372 | 5.76% | 30 | New Hampshire | 58 | 0.90% |
| 6 | Kansas | 331 | 5.12% | 31 | Maryland | 51 | 0.79% |
| 7 | Indiana | 327 | 5.06% | 32 | Connecticut | 50 | 0.77% |
| 8 | Louisiana | 247 | 3.82% | 33 | New Mexico | 47 | 0.73% |
| 9 | Wisconsin | 213 | 3.30% | 34 | Colorado | 45 | 0.70% |
| 10 | Arkansas | 201 | 3.11% | 34 | North Carolina | 45 | 0.70% |
| 11 | Massachusetts | 194 | 3.00% | 36 | New York | 38 | 0.59% |
| 12 | Missouri | 190 | 2.94% | 37 | Utah | 31 | 0.48% |
| 13 | Nebraska | 187 | 2.89% | 38 | Rhode Island | 29 | 0.45% |
| 14 | California | 165 | 2.55% | 39 | Vermont | 27 | 0.42% |
| 15 | Tennessee | 155 | 2.40% | 40 | South Carolina | 18 | 0.28% |
| 16 | Georgia | 148 | 2.29% | 41 | North Dakota | 16 | 0.25% |
| 17 | Kentucky | 137 | 2.12% | 42 | Hawaii | 13 | 0.20% |
| 18 | Maine | 123 | 1.90% | 43 | Wyoming | 12 | 0.19% |
| 19 | Michigan | 120 | 1.86% | 44 | Alabama | 11 | 0.17% |
| 20 | Virginia | 119 | 1.84% | 45 | Montana | 9 | 0.14% |
| 21 | Mississippi | 118 | 1.83% | 46 | Alaska | 7 | 0.11% |
| 22 | Washington | 106 | 1.64% | 46 | Delaware | 7 | 0.11% |
| 23 | Minnesota | 91 | 1.41% | 48 | Arizona | 4 | 0.06% |
| 24 | South Dakota | 87 | 1.35% | 49 | Nevada | 2 | 0.03% |
| 25 | Pennsylvania | 80 | 1.24% | 50 | Idaho | 0 | 0.00% |
|  |  |  |  |  | District of Columbia | 5 | 0.08% |

Source: U.S. Department of Health and Human Services, Health Care Financing Administration and the U.S. Bureau of the Census
unpublished data

# Beds in Certified Nursing Care Facilities in 1991

## National Total = 1,690,481 Beds*

| RANK | STATE | BEDS | % | RANK | STATE | BEDS | % |
|---|---|---|---|---|---|---|---|
| 1 | California | 132,032 | 7.81% | 26 | Arkansas | 26,338 | 1.56% |
| 2 | Texas | 115,148 | 6.81% | 27 | Kentucky | 24,211 | 1.43% |
| 3 | New York | 103,516 | 6.12% | 28 | Alabama | 22,289 | 1.32% |
| 4 | Illinois | 100,587 | 5.95% | 29 | Colorado | 19,854 | 1.17% |
| 5 | Ohio | 92,518 | 5.47% | 30 | Nebraska | 18,464 | 1.09% |
| 6 | Pennsylvania | 88,591 | 5.24% | 31 | Arizona | 15,595 | 0.92% |
| 7 | Florida | 65,837 | 3.89% | 32 | Oregon | 15,165 | 0.90% |
| 8 | Indiana | 64,263 | 3.80% | 33 | Mississippi | 14,691 | 0.87% |
| 9 | Massachusetts | 51,594 | 3.05% | 34 | South Carolina | 14,099 | 0.83% |
| 10 | Michigan | 49,927 | 2.95% | 35 | West Virginia | 10,849 | 0.64% |
| 11 | Wisconsin | 49,297 | 2.92% | 36 | Maine | 10,080 | 0.60% |
| 12 | Minnesota | 48,403 | 2.86% | 37 | Rhode Island | 9,808 | 0.58% |
| 13 | Missouri | 47,446 | 2.81% | 38 | South Dakota | 8,530 | 0.50% |
| 14 | Iowa | 44,950 | 2.66% | 39 | New Hampshire | 7,321 | 0.43% |
| 15 | New Jersey | 44,317 | 2.62% | 40 | North Dakota | 7,123 | 0.42% |
| 16 | Georgia | 38,528 | 2.28% | 41 | Montana | 7,056 | 0.42% |
| 17 | Louisiana | 36,681 | 2.17% | 42 | Utah | 6,913 | 0.41% |
| 18 | Tennessee | 35,551 | 2.10% | 43 | New Mexico | 6,558 | 0.39% |
| 19 | Oklahoma | 33,758 | 2.00% | 44 | Idaho | 5,659 | 0.33% |
| 20 | Virginia | 30,989 | 1.83% | 45 | Delaware | 4,471 | 0.26% |
| 21 | Kansas | 29,767 | 1.76% | 46 | Vermont | 3,585 | 0.21% |
| 22 | North Carolina | 29,658 | 1.75% | 47 | Hawaii | 3,505 | 0.21% |
| 23 | Connecticut | 28,669 | 1.70% | 48 | Nevada | 3,497 | 0.21% |
| 24 | Washington | 28,256 | 1.67% | 49 | Wyoming | 2,859 | 0.17% |
| 25 | Maryland | 27,665 | 1.64% | 50 | Alaska | 875 | 0.05% |
| | | | | | District of Columbia | 3,138 | 0.19% |

*Source: U.S. Department of Health and Human Services, Health Care Financing Administration and the U.S. Bureau of the Census unpublished data*

*Beds in Medicare or Medicaid certified facilities.

# Beds in Certified Nursing Care Facilities per 1,000 Adults Age 65 and Older in 1991

## National Rate = 52.8 Beds per 1,000 Adults Age 65 and Older*

| RANK | STATE | RATE | RANK | STATE | RATE |
|---|---|---|---|---|---|
| 1 | Iowa | 108.3 | 26 | Vermont | 53.3 |
| 2 | Indiana | 92.2 | 27 | Delaware | 52.7 |
| 3 | Minnesota | 87.4 | 28 | Maryland | 51.5 |
| 4 | Kansas | 85.5 | 29 | Kentucky | 51.1 |
| 5 | South Dakota | 84.1 | 30 | Washington | 50.6 |
| 6 | Nebraska | 82.1 | 31 | Idaho | 48.2 |
| 7 | North Dakota | 80.8 | 31 | Pennsylvania | 48.2 |
| 8 | Oklahoma | 78.7 | 33 | Utah | 47.3 |
| 9 | Wisconsin | 76.1 | 34 | Michigan | 45.0 |
| 10 | Louisiana | 75.6 | 35 | Virginia | 44.9 |
| 11 | Arkansas | 72.4 | 36 | Mississippi | 43.9 |
| 12 | Illinois | 69.3 | 37 | New York | 43.0 |
| 13 | Montana | 69.2 | 38 | Alabama | 41.8 |
| 14 | Wyoming | 68.1 | 39 | New Jersey | 40.8 |
| 15 | Ohio | 65.6 | 39 | Oregon | 40.8 |
| 16 | Rhode Island | 64.9 | 41 | West Virginia | 40.7 |
| 17 | Missouri | 64.8 | 42 | California | 40.2 |
| 18 | Texas | 64.0 | 43 | New Mexico | 38.6 |
| 19 | Connecticut | 62.2 | 44 | Alaska | 38.4 |
| 20 | Massachusetts | 61.5 | 45 | North Carolina | 35.3 |
| 21 | Maine | 60.6 | 46 | South Carolina | 34.9 |
| 22 | Colorado | 59.8 | 47 | Arizona | 30.4 |
| 23 | Georgia | 55.6 | 48 | Nevada | 29.9 |
| 24 | Tennessee | 55.2 | 49 | Florida | 26.3 |
| 25 | New Hampshire | 55.0 | 50 | Hawaii | 26.2 |
| | | | | District of Columbia | 39.3 |

Source: U.S. Department of Health and Human Services, Health Care Financing Administration and the U.S. Bureau of the Census
   unpublished data

*Beds in Medicare or Medicaid certified facilities.

# Beds in Certified Nursing Care Facilities per 1,000 Adults Age 85 and Older in 1991

## National Rate = 499.3 Beds per 1,000 Adults Age 85 and Older*

| RANK | STATE | RATE | RANK | STATE | RATE |
|------|-------|------|------|-------|------|
| 1 | Alaska | 875.0 | 26 | Massachusetts | 515.9 |
| 2 | Indiana | 828.1 | 27 | New Hampshire | 501.4 |
| 3 | Iowa | 772.3 | 28 | Maine | 489.3 |
| 4 | Louisiana | 754.8 | 29 | Kentucky | 476.6 |
| 5 | Oklahoma | 680.6 | 30 | Nevada | 472.6 |
| 6 | Minnesota | 654.1 | 31 | Pennsylvania | 469.7 |
| 7 | Arkansas | 648.7 | 32 | Utah | 467.1 |
| 8 | Kansas | 644.3 | 33 | Washington | 460.2 |
| 9 | South Dakota | 636.6 | 34 | Idaho | 456.4 |
| 10 | Illinois | 631.0 | 35 | Virginia | 455.7 |
| 11 | North Dakota | 624.8 | 36 | Vermont | 437.2 |
| 12 | Texas | 621.1 | 37 | Michigan | 428.2 |
| 13 | Montana | 618.9 | 38 | New Jersey | 418.9 |
| 14 | Wisconsin | 614.7 | 39 | New Mexico | 415.1 |
| 15 | Ohio | 605.5 | 40 | Alabama | 409.7 |
| 16 | Nebraska | 584.3 | 41 | California | 402.0 |
| 17 | Rhode Island | 583.8 | 42 | Mississippi | 401.4 |
| 18 | Wyoming | 571.8 | 43 | New York | 393.0 |
| 19 | Georgia | 569.9 | 44 | South Carolina | 391.6 |
| 20 | Connecticut | 564.4 | 45 | West Virginia | 376.7 |
| 21 | Colorado | 560.8 | 46 | Arizona | 371.3 |
| 22 | Missouri | 539.2 | 47 | North Carolina | 369.8 |
| 23 | Delaware | 532.3 | 48 | Oregon | 362.8 |
| 24 | Tennessee | 524.4 | 49 | Hawaii | 324.5 |
| 25 | Maryland | 520.0 | 50 | Florida | 279.7 |
| | | | | District of Columbia | 373.6 |

Source: U.S. Department of Health and Human Services, Health Care Financing Administration and the U.S. Bureau of the Census
   unpublished data

*Beds in Medicare or Medicaid certified facilities.

# Nursing Home Population in 1990

## National Total = 1,772,032 Persons in Nursing Homes

| RANK | STATE | POPULATION | % |
|------|-------|------------|---|
| 1 | California | 148,362 | 8.37% |
| 2 | New York | 126,175 | 7.12% |
| 3 | Pennsylvania | 106,454 | 6.01% |
| 4 | Texas | 101,005 | 5.70% |
| 5 | Ohio | 93,769 | 5.29% |
| 6 | Illinois | 93,662 | 5.29% |
| 7 | Florida | 80,298 | 4.53% |
| 8 | Michigan | 57,622 | 3.25% |
| 9 | Massachusetts | 55,662 | 3.14% |
| 10 | Missouri | 52,060 | 2.94% |
| 11 | Indiana | 50,845 | 2.87% |
| 12 | Wisconsin | 50,345 | 2.84% |
| 13 | New Jersey | 47,054 | 2.66% |
| 14 | Minnesota | 47,051 | 2.66% |
| 15 | North Carolina | 47,014 | 2.65% |
| 16 | Virginia | 37,762 | 2.13% |
| 17 | Georgia | 36,549 | 2.06% |
| 18 | Iowa | 36,455 | 2.06% |
| 19 | Tennessee | 35,192 | 1.99% |
| 20 | Washington | 32,840 | 1.85% |
| 21 | Louisiana | 32,072 | 1.81% |
| 22 | Connecticut | 30,962 | 1.75% |
| 23 | Oklahoma | 29,666 | 1.67% |
| 24 | Kentucky | 27,874 | 1.57% |
| 25 | Maryland | 26,884 | 1.52% |

| RANK | STATE | POPULATION | % |
|------|-------|------------|---|
| 26 | Kansas | 26,155 | 1.48% |
| 27 | Alabama | 24,031 | 1.36% |
| 28 | Arkansas | 21,809 | 1.23% |
| 29 | Nebraska | 19,171 | 1.08% |
| 30 | Colorado | 18,506 | 1.04% |
| 31 | South Carolina | 18,228 | 1.03% |
| 32 | Oregon | 18,200 | 1.03% |
| 33 | Mississippi | 15,803 | 0.89% |
| 34 | Arizona | 14,472 | 0.82% |
| 35 | West Virginia | 12,591 | 0.71% |
| 36 | Rhode Island | 10,156 | 0.57% |
| 37 | Maine | 9,855 | 0.56% |
| 38 | South Dakota | 9,356 | 0.53% |
| 39 | New Hampshire | 8,202 | 0.46% |
| 40 | North Dakota | 8,159 | 0.46% |
| 41 | Montana | 7,764 | 0.44% |
| 42 | Idaho | 6,318 | 0.36% |
| 43 | New Mexico | 6,276 | 0.35% |
| 44 | Utah | 6,222 | 0.35% |
| 45 | Vermont | 4,809 | 0.27% |
| 46 | Delaware | 4,596 | 0.26% |
| 47 | Nevada | 3,605 | 0.20% |
| 48 | Hawaii | 3,225 | 0.18% |
| 49 | Wyoming | 2,679 | 0.15% |
| 50 | Alaska | 1,202 | 0.07% |

| | District of Columbia | 7,008 | 0.40% |

*Source: U.S. Bureau of the Census*
*unpublished data*

# Percent of Population in Nursing Homes in 1990

## National Rate = 0.71% of Population in Nursing Homes*

| RANK | STATE | PERCENT | RANK | STATE | PERCENT |
|------|-------|---------|------|-------|---------|
| 1 | South Dakota | 1.34 | 26 | New York | 0.70 |
| 2 | Iowa | 1.31 | 26 | West Virginia | 0.70 |
| 3 | North Dakota | 1.28 | 28 | Delaware | 0.69 |
| 4 | Nebraska | 1.21 | 29 | Washington | 0.67 |
| 5 | Minnesota | 1.08 | 30 | Oregon | 0.64 |
| 6 | Kansas | 1.06 | 31 | Idaho | 0.63 |
| 7 | Wisconsin | 1.03 | 32 | Florida | 0.62 |
| 8 | Missouri | 1.02 | 32 | Michigan | 0.62 |
| 9 | Rhode Island | 1.01 | 34 | Mississippi | 0.61 |
| 10 | Montana | 0.97 | 34 | New Jersey | 0.61 |
| 11 | Connecticut | 0.94 | 34 | Virginia | 0.61 |
| 11 | Oklahoma | 0.94 | 37 | Alabama | 0.59 |
| 13 | Arkansas | 0.93 | 37 | Texas | 0.59 |
| 13 | Massachusetts | 0.93 | 37 | Wyoming | 0.59 |
| 15 | Indiana | 0.92 | 40 | Colorado | 0.56 |
| 16 | Pennsylvania | 0.90 | 40 | Georgia | 0.56 |
| 17 | Ohio | 0.86 | 40 | Maryland | 0.56 |
| 18 | Vermont | 0.85 | 43 | South Carolina | 0.52 |
| 19 | Illinois | 0.82 | 44 | California | 0.50 |
| 20 | Maine | 0.80 | 45 | New Mexico | 0.41 |
| 21 | Kentucky | 0.76 | 46 | Arizona | 0.39 |
| 21 | Louisiana | 0.76 | 47 | Utah | 0.36 |
| 23 | New Hampshire | 0.74 | 48 | Nevada | 0.30 |
| 24 | Tennessee | 0.72 | 49 | Hawaii | 0.29 |
| 25 | North Carolina | 0.71 | 50 | Alaska | 0.22 |

District of Columbia     1.15

Source: U.S. Bureau of the Census
   unpublished data

*Rates calculated by the editors using 1990 Census resident population figures.

# Nursing Home Population in 1980

## National Total = 1,426,371 Persons in Nursing Homes

| RANK | STATE | POPULATION | % | RANK | STATE | POPULATION | % |
|---|---|---|---|---|---|---|---|
| 1 | California | 134,756 | 9.45% | 26 | Maryland | 19,821 | 1.39% |
| 2 | New York | 114,276 | 8.01% | 27 | Alabama | 18,702 | 1.31% |
| 3 | Texas | 89,275 | 6.26% | 28 | Arkansas | 18,631 | 1.31% |
| 4 | Illinois | 80,410 | 5.64% | 29 | Nebraska | 17,650 | 1.24% |
| 5 | Pennsylvania | 72,285 | 5.07% | 30 | Colorado | 16,109 | 1.13% |
| 6 | Ohio | 71,479 | 5.01% | 31 | Oregon | 16,052 | 1.13% |
| 7 | Michigan | 55,805 | 3.91% | 32 | Mississippi | 12,753 | 0.89% |
| 8 | Massachusetts | 49,728 | 3.49% | 33 | South Carolina | 11,666 | 0.82% |
| 9 | Wisconsin | 48,282 | 3.38% | 34 | Maine | 9,570 | 0.67% |
| 10 | Minnesota | 44,553 | 3.12% | 35 | Arizona | 8,424 | 0.59% |
| 11 | Indiana | 40,112 | 2.81% | 36 | Rhode Island | 8,146 | 0.57% |
| 12 | Missouri | 37,942 | 2.66% | 37 | South Dakota | 8,087 | 0.57% |
| 13 | Florida | 36,306 | 2.55% | 38 | North Dakota | 7,486 | 0.52% |
| 14 | Iowa | 36,217 | 2.54% | 39 | New Hampshire | 6,673 | 0.47% |
| 15 | New Jersey | 34,414 | 2.41% | 40 | West Virginia | 6,355 | 0.45% |
| 16 | North Carolina | 29,596 | 2.07% | 41 | Montana | 5,479 | 0.38% |
| 17 | Georgia | 29,376 | 2.06% | 42 | Idaho | 5,084 | 0.36% |
| 18 | Washington | 27,970 | 1.96% | 43 | Utah | 4,921 | 0.35% |
| 19 | Connecticut | 27,873 | 1.95% | 44 | Vermont | 4,354 | 0.31% |
| 20 | Oklahoma | 25,732 | 1.80% | 45 | Hawaii | 3,159 | 0.22% |
| 21 | Kansas | 24,545 | 1.72% | 46 | Delaware | 2,771 | 0.19% |
| 22 | Virginia | 24,323 | 1.71% | 47 | New Mexico | 2,585 | 0.18% |
| 23 | Kentucky | 23,591 | 1.65% | 48 | Nevada | 2,339 | 0.16% |
| 24 | Louisiana | 22,776 | 1.60% | 49 | Wyoming | 2,198 | 0.15% |
| 25 | Tennessee | 22,014 | 1.54% | 50 | Alaska | 854 | 0.06% |
| | | | | | District of Columbia | 2,866 | 0.20% |

Source: U.S. Bureau of the Census
"Nursing Homes Persons in Institutions and Other Group Quarters" (PC80-2-4D)

# Percent of Population in Nursing Homes in 1980

## National Rate = 0.63% of the Population in Nursing Homes*

| RANK | STATE | PERCENT | | RANK | STATE | PERCENT |
|------|-------|---------|---|------|-------|---------|
| 1 | Iowa | 1.24 | | 25 | Pennsylvania | 0.61 |
| 2 | South Dakota | 1.17 | | 27 | Michigan | 0.60 |
| 3 | North Dakota | 1.15 | | 28 | California | 0.57 |
| 4 | Nebraska | 1.12 | | 29 | Colorado | 0.56 |
| 5 | Minnesota | 1.09 | | 30 | Georgia | 0.54 |
| 6 | Kansas | 1.04 | | 30 | Idaho | 0.54 |
| 7 | Wisconsin | 1.03 | | 30 | Louisiana | 0.54 |
| 8 | Connecticut | 0.90 | | 33 | Mississippi | 0.51 |
| 9 | Massachusetts | 0.87 | | 34 | North Carolina | 0.50 |
| 10 | Rhode Island | 0.86 | | 35 | Alabama | 0.48 |
| 11 | Maine | 0.85 | | 35 | Tennessee | 0.48 |
| 11 | Oklahoma | 0.85 | | 37 | Delaware | 0.47 |
| 11 | Vermont | 0.85 | | 37 | Maryland | 0.47 |
| 14 | Arkansas | 0.81 | | 37 | New Jersey | 0.47 |
| 15 | Missouri | 0.77 | | 37 | Wyoming | 0.47 |
| 16 | Indiana | 0.73 | | 41 | Virginia | 0.45 |
| 17 | New Hampshire | 0.72 | | 42 | Florida | 0.37 |
| 18 | Illinois | 0.70 | | 42 | South Carolina | 0.37 |
| 18 | Montana | 0.70 | | 44 | Utah | 0.34 |
| 20 | Washington | 0.68 | | 45 | Hawaii | 0.33 |
| 21 | Ohio | 0.66 | | 45 | West Virginia | 0.33 |
| 22 | New York | 0.65 | | 47 | Arizona | 0.31 |
| 23 | Kentucky | 0.64 | | 48 | Nevada | 0.29 |
| 24 | Texas | 0.63 | | 49 | Alaska | 0.21 |
| 25 | Oregon | 0.61 | | 50 | New Mexico | 0.20 |

District of Columbia                                    0.45

Source: U.S. Bureau of the Census

  *"Nursing Homes Persons in Institutions and Other Group Quarters" (PC80-2-4D)*

*Rates calculated by the editors using 1980 Census resident population figures.*

# Change in Nursing Home Population: 1980 to 1990

## National Change = 345,661 Increase in Nursing Home Population

| RANK | STATE | INCREASE | % | RANK | STATE | INCREASE | % |
|---|---|---|---|---|---|---|---|
| 1 | Florida | 43,992 | 12.73% | 26 | Arkansas | 3,178 | 0.92% |
| 2 | Pennsylvania | 34,169 | 9.89% | 27 | Connecticut | 3,089 | 0.89% |
| 3 | Ohio | 22,290 | 6.45% | 28 | Mississippi | 3,050 | 0.88% |
| 4 | North Carolina | 17,418 | 5.04% | 29 | Minnesota | 2,498 | 0.72% |
| 5 | Missouri | 14,118 | 4.08% | 30 | Colorado | 2,397 | 0.69% |
| 6 | California | 13,606 | 3.94% | 31 | Montana | 2,285 | 0.66% |
| 7 | Virginia | 13,439 | 3.89% | 32 | Oregon | 2,148 | 0.62% |
| 8 | Illinois | 13,252 | 3.83% | 33 | Wisconsin | 2,063 | 0.60% |
| 9 | Tennessee | 13,178 | 3.81% | 34 | Rhode Island | 2,010 | 0.58% |
| 10 | New Jersey | 12,640 | 3.66% | 35 | Delaware | 1,825 | 0.53% |
| 11 | New York | 11,899 | 3.44% | 36 | Michigan | 1,817 | 0.53% |
| 12 | Texas | 11,730 | 3.39% | 37 | Kansas | 1,610 | 0.47% |
| 13 | Indiana | 10,733 | 3.11% | 38 | New Hampshire | 1,529 | 0.44% |
| 14 | Louisiana | 9,296 | 2.69% | 39 | Nebraska | 1,521 | 0.44% |
| 15 | Georgia | 7,173 | 2.08% | 40 | Utah | 1,301 | 0.38% |
| 16 | Maryland | 7,063 | 2.04% | 41 | South Dakota | 1,269 | 0.37% |
| 17 | South Carolina | 6,562 | 1.90% | 42 | Nevada | 1,266 | 0.37% |
| 18 | West Virginia | 6,236 | 1.80% | 43 | Idaho | 1,234 | 0.36% |
| 19 | Arizona | 6,048 | 1.75% | 44 | North Dakota | 673 | 0.19% |
| 20 | Massachusetts | 5,934 | 1.72% | 45 | Wyoming | 481 | 0.14% |
| 21 | Alabama | 5,329 | 1.54% | 46 | Vermont | 455 | 0.13% |
| 22 | Washington | 4,870 | 1.41% | 47 | Alaska | 348 | 0.10% |
| 23 | Kentucky | 4,283 | 1.24% | 48 | Maine | 285 | 0.08% |
| 24 | Oklahoma | 3,934 | 1.14% | 49 | Iowa | 238 | 0.07% |
| 25 | New Mexico | 3,691 | 1.07% | 50 | Hawaii | 66 | 0.02% |
| | | | | | District of Columbia | 4,142 | 1.20% |

*Source: U.S. Bureau of the Census*
*unpublished data*

# Percent Change in Nursing Home Population: 1980 to 1990

## National Percent Change = 24.2% Increase in Nursing Home Population*

| RANK | STATE | PERCENT INCREASE | RANK | STATE | PERCENT INCREASE |
|---|---|---|---|---|---|
| 1 | New Mexico | 142.8 | 26 | New Hampshire | 22.9 |
| 2 | Florida | 121.2 | 27 | Wyoming | 21.9 |
| 3 | West Virginia | 98.1 | 28 | Kentucky | 18.2 |
| 4 | Arizona | 71.8 | 29 | Washington | 17.4 |
| 5 | Delaware | 65.9 | 30 | Arkansas | 17.1 |
| 6 | Tennessee | 59.9 | 31 | Illinois | 16.5 |
| 7 | North Carolina | 58.9 | 32 | South Dakota | 15.7 |
| 8 | South Carolina | 56.2 | 33 | Oklahoma | 15.3 |
| 9 | Virginia | 55.3 | 34 | Colorado | 14.9 |
| 10 | Nevada | 54.1 | 35 | Oregon | 13.4 |
| 11 | Pennsylvania | 47.3 | 36 | Texas | 13.1 |
| 12 | Montana | 41.7 | 37 | Massachusetts | 11.9 |
| 13 | Louisiana | 40.8 | 38 | Connecticut | 11.1 |
| 14 | Alaska | 40.7 | 39 | Vermont | 10.5 |
| 15 | Missouri | 37.2 | 40 | New York | 10.4 |
| 16 | New Jersey | 36.7 | 41 | California | 10.1 |
| 17 | Maryland | 35.6 | 42 | North Dakota | 9.0 |
| 18 | Ohio | 31.2 | 43 | Nebraska | 8.6 |
| 19 | Alabama | 28.5 | 44 | Kansas | 6.6 |
| 20 | Indiana | 26.8 | 45 | Minnesota | 5.6 |
| 21 | Utah | 26.4 | 46 | Wisconsin | 4.3 |
| 22 | Rhode Island | 24.7 | 47 | Michigan | 3.3 |
| 23 | Georgia | 24.4 | 48 | Maine | 3.0 |
| 24 | Idaho | 24.3 | 49 | Hawaii | 2.1 |
| 25 | Mississippi | 23.9 | 50 | Iowa | 0.7 |

District of Columbia          144.5

Source: U.S. Bureau of the Census
    unpublished data
*Total U.S. resident population increased 9.78% from 1980 to 1990.

# Pharmacies in 1991–1992

## National Total = 63,352 Licensed Pharmacies*

| RANK | STATE | PHARMACIES | % | RANK | STATE | PHARMACIES | % |
|------|-------|-----------|-----|------|-------|-----------|-----|
| 1 | Ohio | 7,145 | 11.28% | 26 | Mississippi | 841 | 1.33% |
| 2 | California | 5,894 | 9.30% | 27 | Kansas | 804 | 1.27% |
| 3 | New York | 4,609 | 7.28% | 28 | Arizona | 781 | 1.23% |
| 4 | Pennsylvania | 3,298 | 5.21% | 29 | Arkansas | 735 | 1.16% |
| 5 | Illinois | 2,804 | 4.43% | 30 | Connecticut | 670 | 1.06% |
| 6 | Colorado | 2,600 | 4.10% | 31 | Nebraska | 612 | 0.97% |
| 7 | Michigan | 2,259 | 3.57% | 32 | West Virginia | 554 | 0.87% |
| 8 | Georgia | 2,200 | 3.47% | 33 | Texas | 521 | 0.82% |
| 9 | North Carolina | 2,023 | 3.19% | 34 | Utah | 455 | 0.72% |
| 10 | New Jersey | 1,982 | 3.13% | 35 | Florida | 383 | 0.60% |
| 11 | Alabama | 1,900 | 3.00% | 36 | Montana | 295 | 0.47% |
| 12 | Tennessee | 1,623 | 2.56% | 37 | New Mexico | 288 | 0.45% |
| 13 | Virginia | 1,510 | 2.38% | 38 | Idaho | 274 | 0.43% |
| 14 | Louisiana | 1,460 | 2.30% | 39 | Maine | 258 | 0.41% |
| 15 | Missouri | 1,344 | 2.12% | 39 | New Hampshire | 258 | 0.41% |
| 16 | Massachusetts | 1,295 | 2.04% | 41 | North Dakota | 250 | 0.39% |
| 17 | Washington | 1,256 | 1.98% | 42 | Nevada | 236 | 0.37% |
| 18 | Kentucky | 1,233 | 1.95% | 43 | South Dakota | 225 | 0.36% |
| 19 | Wisconsin | 1,191 | 1.88% | 44 | Rhode Island | 203 | 0.32% |
| 20 | Minnesota | 1,186 | 1.87% | 45 | Hawaii | 182 | 0.29% |
| 21 | South Carolina | 1,169 | 1.85% | 46 | Vermont | 158 | 0.25% |
| 22 | Oklahoma | 1,005 | 1.59% | 47 | Wyoming | 152 | 0.24% |
| 22 | Oregon | 1,005 | 1.59% | 48 | Delaware | 135 | 0.21% |
| 24 | Maryland | 1,000 | 1.58% | 49 | Alaska | 109 | 0.17% |
| 25 | Iowa | 913 | 1.44% | 50 | Indiana | 69 | 0.11% |

Source: Morgan Quitno Corporation
    unpublished data

*Data gathered by the editors from state licensing agencies. Some data are estimates. Most include out-of-state licenses. National total does not include the District of Columbia.

# IV. FINANCE

# IV. FINANCE (continued)

# IV. FINANCE (continued)

# IV. FINANCE (continued)

# IV. FINANCE (continued)

## Definitions

### The following definitions are from Families USA Foundation of Washington, DC and pertain to charts 189 to 284:

- "Families" are groups of one or more persons related by birth, marriage or adoption and who are residing together.

- "General Taxes" include federal contributions to Medicare, the federal and state components of Medicaid, federal and state government contributions to employer-sponsored insurance, and funding for other federal and state public programs.

- "Health Care Payments" cover expenditures for the delivery of all health services and supplies and the purchase of medical products, including prescription drugs and vision products in retail outlets. It also includes government public health expenditures, the administrative costs of public programs, and the net cost of private insurance.

- "Other Costs" cover worker's compensation and temporary disability and industrial in-plan health benefits.

# Persons Not Covered by Health Insurance in 1991

## National Total = 35,445,000 Uninsured

| RANK | STATE | UNINSURED | % |
|------|-------|-----------|---|
| 1 | California | 5,750,000 | 16.22% |
| 2 | Texas | 3,755,000 | 10.59% |
| 3 | Florida | 2,496,000 | 7.04% |
| 4 | New York | 2,206,000 | 6.22% |
| 5 | Illinois | 1,361,000 | 3.84% |
| 6 | Ohio | 1,147,000 | 3.24% |
| 7 | Virginia | 1,002,000 | 2.83% |
| 8 | North Carolina | 990,000 | 2.79% |
| 9 | Pennsylvania | 954,000 | 2.69% |
| 10 | Georgia | 885,000 | 2.50% |
| 11 | Louisiana | 869,000 | 2.45% |
| 12 | New Jersey | 838,000 | 2.36% |
| 13 | Michigan | 835,000 | 2.36% |
| 14 | Alabama | 749,000 | 2.11% |
| 15 | Indiana | 721,000 | 2.03% |
| 16 | Tennessee | 644,000 | 1.82% |
| 17 | Massachusetts | 633,000 | 1.79% |
| 18 | Maryland | 625,000 | 1.76% |
| 19 | Missouri | 611,000 | 1.72% |
| 20 | Arizona | 607,000 | 1.71% |
| 21 | Oklahoma | 579,000 | 1.63% |
| 22 | Washington | 518,000 | 1.46% |
| 23 | Mississippi | 507,000 | 1.43% |
| 24 | Kentucky | 476,000 | 1.34% |
| 25 | South Carolina | 465,000 | 1.31% |

| RANK | STATE | UNINSURED | % |
|------|-------|-----------|---|
| 26 | Oregon | 422,000 | 1.19% |
| 27 | Minnesota | 406,000 | 1.15% |
| 28 | Wisconsin | 396,000 | 1.12% |
| 29 | Arkansas | 385,000 | 1.09% |
| 30 | New Mexico | 335,000 | 0.95% |
| 31 | Colorado | 334,000 | 0.94% |
| 32 | Kansas | 295,000 | 0.83% |
| 33 | West Virginia | 287,000 | 0.81% |
| 34 | Connecticut | 249,000 | 0.70% |
| 34 | Iowa | 249,000 | 0.70% |
| 36 | Utah | 238,000 | 0.67% |
| 37 | Nevada | 232,000 | 0.65% |
| 38 | Idaho | 184,000 | 0.52% |
| 39 | Nebraska | 137,000 | 0.39% |
| 40 | Maine | 135,000 | 0.38% |
| 41 | New Hampshire | 112,000 | 0.32% |
| 42 | Montana | 104,000 | 0.29% |
| 43 | Rhode Island | 96,000 | 0.27% |
| 44 | Delaware | 94,000 | 0.27% |
| 45 | Hawaii | 82,000 | 0.23% |
| 46 | Vermont | 74,000 | 0.21% |
| 47 | Alaska | 69,000 | 0.19% |
| 48 | South Dakota | 68,000 | 0.19% |
| 49 | Wyoming | 53,000 | 0.15% |
| 50 | North Dakota | 48,000 | 0.14% |
| | District of Columbia | 136,000 | 0.38% |

*Source: U.S. Bureau of the Census*
*unpublished data*

# Percent of Persons Not Covered by Health Insurance in 1991

## National Rate = 14.1% Not Covered by Health Insurance

| RANK | STATE | PERCENT | RANK | STATE | PERCENT |
|------|-------|---------|------|-------|---------|
| 1 | Texas | 22.1 | 26 | Montana | 12.7 |
| 2 | New Mexico | 21.5 | 26 | Vermont | 12.7 |
| 3 | Louisiana | 20.7 | 28 | New York | 12.3 |
| 4 | Mississippi | 18.9 | 29 | Missouri | 12.2 |
| 5 | California | 18.7 | 30 | Illinois | 11.5 |
| 5 | Nevada | 18.7 | 31 | Kansas | 11.4 |
| 7 | Florida | 18.6 | 32 | Wyoming | 11.3 |
| 8 | Oklahoma | 18.2 | 33 | Maine | 11.1 |
| 9 | Alabama | 17.9 | 34 | Massachusetts | 10.9 |
| 10 | Idaho | 17.8 | 35 | New Jersey | 10.8 |
| 11 | Arizona | 16.9 | 36 | Washington | 10.4 |
| 12 | Virginia | 16.3 | 37 | Ohio | 10.3 |
| 13 | Arkansas | 15.7 | 38 | Colorado | 10.1 |
| 13 | West Virginia | 15.7 | 38 | New Hampshire | 10.1 |
| 15 | North Carolina | 14.9 | 38 | Rhode Island | 10.1 |
| 16 | Oregon | 14.2 | 41 | South Dakota | 9.9 |
| 17 | Georgia | 14.1 | 42 | Minnesota | 9.3 |
| 18 | Utah | 13.9 | 43 | Michigan | 9.0 |
| 19 | Tennessee | 13.4 | 44 | Iowa | 8.8 |
| 20 | Delaware | 13.2 | 45 | Nebraska | 8.2 |
| 21 | Alaska | 13.1 | 46 | Wisconsin | 8.0 |
| 21 | Kentucky | 13.1 | 47 | Pennsylvania | 7.8 |
| 21 | Maryland | 13.1 | 48 | North Dakota | 7.6 |
| 21 | South Carolina | 13.1 | 49 | Connecticut | 7.5 |
| 25 | Indiana | 13.0 | 50 | Hawaii | 7.0 |

District of Columbia     25.7

*Source: U.S. Bureau of the Census*
   *"Money Income of Households, Families, and Persons in the United States: 1991" (P-60, No. 180)*

# Persons Covered by Health Insurance in 1991

## National Total = 215,990,000 Insured

| RANK | STATE | INSURED | % | RANK | STATE | INSURED | % |
|---|---|---|---|---|---|---|---|
| 1 | California | 25,006,000 | 11.58% | 26 | Arizona | 2,992,000 | 1.39% |
| 2 | New York | 15,725,000 | 7.28% | 27 | Colorado | 2,988,000 | 1.38% |
| 3 | Texas | 13,251,000 | 6.14% | 28 | Oklahoma | 2,596,000 | 1.20% |
| 4 | Pennsylvania | 11,215,000 | 5.19% | 29 | Iowa | 2,572,000 | 1.19% |
| 5 | Florida | 10,940,000 | 5.07% | 30 | Oregon | 2,549,000 | 1.18% |
| 6 | Illinois | 10,439,000 | 4.83% | 31 | Kansas | 2,286,000 | 1.06% |
| 7 | Ohio | 9,939,000 | 4.60% | 32 | Mississippi | 2,180,000 | 1.01% |
| 8 | Michigan | 8,438,000 | 3.91% | 33 | Arkansas | 2,064,000 | 0.96% |
| 9 | New Jersey | 6,901,000 | 3.20% | 34 | West Virginia | 1,543,000 | 0.71% |
| 10 | North Carolina | 5,654,000 | 2.62% | 35 | Nebraska | 1,527,000 | 0.71% |
| 11 | Georgia | 5,387,000 | 2.49% | 36 | Utah | 1,480,000 | 0.69% |
| 12 | Massachusetts | 5,171,000 | 2.39% | 37 | New Mexico | 1,221,000 | 0.57% |
| 13 | Virginia | 5,145,000 | 2.38% | 38 | Hawaii | 1,083,000 | 0.50% |
| 14 | Indiana | 4,812,000 | 2.23% | 39 | Maine | 1,079,000 | 0.50% |
| 15 | Wisconsin | 4,566,000 | 2.11% | 40 | Nevada | 1,007,000 | 0.47% |
| 16 | Washington | 4,475,000 | 2.07% | 41 | New Hampshire | 1,000,000 | 0.46% |
| 17 | Missouri | 4,382,000 | 2.03% | 42 | Rhode Island | 854,000 | 0.40% |
| 18 | Tennessee | 4,151,000 | 1.92% | 43 | Idaho | 851,000 | 0.39% |
| 19 | Maryland | 4,143,000 | 1.92% | 44 | Montana | 718,000 | 0.33% |
| 20 | Minnesota | 3,978,000 | 1.84% | 45 | South Dakota | 621,000 | 0.29% |
| 21 | Alabama | 3,429,000 | 1.59% | 46 | Delaware | 616,000 | 0.29% |
| 22 | Louisiana | 3,325,000 | 1.54% | 47 | North Dakota | 587,000 | 0.27% |
| 23 | Kentucky | 3,165,000 | 1.47% | 48 | Vermont | 507,000 | 0.23% |
| 24 | Connecticut | 3,092,000 | 1.43% | 49 | Alaska | 456,000 | 0.21% |
| 25 | South Carolina | 3,075,000 | 1.42% | 50 | Wyoming | 418,000 | 0.19% |
| | | | | | District of Columbia | 393,000 | 0.18% |

Source: U.S. Bureau of the Census
unpublished data

# Percent of Population Covered by Health Insurance in 1991

## National Rate = 85.9% Covered by Health Insurance*

| RANK | STATE | PERCENT | RANK | STATE | PERCENT |
|---|---|---|---|---|---|
| 1 | Hawaii | 93.0 | 26 | Indiana | 87.0 |
| 2 | Connecticut | 92.5 | 27 | Alaska | 86.9 |
| 3 | North Dakota | 92.4 | 27 | Kentucky | 86.9 |
| 4 | Pennsylvania | 92.2 | 27 | Maryland | 86.9 |
| 5 | Wisconsin | 92.0 | 27 | South Carolina | 86.9 |
| 6 | Nebraska | 91.8 | 31 | Delaware | 86.8 |
| 7 | Iowa | 91.2 | 32 | Tennessee | 86.6 |
| 8 | Michigan | 91.0 | 33 | Utah | 86.1 |
| 9 | Minnesota | 90.7 | 34 | Georgia | 85.9 |
| 10 | South Dakota | 90.1 | 35 | Oregon | 85.8 |
| 11 | Colorado | 89.9 | 36 | North Carolina | 85.1 |
| 11 | New Hampshire | 89.9 | 37 | Arkansas | 84.3 |
| 11 | Rhode Island | 89.9 | 37 | West Virginia | 84.3 |
| 14 | Ohio | 89.7 | 39 | Virginia | 83.7 |
| 15 | Washington | 89.6 | 40 | Arizona | 83.1 |
| 16 | New Jersey | 89.2 | 41 | Idaho | 82.2 |
| 17 | Massachusetts | 89.1 | 42 | Alabama | 82.1 |
| 18 | Maine | 88.9 | 43 | Oklahoma | 81.8 |
| 19 | Wyoming | 88.7 | 44 | Florida | 81.4 |
| 20 | Kansas | 88.6 | 45 | California | 81.3 |
| 21 | Illinois | 88.5 | 45 | Nevada | 81.3 |
| 22 | Missouri | 87.8 | 47 | Mississippi | 81.1 |
| 23 | New York | 87.7 | 48 | Louisiana | 79.3 |
| 24 | Montana | 87.3 | 49 | New Mexico | 78.5 |
| 24 | Vermont | 87.3 | 50 | Texas | 77.9 |
| | | | | District of Columbia | 74.3 |

Source: U.S. Bureau of the Census

"Money Income of Households, Families, and Persons in the United States: 1991" (P-60, No. 180)

*Percents calculated by the editors using Census figures for percent of population uninsured to obtain percent insured.

# Persons Not Covered by Health Insurance in 1989

## National Total = 33,385,000 Uninsured

| RANK | STATE | UNINSURED | % | | RANK | STATE | UNINSURED | % |
|---|---|---|---|---|---|---|---|---|
| 1 | California | 5,577,000 | 16.71% | | 26 | Mississippi | 436,000 | 1.31% |
| 2 | Texas | 3,770,000 | 11.29% | | 27 | Wisconsin | 414,000 | 1.24% |
| 3 | Florida | 2,169,000 | 6.50% | | 28 | Arkansas | 410,000 | 1.23% |
| 4 | New York | 2,121,000 | 6.35% | | 29 | Oregon | 400,000 | 1.20% |
| 5 | Illinois | 1,162,000 | 3.48% | | 30 | Minnesota | 366,000 | 1.10% |
| 6 | Pennsylvania | 1,088,000 | 3.26% | | 31 | New Mexico | 321,000 | 0.96% |
| 7 | Georgia | 964,000 | 2.89% | | 32 | Connecticut | 260,000 | 0.78% |
| 8 | Ohio | 912,000 | 2.73% | | 33 | West Virginia | 250,000 | 0.75% |
| 9 | North Carolina | 889,000 | 2.66% | | 34 | Kansas | 229,000 | 0.69% |
| 10 | New Jersey | 782,000 | 2.34% | | 35 | Iowa | 206,000 | 0.62% |
| 11 | Michigan | 776,000 | 2.32% | | 36 | Nevada | 176,000 | 0.53% |
| 12 | Louisiana | 732,000 | 2.19% | | 37 | Nebraska | 162,000 | 0.49% |
| 13 | Virginia | 698,000 | 2.09% | | 38 | Idaho | 158,000 | 0.47% |
| 14 | Indiana | 668,000 | 2.00% | | 39 | Utah | 151,000 | 0.45% |
| 15 | Alabama | 665,000 | 1.99% | | 40 | New Hampshire | 141,000 | 0.42% |
| 16 | Oklahoma | 630,000 | 1.89% | | 41 | Montana | 120,000 | 0.36% |
| 17 | Tennessee | 619,000 | 1.85% | | 42 | Maine | 113,000 | 0.34% |
| 18 | Missouri | 614,000 | 1.84% | | 43 | Delaware | 104,000 | 0.31% |
| 19 | Arizona | 580,000 | 1.74% | | 44 | Alaska | 89,000 | 0.27% |
| 20 | Washington | 562,000 | 1.68% | | 44 | Rhode Island | 89,000 | 0.27% |
| 21 | Massachusetts | 495,000 | 1.48% | | 46 | Hawaii | 79,000 | 0.24% |
| 22 | South Carolina | 491,000 | 1.47% | | 47 | South Dakota | 76,000 | 0.23% |
| 23 | Kentucky | 476,000 | 1.43% | | 48 | Wyoming | 58,000 | 0.17% |
| 24 | Maryland | 467,000 | 1.40% | | 49 | North Dakota | 56,000 | 0.17% |
| 25 | Colorado | 443,000 | 1.33% | | 50 | Vermont | 49,000 | 0.15% |
| | | | | | | District of Columbia | 120,000 | 0.36% |

Source: U.S. Bureau of the Census
   unpublished data

# Percent of Persons Not Covered by Health Insurance in 1989

## National Rate = 13.6% Not Covered by Health Insurance

| RANK | STATE | PERCENT | RANK | STATE | PERCENT |
|------|-------|---------|------|-------|---------|
| 1 | Texas | 22.3 | 26 | Indiana | 12.3 |
| 2 | New Mexico | 21.1 | 27 | Washington | 11.9 |
| 3 | Oklahoma | 20.1 | 28 | Missouri | 11.8 |
| 4 | California | 19.0 | 28 | New York | 11.8 |
| 5 | Alaska | 18.2 | 30 | Virginia | 11.3 |
| 6 | Louisiana | 17.9 | 31 | South Dakota | 10.9 |
| 7 | Florida | 17.0 | 32 | Maryland | 10.2 |
| 8 | Arkansas | 16.9 | 32 | New Jersey | 10.2 |
| 8 | Mississippi | 16.9 | 34 | Nebraska | 10.1 |
| 10 | Alabama | 16.3 | 35 | Illinois | 10.0 |
| 10 | Arizona | 16.3 | 36 | Kansas | 9.4 |
| 12 | Idaho | 15.6 | 37 | Maine | 9.2 |
| 12 | Nevada | 15.6 | 37 | Rhode Island | 9.2 |
| 14 | Georgia | 15.5 | 39 | Pennsylvania | 9.0 |
| 15 | Delaware | 15.4 | 39 | Utah | 9.0 |
| 16 | Montana | 14.7 | 41 | Vermont | 8.8 |
| 17 | South Carolina | 14.2 | 41 | Wisconsin | 8.8 |
| 18 | North Carolina | 14.1 | 43 | North Dakota | 8.7 |
| 19 | West Virginia | 13.9 | 44 | Minnesota | 8.6 |
| 20 | Oregon | 13.7 | 45 | Massachusetts | 8.5 |
| 21 | Colorado | 13.6 | 45 | Ohio | 8.5 |
| 22 | Kentucky | 13.3 | 47 | Connecticut | 8.3 |
| 23 | New Hampshire | 12.8 | 47 | Michigan | 8.3 |
| 23 | Tennessee | 12.8 | 49 | Hawaii | 7.3 |
| 25 | Wyoming | 12.6 | 49 | Iowa | 7.3 |

District of Columbia     21.1

Source: U.S. Bureau of the Census

*"Money Income of Households, Families, and Persons in the United States: 1991"* (P-60, No. 180)

# Change in Number of Persons Uninsured: 1989 to 1991

## National Change = 2,060,000 Increase in Persons Uninsured*

| RANK | STATE | CHANGE | | RANK | STATE | CHANGE |
|------|-------|--------|---|------|-------|--------|
| 1 | Florida | 327,000 | | 26 | Maine | 22,000 |
| 2 | Virginia | 304,000 | | 26 | Oregon | 22,000 |
| 3 | Ohio | 235,000 | | 28 | New Mexico | 14,000 |
| 4 | Illinois | 199,000 | | 29 | Rhode Island | 7,000 |
| 5 | California | 173,000 | | 30 | Hawaii | 3,000 |
| 6 | Maryland | 158,000 | | 31 | Kentucky | 0 |
| 7 | Massachusetts | 138,000 | | 32 | Missouri | (3,000) |
| 8 | Louisiana | 137,000 | | 33 | Wyoming | (5,000) |
| 9 | North Carolina | 101,000 | | 34 | North Dakota | (8,000) |
| 10 | Utah | 87,000 | | 34 | South Dakota | (8,000) |
| 11 | New York | 85,000 | | 36 | Delaware | (10,000) |
| 12 | Alabama | 84,000 | | 37 | Connecticut | (11,000) |
| 13 | Mississippi | 71,000 | | 38 | Texas | (15,000) |
| 14 | Kansas | 66,000 | | 39 | Montana | (16,000) |
| 15 | Michigan | 59,000 | | 40 | Wisconsin | (18,000) |
| 16 | Nevada | 56,000 | | 41 | Alaska | (20,000) |
| 16 | New Jersey | 56,000 | | 42 | Arkansas | (25,000) |
| 18 | Indiana | 53,000 | | 42 | Nebraska | (25,000) |
| 19 | Iowa | 43,000 | | 44 | South Carolina | (26,000) |
| 20 | Minnesota | 40,000 | | 45 | New Hampshire | (29,000) |
| 21 | West Virginia | 37,000 | | 46 | Washington | (44,000) |
| 22 | Arizona | 27,000 | | 47 | Oklahoma | (51,000) |
| 23 | Idaho | 26,000 | | 48 | Georgia | (79,000) |
| 24 | Tennessee | 25,000 | | 49 | Colorado | (109,000) |
| 24 | Vermont | 25,000 | | 50 | Pennsylvania | (134,000) |

District of Columbia 16,000

Source: U.S. Bureau of the Census
   unpublished data
*Calculated by the editors.

# Percent Change in Number of Uninsured: 1989 to 1991

## National Rate = 6.17% Increase*

| RANK | STATE | PERCENT CHANGE | RANK | STATE | PERCENT CHANGE |
|------|-------|----------------|------|-------|----------------|
| 1 | Utah | 57.62 | 26 | New Mexico | 4.36 |
| 2 | Vermont | 51.02 | 27 | Tennessee | 4.04 |
| 3 | Virginia | 43.55 | 28 | New York | 4.01 |
| 4 | Maryland | 33.83 | 29 | Hawaii | 3.80 |
| 5 | Nevada | 31.82 | 30 | California | 3.10 |
| 6 | Kansas | 28.82 | 31 | Kentucky | 0.00 |
| 7 | Massachusetts | 27.88 | 32 | Texas | (0.40) |
| 8 | Ohio | 25.77 | 33 | Missouri | (0.49) |
| 9 | Iowa | 20.87 | 34 | Connecticut | (4.23) |
| 10 | Maine | 19.47 | 35 | Wisconsin | (4.35) |
| 11 | Louisiana | 18.72 | 36 | South Carolina | (5.30) |
| 12 | Illinois | 17.13 | 37 | Arkansas | (6.10) |
| 13 | Idaho | 16.46 | 38 | Washington | (7.83) |
| 14 | Mississippi | 16.28 | 39 | Oklahoma | (8.10) |
| 15 | Florida | 15.08 | 40 | Georgia | (8.20) |
| 16 | West Virginia | 14.80 | 41 | Wyoming | (8.62) |
| 17 | Alabama | 12.63 | 42 | Delaware | (9.62) |
| 18 | North Carolina | 11.36 | 43 | South Dakota | (10.53) |
| 19 | Minnesota | 10.93 | 44 | Pennsylvania | (12.32) |
| 20 | Indiana | 7.93 | 45 | Montana | (13.33) |
| 21 | Rhode Island | 7.87 | 46 | North Dakota | (14.29) |
| 22 | Michigan | 7.60 | 47 | Nebraska | (15.43) |
| 23 | New Jersey | 7.16 | 48 | New Hampshire | (20.57) |
| 24 | Oregon | 5.50 | 49 | Alaska | (22.47) |
| 25 | Arizona | 4.66 | 50 | Colorado | (24.60) |

District of Columbia     13.33

Source: U.S. Bureau of the Census
    unpublished data
*Calculated by the editors.

# Number of Health Maintenance Organizations (HMOs) in 1991

## National Total = 550 HMOs*

| RANK | STATE | HMOs | % | RANK | STATE | HMOs | % |
|------|-------|------|------|------|-------|------|------|
| 1 | California | 50 | 9.09% | 22 | Washington | 9 | 1.64% |
| 2 | New York | 36 | 6.55% | 27 | Georgia | 8 | 1.45% |
| 3 | Ohio | 34 | 6.18% | 27 | Utah | 8 | 1.45% |
| 4 | Florida | 33 | 6.00% | 29 | Hawaii | 6 | 1.09% |
| 5 | Wisconsin | 28 | 5.09% | 29 | Kentucky | 6 | 1.09% |
| 6 | Texas | 25 | 4.55% | 29 | Oklahoma | 6 | 1.09% |
| 7 | Illinois | 24 | 4.36% | 32 | Iowa | 5 | 0.91% |
| 8 | Pennsylvania | 20 | 3.64% | 32 | Nebraska | 5 | 0.91% |
| 9 | Michigan | 18 | 3.27% | 32 | New Mexico | 5 | 0.91% |
| 10 | Arizona | 16 | 2.91% | 35 | Delaware | 4 | 0.73% |
| 10 | Missouri | 16 | 2.91% | 35 | South Carolina | 4 | 0.73% |
| 12 | Massachusetts | 15 | 2.73% | 37 | Arkansas | 3 | 0.55% |
| 13 | Colorado | 14 | 2.55% | 37 | Maine | 3 | 0.55% |
| 13 | Maryland | 14 | 2.55% | 37 | Nevada | 3 | 0.55% |
| 15 | Connecticut | 12 | 2.18% | 37 | New Hampshire | 3 | 0.55% |
| 15 | Indiana | 12 | 2.18% | 41 | Idaho | 2 | 0.36% |
| 15 | New Jersey | 12 | 2.18% | 41 | North Dakota | 2 | 0.36% |
| 15 | Virginia | 12 | 2.18% | 41 | Rhode Island | 2 | 0.36% |
| 19 | Kansas | 10 | 1.82% | 44 | Montana | 1 | 0.18% |
| 19 | Minnesota | 10 | 1.82% | 44 | South Dakota | 1 | 0.18% |
| 19 | North Carolina | 10 | 1.82% | 44 | Vermont | 1 | 0.18% |
| 22 | Alabama | 9 | 1.64% | 47 | Alaska | 0 | 0.00% |
| 22 | Louisiana | 9 | 1.64% | 47 | Mississippi | 0 | 0.00% |
| 22 | Oregon | 9 | 1.64% | 47 | West Virginia | 0 | 0.00% |
| 22 | Tennessee | 9 | 1.64% | 47 | Wyoming | 0 | 0.00% |
| | | | | | District of Columbia | 5 | 0.91% |

Source: Group Health Association of America

"National Directory of HMOs-1992" (Reprinted with permission of GHAA, 1129 20th Street, NW, Washington, DC 20036)

*As of December 31, 1991. Total includes two HMOs in Guam.

# Enrollees in Health Maintenance Organizations (HMOs) in 1991

## National Total = 38,615,611 Enrollees*

| RANK | STATE | ENROLLEES | % | RANK | STATE | ENROLLEES | % |
|------|-------|-----------|---|------|-------|-----------|---|
| 1 | California | 10,148,982 | 26.28% | 26 | Alabama | 270,938 | 0.70% |
| 2 | New York | 3,016,126 | 7.81% | 27 | Utah | 266,033 | 0.69% |
| 3 | Massachusetts | 1,855,534 | 4.81% | 28 | Hawaii | 259,790 | 0.67% |
| 4 | Pennsylvania | 1,732,196 | 4.49% | 29 | New Mexico | 227,881 | 0.59% |
| 5 | Florida | 1,651,363 | 4.28% | 30 | Kentucky | 225,383 | 0.58% |
| 6 | Michigan | 1,541,500 | 3.99% | 31 | Oklahoma | 215,577 | 0.56% |
| 7 | Illinois | 1,531,771 | 3.97% | 32 | Tennessee | 206,692 | 0.54% |
| 8 | Texas | 1,455,712 | 3.77% | 33 | Kansas | 204,083 | 0.53% |
| 9 | Ohio | 1,445,891 | 3.74% | 34 | Rhode Island | 152,885 | 0.40% |
| 10 | Minnesota | 1,255,913 | 3.25% | 35 | Nevada | 125,631 | 0.33% |
| 11 | Wisconsin | 1,117,307 | 2.89% | 36 | Delaware | 115,132 | 0.30% |
| 12 | Maryland | 1,082,819 | 2.80% | 37 | New Hampshire | 114,216 | 0.30% |
| 13 | New Jersey | 934,028 | 2.42% | 38 | Nebraska | 91,766 | 0.24% |
| 14 | Arizona | 933,847 | 2.42% | 39 | South Carolina | 88,566 | 0.23% |
| 15 | Oregon | 770,854 | 2.00% | 40 | Vermont | 49,691 | 0.13% |
| 16 | Washington | 743,546 | 1.93% | 41 | Arkansas | 48,705 | 0.13% |
| 17 | Colorado | 740,793 | 1.92% | 42 | Maine | 35,273 | 0.09% |
| 18 | Connecticut | 680,610 | 1.76% | 43 | South Dakota | 21,868 | 0.06% |
| 19 | Missouri | 582,036 | 1.51% | 44 | Idaho | 21,400 | 0.06% |
| 20 | Georgia | 410,409 | 1.06% | 45 | Montana | 9,664 | 0.03% |
| 21 | Virginia | 382,041 | 0.99% | 46 | North Dakota | 6,057 | 0.02% |
| 22 | Indiana | 362,231 | 0.94% | 47 | Alaska | 0 | 0.00% |
| 23 | North Carolina | 321,652 | 0.83% | 47 | Mississippi | 0 | 0.00% |
| 24 | Iowa | 299,710 | 0.78% | 47 | West Virginia | 0 | 0.00% |
| 25 | Louisiana | 293,012 | 0.76% | 47 | Wyoming | 0 | 0.00% |
| | | | | | District of Columbia | 499,897 | 1.29% |

Source: Group Health Association of America

*"National Directory of HMOs-1992" (Reprinted with permission of GHAA, 1129 20th Street, NW, Washington, DC 20036)*

*As of December 31, 1991. Total includes 68,600 enrollees in Guam.*

# Percent of Population Enrolled in Health Maintenance Organizations (HMOs) in 1991

## National Rate = 15.3% Enrolled in HMOs*

| RANK | STATE | PERCENT | RANK | STATE | PERCENT |
|------|-------|---------|------|-------|---------|
| 1 | California | 33.4 | 26 | Nevada | 9.8 |
| 2 | Massachusetts | 30.9 | 27 | Vermont | 8.8 |
| 3 | Minnesota | 28.3 | 28 | Texas | 8.4 |
| 4 | Oregon | 26.4 | 29 | Kansas | 8.2 |
| 5 | Arizona | 24.9 | 30 | Louisiana | 6.9 |
| 6 | Hawaii | 22.9 | 31 | Oklahoma | 6.8 |
| 7 | Wisconsin | 22.5 | 32 | Alabama | 6.6 |
| 8 | Maryland | 22.3 | 33 | Indiana | 6.5 |
| 9 | Colorado | 21.9 | 34 | Georgia | 6.2 |
| 10 | Connecticut | 20.7 | 35 | Kentucky | 6.1 |
| 11 | Delaware | 16.9 | 35 | Virginia | 6.1 |
| 12 | New York | 16.7 | 37 | Nebraska | 5.8 |
| 13 | Michigan | 16.5 | 38 | North Carolina | 4.8 |
| 14 | Rhode Island | 15.2 | 39 | Tennessee | 4.2 |
| 15 | Utah | 15.0 | 40 | South Dakota | 3.1 |
| 16 | Washington | 14.8 | 41 | Maine | 2.9 |
| 17 | New Mexico | 14.7 | 42 | South Carolina | 2.5 |
| 18 | Pennsylvania | 14.5 | 43 | Arkansas | 2.1 |
| 19 | Illinois | 13.3 | 43 | Idaho | 2.1 |
| 20 | Ohio | 13.2 | 45 | Montana | 1.2 |
| 21 | Florida | 12.4 | 46 | North Dakota | 1.0 |
| 22 | New Jersey | 12.0 | 47 | Alaska | 0.0 |
| 23 | Missouri | 11.3 | 47 | Mississippi | 0.0 |
| 24 | Iowa | 10.7 | 47 | West Virginia | 0.0 |
| 25 | New Hampshire | 10.3 | 47 | Wyoming | 0.0 |

District of Columbia 83.6

Source: Group Health Association of America

"National Directory of HMOs-1992" (Reprinted with permission of GHAA, 1129 20th Street, NW, Washington, DC 20036)

*As of December 31, 1991.

# Percent of Insured Population Enrolled in Health Maintenance Organizations (HMOs) in 1991

## National Rate = 17.8% of Insured Enrolled in HMOs*

| RANK | STATE | PERCENT | RANK | STATE | PERCENT |
|------|-------|---------|------|-------|---------|
| 1 | California | 41.3 | 26 | New Hampshire | 11.5 |
| 2 | Massachusetts | 34.0 | 27 | Texas | 10.6 |
| 3 | Minnesota | 31.1 | 28 | Vermont | 9.7 |
| 4 | Oregon | 30.1 | 29 | Kansas | 9.2 |
| 5 | Arizona | 29.5 | 30 | Louisiana | 8.6 |
| 6 | Colorado | 25.7 | 31 | Oklahoma | 8.3 |
| 7 | Maryland | 25.5 | 32 | Alabama | 8.0 |
| 8 | Hawaii | 24.7 | 33 | Georgia | 7.3 |
| 9 | Wisconsin | 24.2 | 34 | Indiana | 7.2 |
| 10 | Connecticut | 22.2 | 34 | Virginia | 7.2 |
| 11 | Delaware | 19.7 | 36 | Kentucky | 7.0 |
| 12 | New York | 19.0 | 37 | Nebraska | 6.3 |
| 13 | New Mexico | 18.9 | 38 | North Carolina | 5.5 |
| 14 | Michigan | 18.2 | 39 | Tennessee | 4.8 |
| 15 | Rhode Island | 17.1 | 40 | South Dakota | 3.5 |
| 16 | Washington | 16.7 | 41 | Maine | 3.2 |
| 17 | Utah | 16.5 | 42 | South Carolina | 3.0 |
| 18 | Pennsylvania | 16.1 | 43 | Arkansas | 2.5 |
| 19 | Florida | 15.2 | 44 | Idaho | 2.4 |
| 20 | Illinois | 14.9 | 45 | Montana | 1.4 |
| 21 | Ohio | 14.7 | 46 | North Dakota | 1.0 |
| 22 | New Jersey | 13.4 | 47 | Alaska | 0.0 |
| 23 | Missouri | 12.9 | 47 | Mississippi | 0.0 |
| 24 | Iowa | 11.7 | 47 | West Virginia | 0.0 |
| 24 | Nevada | 11.7 | 47 | Wyoming | 0.0 |

District of Columbia     100.0

Source: Group Health Association of America

"National Directory of HMOs-1992" (Reprinted with permission of GHAA, 1129 20th Street, NW, Washington, DC 20036)

*As of December 31, 1991.

# Preferred Provider Organizations (PPOs) in 1990

## National Total = 814 PPOs

| RANK | STATE | PPOs | % | RANK | STATE | PPOs | % |
|------|-------|------|------|------|-------|------|------|
| 1 | California | 119 | 14.62% | 26 | Alabama | 10 | 1.23% |
| 2 | Ohio | 54 | 6.63% | 27 | Kentucky | 9 | 1.11% |
| 3 | Florida | 53 | 6.51% | 27 | Nevada | 9 | 1.11% |
| 4 | Texas | 49 | 6.02% | 29 | Utah | 8 | 0.98% |
| 5 | Colorado | 42 | 5.16% | 30 | Connecticut | 6 | 0.74% |
| 5 | Pennsylvania | 42 | 5.16% | 31 | Nebraska | 5 | 0.61% |
| 7 | Illinois | 35 | 4.30% | 31 | New Jersey | 5 | 0.61% |
| 8 | Arizona | 29 | 3.56% | 31 | West Virginia | 5 | 0.61% |
| 9 | Michigan | 28 | 3.44% | 34 | New Mexico | 4 | 0.49% |
| 10 | Missouri | 27 | 3.32% | 34 | South Carolina | 4 | 0.49% |
| 11 | Tennessee | 24 | 2.95% | 36 | Iowa | 3 | 0.37% |
| 12 | Massachusetts | 23 | 2.83% | 37 | Arkansas | 2 | 0.25% |
| 13 | Maryland | 22 | 2.70% | 37 | Hawaii | 2 | 0.25% |
| 14 | Washington | 21 | 2.58% | 37 | Mississippi | 2 | 0.25% |
| 15 | North Carolina | 20 | 2.46% | 40 | Maine | 1 | 0.12% |
| 16 | Georgia | 19 | 2.33% | 40 | New Hampshire | 1 | 0.12% |
| 17 | New York | 18 | 2.21% | 40 | Rhode Island | 1 | 0.12% |
| 18 | Minnesota | 15 | 1.84% | 40 | South Dakota | 1 | 0.12% |
| 19 | Kansas | 14 | 1.72% | 40 | Wyoming | 1 | 0.12% |
| 20 | Indiana | 13 | 1.60% | 45 | Alaska | 0 | 0.00% |
| 20 | Virginia | 13 | 1.60% | 45 | Delaware | 0 | 0.00% |
| 20 | Wisconsin | 13 | 1.60% | 45 | Idaho | 0 | 0.00% |
| 23 | Oregon | 12 | 1.47% | 45 | Montana | 0 | 0.00% |
| 24 | Louisiana | 11 | 1.35% | 45 | North Dakota | 0 | 0.00% |
| 24 | Oklahoma | 11 | 1.35% | 45 | Vermont | 0 | 0.00% |
| | | | | | District of Columbia | 7 | 0.86% |

*Source: American Managed Care and Review Association, Washington D.C. (Reprinted with permission)*
    *"Directory of Preferred Provider Organizations and the Industry Report on PPO Development," January 1990 (Copyright 1988)*

# Total Health Care Payments in 1991

## National Total = $693,696,000,000*

| RANK | STATE | PAYMENTS | % | RANK | STATE | PAYMENTS | % |
|------|-------|----------|---|------|-------|----------|---|
| 1 | California | $92,583,000,000 | 13.35% | 26 | Iowa | $7,571,000,000 | 1.09% |
| 2 | New York | 62,911,000,000 | 9.07% | 27 | Oregon | 7,506,000,000 | 1.08% |
| 3 | Texas | 41,397,000,000 | 5.97% | 28 | Kansas | 7,357,000,000 | 1.06% |
| 4 | Illinois | 36,158,000,000 | 5.21% | 29 | Kentucky | 7,187,000,000 | 1.04% |
| 5 | Pennsylvania | 34,334,000,000 | 4.95% | 30 | Oklahoma | 6,970,000,000 | 1.00% |
| 6 | Florida | 32,532,000,000 | 4.69% | 31 | South Carolina | 6,658,000,000 | 0.96% |
| 7 | Ohio | 31,580,000,000 | 4.55% | 32 | Arkansas | 4,827,000,000 | 0.70% |
| 8 | Michigan | 28,124,000,000 | 4.05% | 33 | Nebraska | 4,555,000,000 | 0.66% |
| 9 | New Jersey | 24,458,000,000 | 3.53% | 34 | Mississippi | 4,443,000,000 | 0.64% |
| 10 | Massachusetts | 22,088,000,000 | 3.18% | 35 | West Virginia | 3,811,000,000 | 0.55% |
| 11 | Georgia | 15,471,000,000 | 2.23% | 36 | Nevada | 3,488,000,000 | 0.50% |
| 12 | Virginia | 15,263,000,000 | 2.20% | 37 | Utah | 3,486,000,000 | 0.50% |
| 13 | Missouri | 14,759,000,000 | 2.13% | 38 | Hawaii | 3,252,000,000 | 0.47% |
| 14 | Indiana | 14,254,000,000 | 2.05% | 39 | Rhode Island | 3,237,000,000 | 0.47% |
| 15 | North Carolina | 14,230,000,000 | 2.05% | 40 | Maine | 3,175,000,000 | 0.46% |
| 16 | Minnesota | 13,897,000,000 | 2.00% | 41 | New Hampshire | 3,121,000,000 | 0.45% |
| 17 | Wisconsin | 13,827,000,000 | 1.99% | 42 | New Mexico | 3,010,000,000 | 0.43% |
| 18 | Maryland | 13,139,000,000 | 1.89% | 43 | Delaware | 2,010,000,000 | 0.29% |
| 19 | Connecticut | 12,750,000,000 | 1.84% | 44 | Idaho | 1,916,000,000 | 0.28% |
| 20 | Washington | 12,713,000,000 | 1.83% | 45 | North Dakota | 1,789,000,000 | 0.26% |
| 21 | Tennessee | 11,534,000,000 | 1.66% | 46 | Montana | 1,725,000,000 | 0.25% |
| 22 | Louisiana | 9,742,000,000 | 1.40% | 47 | South Dakota | 1,715,000,000 | 0.25% |
| 23 | Alabama | 9,385,000,000 | 1.35% | 48 | Alaska | 1,694,000,000 | 0.24% |
| 24 | Colorado | 9,316,000,000 | 1.34% | 49 | Vermont | 1,387,000,000 | 0.20% |
| 25 | Arizona | 8,486,000,000 | 1.22% | 50 | Wyoming | 1,004,000,000 | 0.14% |
| | | | | | District of Columbia | 1,868,000,000 | 0.27% |

Source: Families USA Foundation

"Health Spending: The Growing Threat to the Family Budget" (December 1991) (Reprinted with permission)

*Expenditures by both families and business for health care. See beginning of this chapter for definitions.

# Total Health Care Payments in 1980

## National Total = $229,600,000,000*

| RANK | STATE | PAYMENTS | % | RANK | STATE | PAYMENTS | % |
|------|-------|----------|---|------|-------|----------|---|
| 1 | California | $25,816,000,000 | 11.24% | 26 | Kentucky | $2,856,000,000 | 1.24% |
| 2 | New York | 21,568,000,000 | 9.39% | 27 | Oklahoma | 2,685,000,000 | 1.17% |
| 3 | Texas | 13,728,000,000 | 5.98% | 28 | Kansas | 2,500,000,000 | 1.09% |
| 4 | Illinois | 13,117,000,000 | 5.71% | 29 | Oregon | 2,469,000,000 | 1.08% |
| 5 | Pennsylvania | 12,400,000,000 | 5.40% | 30 | Arizona | 2,324,000,000 | 1.01% |
| 6 | Ohio | 11,987,000,000 | 5.22% | 31 | South Carolina | 2,155,000,000 | 0.94% |
| 7 | Michigan | 10,515,000,000 | 4.58% | 32 | Arkansas | 1,692,000,000 | 0.74% |
| 8 | Florida | 8,604,000,000 | 3.75% | 33 | Nebraska | 1,635,000,000 | 0.71% |
| 9 | New Jersey | 7,779,000,000 | 3.39% | 34 | Mississippi | 1,630,000,000 | 0.71% |
| 10 | Massachusetts | 7,006,000,000 | 3.05% | 35 | West Virginia | 1,624,000,000 | 0.71% |
| 11 | Indiana | 5,394,000,000 | 2.35% | 36 | Rhode Island | 1,084,000,000 | 0.47% |
| 12 | Wisconsin | 5,107,000,000 | 2.22% | 37 | Utah | 1,053,000,000 | 0.46% |
| 13 | Missouri | 5,033,000,000 | 2.19% | 38 | Hawaii | 946,000,000 | 0.41% |
| 14 | Minnesota | 4,742,000,000 | 2.07% | 39 | Maine | 944,000,000 | 0.41% |
| 15 | Virginia | 4,729,000,000 | 2.06% | 40 | New Mexico | 924,000,000 | 0.40% |
| 16 | Georgia | 4,606,000,000 | 2.01% | 41 | Nevada | 865,000,000 | 0.38% |
| 17 | North Carolina | 4,569,000,000 | 1.99% | 42 | New Hampshire | 837,000,000 | 0.36% |
| 18 | Maryland | 4,353,000,000 | 1.90% | 43 | North Dakota | 680,000,000 | 0.30% |
| 19 | Tennessee | 4,054,000,000 | 1.77% | 44 | Idaho | 659,000,000 | 0.29% |
| 20 | Washington | 3,998,000,000 | 1.74% | 45 | Montana | 639,000,000 | 0.28% |
| 21 | Connecticut | 3,993,000,000 | 1.74% | 46 | South Dakota | 623,000,000 | 0.27% |
| 22 | Louisiana | 3,973,000,000 | 1.73% | 47 | Delaware | 596,000,000 | 0.26% |
| 23 | Alabama | 3,257,000,000 | 1.42% | 48 | Alaska | 428,000,000 | 0.19% |
| 24 | Iowa | 2,995,000,000 | 1.30% | 49 | Vermont | 418,000,000 | 0.18% |
| 25 | Colorado | 2,918,000,000 | 1.27% | 50 | Wyoming | 386,000,000 | 0.17% |
| | | | | | District of Columbia | 709,000,000 | 0.31% |

Source: Families USA Foundation

"Health Spending: The Growing Threat to the Family Budget" (December 1991) (Reprinted with permission)

*Expenditures by both families and business for health care. See beginning of this chapter for definitions.

# Projected Total Health Care Payments in 2000

## Projected National Total = $1,576,100,000,000*

| RANK | STATE | PAYMENTS | % | RANK | STATE | PAYMENTS | % |
|---|---|---|---|---|---|---|---|
| 1 | California | $224,830,000,000 | 14.26% | 26 | Oregon | $16,609,000,000 | 1.05% |
| 2 | New York | 135,639,000,000 | 8.61% | 27 | South Carolina | 15,829,000,000 | 1.00% |
| 3 | Texas | 101,336,000,000 | 6.43% | 28 | Kentucky | 15,582,000,000 | 0.99% |
| 4 | Florida | 83,480,000,000 | 5.30% | 29 | Kansas | 15,572,000,000 | 0.99% |
| 5 | Illinois | 75,744,000,000 | 4.81% | 30 | Oklahoma | 15,461,000,000 | 0.98% |
| 6 | Pennsylvania | 70,434,000,000 | 4.47% | 31 | Iowa | 14,562,000,000 | 0.92% |
| 7 | Ohio | 65,476,000,000 | 4.15% | 32 | Arkansas | 10,729,000,000 | 0.68% |
| 8 | Michigan | 59,108,000,000 | 3.75% | 33 | Mississippi | 10,316,000,000 | 0.65% |
| 9 | New Jersey | 56,976,000,000 | 3.61% | 34 | Nebraska | 9,232,000,000 | 0.59% |
| 10 | Massachusetts | 48,650,000,000 | 3.09% | 35 | Nevada | 8,824,000,000 | 0.56% |
| 11 | Georgia | 39,882,000,000 | 2.53% | 36 | Utah | 8,338,000,000 | 0.53% |
| 12 | Virginia | 36,884,000,000 | 2.34% | 37 | Hawaii | 8,182,000,000 | 0.52% |
| 13 | North Carolina | 34,222,000,000 | 2.17% | 38 | New Mexico | 8,070,000,000 | 0.51% |
| 14 | Missouri | 32,037,000,000 | 2.03% | 39 | New Hampshire | 7,805,000,000 | 0.50% |
| 15 | Maryland | 31,620,000,000 | 2.01% | 40 | West Virginia | 7,673,000,000 | 0.49% |
| 16 | Indiana | 29,794,000,000 | 1.89% | 41 | Rhode Island | 7,210,000,000 | 0.46% |
| 17 | Minnesota | 29,563,000,000 | 1.88% | 42 | Maine | 7,062,000,000 | 0.45% |
| 18 | Washington | 29,088,000,000 | 1.85% | 43 | Delaware | 4,350,000,000 | 0.28% |
| 19 | Connecticut | 28,992,000,000 | 1.84% | 44 | Idaho | 4,194,000,000 | 0.27% |
| 20 | Wisconsin | 28,540,000,000 | 1.81% | 45 | Alaska | 4,171,000,000 | 0.26% |
| 21 | Tennessee | 26,205,000,000 | 1.66% | 46 | Montana | 3,692,000,000 | 0.23% |
| 22 | Arizona | 22,632,000,000 | 1.44% | 47 | North Dakota | 3,557,000,000 | 0.23% |
| 23 | Colorado | 22,299,000,000 | 1.41% | 48 | South Dakota | 3,555,000,000 | 0.23% |
| 24 | Louisiana | 21,531,000,000 | 1.37% | 49 | Vermont | 3,063,000,000 | 0.19% |
| 25 | Alabama | 21,368,000,000 | 1.36% | 50 | Wyoming | 2,188,000,000 | 0.14% |
| | | | | | District of Columbia | 3,944,000,000 | 0.25% |

Source: Families USA Foundation

"Health Spending: The Growing Threat to the Family Budget" (December 1991) (Reprinted with permission)

*Expenditures by both families and business for health care. See beginning of this chapter for definitions.

# Change in Total Health Care Payments: 1980 to 1991

## National Change = $464,096,000,000 Increase*

| RANK | STATE | INCREASE | % | RANK | STATE | INCREASE | % |
|---|---|---|---|---|---|---|---|
| 1 | California | $66,767,000,000 | 14.39% | 26 | Oregon | $5,037,000,000 | 1.09% |
| 2 | New York | 41,343,000,000 | 8.91% | 27 | Kansas | 4,857,000,000 | 1.05% |
| 3 | Texas | 27,669,000,000 | 5.96% | 28 | Iowa | 4,576,000,000 | 0.99% |
| 4 | Florida | 23,928,000,000 | 5.16% | 29 | South Carolina | 4,503,000,000 | 0.97% |
| 5 | Illinois | 23,041,000,000 | 4.96% | 30 | Kentucky | 4,331,000,000 | 0.93% |
| 6 | Pennsylvania | 21,934,000,000 | 4.73% | 31 | Oklahoma | 4,285,000,000 | 0.92% |
| 7 | Ohio | 19,593,000,000 | 4.22% | 32 | Arkansas | 3,135,000,000 | 0.68% |
| 8 | Michigan | 17,609,000,000 | 3.79% | 33 | Nebraska | 2,920,000,000 | 0.63% |
| 9 | New Jersey | 16,679,000,000 | 3.59% | 34 | Mississippi | 2,813,000,000 | 0.61% |
| 10 | Massachusetts | 15,082,000,000 | 3.25% | 35 | Nevada | 2,623,000,000 | 0.57% |
| 11 | Georgia | 10,865,000,000 | 2.34% | 36 | Utah | 2,433,000,000 | 0.52% |
| 12 | Virginia | 10,534,000,000 | 2.27% | 37 | Hawaii | 2,306,000,000 | 0.50% |
| 13 | Missouri | 9,726,000,000 | 2.10% | 38 | New Hampshire | 2,284,000,000 | 0.49% |
| 14 | North Carolina | 9,661,000,000 | 2.08% | 39 | Maine | 2,231,000,000 | 0.48% |
| 15 | Minnesota | 9,155,000,000 | 1.97% | 40 | West Virginia | 2,187,000,000 | 0.47% |
| 16 | Indiana | 8,860,000,000 | 1.91% | 41 | Rhode Island | 2,153,000,000 | 0.46% |
| 17 | Maryland | 8,786,000,000 | 1.89% | 42 | New Mexico | 2,086,000,000 | 0.45% |
| 18 | Connecticut | 8,757,000,000 | 1.89% | 43 | Delaware | 1,414,000,000 | 0.30% |
| 19 | Wisconsin | 8,720,000,000 | 1.88% | 44 | Alaska | 1,266,000,000 | 0.27% |
| 20 | Washington | 8,715,000,000 | 1.88% | 45 | Idaho | 1,257,000,000 | 0.27% |
| 21 | Tennessee | 7,480,000,000 | 1.61% | 46 | North Dakota | 1,109,000,000 | 0.24% |
| 22 | Colorado | 6,398,000,000 | 1.38% | 47 | South Dakota | 1,092,000,000 | 0.24% |
| 23 | Arizona | 6,162,000,000 | 1.33% | 48 | Montana | 1,086,000,000 | 0.23% |
| 24 | Alabama | 6,128,000,000 | 1.32% | 49 | Vermont | 969,000,000 | 0.21% |
| 25 | Louisiana | 5,769,000,000 | 1.24% | 50 | Wyoming | 618,000,000 | 0.13% |
|  |  |  |  |  | District of Columbia | 1,159,000,000 | 0.25% |

Source: Families USA Foundation

"Health Spending: The Growing Threat to the Family Budget" (December 1991) (Reprinted with permission)

*Calculated by the editors. Expenditures by both families and business for health care. See beginning of this chapter for definitions.

# Percent Change in Health Care Payments: 1980 to 1991

## National Rate = 202.13% Increase*

| RANK | STATE | PERCENT INCREASE | RANK | STATE | PERCENT INCREASE |
|------|-------|------------------|------|-------|------------------|
| 1 | Nevada | 303.24 | 26 | Kansas | 194.28 |
| 2 | Alaska | 295.79 | 27 | Missouri | 193.24 |
| 3 | Florida | 278.10 | 28 | Minnesota | 193.06 |
| 4 | New Hampshire | 272.88 | 29 | New York | 191.69 |
| 5 | Arizona | 265.15 | 30 | Idaho | 190.74 |
| 6 | California | 258.63 | 31 | Alabama | 188.15 |
| 7 | Hawaii | 243.76 | 32 | Arkansas | 185.28 |
| 8 | Delaware | 237.25 | 33 | Tennessee | 184.51 |
| 9 | Maine | 236.33 | 34 | Nebraska | 178.59 |
| 10 | Georgia | 235.89 | 35 | Pennsylvania | 176.89 |
| 11 | Vermont | 231.82 | 36 | Illinois | 175.66 |
| 12 | Utah | 231.05 | 37 | South Dakota | 175.28 |
| 13 | New Mexico | 225.76 | 38 | Mississippi | 172.58 |
| 14 | Virginia | 222.75 | 39 | Wisconsin | 170.75 |
| 15 | Connecticut | 219.31 | 40 | Montana | 169.95 |
| 16 | Colorado | 219.26 | 41 | Michigan | 167.47 |
| 17 | Washington | 217.98 | 42 | Indiana | 164.26 |
| 18 | Massachusetts | 215.27 | 43 | Ohio | 163.45 |
| 19 | New Jersey | 214.41 | 44 | North Dakota | 163.09 |
| 20 | North Carolina | 211.45 | 45 | Wyoming | 160.10 |
| 21 | South Carolina | 208.96 | 46 | Oklahoma | 159.59 |
| 22 | Oregon | 204.01 | 47 | Iowa | 152.79 |
| 23 | Maryland | 201.84 | 48 | Kentucky | 151.65 |
| 24 | Texas | 201.55 | 49 | Louisiana | 145.21 |
| 25 | Rhode Island | 198.62 | 50 | West Virginia | 134.67 |
| | | | | District of Columbia | 163.47 |

Source: Families USA Foundation

"Health Spending: The Growing Threat to the Family Budget" (December 1991) (Reprinted with permission)

*Calculated by the editors. Expenditures by both families and business for health care. See beginning of this chapter for definitions.

# Annual Percent Change in Total Health Care Payments: 1980 to 1991

## National Change = 10.57% Annual Increase*

| RANK | STATE | PERCENT | RANK | STATE | PERCENT |
|------|-------|---------|------|-------|---------|
| 1 | Nevada | 13.51 | 26 | Kansas | 10.31 |
| 2 | Alaska | 13.32 | 27 | Minnesota | 10.27 |
| 3 | Florida | 12.85 | 27 | Missouri | 10.27 |
| 4 | New Hampshire | 12.71 | 29 | New York | 10.22 |
| 5 | Arizona | 12.50 | 30 | Idaho | 10.19 |
| 6 | California | 12.31 | 31 | Alabama | 10.10 |
| 7 | Hawaii | 11.88 | 32 | Arkansas | 10.00 |
| 8 | Delaware | 11.69 | 33 | Tennessee | 9.97 |
| 9 | Maine | 11.66 | 34 | Nebraska | 9.76 |
| 10 | Georgia | 11.64 | 35 | Pennsylvania | 9.70 |
| 11 | Vermont | 11.52 | 36 | Illinois | 9.66 |
| 12 | Utah | 11.50 | 37 | South Dakota | 9.64 |
| 13 | New Mexico | 11.33 | 38 | Mississippi | 9.54 |
| 14 | Virginia | 11.24 | 39 | Wisconsin | 9.48 |
| 15 | Colorado | 11.13 | 40 | Montana | 9.45 |
| 15 | Connecticut | 11.13 | 41 | Michigan | 9.36 |
| 17 | Washington | 11.09 | 42 | Indiana | 9.24 |
| 18 | Massachusetts | 11.00 | 43 | Ohio | 9.21 |
| 19 | New Jersey | 10.98 | 44 | North Dakota | 9.19 |
| 20 | North Carolina | 10.88 | 45 | Wyoming | 9.08 |
| 21 | South Carolina | 10.80 | 46 | Oklahoma | 9.06 |
| 22 | Oregon | 10.64 | 47 | Iowa | 8.80 |
| 23 | Maryland | 10.56 | 48 | Kentucky | 8.75 |
| 24 | Texas | 10.55 | 49 | Louisiana | 8.50 |
| 25 | Rhode Island | 10.46 | 50 | West Virginia | 8.06 |
| | | | | District of Columbia | 9.21 |

Source: Families USA Foundation

"Health Spending: The Growing Threat to the Family Budget" (December 1991) (Reprinted with permission)

*Calculated by the editors. Expenditures by both families and business for health care. See beginning of this chapter for definitions.

# Projected Change in Total Health Care Payments: 1991 to 2000

## Projected National Change = $882,404,000,000 Increase*

| RANK | STATE | INCREASE | % | RANK | STATE | INCREASE | % |
|---|---|---|---|---|---|---|---|
| 1 | California | $132,247,000,000 | 14.99% | 26 | South Carolina | $9,171,000,000 | 1.04% |
| 2 | New York | 72,728,000,000 | 8.24% | 27 | Oregon | 9,103,000,000 | 1.03% |
| 3 | Texas | 59,939,000,000 | 6.79% | 28 | Oklahoma | 8,491,000,000 | 0.96% |
| 4 | Florida | 50,948,000,000 | 5.77% | 29 | Kentucky | 8,395,000,000 | 0.95% |
| 5 | Illinois | 39,586,000,000 | 4.49% | 30 | Kansas | 8,215,000,000 | 0.93% |
| 6 | Pennsylvania | 36,100,000,000 | 4.09% | 31 | Iowa | 6,991,000,000 | 0.79% |
| 7 | Ohio | 33,896,000,000 | 3.84% | 32 | Arkansas | 5,902,000,000 | 0.67% |
| 8 | New Jersey | 32,518,000,000 | 3.69% | 33 | Mississippi | 5,873,000,000 | 0.67% |
| 9 | Michigan | 30,984,000,000 | 3.51% | 34 | Nevada | 5,336,000,000 | 0.60% |
| 10 | Massachusetts | 26,562,000,000 | 3.01% | 35 | New Mexico | 5,060,000,000 | 0.57% |
| 11 | Georgia | 24,411,000,000 | 2.77% | 36 | Hawaii | 4,930,000,000 | 0.56% |
| 12 | Virginia | 21,621,000,000 | 2.45% | 37 | Utah | 4,852,000,000 | 0.55% |
| 13 | North Carolina | 19,992,000,000 | 2.27% | 38 | New Hampshire | 4,684,000,000 | 0.53% |
| 14 | Maryland | 18,481,000,000 | 2.09% | 39 | Nebraska | 4,677,000,000 | 0.53% |
| 15 | Missouri | 17,278,000,000 | 1.96% | 40 | Rhode Island | 3,973,000,000 | 0.45% |
| 16 | Washington | 16,375,000,000 | 1.86% | 41 | Maine | 3,887,000,000 | 0.44% |
| 17 | Connecticut | 16,242,000,000 | 1.84% | 42 | West Virginia | 3,862,000,000 | 0.44% |
| 18 | Minnesota | 15,666,000,000 | 1.78% | 43 | Alaska | 2,477,000,000 | 0.28% |
| 19 | Indiana | 15,540,000,000 | 1.76% | 44 | Delaware | 2,340,000,000 | 0.27% |
| 20 | Wisconsin | 14,713,000,000 | 1.67% | 45 | Idaho | 2,278,000,000 | 0.26% |
| 21 | Tennessee | 14,671,000,000 | 1.66% | 46 | Montana | 1,967,000,000 | 0.22% |
| 22 | Arizona | 14,146,000,000 | 1.60% | 47 | South Dakota | 1,840,000,000 | 0.21% |
| 23 | Colorado | 12,983,000,000 | 1.47% | 48 | North Dakota | 1,768,000,000 | 0.20% |
| 24 | Alabama | 11,983,000,000 | 1.36% | 49 | Vermont | 1,676,000,000 | 0.19% |
| 25 | Louisiana | 11,789,000,000 | 1.34% | 50 | Wyoming | 1,184,000,000 | 0.13% |
|  |  |  |  |  | District of Columbia | 2,076,000,000 | 0.24% |

Source: Families USA Foundation

"Health Spending: The Growing Threat to the Family Budget" (December 1991) (Reprinted with permission)

*Calculated by the editors. Expenditures by both families and business for health care. See beginning of this chapter for definitions.

# Projected Percent Change in Total Health Care Payments: 1991 to 2000

## Projected National Rate = 127.20% Increase*

| RANK | STATE | PERCENT INCREASE | RANK | STATE | PERCENT INCREASE |
|---|---|---|---|---|---|
| 1 | New Mexico | 168.11 | 26 | Oklahoma | 121.82 |
| 2 | Arizona | 166.70 | 27 | Oregon | 121.28 |
| 3 | Georgia | 157.79 | 28 | Louisiana | 121.01 |
| 4 | Florida | 156.61 | 29 | Vermont | 120.84 |
| 5 | Nevada | 152.98 | 30 | Massachusetts | 120.26 |
| 6 | Hawaii | 151.60 | 31 | Idaho | 118.89 |
| 7 | New Hampshire | 150.08 | 32 | Wyoming | 117.93 |
| 8 | Alaska | 146.22 | 33 | Missouri | 117.07 |
| 9 | Texas | 144.79 | 34 | Kentucky | 116.81 |
| 10 | California | 142.84 | 35 | Delaware | 116.42 |
| 11 | Virginia | 141.66 | 36 | New York | 115.60 |
| 12 | Maryland | 140.66 | 37 | Montana | 114.03 |
| 13 | North Carolina | 140.49 | 38 | Minnesota | 112.73 |
| 14 | Colorado | 139.36 | 39 | Kansas | 111.66 |
| 15 | Utah | 139.19 | 40 | Michigan | 110.17 |
| 16 | South Carolina | 137.74 | 41 | Illinois | 109.48 |
| 17 | New Jersey | 132.95 | 42 | Indiana | 109.02 |
| 18 | Mississippi | 132.19 | 43 | Ohio | 107.33 |
| 19 | Washington | 128.81 | 44 | South Dakota | 107.29 |
| 20 | Alabama | 127.68 | 45 | Wisconsin | 106.41 |
| 21 | Connecticut | 127.39 | 46 | Pennsylvania | 105.14 |
| 22 | Tennessee | 127.20 | 47 | Nebraska | 102.68 |
| 23 | Rhode Island | 122.74 | 48 | West Virginia | 101.34 |
| 24 | Maine | 122.43 | 49 | North Dakota | 98.83 |
| 25 | Arkansas | 122.27 | 50 | Iowa | 92.34 |
| | | | | District of Columbia | 111.13 |

Source: Families USA Foundation

"Health Spending: The Growing Threat to the Family Budget" (December 1991) (Reprinted with permission)

*Calculated by the editors. Expenditures by both families and business for health care. See beginning of this chapter for definitions.

# Projected Annual Percent Change in Total Health Care Payments: 1991 to 2000

## Projected National Change = 9.55% Annual Increase*

| RANK | STATE | PERCENT | RANK | STATE | PERCENT |
|---|---|---|---|---|---|
| 1 | New Mexico | 11.58 | 26 | Oklahoma | 9.26 |
| 2 | Arizona | 11.52 | 27 | Oregon | 9.23 |
| 3 | Georgia | 11.10 | 28 | Louisiana | 9.21 |
| 4 | Florida | 11.04 | 29 | Vermont | 9.20 |
| 5 | Nevada | 10.86 | 30 | Massachusetts | 9.17 |
| 6 | Hawaii | 10.80 | 31 | Idaho | 9.09 |
| 7 | New Hampshire | 10.72 | 32 | Wyoming | 9.04 |
| 8 | Alaska | 10.53 | 33 | Missouri | 8.99 |
| 9 | Texas | 10.46 | 34 | Kentucky | 8.98 |
| 10 | California | 10.36 | 35 | Delaware | 8.96 |
| 11 | Virginia | 10.30 | 36 | New York | 8.91 |
| 12 | Maryland | 10.25 | 37 | Montana | 8.82 |
| 13 | North Carolina | 10.24 | 38 | Minnesota | 8.75 |
| 14 | Colorado | 10.18 | 39 | Kansas | 8.69 |
| 15 | Utah | 10.17 | 40 | Michigan | 8.60 |
| 16 | South Carolina | 10.10 | 41 | Illinois | 8.56 |
| 17 | New Jersey | 9.85 | 42 | Indiana | 8.54 |
| 18 | Mississippi | 9.81 | 43 | Ohio | 8.44 |
| 19 | Washington | 9.63 | 43 | South Dakota | 8.44 |
| 20 | Alabama | 9.57 | 45 | Wisconsin | 8.39 |
| 21 | Connecticut | 9.56 | 46 | Pennsylvania | 8.31 |
| 22 | Tennessee | 9.55 | 47 | Nebraska | 8.17 |
| 23 | Rhode Island | 9.31 | 48 | West Virginia | 8.09 |
| 24 | Maine | 9.29 | 49 | North Dakota | 7.94 |
| 25 | Arkansas | 9.28 | 50 | Iowa | 7.54 |

| | | | | | |
|---|---|---|---|---|---|
| | | | | District of Columbia | 8.66 |

Source: Families USA Foundation

"Health Spending: The Growing Threat to the Family Budget" (December 1991) (Reprinted with permission)

*Calculated by the editors. Expenditures by both families and business for health care. See beginning of this chapter for definitions.

# Total Health Care Payments per Family in 1991

## National Figure = $6,535 per Family*

| RANK | STATE | PER FAMILY | | RANK | STATE | PER FAMILY |
|------|-------|------------|---|------|-------|------------|
| 1 | Connecticut | $9,312 | | 26 | Oregon | $6,045 |
| 2 | Massachusetts | 8,484 | | 27 | Indiana | 5,930 |
| 3 | New York | 8,210 | | 28 | South Dakota | 5,919 |
| 4 | Alaska | 7,756 | | 29 | Virginia | 5,906 |
| 5 | Rhode Island | 7,647 | | 30 | Texas | 5,891 |
| 6 | New Jersey | 7,586 | | 31 | Washington | 5,826 |
| 7 | Illinois | 7,370 | | 32 | Georgia | 5,792 |
| 8 | Michigan | 7,337 | | 33 | Utah | 5,699 |
| 9 | Minnesota | 7,252 | | 34 | Louisiana | 5,677 |
| 10 | Hawaii | 7,190 | | 35 | Tennessee | 5,639 |
| 11 | California | 7,141 | | 36 | Alabama | 5,604 |
| 12 | Ohio | 7,005 | | 37 | Vermont | 5,598 |
| 13 | Kansas | 6,959 | | 38 | Florida | 5,556 |
| 14 | Pennsylvania | 6,825 | | 39 | Arizona | 5,321 |
| 15 | Missouri | 6,715 | | 40 | Wyoming | 5,284 |
| 16 | Wisconsin | 6,651 | | 41 | Oklahoma | 5,179 |
| 17 | Delaware | 6,573 | | 42 | North Carolina | 5,101 |
| 18 | New Hampshire | 6,561 | | 43 | West Virginia | 5,096 |
| 19 | Nebraska | 6,554 | | 44 | Montana | 4,910 |
| 20 | North Dakota | 6,528 | | 45 | New Mexico | 4,815 |
| 21 | Nevada | 6,290 | | 46 | Arkansas | 4,781 |
| 22 | Maine | 6,268 | | 47 | South Carolina | 4,722 |
| 23 | Maryland | 6,181 | | 48 | Idaho | 4,599 |
| 24 | Iowa | 6,148 | | 49 | Kentucky | 4,535 |
| 25 | Colorado | 6,073 | | 50 | Mississippi | 4,158 |
| | | | | | District of Columbia | 6,054 |

*Source: Families USA Foundation*

   *"Health Spending: The Growing Threat to the Family Budget" (December 1991) (Reprinted with permission)*

*Expenditures by both families and business for health care.  See beginning of this chapter for definitions.*

# Total Health Care Payments per Family in 1980

## National Average = $2,572 per Family*

| RANK | STATE | PER FAMILY | RANK | STATE | PER FAMILY |
|---|---|---|---|---|---|
| 1 | Connecticut | $3,252 | 26 | South Dakota | $2,367 |
| 2 | New York | 3,135 | 27 | Nevada | 2,338 |
| 3 | Massachusetts | 3,088 | 28 | Tennessee | 2,313 |
| 4 | Illinois | 3,069 | 29 | Alabama | 2,287 |
| 5 | Michigan | 2,957 | 30 | Georgia | 2,283 |
| 6 | Rhode Island | 2,946 | 31 | New Hampshire | 2,244 |
| 7 | Minnesota | 2,936 | 31 | Washington | 2,244 |
| 8 | New Jersey | 2,926 | 33 | West Virginia | 2,217 |
| 9 | Ohio | 2,883 | 34 | Virginia | 2,216 |
| 10 | Maryland | 2,812 | 35 | Maine | 2,213 |
| 11 | Alaska | 2,798 | 36 | Oklahoma | 2,184 |
| 12 | Wisconsin | 2,751 | 37 | Oregon | 2,176 |
| 13 | North Dakota | 2,713 | 38 | Kentucky | 2,146 |
| 14 | Iowa | 2,708 | 39 | North Carolina | 2,085 |
| 15 | Hawaii | 2,701 | 40 | Utah | 2,082 |
| 16 | Kansas | 2,696 | 41 | Montana | 2,009 |
| 17 | Pennsylvania | 2,675 | 42 | Wyoming | 2,002 |
| 18 | Nebraska | 2,658 | 43 | Arizona | 1,995 |
| 19 | Delaware | 2,642 | 44 | Florida | 1,973 |
| 20 | Missouri | 2,556 | 45 | Vermont | 1,969 |
| 21 | California | 2,553 | 46 | Arkansas | 1,951 |
| 22 | Louisiana | 2,493 | 47 | New Mexico | 1,878 |
| 23 | Colorado | 2,483 | 48 | South Carolina | 1,847 |
| 23 | Texas | 2,483 | 49 | Mississippi | 1,808 |
| 25 | Indiana | 2,457 | 50 | Idaho | 1,806 |
| | | | | District of Columbia | 2,247 |

Source: Families USA Foundation

"Health Spending: The Growing Threat to the Family Budget" (December 1991) (Reprinted with permission)

*Expenditures by both families and business for health care. See beginning of this chapter for definitions.

# Projected Total Health Care Payments per Family in 2000

## Projected National Figure = $13,911 per Family*

| RANK | STATE | PER FAMILY |
|------|-------|------------|
| 1 | Connecticut | $20,174 |
| 2 | Massachusetts | 18,385 |
| 3 | New York | 17,999 |
| 4 | Rhode Island | 16,459 |
| 5 | New Jersey | 16,249 |
| 6 | Illinois | 15,897 |
| 7 | Michigan | 15,684 |
| 8 | California | 15,300 |
| 9 | Minnesota | 15,144 |
| 10 | Alaska | 15,081 |
| 11 | Ohio | 15,009 |
| 12 | Hawaii | 14,951 |
| 13 | Kansas | 14,854 |
| 14 | Pennsylvania | 14,700 |
| 15 | Wisconsin | 14,175 |
| 16 | Missouri | 14,144 |
| 17 | North Dakota | 14,077 |
| 18 | Nebraska | 13,953 |
| 19 | New Hampshire | 13,623 |
| 20 | Maine | 13,422 |
| 21 | Iowa | 13,344 |
| 22 | Maryland | 13,274 |
| 23 | Nevada | 13,254 |
| 24 | Oregon | 13,199 |
| 25 | Delaware | 13,021 |

| RANK | STATE | PER FAMILY |
|------|-------|------------|
| 26 | Colorado | $12,866 |
| 27 | Washington | 12,738 |
| 28 | Virginia | 12,735 |
| 29 | Indiana | 12,699 |
| 30 | South Dakota | 12,547 |
| 31 | Louisiana | 12,531 |
| 32 | Texas | 12,456 |
| 33 | Utah | 12,328 |
| 34 | Georgia | 12,164 |
| 35 | Alabama | 12,041 |
| 36 | Tennessee | 12,031 |
| 37 | Vermont | 11,909 |
| 38 | Wyoming | 11,744 |
| 39 | Florida | 11,512 |
| 40 | West Virginia | 11,282 |
| 41 | Oklahoma | 11,227 |
| 42 | Arizona | 10,919 |
| 43 | Montana | 10,841 |
| 44 | North Carolina | 10,722 |
| 45 | Arkansas | 10,213 |
| 46 | New Mexico | 10,199 |
| 47 | South Carolina | 10,112 |
| 48 | Idaho | 10,011 |
| 49 | Kentucky | 9,952 |
| 50 | Mississippi | 9,011 |

| | | |
|--|--|--|
| | District of Columbia | 12,685 |

Source: Families USA Foundation

"Health Spending: The Growing Threat to the Family Budget" (December 1991) (Reprinted with permission)

*Expenditures by both families and business for health care. See beginning of this chapter for definitions.

# Per Capita Total Health Care Payments in 1991

## National Per Capita = $2,751*

| RANK | STATE | PER CAPITA |
|------|-------|-----------|
| 1 | Connecticut | $3,874 |
| 2 | Massachusetts | 3,684 |
| 3 | New York | 3,484 |
| 4 | Rhode Island | 3,224 |
| 5 | New Jersey | 3,152 |
| 6 | Minnesota | 3,136 |
| 7 | Illinois | 3,132 |
| 8 | California | 3,047 |
| 9 | Michigan | 3,002 |
| 10 | Alaska | 2,972 |
| 11 | Delaware | 2,956 |
| 12 | Kansas | 2,949 |
| 13 | Ohio | 2,887 |
| 14 | Pennsylvania | 2,870 |
| 15 | Hawaii | 2,865 |
| 16 | Missouri | 2,861 |
| 17 | Nebraska | 2,859 |
| 18 | New Hampshire | 2,824 |
| 19 | North Dakota | 2,817 |
| 20 | Wisconsin | 2,791 |
| 21 | Colorado | 2,759 |
| 22 | Nevada | 2,717 |
| 23 | Iowa | 2,709 |
| 24 | Maryland | 2,703 |
| 25 | Maine | 2,571 |

| RANK | STATE | PER CAPITA |
|------|-------|-----------|
| 26 | Oregon | $2,569 |
| 27 | Indiana | 2,541 |
| 28 | Washington | 2,533 |
| 29 | Florida | 2,450 |
| 30 | Vermont | 2,446 |
| 31 | South Dakota | 2,440 |
| 32 | Virginia | 2,428 |
| 33 | Texas | 2,386 |
| 34 | Georgia | 2,336 |
| 35 | Tennessee | 2,329 |
| 36 | Alabama | 2,295 |
| 37 | Louisiana | 2,291 |
| 38 | Arizona | 2,263 |
| 39 | Oklahoma | 2,195 |
| 40 | Wyoming | 2,183 |
| 41 | Montana | 2,135 |
| 42 | West Virginia | 2,116 |
| 43 | North Carolina | 2,112 |
| 44 | Arkansas | 2,035 |
| 45 | Utah | 1,969 |
| 46 | New Mexico | 1,944 |
| 47 | Kentucky | 1,936 |
| 48 | South Carolina | 1,870 |
| 49 | Idaho | 1,844 |
| 50 | Mississippi | 1,714 |

| | District of Columbia | 3,124 |

Source: Families USA Foundation

"Health Spending: The Growing Threat to the Family Budget" (December 1991) (Reprinted with permission)

*Calculated by the editors using 1991 Census resident population figures. Expenditures by both families and business for health care. See beginning of this chapter for definitions.

# Per Capita Total Health Care Payments in 1980

## National Per Capita = $1,014*

| RANK | STATE | PER CAPITA | | RANK | STATE | PER CAPITA |
|---|---|---|---|---|---|---|
| 1 | Connecticut | $1,285 | | 26 | Texas | $965 |
| 2 | New York | 1,228 | | 27 | Louisiana | 945 |
| 3 | Massachusetts | 1,221 | | 28 | Oregon | 938 |
| 4 | Minnesota | 1,163 | | 29 | New Hampshire | 909 |
| 5 | Illinois | 1,148 | | 30 | South Dakota | 902 |
| 6 | Rhode Island | 1,144 | | 31 | Oklahoma | 888 |
| 7 | Michigan | 1,135 | | 32 | Virginia | 884 |
| 8 | Ohio | 1,110 | | 33 | Florida | 883 |
| 9 | California | 1,091 | | 33 | Tennessee | 883 |
| 10 | Wisconsin | 1,085 | | 35 | Arizona | 855 |
| 11 | Nevada | 1,081 | | 36 | Georgia | 843 |
| 12 | Alaska | 1,065 | | 37 | Maine | 839 |
| 13 | Kansas | 1,058 | | 38 | Alabama | 836 |
| 14 | New Jersey | 1,056 | | 39 | West Virginia | 833 |
| 15 | Pennsylvania | 1,045 | | 40 | Wyoming | 822 |
| 16 | Nebraska | 1,042 | | 41 | Vermont | 817 |
| 16 | North Dakota | 1,042 | | 42 | Montana | 812 |
| 18 | Maryland | 1,032 | | 43 | Kentucky | 780 |
| 19 | Iowa | 1,028 | | 44 | North Carolina | 777 |
| 20 | Missouri | 1,024 | | 45 | Arkansas | 740 |
| 21 | Colorado | 1,010 | | 46 | Utah | 721 |
| 22 | Delaware | 1,003 | | 47 | New Mexico | 709 |
| 23 | Indiana | 982 | | 48 | Idaho | 698 |
| 24 | Hawaii | 981 | | 49 | South Carolina | 690 |
| 25 | Washington | 968 | | 50 | Mississippi | 647 |

District of Columbia     1,111

*Source: Families USA Foundation*

*"Health Spending: The Growing Threat to the Family Budget" (December 1991) (Reprinted with permission)*

*\*Calculated by the editors using 1980 Census resident population figures. Expenditures by both families and business for health care. See beginning of this chapter for definitions.*

# Projected Per Capita Health Care Payments in 2000

## Projected National Per Capita = $5,887*

| RANK | STATE | PER CAPITA | | RANK | STATE | PER CAPITA |
|------|-------|------------|---|------|-------|------------|
| 1 | Connecticut | $8,416 | | 26 | North Dakota | $5,655 |
| 2 | Massachusetts | 7,992 | | 27 | Maine | 5,556 |
| 3 | New York | 7,541 | | 28 | Florida | 5,416 |
| 4 | Rhode Island | 6,873 | | 29 | Indiana | 5,415 |
| 5 | Nevada | 6,772 | | 30 | Virginia | 5,363 |
| 6 | California | 6,711 | | 31 | Vermont | 5,183 |
| 7 | New Jersey | 6,667 | | 32 | Texas | 5,014 |
| 8 | Minnesota | 6,584 | | 33 | Georgia | 5,012 |
| 9 | Illinois | 6,541 | | 34 | South Dakota | 4,979 |
| 10 | Michigan | 6,390 | | 35 | Tennessee | 4,976 |
| 11 | Ohio | 6,160 | | 36 | Arizona | 4,901 |
| 12 | Kansas | 6,157 | | 37 | Alabama | 4,845 |
| 13 | Pennsylvania | 6,123 | | 38 | Louisiana | 4,768 |
| 14 | Hawaii | 6,083 | | 39 | Montana | 4,650 |
| 15 | Alaska | 6,071 | | 40 | Oklahoma | 4,580 |
| 16 | Maryland | 5,995 | | 41 | North Carolina | 4,573 |
| 17 | Wisconsin | 5,966 | | 42 | Wyoming | 4,474 |
| 18 | Missouri | 5,952 | | 43 | West Virginia | 4,456 |
| 19 | Nebraska | 5,933 | | 44 | Arkansas | 4,242 |
| 20 | Delaware | 5,926 | | 45 | Utah | 4,188 |
| 21 | New Hampshire | 5,855 | | 46 | Kentucky | 4,174 |
| 22 | Colorado | 5,848 | | 47 | New Mexico | 4,101 |
| 23 | Washington | 5,828 | | 48 | South Carolina | 4,052 |
| 24 | Oregon | 5,773 | | 49 | Idaho | 4,006 |
| 25 | Iowa | 5,713 | | 50 | Mississippi | 3,586 |

District of Columbia     6,221

Source: Families USA Foundation

"Health Spending: The Growing Threat to the Family Budget" (December 1991) (Reprinted with permission)

*Calculated by the editors using Census projected resident population figures for 2000. Expenditures by both families and business for health care. See beginning of this chapter for definitions.

# Change in Per Capita Health Care Payments: 1980 to 1991

## National Per Capita Change = $1,737 Increase*

| RANK | STATE | INCREASE | RANK | STATE | INCREASE |
|------|-------|----------|------|-------|----------|
| 1 | Connecticut | $2,589 | 26 | Oregon | $1,631 |
| 2 | Massachusetts | 2,463 | 27 | Vermont | 1,629 |
| 3 | New York | 2,256 | 28 | Florida | 1,567 |
| 4 | New Jersey | 2,096 | 29 | Washington | 1,565 |
| 5 | Rhode Island | 2,080 | 30 | Indiana | 1,559 |
| 6 | Illinois | 1,984 | 31 | Virginia | 1,544 |
| 7 | Minnesota | 1,973 | 32 | South Dakota | 1,538 |
| 8 | California | 1,956 | 33 | Georgia | 1,493 |
| 9 | Delaware | 1,953 | 34 | Alabama | 1,459 |
| 10 | New Hampshire | 1,915 | 35 | Tennessee | 1,446 |
| 11 | Alaska | 1,907 | 36 | Texas | 1,421 |
| 12 | Kansas | 1,891 | 37 | Arizona | 1,408 |
| 13 | Hawaii | 1,884 | 38 | Wyoming | 1,361 |
| 14 | Michigan | 1,867 | 39 | Louisiana | 1,346 |
| 15 | Missouri | 1,837 | 40 | North Carolina | 1,335 |
| 16 | Pennsylvania | 1,825 | 41 | Montana | 1,323 |
| 17 | Nebraska | 1,817 | 42 | Oklahoma | 1,307 |
| 18 | Ohio | 1,777 | 43 | Arkansas | 1,295 |
| 19 | North Dakota | 1,775 | 44 | West Virginia | 1,283 |
| 20 | Colorado | 1,749 | 45 | Utah | 1,248 |
| 21 | Maine | 1,732 | 46 | New Mexico | 1,235 |
| 22 | Wisconsin | 1,706 | 47 | South Carolina | 1,180 |
| 23 | Iowa | 1,681 | 48 | Kentucky | 1,156 |
| 24 | Maryland | 1,671 | 49 | Idaho | 1,146 |
| 25 | Nevada | 1,636 | 50 | Mississippi | 1,067 |

District of Columbia     2,013

Source: Families USA Foundation

*"Health Spending: The Growing Threat to the Family Budget" (December 1991) (Reprinted with permission)*

*Calculated by the editors using Census resident population figures. Expenditures by both families and business for health care. See beginning of this chapter for definitions.*

## Percent Change in Per Capita Health Care Payments: 1980 to 1991

## National Change = 171.30% Increase*

| RANK | STATE | PERCENT INCREASE | RANK | STATE | PERCENT INCREASE |
|---|---|---|---|---|---|
| 1 | New Hampshire | 210.67 | 26 | Illinois | 172.82 |
| 2 | Maine | 206.44 | 27 | North Carolina | 171.81 |
| 3 | Massachusetts | 201.72 | 28 | South Carolina | 171.01 |
| 4 | Connecticut | 201.48 | 29 | South Dakota | 170.51 |
| 5 | Vermont | 199.39 | 30 | North Dakota | 170.35 |
| 6 | New Jersey | 198.48 | 31 | Minnesota | 169.65 |
| 7 | Delaware | 194.72 | 32 | Wyoming | 165.57 |
| 8 | Hawaii | 192.05 | 33 | Mississippi | 164.91 |
| 9 | New York | 183.71 | 34 | Arizona | 164.68 |
| 10 | Rhode Island | 181.82 | 35 | Michigan | 164.49 |
| 11 | Missouri | 179.39 | 36 | Idaho | 164.18 |
| 12 | California | 179.29 | 37 | Tennessee | 163.76 |
| 13 | Alaska | 179.06 | 38 | Iowa | 163.52 |
| 14 | Kansas | 178.73 | 39 | Montana | 162.93 |
| 15 | Florida | 177.46 | 40 | Maryland | 161.92 |
| 16 | Georgia | 177.11 | 41 | Washington | 161.67 |
| 17 | Arkansas | 175.00 | 42 | Ohio | 160.09 |
| 18 | Virginia | 174.66 | 43 | Indiana | 158.76 |
| 19 | Pennsylvania | 174.64 | 44 | Wisconsin | 157.24 |
| 20 | Alabama | 174.52 | 45 | West Virginia | 154.02 |
| 21 | Nebraska | 174.38 | 46 | Nevada | 151.34 |
| 22 | New Mexico | 174.19 | 47 | Kentucky | 148.21 |
| 23 | Oregon | 173.88 | 48 | Texas | 147.25 |
| 24 | Colorado | 173.17 | 49 | Oklahoma | 147.18 |
| 25 | Utah | 173.09 | 50 | Louisiana | 142.43 |
| | | | | District of Columbia | 181.19 |

Source: Families USA Foundation

"Health Spending: The Growing Threat to the Family Budget" (December 1991) (Reprinted with permission)

*Calculated by the editors using Census resident population figures. Expenditures by both families and business for health care. See beginning of this chapter for definitions.

# Annual Percent Change in Per Capita Health Care Payments: 1980 to 1991

## National Change = 9.50% Annual Increase*

| RANK | STATE | PERCENT INCREASE | RANK | STATE | PERCENT INCREASE |
|------|-------|------------------|------|-------|------------------|
| 1 | New Hampshire | 10.85 | 26 | Illinois | 9.55 |
| 2 | Maine | 10.72 | 27 | North Carolina | 9.52 |
| 3 | Massachusetts | 10.56 | 28 | South Carolina | 9.49 |
| 4 | Connecticut | 10.55 | 29 | South Dakota | 9.47 |
| 5 | Vermont | 10.48 | 30 | North Dakota | 9.46 |
| 6 | New Jersey | 10.45 | 31 | Minnesota | 9.44 |
| 7 | Delaware | 10.32 | 32 | Wyoming | 9.29 |
| 8 | Hawaii | 10.23 | 33 | Mississippi | 9.26 |
| 9 | New York | 9.94 | 34 | Arizona | 9.25 |
| 10 | Rhode Island | 9.88 | 35 | Michigan | 9.24 |
| 11 | California | 9.79 | 36 | Idaho | 9.23 |
| 11 | Missouri | 9.79 | 37 | Tennessee | 9.22 |
| 13 | Alaska | 9.78 | 38 | Iowa | 9.21 |
| 14 | Kansas | 9.77 | 39 | Montana | 9.19 |
| 15 | Florida | 9.72 | 40 | Maryland | 9.15 |
| 16 | Georgia | 9.71 | 41 | Washington | 9.14 |
| 17 | Arkansas | 9.63 | 42 | Ohio | 9.08 |
| 18 | Alabama | 9.62 | 43 | Indiana | 9.03 |
| 18 | Pennsylvania | 9.62 | 44 | Wisconsin | 8.97 |
| 18 | Virginia | 9.62 | 45 | West Virginia | 8.84 |
| 21 | Nebraska | 9.61 | 46 | Nevada | 8.74 |
| 22 | New Mexico | 9.60 | 47 | Kentucky | 8.62 |
| 23 | Oregon | 9.59 | 48 | Texas | 8.58 |
| 24 | Colorado | 9.57 | 49 | Oklahoma | 8.57 |
| 25 | Utah | 9.56 | 50 | Louisiana | 8.38 |
| | | | | District of Columbia | 9.85 |

Source: Families USA Foundation

"Health Spending: The Growing Threat to the Family Budget" (December 1991) (Reprinted with permission)

*Calculated by the editors using Census resident population figures. Expenditures by both families and business for health care. See beginning of this chapter for definitions.

# Projected Change in Per Capita Health Care Payments: 1991 to 2000

## Projected National Per Capita Change = $3,136 Increase*

| RANK | STATE | INCREASE | | RANK | STATE | INCREASE |
|---|---|---|---|---|---|---|
| 1 | Connecticut | $4,542 | | 26 | Delaware | $2,970 |
| 2 | Massachusetts | 4,308 | | 27 | Florida | 2,966 |
| 3 | New York | 4,057 | | 28 | Virginia | 2,935 |
| 4 | Nevada | 4,055 | | 29 | Indiana | 2,874 |
| 5 | California | 3,664 | | 30 | North Dakota | 2,838 |
| 6 | Rhode Island | 3,649 | | 31 | Vermont | 2,737 |
| 7 | New Jersey | 3,515 | | 32 | Georgia | 2,676 |
| 8 | Minnesota | 3,448 | | 33 | Tennessee | 2,647 |
| 9 | Illinois | 3,409 | | 34 | Arizona | 2,638 |
| 10 | Michigan | 3,388 | | 35 | Texas | 2,628 |
| 11 | Washington | 3,295 | | 36 | Alabama | 2,550 |
| 12 | Maryland | 3,292 | | 37 | South Dakota | 2,539 |
| 13 | Ohio | 3,273 | | 38 | Montana | 2,515 |
| 14 | Pennsylvania | 3,253 | | 39 | Louisiana | 2,477 |
| 15 | Hawaii | 3,218 | | 40 | North Carolina | 2,461 |
| 16 | Kansas | 3,208 | | 41 | Oklahoma | 2,385 |
| 17 | Oregon | 3,204 | | 42 | West Virginia | 2,340 |
| 18 | Wisconsin | 3,175 | | 43 | Wyoming | 2,291 |
| 19 | Alaska | 3,099 | | 44 | Kentucky | 2,238 |
| 20 | Missouri | 3,091 | | 45 | Utah | 2,219 |
| 21 | Colorado | 3,089 | | 46 | Arkansas | 2,207 |
| 22 | Nebraska | 3,074 | | 47 | South Carolina | 2,182 |
| 23 | New Hampshire | 3,031 | | 48 | Idaho | 2,162 |
| 24 | Iowa | 3,004 | | 49 | New Mexico | 2,157 |
| 25 | Maine | 2,985 | | 50 | Mississippi | 1,872 |
| | | | | | District of Columbia | 3,097 |

Source: Families USA Foundation

"Health Spending: The Growing Threat to the Family Budget" (December 1991) (Reprinted with permission)

*Calculated by the editors using Census resident population figures. Expenditures by both families and business for health care. See beginning of this chapter for definitions.

# Projected Percent Change in Per Capita Health Care Payments: 1991 to 2000

## Projected National Change = 113.99% Increase*

| RANK | STATE | PERCENT INCREASE | | RANK | STATE | PERCENT INCREASE |
|---|---|---|---|---|---|---|
| 1 | Nevada | 149.25 | | 26 | Utah | 112.70 |
| 2 | Washington | 130.08 | | 27 | Hawaii | 112.32 |
| 3 | Oregon | 124.72 | | 28 | Colorado | 111.96 |
| 4 | Maryland | 121.79 | | 29 | Vermont | 111.90 |
| 5 | Florida | 121.06 | | 30 | New Jersey | 111.52 |
| 6 | Virginia | 120.88 | | 31 | Alabama | 111.11 |
| 7 | California | 120.25 | | 32 | New Mexico | 110.96 |
| 8 | Montana | 117.80 | | 33 | Iowa | 110.89 |
| 9 | Idaho | 117.25 | | 34 | West Virginia | 110.59 |
| 10 | Connecticut | 117.24 | | 35 | Texas | 110.14 |
| 11 | Massachusetts | 116.94 | | 36 | Minnesota | 109.95 |
| 12 | South Carolina | 116.68 | | 37 | Mississippi | 109.22 |
| 13 | Arizona | 116.57 | | 38 | Illinois | 108.84 |
| 14 | North Carolina | 116.52 | | 39 | Kansas | 108.78 |
| 15 | New York | 116.45 | | 40 | Oklahoma | 108.66 |
| 16 | Maine | 116.10 | | 41 | Arkansas | 108.45 |
| 17 | Kentucky | 115.60 | | 42 | Louisiana | 108.12 |
| 18 | Georgia | 114.55 | | 43 | Missouri | 108.04 |
| 19 | Wisconsin | 113.76 | | 44 | Nebraska | 107.52 |
| 20 | Tennessee | 113.65 | | 45 | New Hampshire | 107.33 |
| 21 | Ohio | 113.37 | | 46 | Wyoming | 104.95 |
| 22 | Pennsylvania | 113.34 | | 47 | Alaska | 104.27 |
| 23 | Rhode Island | 113.18 | | 48 | South Dakota | 104.06 |
| 24 | Indiana | 113.11 | | 49 | North Dakota | 100.75 |
| 25 | Michigan | 112.86 | | 50 | Delaware | 100.47 |
| | | | | | District of Columbia | 99.14 |

Source: Families USA Foundation

"Health Spending: The Growing Threat to the Family Budget" (December 1991) (Reprinted with permission)

*Calculated by the editors using Census resident population figures. Expenditures by both families and business for health care. See beginning of this chapter for definitions.

# Projected Annual Percent Change in Per Capita Health Care Payments: 1991 to 2000

## Projected National Change = 8.88% Annual Increase*

| RANK | STATE | PERCENT INCREASE | RANK | STATE | PERCENT INCREASE |
|------|-------|------------------|------|-------|------------------|
| 1 | Nevada | 10.68 | 26 | Utah | 8.75 |
| 2 | Washington | 9.70 | 27 | Hawaii | 8.73 |
| 3 | Oregon | 9.41 | 28 | Colorado | 8.71 |
| 4 | Maryland | 9.25 | 29 | Vermont | 8.70 |
| 5 | Florida | 9.21 | 30 | New Jersey | 8.68 |
| 6 | Virginia | 9.20 | 31 | Alabama | 8.66 |
| 7 | California | 9.17 | 32 | New Mexico | 8.65 |
| 8 | Montana | 9.03 | 33 | Iowa | 8.64 |
| 9 | Connecticut | 9.00 | 34 | West Virginia | 8.63 |
| 9 | Idaho | 9.00 | 35 | Texas | 8.60 |
| 11 | Massachusetts | 8.99 | 36 | Minnesota | 8.59 |
| 12 | Arizona | 8.97 | 37 | Mississippi | 8.55 |
| 12 | South Carolina | 8.97 | 38 | Illinois | 8.53 |
| 14 | New York | 8.96 | 39 | Kansas | 8.52 |
| 14 | North Carolina | 8.96 | 39 | Oklahoma | 8.52 |
| 16 | Maine | 8.94 | 41 | Arkansas | 8.50 |
| 17 | Kentucky | 8.91 | 42 | Louisiana | 8.48 |
| 18 | Georgia | 8.85 | 42 | Missouri | 8.48 |
| 19 | Wisconsin | 8.81 | 44 | Nebraska | 8.45 |
| 20 | Tennessee | 8.80 | 45 | New Hampshire | 8.44 |
| 21 | Ohio | 8.79 | 46 | Wyoming | 8.30 |
| 22 | Pennsylvania | 8.78 | 47 | Alaska | 8.26 |
| 23 | Indiana | 8.77 | 48 | South Dakota | 8.25 |
| 23 | Rhode Island | 8.77 | 49 | North Dakota | 8.05 |
| 25 | Michigan | 8.76 | 50 | Delaware | 8.03 |
| | | | | District of Columbia | 7.95 |

Source: Families USA Foundation

"Health Spending: The Growing Threat to the Family Budget" (December 1991) (Reprinted with permission)

*Calculated by the editors using Census resident population figures. Expenditures by both families and business for health care. See beginning of this chapter for definitions.

# Health Care Payments Paid by Families in 1991

## National Total = $456,055,000,000*

| RANK | STATE | PAYMENTS | % | RANK | STATE | PAYMENTS | % |
|---|---|---|---|---|---|---|---|
| 1 | California | $57,474,000,000 | 12.60% | 26 | Oklahoma | $5,095,000,000 | 1.12% |
| 2 | New York | 42,794,000,000 | 9.38% | 27 | Kentucky | 5,081,000,000 | 1.11% |
| 3 | Texas | 28,778,000,000 | 6.31% | 28 | Iowa | 4,958,000,000 | 1.09% |
| 4 | Florida | 23,026,000,000 | 5.05% | 29 | Oregon | 4,842,000,000 | 1.06% |
| 5 | Illinois | 22,910,000,000 | 5.02% | 30 | South Carolina | 4,814,000,000 | 1.06% |
| 6 | Pennsylvania | 21,634,000,000 | 4.74% | 31 | Kansas | 4,738,000,000 | 1.04% |
| 7 | Ohio | 20,168,000,000 | 4.42% | 32 | Arkansas | 3,514,000,000 | 0.77% |
| 8 | Michigan | 17,515,000,000 | 3.84% | 33 | Mississippi | 3,215,000,000 | 0.70% |
| 9 | New Jersey | 15,681,000,000 | 3.44% | 34 | Nebraska | 2,966,000,000 | 0.65% |
| 10 | Massachusetts | 13,852,000,000 | 3.04% | 35 | West Virginia | 2,575,000,000 | 0.56% |
| 11 | Virginia | 11,264,000,000 | 2.47% | 36 | Utah | 2,252,000,000 | 0.49% |
| 12 | Georgia | 11,110,000,000 | 2.44% | 37 | Nevada | 2,161,000,000 | 0.47% |
| 13 | North Carolina | 10,126,000,000 | 2.22% | 38 | Rhode Island | 2,080,000,000 | 0.46% |
| 14 | Missouri | 9,587,000,000 | 2.10% | 39 | Hawaii | 2,079,000,000 | 0.46% |
| 15 | Indiana | 9,549,000,000 | 2.09% | 40 | New Mexico | 2,061,000,000 | 0.45% |
| 16 | Maryland | 9,532,000,000 | 2.09% | 41 | Maine | 1,999,000,000 | 0.44% |
| 17 | Wisconsin | 8,825,000,000 | 1.94% | 42 | New Hampshire | 1,836,000,000 | 0.40% |
| 18 | Minnesota | 8,753,000,000 | 1.92% | 43 | Delaware | 1,343,000,000 | 0.29% |
| 19 | Washington | 8,094,000,000 | 1.77% | 44 | Idaho | 1,252,000,000 | 0.27% |
| 20 | Connecticut | 7,423,000,000 | 1.63% | 45 | North Dakota | 1,149,000,000 | 0.25% |
| 21 | Tennessee | 7,132,000,000 | 1.56% | 46 | South Dakota | 1,119,000,000 | 0.25% |
| 22 | Alabama | 6,805,000,000 | 1.49% | 47 | Montana | 1,108,000,000 | 0.24% |
| 23 | Louisiana | 6,536,000,000 | 1.43% | 48 | Vermont | 904,000,000 | 0.20% |
| 24 | Colorado | 6,032,000,000 | 1.32% | 49 | Alaska | 840,000,000 | 0.18% |
| 25 | Arizona | 5,484,000,000 | 1.20% | 50 | Wyoming | 660,000,000 | 0.14% |
|  |  |  |  |  | District of Columbia | 1,327,000,000 | 0.29% |

Source: Families USA Foundation

"Health Spending: The Growing Threat to the Family Budget" (December 1991) (Reprinted with permission)

*Reflects payments made directly by families and does not inlcude payments made by business.  See beginning of this chapter for definitions.

# Percent of Health Care Payments Paid by Families in 1991

## National Rate = 65.7% Paid by Families*

| RANK | STATE | PERCENT | RANK | STATE | PERCENT |
|------|-------|---------|------|-------|---------|
| 1 | Virginia | 73.8 | 26 | Colorado | 64.8 |
| 2 | Oklahoma | 73.1 | 27 | Arizona | 64.6 |
| 3 | Arkansas | 72.8 | 27 | Utah | 64.6 |
| 4 | Alabama | 72.5 | 29 | Oregon | 64.5 |
| 4 | Maryland | 72.5 | 30 | Kansas | 64.4 |
| 6 | Mississippi | 72.4 | 31 | Rhode Island | 64.3 |
| 7 | South Carolina | 72.3 | 32 | Montana | 64.2 |
| 8 | Georgia | 71.8 | 32 | North Dakota | 64.2 |
| 9 | North Carolina | 71.2 | 34 | New Jersey | 64.1 |
| 10 | Florida | 70.8 | 35 | Hawaii | 63.9 |
| 11 | Kentucky | 70.7 | 35 | Ohio | 63.9 |
| 12 | Texas | 69.5 | 37 | Wisconsin | 63.8 |
| 13 | New Mexico | 68.5 | 38 | Washington | 63.7 |
| 14 | New York | 68.0 | 39 | Illinois | 63.4 |
| 15 | West Virginia | 67.6 | 40 | Maine | 63.0 |
| 16 | Louisiana | 67.1 | 40 | Minnesota | 63.0 |
| 17 | Indiana | 67.0 | 40 | Pennsylvania | 63.0 |
| 18 | Delaware | 66.8 | 43 | Massachusetts | 62.7 |
| 19 | Wyoming | 65.7 | 44 | Michigan | 62.3 |
| 20 | Iowa | 65.5 | 45 | California | 62.1 |
| 21 | Idaho | 65.3 | 46 | Nevada | 62.0 |
| 21 | South Dakota | 65.3 | 47 | Tennessee | 61.8 |
| 23 | Vermont | 65.2 | 48 | New Hampshire | 58.8 |
| 24 | Nebraska | 65.1 | 49 | Connecticut | 58.2 |
| 25 | Missouri | 65.0 | 50 | Alaska | 49.6 |

District of Columbia                71.0

*Source: Families USA Foundation*

*"Health Spending: The Growing Threat to the Family Budget" (December 1991) (Reprinted with permission)*

*\*As a percent of total health care payments by business and families. See beginning of this chapter for definitions.*

# Health Care Payments Paid by Families in 1980

## National Total = $155,517,000,000*

| RANK | STATE | PAYMENTS | % | RANK | STATE | PAYMENTS | % |
|---|---|---|---|---|---|---|---|
| 1 | California | $16,845,000,000 | 10.83% | 26 | Oklahoma | $1,985,000,000 | 1.28% |
| 2 | New York | 14,851,000,000 | 9.55% | 27 | Colorado | 1,949,000,000 | 1.25% |
| 3 | Texas | 9,918,000,000 | 6.38% | 28 | Kansas | 1,670,000,000 | 1.07% |
| 4 | Illinois | 8,554,000,000 | 5.50% | 29 | Oregon | 1,609,000,000 | 1.03% |
| 5 | Pennsylvania | 8,109,000,000 | 5.21% | 30 | South Carolina | 1,605,000,000 | 1.03% |
| 6 | Ohio | 7,672,000,000 | 4.93% | 31 | Arizona | 1,524,000,000 | 0.98% |
| 7 | Michigan | 6,683,000,000 | 4.30% | 32 | Arkansas | 1,252,000,000 | 0.81% |
| 8 | Florida | 6,377,000,000 | 4.10% | 33 | Mississippi | 1,175,000,000 | 0.76% |
| 9 | New Jersey | 5,156,000,000 | 3.32% | 34 | West Virginia | 1,166,000,000 | 0.75% |
| 10 | Massachusetts | 4,678,000,000 | 3.01% | 35 | Nebraska | 1,110,000,000 | 0.71% |
| 11 | Indiana | 3,607,000,000 | 2.32% | 36 | Utah | 729,000,000 | 0.47% |
| 12 | Virginia | 3,554,000,000 | 2.29% | 37 | Rhode Island | 699,000,000 | 0.45% |
| 13 | Missouri | 3,432,000,000 | 2.21% | 38 | Hawaii | 641,000,000 | 0.41% |
| 14 | Georgia | 3,361,000,000 | 2.16% | 39 | Maine | 634,000,000 | 0.41% |
| 15 | Wisconsin | 3,343,000,000 | 2.15% | 40 | New Mexico | 595,000,000 | 0.38% |
| 16 | North Carolina | 3,332,000,000 | 2.14% | 41 | Nevada | 559,000,000 | 0.36% |
| 17 | Maryland | 3,173,000,000 | 2.04% | 42 | New Hampshire | 518,000,000 | 0.33% |
| 18 | Minnesota | 3,102,000,000 | 1.99% | 43 | North Dakota | 450,000,000 | 0.29% |
| 19 | Louisiana | 2,663,000,000 | 1.71% | 44 | Idaho | 439,000,000 | 0.28% |
| 20 | Washington | 2,652,000,000 | 1.71% | 45 | Delaware | 432,000,000 | 0.28% |
| 21 | Tennessee | 2,582,000,000 | 1.66% | 46 | South Dakota | 430,000,000 | 0.28% |
| 22 | Connecticut | 2,474,000,000 | 1.59% | 47 | Montana | 428,000,000 | 0.28% |
| 23 | Alabama | 2,431,000,000 | 1.56% | 48 | Vermont | 282,000,000 | 0.18% |
| 24 | Kentucky | 2,029,000,000 | 1.30% | 49 | Wyoming | 267,000,000 | 0.17% |
| 25 | Iowa | 2,019,000,000 | 1.30% | 50 | Alaska | 243,000,000 | 0.16% |
| | | | | | District of Columbia | 529,000,000 | 0.34% |

*Source: Families USA Foundation*

*"Health Spending: The Growing Threat to the Family Budget" (December 1991) (Reprinted with permission)*

*\*Reflects payments made directly by families and does not inlcude payments made by business. See beginning of this chapter for definitions.*

# Percent of Health Care Payments Paid by Families in 1980

## National Rate = 67.7% Paid by Families*

| RANK | STATE | PERCENT | RANK | STATE | PERCENT |
|------|-------|---------|------|-------|---------|
| 1 | Virginia | 75.2 | 25 | Montana | 67.0 |
| 2 | Alabama | 74.6 | 27 | Indiana | 66.9 |
| 3 | South Carolina | 74.5 | 28 | Colorado | 66.8 |
| 4 | Florida | 74.1 | 28 | Kansas | 66.8 |
| 5 | Arkansas | 74.0 | 28 | Massachusetts | 66.8 |
| 6 | Oklahoma | 73.9 | 31 | Idaho | 66.6 |
| 7 | Georgia | 73.0 | 32 | New Jersey | 66.3 |
| 8 | Maryland | 72.9 | 32 | Washington | 66.3 |
| 8 | North Carolina | 72.9 | 34 | North Dakota | 66.2 |
| 10 | Delaware | 72.4 | 35 | Arizona | 65.6 |
| 11 | Texas | 72.2 | 36 | Wisconsin | 65.5 |
| 12 | Mississippi | 72.1 | 37 | Minnesota | 65.4 |
| 13 | West Virginia | 71.8 | 37 | Pennsylvania | 65.4 |
| 14 | Kentucky | 71.0 | 39 | California | 65.2 |
| 15 | Utah | 69.2 | 39 | Illinois | 65.2 |
| 15 | Wyoming | 69.2 | 39 | Oregon | 65.2 |
| 17 | South Dakota | 69.0 | 42 | Nevada | 64.6 |
| 18 | New York | 68.9 | 43 | Rhode Island | 64.5 |
| 19 | Missouri | 68.2 | 44 | New Mexico | 64.4 |
| 20 | Nebraska | 67.9 | 45 | Ohio | 64.0 |
| 21 | Hawaii | 67.7 | 46 | Tennessee | 63.7 |
| 22 | Vermont | 67.5 | 47 | Michigan | 63.6 |
| 23 | Iowa | 67.4 | 48 | Connecticut | 62.0 |
| 24 | Maine | 67.2 | 49 | New Hampshire | 61.9 |
| 25 | Louisiana | 67.0 | 50 | Alaska | 56.8 |
|  |  |  |  | District of Columbia | 74.6 |

*Source: Families USA Foundation*

*"Health Spending: The Growing Threat to the Family Budget" (December 1991) (Reprinted with permission)*

*As a percent of total health care payments by business and families. See beginning of this chapter for definitions.*

# Projected Health Care Payments Paid by Families in 2000

## Projected National Total = $1,064,661,000,000*

| RANK | STATE | PAYMENTS | % | RANK | STATE | PAYMENTS | % |
|---|---|---|---|---|---|---|---|
| 1 | California | $143,496,000,000 | 13.48% | 26 | South Carolina | $11,699,000,000 | 1.10% |
| 2 | New York | 95,633,000,000 | 8.98% | 27 | Oklahoma | 11,519,000,000 | 1.08% |
| 3 | Texas | 71,498,000,000 | 6.72% | 28 | Kentucky | 11,236,000,000 | 1.06% |
| 4 | Florida | 59,720,000,000 | 5.61% | 29 | Oregon | 11,038,000,000 | 1.04% |
| 5 | Illinois | 49,662,000,000 | 4.66% | 30 | Kansas | 10,313,000,000 | 0.97% |
| 6 | Pennsylvania | 45,858,000,000 | 4.31% | 31 | Iowa | 9,844,000,000 | 0.92% |
| 7 | Ohio | 43,184,000,000 | 4.06% | 32 | Arkansas | 7,959,000,000 | 0.75% |
| 8 | Michigan | 37,889,000,000 | 3.56% | 33 | Mississippi | 7,542,000,000 | 0.71% |
| 9 | New Jersey | 37,701,000,000 | 3.54% | 34 | Nebraska | 6,185,000,000 | 0.58% |
| 10 | Massachusetts | 31,580,000,000 | 2.97% | 35 | New Mexico | 5,625,000,000 | 0.53% |
| 11 | Georgia | 29,129,000,000 | 2.74% | 36 | Nevada | 5,589,000,000 | 0.52% |
| 12 | Virginia | 27,895,000,000 | 2.62% | 37 | Utah | 5,536,000,000 | 0.52% |
| 13 | North Carolina | 24,876,000,000 | 2.34% | 38 | Hawaii | 5,466,000,000 | 0.51% |
| 14 | Maryland | 23,530,000,000 | 2.21% | 39 | West Virginia | 5,241,000,000 | 0.49% |
| 15 | Missouri | 21,355,000,000 | 2.01% | 40 | Rhode Island | 4,758,000,000 | 0.45% |
| 16 | Indiana | 20,575,000,000 | 1.93% | 41 | New Hampshire | 4,612,000,000 | 0.43% |
| 17 | Minnesota | 19,255,000,000 | 1.81% | 42 | Maine | 4,546,000,000 | 0.43% |
| 18 | Washington | 19,094,000,000 | 1.79% | 43 | Delaware | 3,025,000,000 | 0.28% |
| 19 | Wisconsin | 18,799,000,000 | 1.77% | 44 | Idaho | 2,818,000,000 | 0.26% |
| 20 | Connecticut | 17,388,000,000 | 1.63% | 45 | Montana | 2,435,000,000 | 0.23% |
| 21 | Tennessee | 16,120,000,000 | 1.51% | 46 | South Dakota | 2,370,000,000 | 0.22% |
| 22 | Alabama | 15,781,000,000 | 1.48% | 47 | North Dakota | 2,332,000,000 | 0.22% |
| 23 | Arizona | 14,970,000,000 | 1.41% | 48 | Vermont | 2,051,000,000 | 0.19% |
| 24 | Colorado | 14,885,000,000 | 1.40% | 49 | Alaska | 2,008,000,000 | 0.19% |
| 25 | Louisiana | 14,624,000,000 | 1.37% | 50 | Wyoming | 1,480,000,000 | 0.14% |
| | | | | | District of Columbia | 2,937,000,000 | 0.28% |

Source: Families USA Foundation

"Health Spending: The Growing Threat to the Family Budget" (December 1991) (Reprinted with permission)

*Reflects payments made directly by families and does not inlcude payments made by business. See beginning of this chapter for definitions.

# Projected Percent of Health Care Payments Paid by Families in 2000

## Projected National Rate = 67.6% Paid by Families*

| RANK | STATE | PERCENT | RANK | STATE | PERCENT |
|------|-------|---------|------|-------|---------|
| 1 | Virginia | 75.6 | 26 | Missouri | 66.7 |
| 2 | Oklahoma | 74.5 | 26 | South Dakota | 66.7 |
| 3 | Maryland | 74.4 | 28 | Oregon | 66.5 |
| 4 | Arkansas | 74.2 | 29 | Utah | 66.4 |
| 5 | Alabama | 73.9 | 30 | Kansas | 66.2 |
| 5 | South Carolina | 73.9 | 30 | New Jersey | 66.2 |
| 7 | Mississippi | 73.1 | 32 | Arizona | 66.1 |
| 8 | Georgia | 73.0 | 33 | Montana | 66.0 |
| 9 | North Carolina | 72.7 | 33 | Ohio | 66.0 |
| 10 | Kentucky | 72.1 | 33 | Rhode Island | 66.0 |
| 11 | Florida | 71.5 | 36 | Wisconsin | 65.9 |
| 12 | Texas | 70.6 | 37 | Illinois | 65.6 |
| 13 | New York | 70.5 | 37 | North Dakota | 65.6 |
| 14 | New Mexico | 69.7 | 37 | Washington | 65.6 |
| 15 | Delaware | 69.5 | 40 | Minnesota | 65.1 |
| 16 | Indiana | 69.1 | 40 | Pennsylvania | 65.1 |
| 17 | West Virginia | 68.3 | 42 | Massachusetts | 64.9 |
| 18 | Louisiana | 67.9 | 43 | Maine | 64.4 |
| 19 | Wyoming | 67.7 | 44 | Michigan | 64.1 |
| 20 | Iowa | 67.6 | 45 | California | 63.8 |
| 21 | Idaho | 67.2 | 46 | Nevada | 63.3 |
| 22 | Nebraska | 67.0 | 47 | Tennessee | 61.5 |
| 22 | Vermont | 67.0 | 48 | Connecticut | 60.0 |
| 24 | Colorado | 66.8 | 49 | New Hampshire | 59.1 |
| 24 | Hawaii | 66.8 | 50 | Alaska | 48.1 |

District of Columbia     74.5

Source: Families USA Foundation

*"Health Spending: The Growing Threat to the Family Budget"* (December 1991) (Reprinted with permission)

*As a percent of total health care payments by business and families. See beginning of this chapter for definitions.

# Percent of Average Family Income Spent on Health Care in 1991

## National Rate = 11.7% of Family Income*

| RANK | STATE | PERCENT OF INCOME | RANK | STATE | PERCENT OF INCOME |
|---|---|---|---|---|---|
| 1 | North Dakota | 14.1 | 26 | Oklahoma | 11.5 |
| 2 | Alabama | 14.0 | 27 | Oregon | 11.4 |
| 3 | New York | 13.9 | 28 | Tennessee | 11.3 |
| 4 | South Dakota | 13.1 | 29 | Colorado | 11.2 |
| 5 | Rhode Island | 13.0 | 30 | California | 11.1 |
| 6 | Nebraska | 12.9 | 31 | Maine | 11.0 |
| 7 | Missouri | 12.8 | 31 | North Carolina | 11.0 |
| 8 | Iowa | 12.7 | 33 | Connecticut | 10.9 |
| 8 | Kansas | 12.7 | 33 | Kentucky | 10.9 |
| 10 | Louisiana | 12.6 | 33 | Mississippi | 10.9 |
| 10 | Minnesota | 12.6 | 33 | New Hampshire | 10.9 |
| 12 | Indiana | 12.4 | 37 | Maryland | 10.8 |
| 12 | Ohio | 12.4 | 37 | Montana | 10.8 |
| 14 | Arkansas | 12.3 | 39 | New Jersey | 10.3 |
| 14 | Delaware | 12.3 | 39 | New Mexico | 10.3 |
| 14 | Massachusetts | 12.3 | 39 | South Carolina | 10.3 |
| 14 | Michigan | 12.3 | 39 | Virginia | 10.3 |
| 14 | West Virginia | 12.3 | 43 | Utah | 10.2 |
| 19 | Wisconsin | 12.2 | 44 | Hawaii | 10.0 |
| 20 | Texas | 12.1 | 44 | Washington | 10.0 |
| 21 | Illinois | 12.0 | 46 | Arizona | 9.9 |
| 22 | Florida | 11.9 | 47 | Idaho | 9.8 |
| 23 | Georgia | 11.7 | 47 | Vermont | 9.8 |
| 24 | Nevada | 11.6 | 49 | Wyoming | 9.7 |
| 24 | Pennsylvania | 11.6 | 50 | Alaska | 9.0 |
|  |  |  |  | District of Columbia | 12.6 |

Source: Families USA Foundation

*"Health Spending: The Growing Threat to the Family Budget" (December 1991) (Reprinted with permission)*

*See beginning of this chapter for definitions.*

# Percent of Average Family Income Spent on Health Care in 1980

## National Rate = 9.0% of Family Income*

| RANK | STATE | PERCENT OF INCOME | RANK | STATE | PERCENT OF INCOME |
|------|-------|-------------------|------|-------|-------------------|
| 1 | New York | 11.2 | 25 | Tennessee | 8.8 |
| 2 | Alabama | 10.5 | 27 | Florida | 8.7 |
| 3 | North Dakota | 10.3 | 27 | New Jersey | 8.7 |
| 3 | Rhode Island | 10.3 | 29 | Kentucky | 8.6 |
| 5 | Nebraska | 10.1 | 29 | Maryland | 8.6 |
| 6 | Massachusetts | 10.0 | 29 | Mississippi | 8.6 |
| 6 | Minnesota | 10.0 | 32 | Georgia | 8.5 |
| 6 | South Dakota | 10.0 | 32 | South Carolina | 8.5 |
| 9 | West Virginia | 9.8 | 34 | Virginia | 8.4 |
| 10 | Missouri | 9.7 | 35 | North Carolina | 8.3 |
| 11 | Arkansas | 9.5 | 36 | Hawaii | 8.2 |
| 11 | Louisiana | 9.5 | 37 | California | 8.1 |
| 13 | Indiana | 9.4 | 38 | Colorado | 7.8 |
| 13 | Iowa | 9.4 | 39 | Vermont | 7.7 |
| 13 | Michigan | 9.4 | 39 | Washington | 7.7 |
| 16 | Connecticut | 9.3 | 41 | Nevada | 7.6 |
| 16 | Kansas | 9.3 | 42 | Montana | 7.5 |
| 18 | Delaware | 9.2 | 42 | Oregon | 7.5 |
| 18 | Illinois | 9.2 | 44 | Idaho | 7.3 |
| 18 | Ohio | 9.2 | 45 | Utah | 7.2 |
| 18 | Texas | 9.2 | 46 | Arizona | 7.0 |
| 18 | Wisconsin | 9.2 | 47 | New Hampshire | 6.9 |
| 23 | Pennsylvania | 9.1 | 47 | New Mexico | 6.9 |
| 24 | Maine | 9.0 | 49 | Wyoming | 6.8 |
| 25 | Oklahoma | 8.8 | 50 | Alaska | 6.2 |
| | | | | District of Columbia | 9.8 |

Source: Families USA Foundation

"Health Spending: The Growing Threat to the Family Budget" (December 1991) (Reprinted with permission)

*See beginning of this chapter for definitions.

# Average Annual Health Care Payments Paid by Families in 1991

## National Average = $4,296*

| RANK | STATE | AVERAGE PAYMENTS | RANK | STATE | AVERAGE PAYMENTS |
|------|-------|------------------|------|-------|------------------|
| 1 | New York | $5,585 | 26 | Maine | $3,946 |
| 2 | Connecticut | 5,421 | 27 | Colorado | 3,933 |
| 3 | Massachusetts | 5,321 | 28 | Florida | 3,932 |
| 4 | Rhode Island | 4,914 | 29 | Oregon | 3,900 |
| 5 | New Jersey | 4,863 | 30 | Nevada | 3,897 |
| 6 | Illinois | 4,670 | 31 | South Dakota | 3,863 |
| 7 | Hawaii | 4,596 | 32 | New Hampshire | 3,860 |
| 8 | Michigan | 4,569 | 33 | Alaska | 3,846 |
| 9 | Minnesota | 4,568 | 34 | Louisiana | 3,809 |
| 10 | Maryland | 4,484 | 35 | Oklahoma | 3,786 |
| 11 | Kansas | 4,481 | 36 | Washington | 3,710 |
| 12 | Ohio | 4,474 | 37 | Utah | 3,682 |
| 13 | California | 4,433 | 38 | Vermont | 3,649 |
| 14 | Delaware | 4,393 | 39 | North Carolina | 3,630 |
| 15 | Missouri | 4,362 | 40 | Tennessee | 3,487 |
| 16 | Virginia | 4,358 | 41 | Arkansas | 3,480 |
| 17 | Pennsylvania | 4,300 | 42 | Wyoming | 3,474 |
| 18 | Nebraska | 4,268 | 43 | West Virginia | 3,443 |
| 19 | Wisconsin | 4,245 | 44 | Arizona | 3,439 |
| 20 | North Dakota | 4,193 | 45 | South Carolina | 3,414 |
| 21 | Georgia | 4,159 | 46 | New Mexico | 3,297 |
| 22 | Texas | 4,095 | 47 | Kentucky | 3,206 |
| 23 | Alabama | 4,064 | 48 | Montana | 3,154 |
| 24 | Iowa | 4,026 | 49 | Mississippi | 3,009 |
| 25 | Indiana | 3,972 | 50 | Idaho | 3,005 |

District of Columbia   4,300

*Source: Families USA Foundation*

*"Health Spending: The Growing Threat to the Family Budget" (December 1991) (Reprinted with permission)*

*This is an average paid directly by each family and does not include payments made by business. See beginning of this chapter for definitions.*

# Average Annual Health Payments Paid by Families in 1980

## National Average = $1,742*

| RANK | STATE | AVERAGE PAYMENTS | RANK | STATE | AVERAGE PAYMENTS |
|---|---|---|---|---|---|
| 1 | New York | $2,159 | 26 | Colorado | $1,658 |
| 2 | Massachusetts | 2,062 | 27 | Indiana | 1,643 |
| 3 | Maryland | 2,049 | 28 | South Dakota | 1,632 |
| 4 | Connecticut | 2,015 | 29 | Oklahoma | 1,614 |
| 5 | Illinois | 2,002 | 30 | West Virginia | 1,592 |
| 6 | New Jersey | 1,940 | 31 | Alaska | 1,590 |
| 7 | Minnesota | 1,920 | 32 | Kentucky | 1,524 |
| 8 | Delaware | 1,913 | 33 | North Carolina | 1,521 |
| 9 | Rhode Island | 1,900 | 34 | Nevada | 1,511 |
| 10 | Michigan | 1,879 | 35 | Washington | 1,489 |
| 11 | Ohio | 1,845 | 36 | Maine | 1,487 |
| 12 | Hawaii | 1,829 | 37 | Tennessee | 1,473 |
| 13 | Iowa | 1,826 | 38 | Florida | 1,463 |
| 14 | Nebraska | 1,804 | 39 | Arkansas | 1,444 |
| 15 | Kansas | 1,801 | 40 | Utah | 1,441 |
| 15 | Wisconsin | 1,801 | 41 | Oregon | 1,418 |
| 17 | North Dakota | 1,795 | 42 | New Hampshire | 1,390 |
| 18 | Texas | 1,794 | 43 | Wyoming | 1,385 |
| 19 | Pennsylvania | 1,749 | 44 | South Carolina | 1,376 |
| 20 | Missouri | 1,743 | 45 | Montana | 1,345 |
| 21 | Alabama | 1,707 | 46 | Vermont | 1,329 |
| 22 | Louisiana | 1,671 | 47 | Arizona | 1,308 |
| 23 | California | 1,666 | 48 | Mississippi | 1,303 |
| 23 | Georgia | 1,666 | 49 | New Mexico | 1,209 |
| 25 | Virginia | 1,665 | 50 | Idaho | 1,202 |
| | | | | District of Columbia | 1,676 |

Source: Families USA Foundation

"Health Spending: The Growing Threat to the Family Budget" (December 1991) (Reprinted with permission)

*This is an average paid directly by each family and does not include payments made by business. See beginning of this chapter for definitions.

# Projected Average Annual Health Payments Paid by Families in 2000

## Projected National Average = $9,397*

| RANK | STATE | AVERAGE PAYMENTS | RANK | STATE | AVERAGE PAYMENTS |
|---|---|---|---|---|---|
| 1 | New York | $12,690 | 26 | Indiana | $8,770 |
| 2 | Connecticut | 12,100 | 27 | Maine | 8,640 |
| 3 | Massachusetts | 11,934 | 28 | Colorado | 8,588 |
| 4 | Rhode Island | 10,862 | 29 | Louisiana | 8,511 |
| 5 | New Jersey | 10,752 | 30 | Nevada | 8,394 |
| 6 | Illinois | 10,423 | 31 | South Dakota | 8,365 |
| 7 | Michigan | 10,054 | 32 | Oklahoma | 8,364 |
| 8 | Hawaii | 9,988 | 33 | Washington | 8,361 |
| 9 | Ohio | 9,899 | 34 | Florida | 8,235 |
| 10 | Maryland | 9,878 | 35 | Utah | 8,184 |
| 11 | Minnesota | 9,864 | 36 | New Hampshire | 8,050 |
| 12 | Kansas | 9,837 | 37 | Vermont | 7,974 |
| 13 | California | 9,765 | 38 | Wyoming | 7,945 |
| 14 | Virginia | 9,631 | 39 | North Carolina | 7,794 |
| 15 | Pennsylvania | 9,571 | 40 | West Virginia | 7,706 |
| 16 | Missouri | 9,428 | 41 | Arkansas | 7,576 |
| 17 | Nebraska | 9,348 | 42 | South Carolina | 7,474 |
| 18 | Wisconsin | 9,337 | 43 | Tennessee | 7,401 |
| 19 | North Dakota | 9,229 | 44 | Alaska | 7,260 |
| 20 | Delaware | 9,055 | 45 | Arizona | 7,222 |
| 21 | Iowa | 9,021 | 46 | Kentucky | 7,177 |
| 22 | Alabama | 8,893 | 47 | Montana | 7,150 |
| 23 | Georgia | 8,884 | 48 | New Mexico | 7,109 |
| 24 | Texas | 8,789 | 49 | Idaho | 6,726 |
| 25 | Oregon | 8,772 | 50 | Mississippi | 6,566 |
| | | | | District of Columbia | 9,445 |

Source: Families USA Foundation

"Health Spending: The Growing Threat to the Family Budget" (December 1991) (Reprinted with permission)

*This is an average paid directly by each family and does not include payments made by business. See beginning of this chapter for definitions.

# Percent Change in Average Annual Health Payments Paid by Families: 1980 to 1991

## National Percent Change = 147% Increase*

| RANK | STATE | PERCENT CHANGE | RANK | STATE | PERCENT CHANGE |
|------|-------|----------------|------|-------|----------------|
| 1 | New Hampshire | 178 | 26 | Michigan | 143 |
| 2 | Oregon | 175 | 27 | Alaska | 142 |
| 2 | Vermont | 175 | 27 | Indiana | 142 |
| 4 | New Mexico | 173 | 27 | Ohio | 142 |
| 5 | Connecticut | 169 | 30 | Arkansas | 141 |
| 5 | Florida | 169 | 31 | North Carolina | 139 |
| 7 | California | 166 | 32 | Alabama | 138 |
| 8 | Maine | 165 | 32 | Minnesota | 138 |
| 9 | Arizona | 163 | 34 | Colorado | 137 |
| 10 | Virginia | 162 | 34 | Nebraska | 137 |
| 11 | New York | 159 | 34 | South Dakota | 137 |
| 11 | Rhode Island | 159 | 34 | Tennessee | 137 |
| 13 | Massachusetts | 158 | 38 | Wisconsin | 136 |
| 13 | Nevada | 158 | 39 | Montana | 135 |
| 15 | Utah | 155 | 40 | North Dakota | 134 |
| 16 | Hawaii | 151 | 40 | Oklahoma | 134 |
| 16 | New Jersey | 151 | 42 | Illinois | 133 |
| 16 | Wyoming | 151 | 43 | Mississippi | 131 |
| 19 | Georgia | 150 | 44 | Delaware | 130 |
| 19 | Idaho | 150 | 45 | Louisiana | 128 |
| 19 | Missouri | 150 | 45 | Texas | 128 |
| 22 | Kansas | 149 | 47 | Iowa | 121 |
| 22 | Washington | 149 | 48 | Maryland | 119 |
| 24 | South Carolina | 148 | 49 | West Virginia | 116 |
| 25 | Pennsylvania | 146 | 50 | Kentucky | 110 |

District of Columbia 157

Source: Families USA Foundation

*"Health Spending: The Growing Threat to the Family Budget" (December 1991) (Reprinted with permission)*

*This is for payments paid directly by each family and does not include payments made by business. See beginning of this chapter for definitions.*

# Projected Percent Change in Average Annual Health Payment by Families: 1991 to 2000

## Projected National Rate = 118.74% Increase*

| RANK | STATE | PERCENT INCREASE | RANK | STATE | PERCENT INCREASE |
|---|---|---|---|---|---|
| 1 | Wyoming | 128.70 | 26 | Kansas | 119.53 |
| 2 | New York | 127.22 | 27 | Nebraska | 119.03 |
| 3 | Montana | 126.70 | 28 | Maine | 118.96 |
| 4 | Washington | 125.36 | 29 | South Carolina | 118.92 |
| 5 | Oregon | 124.92 | 30 | Alabama | 118.82 |
| 6 | Massachusetts | 124.28 | 31 | Vermont | 118.53 |
| 7 | Iowa | 124.07 | 32 | Colorado | 118.36 |
| 8 | Kentucky | 123.86 | 33 | Mississippi | 118.21 |
| 9 | Idaho | 123.83 | 34 | Arkansas | 117.70 |
| 10 | West Virginia | 123.82 | 35 | Hawaii | 117.32 |
| 11 | Louisiana | 123.44 | 36 | South Dakota | 116.54 |
| 12 | Connecticut | 123.21 | 37 | Missouri | 116.14 |
| 13 | Illinois | 123.19 | 38 | Minnesota | 115.94 |
| 14 | Pennsylvania | 122.58 | 39 | New Mexico | 115.62 |
| 15 | Ohio | 121.26 | 40 | Nevada | 115.40 |
| 16 | New Jersey | 121.10 | 41 | North Carolina | 114.71 |
| 17 | Rhode Island | 121.04 | 42 | Texas | 114.63 |
| 18 | Virginia | 121.00 | 43 | Georgia | 113.61 |
| 19 | Oklahoma | 120.92 | 44 | Tennessee | 112.25 |
| 20 | Indiana | 120.80 | 45 | Utah | 110.82 |
| 21 | Maryland | 120.29 | 46 | Arizona | 110.00 |
| 22 | California | 120.28 | 47 | Florida | 109.44 |
| 23 | North Dakota | 120.10 | 48 | New Hampshire | 108.55 |
| 24 | Michigan | 120.05 | 49 | Delaware | 106.12 |
| 25 | Wisconsin | 119.95 | 50 | Alaska | 88.77 |
| | | | | District of Columbia | 119.65 |

Source: Families USA Foundation

"Health Spending: The Growing Threat to the Family Budget" (December 1991) (Reprinted with permission)

*Calculated by the editors. This is for payments paid directly by each family and does not include payments made by business. See beginning of this chapter for definitions.

# Average Annual Health Payments Paid Out-Of-Pocket by Families in 1991

## National Average = $1,362 Per Family*

| RANK | STATE | PAYMENTS | RANK | STATE | PAYMENTS |
|------|-------|----------|------|-------|----------|
| 1 | Massachusetts | $1,526 | 26 | Iowa | $1,332 |
| 1 | Texas | 1,526 | 27 | Delaware | 1,329 |
| 3 | Alabama | 1,503 | 28 | Louisiana | 1,328 |
| 4 | Kansas | 1,499 | 29 | Georgia | 1,327 |
| 5 | Illinois | 1,496 | 30 | West Virginia | 1,313 |
| 6 | Connecticut | 1,488 | 31 | Nevada | 1,303 |
| 6 | Rhode Island | 1,488 | 32 | Arkansas | 1,284 |
| 8 | Missouri | 1,482 | 33 | New Hampshire | 1,282 |
| 9 | Nebraska | 1,458 | 34 | New Jersey | 1,261 |
| 10 | South Dakota | 1,449 | 35 | Indiana | 1,258 |
| 11 | North Dakota | 1,446 | 36 | Colorado | 1,223 |
| 12 | Tennessee | 1,436 | 37 | North Carolina | 1,220 |
| 13 | Florida | 1,432 | 38 | Maine | 1,218 |
| 14 | Pennsylvania | 1,421 | 39 | Oregon | 1,194 |
| 15 | Michigan | 1,420 | 40 | Vermont | 1,166 |
| 16 | Minnesota | 1,415 | 41 | Utah | 1,136 |
| 17 | California | 1,406 | 42 | Arizona | 1,106 |
| 18 | Ohio | 1,382 | 43 | Mississippi | 1,104 |
| 19 | Hawaii | 1,379 | 44 | Kentucky | 1,099 |
| 20 | New York | 1,370 | 45 | Washington | 1,071 |
| 21 | Alaska | 1,349 | 46 | South Carolina | 1,021 |
| 22 | Oklahoma | 1,347 | 47 | New Mexico | 1,010 |
| 23 | Virginia | 1,345 | 48 | Montana | 976 |
| 24 | Wisconsin | 1,339 | 49 | Wyoming | 970 |
| 25 | Maryland | 1,333 | 50 | Idaho | 945 |
| | | | | District of Columbia | 924 |

Source: Families USA Foundation

"Health Spending: The Growing Threat to the Family Budget" (December 1991) (Reprinted with permission)

*This is an average paid directly by each family and does not include payments made by business. It is a subset of average annual family health payments. See beginning of this chapter for definitions.

223

# Percent of Average Annual Health Payments Paid Out-Of-Pocket by Families in 1991

## National Rate = 31.7% Paid Out-Of-Pocket*

| RANK | STATE | PERCENT | RANK | STATE | PERCENT |
|---|---|---|---|---|---|
| 1 | Tennessee | 41.2 | 26 | California | 31.7 |
| 2 | West Virginia | 38.1 | 26 | Indiana | 31.7 |
| 3 | South Dakota | 37.5 | 28 | Idaho | 31.5 |
| 4 | Texas | 37.3 | 28 | Wisconsin | 31.5 |
| 5 | Alabama | 37.0 | 30 | Colorado | 31.1 |
| 6 | Arkansas | 36.9 | 30 | Michigan | 31.1 |
| 7 | Mississippi | 36.7 | 32 | Minnesota | 31.0 |
| 8 | Florida | 36.4 | 33 | Maine | 30.9 |
| 9 | Oklahoma | 35.6 | 33 | Montana | 30.9 |
| 10 | Alaska | 35.1 | 33 | Ohio | 30.9 |
| 11 | Louisiana | 34.9 | 33 | Utah | 30.9 |
| 12 | North Dakota | 34.5 | 33 | Virginia | 30.9 |
| 13 | Kentucky | 34.3 | 38 | New Mexico | 30.6 |
| 14 | Nebraska | 34.2 | 38 | Oregon | 30.6 |
| 15 | Missouri | 34.0 | 40 | Delaware | 30.3 |
| 16 | North Carolina | 33.6 | 40 | Rhode Island | 30.3 |
| 17 | Kansas | 33.5 | 42 | Hawaii | 30.0 |
| 18 | Nevada | 33.4 | 43 | South Carolina | 29.9 |
| 19 | New Hampshire | 33.2 | 44 | Maryland | 29.7 |
| 20 | Iowa | 33.1 | 45 | Washington | 28.9 |
| 21 | Pennsylvania | 33.0 | 46 | Massachusetts | 28.7 |
| 22 | Arizona | 32.2 | 47 | Wyoming | 27.9 |
| 23 | Illinois | 32.0 | 48 | Connecticut | 27.4 |
| 23 | Vermont | 32.0 | 49 | New Jersey | 25.9 |
| 25 | Georgia | 31.9 | 50 | New York | 24.5 |
| | | | | District of Columbia | 21.5 |

Source: Families USA Foundation

"Health Spending: The Growing Threat to the Family Budget" (December 1991) (Reprinted with permission)

*This is a percent paid directly by each family and does not include payments made by business. It is a percent of annual family health payments. See beginning of this chapter for definitions.

# Average Annual Health Payments Paid Out-Of-Pocket by Families in 1980

## National Average = $654 per Family*

| RANK | STATE | PAYMENTS |
|---|---|---|
| 1 | Massachusetts | $800 |
| 2 | Connecticut | 773 |
| 3 | Maryland | 769 |
| 4 | New York | 740 |
| 5 | Alabama | 739 |
| 6 | Illinois | 736 |
| 6 | North Dakota | 736 |
| 8 | Rhode Island | 732 |
| 9 | Tennessee | 727 |
| 10 | Ohio | 716 |
| 11 | Minnesota | 712 |
| 11 | South Dakota | 712 |
| 13 | Texas | 710 |
| 14 | Nebraska | 706 |
| 15 | Missouri | 696 |
| 15 | Pennsylvania | 696 |
| 15 | West Virginia | 696 |
| 18 | Louisiana | 695 |
| 19 | Delaware | 689 |
| 19 | Michigan | 689 |
| 21 | Georgia | 687 |
| 22 | Iowa | 683 |
| 23 | Kansas | 672 |
| 23 | Wisconsin | 672 |
| 25 | New Jersey | 664 |

| RANK | STATE | PAYMENTS |
|---|---|---|
| 26 | Kentucky | $657 |
| 27 | Mississippi | 635 |
| 28 | Oklahoma | 632 |
| 29 | Indiana | 631 |
| 30 | Arkansas | 622 |
| 31 | Maine | 618 |
| 32 | North Carolina | 609 |
| 33 | Virginia | 608 |
| 34 | Florida | 597 |
| 35 | Hawaii | 575 |
| 36 | New Hampshire | 563 |
| 37 | California | 559 |
| 38 | Colorado | 547 |
| 39 | Alaska | 538 |
| 40 | South Carolina | 526 |
| 41 | Vermont | 522 |
| 42 | Nevada | 507 |
| 43 | Utah | 478 |
| 44 | Arizona | 463 |
| 45 | Montana | 461 |
| 46 | Oregon | 455 |
| 47 | Washington | 442 |
| 48 | New Mexico | 430 |
| 49 | Idaho | 399 |
| 50 | Wyoming | 374 |
| | District of Columbia | 494 |

Source: Families USA Foundation

"Health Spending: The Growing Threat to the Family Budget" (December 1991) (Reprinted with permission)

*This is an average paid directly by each family and does not include payments made by business. It is a subset of average annual family health payments. See beginning of this chapter for definitions.

# Percent of Average Annual Health Payments Paid Out–Of–Pocket by Families in 1980

## National Rate = 37.6% Paid Out–Of–Pocket*

| RANK | STATE | PERCENT | RANK | STATE | PERCENT |
|------|-------|---------|------|-------|---------|
| 1 | Tennessee | 49.3 | 26 | South Carolina | 38.2 |
| 2 | Mississippi | 48.8 | 27 | Maryland | 37.5 |
| 3 | West Virginia | 43.7 | 28 | Iowa | 37.4 |
| 4 | South Dakota | 43.6 | 29 | Kansas | 37.3 |
| 5 | Alabama | 43.3 | 29 | Wisconsin | 37.3 |
| 6 | Kentucky | 43.1 | 31 | Minnesota | 37.1 |
| 7 | Arkansas | 43.0 | 32 | Illinois | 36.8 |
| 8 | Louisiana | 41.6 | 33 | Michigan | 36.6 |
| 9 | Maine | 41.5 | 34 | Virginia | 36.5 |
| 10 | Georgia | 41.3 | 35 | Delaware | 36.0 |
| 11 | North Dakota | 41.0 | 36 | New Mexico | 35.5 |
| 12 | Florida | 40.8 | 37 | Arizona | 35.4 |
| 13 | New Hampshire | 40.5 | 38 | Montana | 34.3 |
| 14 | North Carolina | 40.1 | 38 | New York | 34.3 |
| 15 | Missouri | 39.9 | 40 | New Jersey | 34.2 |
| 16 | Pennsylvania | 39.8 | 41 | Alaska | 33.9 |
| 17 | Texas | 39.6 | 42 | California | 33.6 |
| 18 | Vermont | 39.3 | 43 | Nevada | 33.5 |
| 19 | Nebraska | 39.2 | 44 | Idaho | 33.2 |
| 20 | Oklahoma | 39.1 | 44 | Utah | 33.2 |
| 21 | Massachusetts | 38.8 | 46 | Colorado | 33.0 |
| 21 | Ohio | 38.8 | 47 | Oregon | 32.1 |
| 23 | Rhode Island | 38.5 | 48 | Hawaii | 31.5 |
| 24 | Connecticut | 38.4 | 49 | Washington | 29.7 |
| 24 | Indiana | 38.4 | 50 | Wyoming | 27.0 |
| | | | | District of Columbia | 29.5 |

Source: Families USA Foundation

   *"Health Spending: The Growing Threat to the Family Budget" (December 1991) (Reprinted with permission)*

*This is a percent paid directly by each family and does not include payments made by business. It is a percent of annual family health payments. See beginning of this chapter for definitions.*

# Projected Average Annual Health Payments Paid Out-Of-Pocket by Families in 2000

## Projected National Average = $2,562 per Family*

| RANK | STATE | PAYMENTS | RANK | STATE | PAYMENTS |
|------|-------|----------|------|-------|----------|
| 1 | Texas | $2,883 | 26 | Georgia | $2,500 |
| 2 | Massachusetts | 2,875 | 27 | Iowa | 2,499 |
| 3 | Illinois | 2,824 | 28 | Delaware | 2,498 |
| 3 | Kansas | 2,824 | 29 | Louisiana | 2,491 |
| 5 | Alabama | 2,818 | 30 | Nevada | 2,462 |
| 6 | Rhode Island | 2,813 | 31 | West Virginia | 2,460 |
| 7 | Connecticut | 2,798 | 32 | New Hampshire | 2,419 |
| 8 | Missouri | 2,788 | 33 | Arkansas | 2,412 |
| 9 | Nebraska | 2,742 | 34 | New Jersey | 2,373 |
| 10 | South Dakota | 2,735 | 35 | Indiana | 2,361 |
| 11 | North Dakota | 2,723 | 36 | Colorado | 2,293 |
| 12 | Tennessee | 2,686 | 37 | Maine | 2,292 |
| 13 | Florida | 2,682 | 38 | North Carolina | 2,279 |
| 14 | Michigan | 2,671 | 39 | Oregon | 2,258 |
| 15 | California | 2,667 | 40 | Vermont | 2,200 |
| 15 | Minnesota | 2,667 | 41 | Utah | 2,169 |
| 17 | Pennsylvania | 2,662 | 42 | Arizona | 2,074 |
| 18 | Ohio | 2,590 | 43 | Mississippi | 2,062 |
| 19 | Hawaii | 2,584 | 44 | Kentucky | 2,060 |
| 20 | New York | 2,580 | 45 | Washington | 2,023 |
| 21 | Alaska | 2,543 | 46 | New Mexico | 1,910 |
| 22 | Oklahoma | 2,534 | 47 | South Carolina | 1,909 |
| 23 | Virginia | 2,530 | 48 | Wyoming | 1,838 |
| 24 | Wisconsin | 2,517 | 49 | Montana | 1,837 |
| 25 | Maryland | 2,508 | 50 | Idaho | 1,791 |
| | | | | District of Columbia | 1,743 |

Source: Families USA Foundation

"Health Spending: The Growing Threat to the Family Budget" (December 1991) (Reprinted with permission)

*This is an average paid directly by each family and does not include payments made by business. It is a subset of average annual family health payments. See beginning of this chapter for definitions.

# Projected Percent Average Annual Health Payments Paid Out-Of-Pocket by Families in 2000

## Projected National Rate = 27.3% Paid Out-Of-Pocket*

| RANK | STATE | PERCENT | RANK | STATE | PERCENT |
|------|-------|---------|------|-------|---------|
| 1 | Tennessee | 36.3 | 26 | California | 27.3 |
| 2 | Alaska | 35.0 | 27 | Illinois | 27.1 |
| 3 | Texas | 32.8 | 28 | Minnesota | 27.0 |
| 4 | South Dakota | 32.7 | 28 | Wisconsin | 27.0 |
| 5 | Florida | 32.6 | 30 | Indiana | 26.9 |
| 6 | West Virginia | 31.9 | 30 | New Mexico | 26.9 |
| 7 | Arkansas | 31.8 | 32 | Colorado | 26.7 |
| 8 | Alabama | 31.7 | 33 | Idaho | 26.6 |
| 9 | Mississippi | 31.6 | 33 | Michigan | 26.6 |
| 10 | Oklahoma | 30.3 | 35 | Maine | 26.5 |
| 11 | New Hampshire | 30.1 | 35 | Utah | 26.5 |
| 12 | Missouri | 29.6 | 37 | Virginia | 26.3 |
| 13 | North Dakota | 29.5 | 38 | Ohio | 26.2 |
| 14 | Louisiana | 29.3 | 39 | Hawaii | 25.9 |
| 14 | Nebraska | 29.3 | 39 | Rhode Island | 25.9 |
| 14 | Nevada | 29.3 | 41 | Montana | 25.7 |
| 17 | North Carolina | 29.2 | 41 | Oregon | 25.7 |
| 18 | Arizona | 28.7 | 43 | South Carolina | 25.5 |
| 18 | Kansas | 28.7 | 44 | Maryland | 25.4 |
| 18 | Kentucky | 28.7 | 45 | Washington | 24.2 |
| 21 | Georgia | 28.1 | 46 | Massachusetts | 24.1 |
| 22 | Pennsylvania | 27.8 | 47 | Connecticut | 23.1 |
| 23 | Iowa | 27.7 | 47 | Wyoming | 23.1 |
| 24 | Delaware | 27.6 | 49 | New Jersey | 22.1 |
| 24 | Vermont | 27.6 | 50 | New York | 20.3 |
| | | | | District of Columbia | 18.4 |

*Source: Families USA Foundation*

*"Health Spending: The Growing Threat to the Family Budget" (December 1991) (Reprinted with permission)*

*This is a percent paid directly by each family and does not include payments made by business. It is a percent of annual family health payments. See beginning of this chapter for definitions.*

# Average Annual Family Health Payments Paid through Insurance in 1991

## National Average = $739 per Family*

| RANK | STATE | PAYMENTS | | RANK | STATE | PAYMENTS |
|------|-------|----------|---|------|-------|----------|
| 1 | Kansas | $1,031 | | 26 | Colorado | $673 |
| 2 | Michigan | 1,014 | | 27 | Utah | 669 |
| 3 | North Dakota | 1,013 | | 28 | Oregon | 648 |
| 4 | Connecticut | 1,012 | | 29 | Alabama | 627 |
| 5 | Illinois | 997 | | 30 | Tennessee | 612 |
| 6 | Nebraska | 989 | | 31 | Maryland | 591 |
| 7 | Missouri | 987 | | 32 | Delaware | 589 |
| 8 | Ohio | 973 | | 33 | Washington | 587 |
| 9 | Minnesota | 968 | | 34 | Texas | 580 |
| 10 | Wisconsin | 959 | | 35 | Virginia | 571 |
| 11 | Massachusetts | 950 | | 36 | Arizona | 556 |
| 12 | Iowa | 934 | | 36 | Georgia | 556 |
| 13 | South Dakota | 912 | | 38 | Florida | 553 |
| 14 | Pennsylvania | 892 | | 39 | Wyoming | 548 |
| 15 | Rhode Island | 875 | | 40 | West Virginia | 542 |
| 16 | Indiana | 850 | | 41 | Louisiana | 537 |
| 17 | Maine | 813 | | 42 | Oklahoma | 522 |
| 18 | New York | 809 | | 43 | North Carolina | 510 |
| 19 | New Jersey | 769 | | 44 | Idaho | 497 |
| 20 | Hawaii | 757 | | 45 | South Carolina | 490 |
| 21 | California | 732 | | 46 | Montana | 483 |
| 22 | New Hampshire | 704 | | 47 | New Mexico | 478 |
| 23 | Alaska | 699 | | 48 | Arkansas | 474 |
| 24 | Vermont | 694 | | 49 | Kentucky | 443 |
| 25 | Nevada | 689 | | 50 | Mississippi | 409 |
| | | | | | District of Columbia | 360 |

Source: Families USA Foundation

"Health Spending: The Growing Threat to the Family Budget" (December 1991) (Reprinted with permission)

*This is an average paid directly by each family and does not include payments made by business. It is a subset of average annual family health payments. See beginning of this chapter for definitions.

# Percent of Average Annual Family Health Payments Paid through Insurance in 1991

## National Rate = 17.2% Paid through Insurance*

| RANK | STATE | PERCENT | RANK | STATE | PERCENT |
|------|-------|---------|------|-------|---------|
| 1 | North Dakota | 24.2 | 26 | California | 16.5 |
| 2 | South Dakota | 23.6 | 26 | Hawaii | 16.5 |
| 3 | Iowa | 23.2 | 26 | Idaho | 16.5 |
| 3 | Nebraska | 23.2 | 29 | Arizona | 16.2 |
| 5 | Kansas | 23.0 | 30 | New Jersey | 15.8 |
| 6 | Missouri | 22.6 | 30 | Washington | 15.8 |
| 6 | Wisconsin | 22.6 | 30 | Wyoming | 15.8 |
| 8 | Michigan | 22.2 | 33 | West Virginia | 15.7 |
| 9 | Ohio | 21.8 | 34 | Alabama | 15.4 |
| 10 | Illinois | 21.4 | 35 | Montana | 15.3 |
| 10 | Indiana | 21.4 | 36 | New Mexico | 14.5 |
| 12 | Minnesota | 21.2 | 36 | New York | 14.5 |
| 13 | Pennsylvania | 20.7 | 38 | South Carolina | 14.4 |
| 14 | Maine | 20.6 | 39 | Texas | 14.2 |
| 15 | Vermont | 19.0 | 40 | Florida | 14.1 |
| 16 | Connecticut | 18.7 | 40 | Louisiana | 14.1 |
| 17 | Alaska | 18.2 | 40 | North Carolina | 14.1 |
| 17 | New Hampshire | 18.2 | 43 | Kentucky | 13.8 |
| 17 | Utah | 18.2 | 43 | Oklahoma | 13.8 |
| 20 | Massachusetts | 17.9 | 45 | Arkansas | 13.6 |
| 21 | Rhode Island | 17.8 | 45 | Mississippi | 13.6 |
| 22 | Nevada | 17.7 | 47 | Delaware | 13.4 |
| 23 | Tennessee | 17.6 | 47 | Georgia | 13.4 |
| 24 | Colorado | 17.1 | 49 | Maryland | 13.2 |
| 25 | Oregon | 16.6 | 50 | Virginia | 13.1 |
| | | | | District of Columbia | 8.4 |

Source: Families USA Foundation

"Health Spending: The Growing Threat to the Family Budget" (December 1991) (Reprinted with permission)

*This is a percent paid directly by each family and does not include payments made by business. It is a percent of annual family health payments. See beginning of this chapter for definitions.

# Average Annual Family Health Payments Paid through Insurance in 1980

## National Average = $259 per Family*

| RANK | STATE | PAYMENTS | | RANK | STATE | PAYMENTS |
|---|---|---|---|---|---|---|
| 1 | Ohio | $378 | | 26 | Louisiana | $209 |
| 2 | North Dakota | 375 | | 27 | Kentucky | 207 |
| 3 | Minnesota | 366 | | 28 | West Virginia | 206 |
| 4 | Illinois | 365 | | 29 | Georgia | 203 |
| 5 | Wisconsin | 358 | | 30 | Texas | 201 |
| 6 | Michigan | 352 | | 31 | Hawaii | 200 |
| 7 | Connecticut | 351 | | 32 | Colorado | 194 |
| 7 | Iowa | 351 | | 33 | Virginia | 192 |
| 7 | Kansas | 351 | | 34 | California | 187 |
| 7 | Nebraska | 351 | | 35 | Oklahoma | 186 |
| 11 | Missouri | 349 | | 36 | North Carolina | 182 |
| 12 | Rhode Island | 348 | | 37 | Alaska | 179 |
| 13 | Massachusetts | 345 | | 38 | Nevada | 177 |
| 14 | South Dakota | 337 | | 39 | Florida | 172 |
| 15 | New York | 326 | | 40 | Utah | 169 |
| 16 | Pennsylvania | 318 | | 41 | Arkansas | 166 |
| 17 | Indiana | 315 | | 42 | Oregon | 161 |
| 18 | New Jersey | 313 | | 43 | Arizona | 160 |
| 19 | Maine | 281 | | 44 | Washington | 154 |
| 20 | Maryland | 253 | | 45 | Montana | 153 |
| 20 | New Hampshire | 253 | | 46 | South Carolina | 140 |
| 22 | Vermont | 237 | | 47 | Idaho | 137 |
| 23 | Tennessee | 221 | | 48 | Wyoming | 136 |
| 24 | Delaware | 220 | | 49 | New Mexico | 133 |
| 25 | Alabama | 212 | | 50 | Mississippi | 77 |
| | | | | | District of Columbia | 150 |

Source: Families USA Foundation

"Health Spending: The Growing Threat to the Family Budget" (December 1991) (Reprinted with permission)

*This is an average paid directly by each family and does not include payments made by business. It is a subset of average annual family health payments. See beginning of this chapter for definitions.

# Percent of Average Annual Family Health Payments Paid through Insurance in 1980

## National Rate = 14.9% Paid through Insurance*

| RANK | STATE | PERCENT | RANK | STATE | PERCENT |
|------|-------|---------|------|-------|---------|
| 1 | North Dakota | 20.9 | 26 | Alabama | 12.4 |
| 2 | South Dakota | 20.6 | 27 | Maryland | 12.3 |
| 3 | Ohio | 20.5 | 28 | Arizona | 12.2 |
| 4 | Missouri | 20.0 | 28 | Georgia | 12.2 |
| 5 | Wisconsin | 19.9 | 30 | North Carolina | 12.0 |
| 6 | Kansas | 19.5 | 31 | Colorado | 11.7 |
| 7 | Nebraska | 19.4 | 31 | Florida | 11.7 |
| 8 | Iowa | 19.3 | 31 | Nevada | 11.7 |
| 9 | Indiana | 19.1 | 31 | Utah | 11.7 |
| 9 | Minnesota | 19.1 | 35 | Arkansas | 11.5 |
| 11 | Maine | 18.9 | 35 | Delaware | 11.5 |
| 12 | Michigan | 18.8 | 35 | Oklahoma | 11.5 |
| 13 | Rhode Island | 18.3 | 35 | Virginia | 11.5 |
| 14 | Illinois | 18.2 | 39 | Idaho | 11.4 |
| 14 | New Hampshire | 18.2 | 39 | Montana | 11.4 |
| 14 | Pennsylvania | 18.2 | 39 | Oregon | 11.4 |
| 17 | Vermont | 17.8 | 42 | Alaska | 11.2 |
| 18 | Connecticut | 17.4 | 42 | California | 11.2 |
| 19 | Massachusetts | 16.7 | 42 | Texas | 11.2 |
| 20 | New Jersey | 16.1 | 45 | New Mexico | 11.0 |
| 21 | New York | 15.1 | 46 | Hawaii | 10.9 |
| 22 | Tennessee | 15.0 | 47 | Washington | 10.3 |
| 23 | Kentucky | 13.6 | 48 | South Carolina | 10.2 |
| 24 | West Virginia | 13.0 | 49 | Wyoming | 9.8 |
| 25 | Louisiana | 12.5 | 50 | Mississippi | 5.9 |

District of Columbia     9.0

Source: Families USA Foundation

"Health Spending: The Growing Threat to the Family Budget" (December 1991) (Reprinted with permission)

*This is a percent paid directly by each family and does not include payments made by business. It is a percent of annual family health payments. See beginning of this chapter for definitions.

# Projected Average Annual Family Health Payments Paid through Insurance in 2000

## Projected National Average = $1,610 per Family*

| RANK | STATE | PAYMENTS | RANK | STATE | PAYMENTS |
|------|-------|----------|------|-------|----------|
| 1 | Kansas | $2,236 | 26 | Vermont | $1,529 |
| 2 | Connecticut | 2,234 | 27 | Colorado | 1,498 |
| 3 | Michigan | 2,195 | 28 | Oregon | 1,466 |
| 4 | North Dakota | 2,187 | 29 | Alabama | 1,369 |
| 5 | Illinois | 2,173 | 30 | Tennessee | 1,334 |
| 6 | Missouri | 2,138 | 31 | Washington | 1,330 |
| 7 | Nebraska | 2,133 | 32 | Maryland | 1,298 |
| 8 | Massachusetts | 2,116 | 33 | Delaware | 1,292 |
| 9 | Minnesota | 2,111 | 34 | Texas | 1,279 |
| 10 | Ohio | 2,098 | 35 | Arizona | 1,267 |
| 11 | Wisconsin | 2,078 | 36 | Virginia | 1,258 |
| 12 | Iowa | 2,017 | 37 | Wyoming | 1,242 |
| 13 | South Dakota | 1,990 | 38 | Florida | 1,226 |
| 14 | Pennsylvania | 1,950 | 39 | Georgia | 1,221 |
| 15 | Rhode Island | 1,944 | 40 | West Virginia | 1,189 |
| 16 | Indiana | 1,832 | 41 | Louisiana | 1,183 |
| 17 | New York | 1,793 | 42 | Oklahoma | 1,155 |
| 18 | Maine | 1,785 | 43 | Idaho | 1,138 |
| 19 | New Jersey | 1,718 | 44 | North Carolina | 1,125 |
| 20 | Hawaii | 1,707 | 45 | Montana | 1,103 |
| 21 | California | 1,661 | 46 | New Mexico | 1,085 |
| 22 | New Hampshire | 1,566 | 47 | South Carolina | 1,082 |
| 23 | Alaska | 1,564 | 48 | Arkansas | 1,056 |
| 24 | Nevada | 1,552 | 49 | Kentucky | 989 |
| 25 | Utah | 1,532 | 50 | Mississippi | 916 |
| | | | | District of Columbia | 809 |

Source: Families USA Foundation

"Health Spending: The Growing Threat to the Family Budget" (December 1991) (Reprinted with permission)

*This is an average paid directly by each family and does not include payments made by business. It is a subset of average annual family health payments. See beginning of this chapter for definitions.

233

# Projected Percent of Average Annual Family Health Payments Paid through Insurance in 2000

## Projected National Rate = 17.1% Paid through Insurance*

| RANK | STATE | PERCENT | RANK | STATE | PERCENT |
|------|-------|---------|------|-------|---------|
| 1 | South Dakota | 23.8 | 26 | Hawaii | 17.1 |
| 2 | North Dakota | 23.7 | 27 | California | 17.0 |
| 3 | Nebraska | 22.8 | 28 | Idaho | 16.9 |
| 4 | Kansas | 22.7 | 29 | Oregon | 16.7 |
| 4 | Missouri | 22.7 | 30 | New Jersey | 16.0 |
| 6 | Iowa | 22.4 | 31 | Washington | 15.9 |
| 7 | Wisconsin | 22.3 | 32 | Wyoming | 15.6 |
| 8 | Michigan | 21.8 | 33 | Alabama | 15.4 |
| 9 | Alaska | 21.5 | 33 | Montana | 15.4 |
| 10 | Minnesota | 21.4 | 33 | West Virginia | 15.4 |
| 11 | Ohio | 21.2 | 36 | New Mexico | 15.3 |
| 12 | Indiana | 20.9 | 37 | Florida | 14.9 |
| 13 | Illinois | 20.8 | 38 | South Carolina | 14.5 |
| 14 | Maine | 20.7 | 38 | Texas | 14.5 |
| 15 | Pennsylvania | 20.4 | 40 | North Carolina | 14.4 |
| 16 | New Hampshire | 19.5 | 41 | Delaware | 14.3 |
| 17 | Vermont | 19.2 | 42 | New York | 14.1 |
| 18 | Utah | 18.7 | 43 | Arkansas | 13.9 |
| 19 | Connecticut | 18.5 | 43 | Louisiana | 13.9 |
| 19 | Nevada | 18.5 | 43 | Mississippi | 13.9 |
| 21 | Tennessee | 18.0 | 46 | Kentucky | 13.8 |
| 22 | Rhode Island | 17.9 | 46 | Oklahoma | 13.8 |
| 23 | Massachusetts | 17.7 | 48 | Georgia | 13.7 |
| 24 | Arizona | 17.5 | 49 | Maryland | 13.1 |
| 25 | Colorado | 17.4 | 49 | Virginia | 13.1 |
|  |  |  |  | District of Columbia | 8.6 |

Source: Families USA Foundation

*Source: Families USA Foundation*

    *"Health Spending: The Growing Threat to the Family Budget" (December 1991) (Reprinted with permission)*

*This is a percent paid directly by each family and does not include payments made by business. It is a percent of annual family health payments. See beginning of this chapter for definitions.*

234

# Average Annual Family Health Payments Paid for Medicare Payroll Tax in 1991

## National Average = $369 per Family*

| RANK | STATE | PAYMENTS | | RANK | STATE | PAYMENTS |
|---|---|---|---|---|---|---|
| 1 | Delaware | $708 | | 26 | Iowa | $320 |
| 2 | Connecticut | 567 | | 27 | North Carolina | 317 |
| 3 | New York | 565 | | 28 | Vermont | 316 |
| 4 | Alaska | 546 | | 29 | Texas | 315 |
| 5 | New Jersey | 505 | | 30 | Colorado | 312 |
| 6 | Michigan | 461 | | 31 | Arkansas | 310 |
| 7 | Massachusetts | 449 | | 32 | Washington | 309 |
| 8 | Minnesota | 427 | | 33 | Wyoming | 305 |
| 9 | Illinois | 421 | | 34 | Utah | 298 |
| 10 | Rhode Island | 405 | | 35 | North Dakota | 292 |
| 11 | Ohio | 397 | | 36 | Louisiana | 290 |
| 12 | Wisconsin | 393 | | 37 | Oklahoma | 286 |
| 13 | Pennsylvania | 391 | | 38 | Arizona | 281 |
| 14 | Maryland | 373 | | 39 | Idaho | 277 |
| 15 | Missouri | 365 | | 40 | Alabama | 274 |
| 16 | New Hampshire | 362 | | 41 | South Carolina | 272 |
| 17 | California | 356 | | 42 | Maine | 268 |
| 18 | Nebraska | 353 | | 43 | Florida | 260 |
| 19 | Hawaii | 341 | | 43 | New Mexico | 260 |
| 20 | Georgia | 340 | | 45 | South Dakota | 255 |
| 20 | Kansas | 340 | | 46 | Nevada | 252 |
| 22 | Oregon | 330 | | 47 | Montana | 248 |
| 23 | Indiana | 325 | | 48 | West Virginia | 242 |
| 23 | Virginia | 325 | | 49 | Kentucky | 240 |
| 25 | Tennessee | 322 | | 50 | Mississippi | 208 |

District of Columbia          901

Source: Families USA Foundation

"Health Spending: The Growing Threat to the Family Budget" (December 1991) (Reprinted with permission)

*This is an average paid directly by each family and does not include payments made by business. It is a subset of average annual family health payments. See beginning of this chapter for definitions.

235

# Percent of Average Annual Family Health Payments Paid for Medicare Payroll Tax in 1991

## National Rate = 8.6% Paid for Medicare Payroll Tax*

| RANK | STATE | PERCENT | | RANK | STATE | PERCENT |
|------|-------|---------|---|------|-------|---------|
| 1 | Delaware | 16.1 | | 25 | Georgia | 8.2 |
| 2 | Alaska | 14.2 | | 25 | Indiana | 8.2 |
| 3 | Connecticut | 10.5 | | 25 | Rhode Island | 8.2 |
| 4 | New Jersey | 10.4 | | 29 | Utah | 8.1 |
| 5 | Michigan | 10.1 | | 30 | California | 8.0 |
| 5 | New York | 10.1 | | 30 | South Carolina | 8.0 |
| 7 | New Hampshire | 9.4 | | 32 | Colorado | 7.9 |
| 8 | Minnesota | 9.3 | | 32 | Iowa | 7.9 |
| 8 | Wisconsin | 9.3 | | 32 | Montana | 7.9 |
| 10 | Idaho | 9.2 | | 32 | New Mexico | 7.9 |
| 10 | Tennessee | 9.2 | | 36 | Texas | 7.7 |
| 12 | Pennsylvania | 9.1 | | 37 | Kansas | 7.6 |
| 13 | Illinois | 9.0 | | 37 | Louisiana | 7.6 |
| 14 | Arkansas | 8.9 | | 39 | Kentucky | 7.5 |
| 14 | Ohio | 8.9 | | 39 | Oklahoma | 7.5 |
| 16 | Wyoming | 8.8 | | 39 | Virginia | 7.5 |
| 17 | North Carolina | 8.7 | | 42 | Hawaii | 7.4 |
| 17 | Vermont | 8.7 | | 43 | North Dakota | 7.0 |
| 19 | Oregon | 8.5 | | 43 | West Virginia | 7.0 |
| 20 | Massachusetts | 8.4 | | 45 | Mississippi | 6.9 |
| 20 | Missouri | 8.4 | | 46 | Alabama | 6.8 |
| 22 | Maryland | 8.3 | | 46 | Maine | 6.8 |
| 22 | Nebraska | 8.3 | | 48 | Florida | 6.6 |
| 22 | Washington | 8.3 | | 48 | South Dakota | 6.6 |
| 25 | Arizona | 8.2 | | 50 | Nevada | 6.5 |

District of Columbia      21.0

Source: Families USA Foundation
   "Health Spending: The Growing Threat to the Family Budget" (December 1991) (Reprinted with permission)
*This is a percent paid directly by each family and does not include payments made by business. It is a percent of annual family health payments. See beginning of this chapter for definitions.

# Average Annual Family Health Payments Paid for Medicare Payroll Tax in 1980

## National Average = $132 per Family*

| RANK | STATE | PAYMENTS | | RANK | STATE | PAYMENTS |
|------|-------|----------|---|------|-------|----------|
| 1 | Delaware | $180 | | 25 | Oregon | $118 |
| 2 | New York | 175 | | 27 | Oklahoma | 117 |
| 3 | Michigan | 163 | | 28 | Louisiana | 116 |
| 4 | Connecticut | 161 | | 28 | New Hampshire | 116 |
| 4 | Illinois | 161 | | 30 | Georgia | 115 |
| 6 | Minnesota | 159 | | 31 | North Dakota | 113 |
| 7 | New Jersey | 157 | | 31 | Washington | 113 |
| 8 | Ohio | 147 | | 33 | Alabama | 106 |
| 9 | Wisconsin | 142 | | 33 | South Carolina | 106 |
| 10 | Pennsylvania | 138 | | 35 | South Dakota | 105 |
| 11 | Massachusetts | 135 | | 36 | Wyoming | 104 |
| 12 | Texas | 133 | | 37 | Arizona | 103 |
| 13 | Maryland | 132 | | 37 | Montana | 103 |
| 13 | Rhode Island | 132 | | 37 | New Mexico | 103 |
| 15 | Indiana | 131 | | 37 | Virginia | 103 |
| 16 | Missouri | 129 | | 41 | Nevada | 102 |
| 17 | Hawaii | 128 | | 41 | West Virginia | 102 |
| 17 | Iowa | 128 | | 43 | Kentucky | 99 |
| 19 | Nebraska | 127 | | 44 | Arkansas | 98 |
| 20 | California | 125 | | 44 | Utah | 98 |
| 21 | Colorado | 124 | | 44 | Vermont | 98 |
| 21 | Kansas | 124 | | 47 | Maine | 95 |
| 23 | Tennessee | 123 | | 48 | Florida | 92 |
| 24 | Idaho | 119 | | 49 | Mississippi | 85 |
| 25 | North Carolina | 118 | | 50 | Alaska | 57 |

District of Columbia                    204

Source: Families USA Foundation

"Health Spending: The Growing Threat to the Family Budget" (December 1991) (Reprinted with permission)

*This is an average paid directly by each family and does not include payments made by business. It is a subset of average annual family health payments. See beginning of this chapter for definitions.

# Percent of Average Annual Family Health Payments Paid for Medicare Payroll Tax in 1980

## National Rate = 7.6% Paid for Medicare Payroll Tax*

| RANK | STATE | PERCENT | | RANK | STATE | PERCENT |
|------|-------|---------|---|------|-------|---------|
| 1 | Idaho | 9.9 | | 25 | Texas | 7.4 |
| 2 | Delaware | 9.4 | | 25 | Vermont | 7.4 |
| 3 | Michigan | 8.7 | | 28 | Oklahoma | 7.2 |
| 4 | New Mexico | 8.5 | | 29 | Nebraska | 7.1 |
| 5 | Tennessee | 8.4 | | 30 | Hawaii | 7.0 |
| 6 | Minnesota | 8.3 | | 30 | Iowa | 7.0 |
| 6 | New Hampshire | 8.3 | | 30 | Rhode Island | 7.0 |
| 6 | Oregon | 8.3 | | 33 | Georgia | 6.9 |
| 9 | New Jersey | 8.1 | | 33 | Kansas | 6.9 |
| 9 | New York | 8.1 | | 33 | Louisiana | 6.9 |
| 11 | Connecticut | 8.0 | | 36 | Arkansas | 6.8 |
| 11 | Illinois | 8.0 | | 36 | Nevada | 6.8 |
| 11 | Indiana | 8.0 | | 36 | Utah | 6.8 |
| 11 | Ohio | 8.0 | | 39 | Kentucky | 6.5 |
| 15 | Arizona | 7.9 | | 39 | Maryland | 6.5 |
| 15 | Pennsylvania | 7.9 | | 39 | Massachusetts | 6.5 |
| 15 | Wisconsin | 7.9 | | 39 | Mississippi | 6.5 |
| 18 | North Carolina | 7.8 | | 43 | Maine | 6.4 |
| 19 | Montana | 7.7 | | 43 | South Dakota | 6.4 |
| 19 | South Carolina | 7.7 | | 43 | West Virginia | 6.4 |
| 21 | Washington | 7.6 | | 46 | Florida | 6.3 |
| 22 | California | 7.5 | | 46 | North Dakota | 6.3 |
| 22 | Colorado | 7.5 | | 48 | Alabama | 6.2 |
| 22 | Wyoming | 7.5 | | 48 | Virginia | 6.2 |
| 25 | Missouri | 7.4 | | 50 | Alaska | 3.6 |

District of Columbia     12.2

Source: Families USA Foundation

"Health Spending: The Growing Threat to the Family Budget" (December 1991) (Reprinted with permission)

*This is a percent paid directly by each family and does not include payments made by business. It is a percent of annual family health payments. See beginning of this chapter for definitions.

# Projected Average Annual Family Health Payments Paid for Medicare Payroll Tax in 2000

## Projected National Average = $605 per Family*

| RANK | STATE | PAYMENTS | RANK | STATE | PAYMENTS |
|------|-------|----------|------|-------|----------|
| 1 | Connecticut | $948 | 26 | Texas | $527 |
| 2 | New York | 944 | 27 | North Carolina | 521 |
| 3 | New Jersey | 844 | 28 | Washington | 519 |
| 4 | Delaware | 825 | 29 | Colorado | 517 |
| 5 | Michigan | 770 | 30 | Arkansas | 516 |
| 6 | Massachusetts | 755 | 31 | Wyoming | 515 |
| 7 | Illinois | 706 | 32 | Utah | 506 |
| 8 | Rhode Island | 686 | 33 | North Dakota | 489 |
| 9 | Ohio | 658 | 34 | Louisiana | 480 |
| 10 | Wisconsin | 656 | 35 | Hawaii | 478 |
| 11 | Pennsylvania | 650 | 36 | Oklahoma | 477 |
| 12 | Maryland | 622 | 37 | Idaho | 467 |
| 13 | Missouri | 610 | 38 | Arizona | 463 |
| 13 | New Hampshire | 610 | 39 | Alabama | 455 |
| 15 | California | 600 | 40 | Maine | 449 |
| 16 | Nebraska | 588 | 40 | South Carolina | 449 |
| 17 | Minnesota | 587 | 42 | New Mexico | 437 |
| 18 | Georgia | 568 | 43 | South Dakota | 429 |
| 18 | Kansas | 568 | 44 | Florida | 428 |
| 20 | Oregon | 559 | 45 | Nevada | 424 |
| 21 | Virginia | 542 | 46 | Montana | 415 |
| 22 | Indiana | 540 | 47 | West Virginia | 402 |
| 23 | Tennessee | 532 | 48 | Kentucky | 397 |
| 24 | Iowa | 531 | 49 | Alaska | 374 |
| 24 | Vermont | 531 | 50 | Mississippi | 348 |

| | | | District of Columbia | 1,221 |
|---|---|---|---|---|

Source: Families USA Foundation

"Health Spending: The Growing Threat to the Family Budget" (December 1991) (Reprinted with permission)

*This is an average paid directly by each family and does not include payments made by business. It is a subset of average annual family health payments. See beginning of this chapter for definitions.

# Projected Percent of Average Annual Family Health Payments Paid for Medicare Payroll Tax in 2000

## Projected National Rate = 6.4% Paid for Medicare Payroll Tax*

| RANK | STATE | PERCENT | RANK | STATE | PERCENT |
|------|-------|---------|------|-------|---------|
| 1 | Delaware | 9.1 | 25 | New Mexico | 6.2 |
| 2 | Connecticut | 7.8 | 25 | Utah | 6.2 |
| 2 | New Jersey | 7.8 | 25 | Washington | 6.2 |
| 4 | Michigan | 7.7 | 29 | California | 6.1 |
| 5 | New Hampshire | 7.6 | 30 | Colorado | 6.0 |
| 6 | New York | 7.4 | 30 | Minnesota | 6.0 |
| 7 | Tennessee | 7.2 | 30 | South Carolina | 6.0 |
| 8 | Wisconsin | 7.0 | 30 | Texas | 6.0 |
| 9 | Idaho | 6.9 | 34 | Iowa | 5.9 |
| 10 | Arkansas | 6.8 | 35 | Kansas | 5.8 |
| 10 | Illinois | 6.8 | 35 | Montana | 5.8 |
| 10 | Pennsylvania | 6.8 | 37 | Oklahoma | 5.7 |
| 13 | North Carolina | 6.7 | 38 | Louisiana | 5.6 |
| 13 | Vermont | 6.7 | 38 | Virginia | 5.6 |
| 15 | Ohio | 6.6 | 40 | Kentucky | 5.5 |
| 16 | Missouri | 6.5 | 41 | Mississippi | 5.3 |
| 16 | Wyoming | 6.5 | 41 | North Dakota | 5.3 |
| 18 | Arizona | 6.4 | 43 | Alaska | 5.2 |
| 18 | Georgia | 6.4 | 43 | Florida | 5.2 |
| 18 | Oregon | 6.4 | 43 | Maine | 5.2 |
| 21 | Maryland | 6.3 | 43 | West Virginia | 5.2 |
| 21 | Massachusetts | 6.3 | 47 | Alabama | 5.1 |
| 21 | Nebraska | 6.3 | 47 | South Dakota | 5.1 |
| 21 | Rhode Island | 6.3 | 49 | Nevada | 5.0 |
| 25 | Indiana | 6.2 | 50 | Hawaii | 4.8 |

District of Columbia    12.9

Source: Families USA Foundation

"Health Spending: The Growing Threat to the Family Budget" (December 1991) (Reprinted with permission)

*This is a percent paid directly by each family and does not include payments made by business. It is a percent of annual family health payments. See beginning of this chapter for definitions.

# Average Annual Family Health Payments Paid for Medicare Premiums in 1991

## National Average = $112 per Family*

| RANK | STATE | PAYMENTS | | RANK | STATE | PAYMENTS |
|------|-------|----------|---|------|-------|----------|
| 1 | Florida | $146 | | 24 | Mississippi | $114 |
| 2 | Pennsylvania | 140 | | 27 | Michigan | 113 |
| 3 | West Virginia | 139 | | 28 | Arizona | 112 |
| 4 | South Dakota | 138 | | 28 | Indiana | 112 |
| 5 | Iowa | 136 | | 28 | Minnesota | 112 |
| 6 | Arkansas | 133 | | 31 | Illinois | 111 |
| 7 | North Dakota | 131 | | 31 | North Carolina | 111 |
| 7 | Rhode Island | 131 | | 33 | Vermont | 107 |
| 9 | Maine | 128 | | 34 | South Carolina | 106 |
| 10 | Missouri | 126 | | 35 | Louisiana | 104 |
| 11 | Kansas | 125 | | 36 | New Hampshire | 103 |
| 11 | Nebraska | 125 | | 37 | Delaware | 102 |
| 13 | Connecticut | 124 | | 38 | Hawaii | 100 |
| 14 | Oregon | 123 | | 38 | Washington | 100 |
| 14 | Wisconsin | 123 | | 40 | New Mexico | 99 |
| 16 | New Jersey | 122 | | 41 | Wyoming | 98 |
| 17 | Ohio | 121 | | 42 | Virginia | 97 |
| 18 | Oklahoma | 120 | | 43 | Georgia | 93 |
| 19 | Alabama | 118 | | 43 | Texas | 93 |
| 19 | Montana | 118 | | 43 | Utah | 93 |
| 21 | Massachusetts | 117 | | 46 | California | 90 |
| 22 | Tennessee | 116 | | 46 | Maryland | 90 |
| 23 | New York | 115 | | 48 | Nevada | 89 |
| 24 | Idaho | 114 | | 49 | Colorado | 82 |
| 24 | Kentucky | 114 | | 50 | Alaska | 38 |
| | | | | | District of Columbia | 85 |

Source: Families USA Foundation

"Health Spending: The Growing Threat to the Family Budget" (December 1991) (Reprinted with permission)

*This is an average paid directly by each family and does not include payments made by business. It is a subset of average annual family health payments. See beginning of this chapter for definitions.

# Percent of Average Annual Family Health Payments Paid for Medicare Premiums in 1991

## National Rate = 2.6% Paid for Medicare Premiums*

| RANK | STATE | PERCENT | RANK | STATE | PERCENT |
|------|-------|---------|------|-------|---------|
| 1 | West Virginia | 4.0 | 25 | Kansas | 2.8 |
| 2 | Arkansas | 3.8 | 25 | Wyoming | 2.8 |
| 2 | Idaho | 3.8 | 28 | Louisiana | 2.7 |
| 2 | Mississippi | 3.8 | 28 | New Hampshire | 2.7 |
| 5 | Florida | 3.7 | 28 | Ohio | 2.7 |
| 5 | Montana | 3.7 | 28 | Rhode Island | 2.7 |
| 7 | Kentucky | 3.6 | 28 | Washington | 2.7 |
| 7 | South Dakota | 3.6 | 33 | Michigan | 2.5 |
| 9 | Iowa | 3.4 | 33 | New Jersey | 2.5 |
| 10 | Arizona | 3.3 | 33 | Utah | 2.5 |
| 10 | Tennessee | 3.3 | 36 | Illinois | 2.4 |
| 12 | Maine | 3.2 | 36 | Minnesota | 2.4 |
| 12 | Oklahoma | 3.2 | 38 | Connecticut | 2.3 |
| 12 | Pennsylvania | 3.2 | 38 | Delaware | 2.3 |
| 15 | North Carolina | 3.1 | 38 | Nevada | 2.3 |
| 15 | North Dakota | 3.1 | 38 | Texas | 2.3 |
| 15 | Oregon | 3.1 | 42 | Georgia | 2.2 |
| 15 | South Carolina | 3.1 | 42 | Hawaii | 2.2 |
| 19 | New Mexico | 3.0 | 42 | Massachusetts | 2.2 |
| 20 | Alabama | 2.9 | 42 | Virginia | 2.2 |
| 20 | Missouri | 2.9 | 46 | Colorado | 2.1 |
| 20 | Nebraska | 2.9 | 46 | New York | 2.1 |
| 20 | Vermont | 2.9 | 48 | California | 2.0 |
| 20 | Wisconsin | 2.9 | 48 | Maryland | 2.0 |
| 25 | Indiana | 2.8 | 50 | Alaska | 1.0 |
| | | | | District of Columbia | 2.0 |

Source: Families USA Foundation

*"Health Spending: The Growing Threat to the Family Budget"* (December 1991) (Reprinted with permission)

*This is a percent paid directly by each family and does not include payments made by business. It is a percent of annual family health payments. See beginning of this chapter for definitions.

# Average Annual Family Health Payments Paid for Medicare Premiums in 1980

## National Average = $34 per Family*

| RANK | STATE | PAYMENTS | | RANK | STATE | PAYMENTS |
|------|-------|----------|---|------|-------|----------|
| 1 | Arkansas | $43 | | 26 | North Carolina | $33 |
| 1 | Florida | 43 | | 26 | Vermont | 33 |
| 3 | Iowa | 41 | | 28 | Delaware | 32 |
| 3 | Rhode Island | 41 | | 28 | Indiana | 32 |
| 3 | West Virginia | 41 | | 28 | Montana | 32 |
| 6 | Maine | 40 | | 28 | New Hampshire | 32 |
| 6 | South Dakota | 40 | | 32 | Georgia | 31 |
| 8 | Mississippi | 39 | | 32 | Idaho | 31 |
| 8 | Missouri | 39 | | 32 | Michigan | 31 |
| 8 | Nebraska | 39 | | 32 | Oregon | 31 |
| 8 | New Jersey | 39 | | 36 | Arizona | 30 |
| 8 | Pennsylvania | 39 | | 36 | South Carolina | 30 |
| 13 | Kansas | 38 | | 38 | Louisiana | 29 |
| 13 | Kentucky | 38 | | 38 | Maryland | 29 |
| 13 | North Dakota | 38 | | 40 | California | 28 |
| 16 | Alabama | 37 | | 40 | New Mexico | 28 |
| 16 | Massachusetts | 37 | | 40 | Texas | 28 |
| 16 | New York | 37 | | 40 | Virginia | 28 |
| 19 | Tennessee | 36 | | 40 | Washington | 28 |
| 19 | Wisconsin | 36 | | 45 | Hawaii | 25 |
| 21 | Connecticut | 35 | | 46 | Colorado | 24 |
| 21 | Minnesota | 35 | | 46 | Utah | 24 |
| 21 | Oklahoma | 35 | | 48 | Wyoming | 23 |
| 24 | Illinois | 34 | | 49 | Nevada | 21 |
| 24 | Ohio | 34 | | 50 | Alaska | 8 |

District of Columbia     25

Source: Families USA Foundation

"Health Spending: The Growing Threat to the Family Budget" (December 1991) (Reprinted with permission)

*This is an average paid directly by each family and does not include payments made by business. It is a subset of average annual family health payments. See beginning of this chapter for definitions.

# Percent of Average Annual Family Health Payments Paid for Medicare Premiums in 1980

## National Rate = 1.9% Paid for Medicare Premiums*

| RANK | STATE | PERCENT | | RANK | STATE | PERCENT |
|------|-------|---------|---|------|-------|---------|
| 1 | Arkansas | 3.0 | | 23 | Rhode Island | 2.1 |
| 1 | Mississippi | 3.0 | | 27 | New Jersey | 2.0 |
| 3 | Florida | 2.9 | | 27 | Wisconsin | 2.0 |
| 4 | Maine | 2.7 | | 29 | Georgia | 1.9 |
| 5 | Idaho | 2.5 | | 29 | Indiana | 1.9 |
| 5 | Kentucky | 2.5 | | 29 | Washington | 1.9 |
| 5 | South Dakota | 2.5 | | 32 | Massachusetts | 1.8 |
| 5 | Vermont | 2.5 | | 32 | Minnesota | 1.8 |
| 5 | West Virginia | 2.5 | | 32 | Ohio | 1.8 |
| 10 | Montana | 2.4 | | 35 | California | 1.7 |
| 10 | Tennessee | 2.4 | | 35 | Connecticut | 1.7 |
| 12 | Arizona | 2.3 | | 35 | Delaware | 1.7 |
| 12 | New Hampshire | 2.3 | | 35 | Illinois | 1.7 |
| 12 | New Mexico | 2.3 | | 35 | Louisiana | 1.7 |
| 15 | Alabama | 2.2 | | 35 | Michigan | 1.7 |
| 15 | Iowa | 2.2 | | 35 | New York | 1.7 |
| 15 | Missouri | 2.2 | | 35 | Utah | 1.7 |
| 15 | North Carolina | 2.2 | | 35 | Virginia | 1.7 |
| 15 | Oklahoma | 2.2 | | 44 | Texas | 1.6 |
| 15 | Oregon | 2.2 | | 44 | Wyoming | 1.6 |
| 15 | Pennsylvania | 2.2 | | 46 | Colorado | 1.5 |
| 15 | South Carolina | 2.2 | | 47 | Hawaii | 1.4 |
| 23 | Kansas | 2.1 | | 47 | Maryland | 1.4 |
| 23 | Nebraska | 2.1 | | 47 | Nevada | 1.4 |
| 23 | North Dakota | 2.1 | | 50 | Alaska | 0.5 |
| | | | | | District of Columbia | 1.5 |

*Source: Families USA Foundation*

   *"Health Spending: The Growing Threat to the Family Budget" (December 1991) (Reprinted with permission)*

*This is a percent paid directly by each family and does not include payments made by business. It is a percent of annual family health payments. See beginning of this chapter for definitions.*

244

# Projected Average Annual Family Health Payments Paid for Medicare Premiums in 2000

## Projected National Average = $219 Paid per Family*

| RANK | STATE | PAYMENTS | RANK | STATE | PAYMENTS |
|------|-------|----------|------|-------|----------|
| 1 | Florida | $292 | 26 | Mississippi | $223 |
| 2 | West Virginia | 272 | 27 | Hawaii | 222 |
| 3 | Pennsylvania | 271 | 27 | Indiana | 222 |
| 4 | Iowa | 267 | 27 | Michigan | 222 |
| 5 | South Dakota | 264 | 30 | Idaho | 220 |
| 6 | Arkansas | 260 | 30 | Massachusetts | 220 |
| 7 | North Dakota | 256 | 32 | Minnesota | 217 |
| 8 | Nebraska | 246 | 33 | Illinois | 215 |
| 9 | Kansas | 244 | 33 | South Carolina | 215 |
| 10 | Missouri | 243 | 35 | Louisiana | 212 |
| 10 | Rhode Island | 243 | 36 | Delaware | 209 |
| 12 | Maine | 242 | 37 | Vermont | 202 |
| 13 | Wisconsin | 240 | 38 | New Mexico | 193 |
| 14 | Ohio | 239 | 38 | Virginia | 193 |
| 15 | Connecticut | 238 | 38 | Washington | 193 |
| 16 | Alabama | 236 | 41 | New Hampshire | 192 |
| 17 | New Jersey | 235 | 42 | Wyoming | 188 |
| 18 | Oklahoma | 234 | 43 | Texas | 187 |
| 18 | Tennessee | 234 | 44 | Utah | 184 |
| 20 | Arizona | 228 | 45 | Georgia | 182 |
| 20 | Kentucky | 228 | 46 | California | 178 |
| 20 | Montana | 228 | 47 | Maryland | 177 |
| 23 | North Carolina | 227 | 48 | Nevada | 173 |
| 23 | Oregon | 227 | 49 | Colorado | 168 |
| 25 | New York | 224 | 50 | Alaska | 82 |
| | | | | District of Columbia | 165 |

*Source: Families USA Foundation*

*"Health Spending: The Growing Threat to the Family Budget" (December 1991) (Reprinted with permission)*

*\*This is an average paid directly by each family and does not include payments made by business. It is a subset of average annual family health payments. See beginning of this chapter for definitions.*

# Projected Percent of Average Annual Family Health Payments Paid for Medicare Premiums in 2000

## Projected National Rate = 2.3% Paid for Medicare Premiums*

| RANK | STATE | PERCENT | RANK | STATE | PERCENT |
|------|-------|---------|------|-------|---------|
| 1 | Florida | 3.5 | 24 | Louisiana | 2.5 |
| 1 | West Virginia | 3.5 | 24 | Vermont | 2.5 |
| 3 | Arkansas | 3.4 | 28 | New Hampshire | 2.4 |
| 3 | Mississippi | 3.4 | 28 | Ohio | 2.4 |
| 5 | Idaho | 3.3 | 28 | Wyoming | 2.4 |
| 6 | Arizona | 3.2 | 31 | Delaware | 2.3 |
| 6 | Kentucky | 3.2 | 31 | Utah | 2.3 |
| 6 | Montana | 3.2 | 31 | Washington | 2.3 |
| 6 | South Dakota | 3.2 | 34 | Hawaii | 2.2 |
| 6 | Tennessee | 3.2 | 34 | Michigan | 2.2 |
| 11 | Iowa | 3.0 | 34 | Minnesota | 2.2 |
| 12 | North Carolina | 2.9 | 34 | New Jersey | 2.2 |
| 12 | South Carolina | 2.9 | 34 | Rhode Island | 2.2 |
| 14 | Maine | 2.8 | 39 | Illinois | 2.1 |
| 14 | North Dakota | 2.8 | 39 | Nevada | 2.1 |
| 14 | Oklahoma | 2.8 | 39 | Texas | 2.1 |
| 14 | Pennsylvania | 2.8 | 42 | Colorado | 2.0 |
| 18 | Alabama | 2.7 | 42 | Connecticut | 2.0 |
| 18 | New Mexico | 2.7 | 42 | Georgia | 2.0 |
| 20 | Missouri | 2.6 | 42 | Virginia | 2.0 |
| 20 | Nebraska | 2.6 | 46 | California | 1.8 |
| 20 | Oregon | 2.6 | 46 | Maryland | 1.8 |
| 20 | Wisconsin | 2.6 | 46 | Massachusetts | 1.8 |
| 24 | Indiana | 2.5 | 46 | New York | 1.8 |
| 24 | Kansas | 2.5 | 50 | Alaska | 1.1 |
| | | | | District of Columbia | 1.7 |

Source: Families USA Foundation

   "Health Spending: The Growing Threat to the Family Budget" (December 1991) (Reprinted with permission)

*This is a percent paid directly by each family and does not include payments made by business.  It is a percent of annual family health payments.  See beginning of this chapter for definitions.

# Average Annual Family Health Payments Paid through General Taxes in 1991

## National Average = $1,715 per Family*

| RANK | STATE | GENERAL TAXES | RANK | STATE | GENERAL TAXES |
|------|-------|---------------|------|-------|---------------|
| 1 | New York | $2,726 | 26 | Maine | $1,520 |
| 2 | Massachusetts | 2,278 | 27 | Oklahoma | 1,512 |
| 3 | Connecticut | 2,230 | 28 | Kansas | 1,486 |
| 4 | New Jersey | 2,207 | 29 | Utah | 1,485 |
| 5 | Maryland | 2,097 | 30 | North Carolina | 1,472 |
| 6 | Hawaii | 2,020 | 31 | Pennsylvania | 1,457 |
| 6 | Virginia | 2,020 | 32 | New Mexico | 1,449 |
| 8 | Rhode Island | 2,014 | 33 | Wisconsin | 1,431 |
| 9 | California | 1,849 | 34 | Indiana | 1,427 |
| 10 | Georgia | 1,843 | 35 | New Hampshire | 1,409 |
| 11 | Delaware | 1,664 | 36 | Missouri | 1,402 |
| 12 | Minnesota | 1,646 | 37 | Arizona | 1,384 |
| 13 | Illinois | 1,644 | 38 | Vermont | 1,367 |
| 14 | Colorado | 1,643 | 39 | Nebraska | 1,344 |
| 15 | Washington | 1,642 | 40 | Montana | 1,329 |
| 16 | Oregon | 1,605 | 41 | North Dakota | 1,311 |
| 17 | Ohio | 1,601 | 42 | Kentucky | 1,310 |
| 18 | Texas | 1,581 | 43 | Iowa | 1,305 |
| 19 | Nevada | 1,564 | 44 | Arkansas | 1,279 |
| 20 | Michigan | 1,561 | 45 | Alaska | 1,214 |
| 21 | Wyoming | 1,552 | 46 | West Virginia | 1,207 |
| 22 | Louisiana | 1,551 | 47 | Mississippi | 1,173 |
| 23 | Alabama | 1,541 | 48 | Idaho | 1,172 |
| 23 | Florida | 1,541 | 49 | South Dakota | 1,109 |
| 25 | South Carolina | 1,525 | 50 | Tennessee | 1,001 |
| | | | | District of Columbia | 2,030 |

Source: Families USA Foundation

"Health Spending: The Growing Threat to the Family Budget" (December 1991) (Reprinted with permission)

*This is an average paid directly by each family and does not include payments made by business. It is a subset of average annual family health payments. See beginning of this chapter for definitions.

# Percent of Average Annual Family Health Payments Paid through General Taxes in 1991

## National Rate = 39.9% Paid through General Taxes*

| RANK | STATE | PERCENT | RANK | STATE | PERCENT |
|------|-------|---------|------|-------|---------|
| 1 | New York | 48.8 | 26 | Idaho | 39.0 |
| 2 | Maryland | 46.8 | 26 | Mississippi | 39.0 |
| 3 | Virginia | 46.4 | 28 | Texas | 38.6 |
| 4 | New Jersey | 45.4 | 29 | Maine | 38.5 |
| 5 | South Carolina | 44.7 | 30 | Alabama | 37.9 |
| 5 | Wyoming | 44.7 | 30 | Delaware | 37.9 |
| 7 | Georgia | 44.3 | 32 | Vermont | 37.4 |
| 7 | Washington | 44.3 | 33 | Arkansas | 36.8 |
| 9 | New Mexico | 44.0 | 34 | New Hampshire | 36.5 |
| 10 | Hawaii | 43.9 | 35 | Minnesota | 36.0 |
| 11 | Massachusetts | 42.8 | 36 | Indiana | 35.9 |
| 12 | Montana | 42.1 | 37 | Ohio | 35.8 |
| 13 | Colorado | 41.8 | 38 | Illinois | 35.2 |
| 14 | California | 41.7 | 39 | West Virginia | 35.1 |
| 15 | Oregon | 41.2 | 40 | Michigan | 34.2 |
| 16 | Connecticut | 41.1 | 41 | Pennsylvania | 33.9 |
| 17 | Rhode Island | 41.0 | 42 | Wisconsin | 33.7 |
| 18 | Kentucky | 40.9 | 43 | Kansas | 33.2 |
| 19 | Louisiana | 40.7 | 44 | Iowa | 32.4 |
| 20 | North Carolina | 40.5 | 45 | Missouri | 32.1 |
| 21 | Arizona | 40.3 | 46 | Alaska | 31.6 |
| 21 | Utah | 40.3 | 47 | Nebraska | 31.5 |
| 23 | Nevada | 40.1 | 48 | North Dakota | 31.3 |
| 24 | Oklahoma | 39.9 | 49 | South Dakota | 28.7 |
| 25 | Florida | 39.2 | 49 | Tennessee | 28.7 |

District of Columbia          47.2

Source: Families USA Foundation

   "Health Spending: The Growing Threat to the Family Budget" (December 1991) (Reprinted with permission)

*This is a percent paid directly by each family and does not include payments made by business.  It is a percent of annual family health payments.  See beginning of this chapter for definitions.

# Average Annual Family Health Payments Paid through General Taxes in 1980

## National Average = $664 per Family*

| RANK | STATE | GENERAL TAXES | | RANK | STATE | GENERAL TAXES |
|------|-------|---------------|---|------|-------|---------------|
| 1 | Hawaii | $901 | | 26 | Kansas | $615 |
| 2 | New York | 881 | | 27 | Alabama | 612 |
| 3 | Maryland | 867 | | 28 | Montana | 596 |
| 4 | Alaska | 808 | | 29 | Wisconsin | 592 |
| 5 | Delaware | 792 | | 30 | Nebraska | 581 |
| 6 | Colorado | 769 | | 31 | North Carolina | 578 |
| 7 | New Jersey | 768 | | 32 | South Carolina | 574 |
| 8 | California | 767 | | 33 | Ohio | 571 |
| 9 | Washington | 751 | | 34 | Florida | 559 |
| 10 | Wyoming | 748 | | 35 | Pennsylvania | 558 |
| 11 | Massachusetts | 746 | | 36 | Arizona | 552 |
| 12 | Virginia | 734 | | 37 | West Virginia | 547 |
| 13 | Texas | 722 | | 38 | Indiana | 535 |
| 14 | Illinois | 706 | | 39 | North Dakota | 533 |
| 15 | Nevada | 704 | | 40 | Missouri | 530 |
| 16 | Connecticut | 695 | | 41 | Kentucky | 524 |
| 17 | Utah | 671 | | 42 | Idaho | 517 |
| 18 | Oregon | 652 | | 43 | Arkansas | 516 |
| 19 | Minnesota | 649 | | 44 | New Mexico | 515 |
| 20 | Rhode Island | 648 | | 45 | Mississippi | 468 |
| 21 | Michigan | 644 | | 46 | Maine | 453 |
| 21 | Oklahoma | 644 | | 47 | Vermont | 440 |
| 23 | Georgia | 629 | | 48 | South Dakota | 439 |
| 24 | Iowa | 622 | | 49 | New Hampshire | 425 |
| 24 | Louisiana | 622 | | 50 | Tennessee | 367 |
| | | | | | District of Columbia | 802 |

Source: Families USA Foundation

"Health Spending: The Growing Threat to the Family Budget" (December 1991) (Reprinted with permission)

*This is an average paid directly by each family and does not include payments made by business. It is a subset of average annual family health payments. See beginning of this chapter for definitions.

## Percent of Average Annual Family Health Payments Paid through General Taxes in 1980

## National Rate = 38.1% Paid through General Taxes*

| RANK | STATE | PERCENT | RANK | STATE | PERCENT |
|---|---|---|---|---|---|
| 1 | Wyoming | 54.0 | 26 | Massachusetts | 36.2 |
| 2 | Alaska | 50.8 | 27 | Alabama | 35.9 |
| 3 | Washington | 50.5 | 27 | Mississippi | 35.9 |
| 4 | Hawaii | 49.3 | 29 | Arkansas | 35.7 |
| 5 | Nevada | 46.6 | 30 | Illinois | 35.3 |
| 5 | Utah | 46.6 | 31 | Connecticut | 34.5 |
| 7 | Colorado | 46.4 | 32 | West Virginia | 34.4 |
| 8 | California | 46.1 | 33 | Kentucky | 34.3 |
| 9 | Oregon | 46.0 | 33 | Michigan | 34.3 |
| 10 | Montana | 44.3 | 35 | Kansas | 34.2 |
| 11 | Virginia | 44.1 | 36 | Iowa | 34.1 |
| 12 | Idaho | 43.0 | 36 | Rhode Island | 34.1 |
| 13 | New Mexico | 42.6 | 38 | Minnesota | 33.8 |
| 14 | Maryland | 42.3 | 39 | Vermont | 33.1 |
| 15 | Arizona | 42.2 | 40 | Wisconsin | 32.9 |
| 16 | South Carolina | 41.7 | 41 | Indiana | 32.6 |
| 17 | Delaware | 41.4 | 42 | Nebraska | 32.2 |
| 18 | New York | 40.8 | 43 | Pennsylvania | 31.9 |
| 19 | Texas | 40.2 | 44 | Ohio | 31.0 |
| 20 | Oklahoma | 39.9 | 45 | New Hampshire | 30.6 |
| 21 | New Jersey | 39.6 | 46 | Maine | 30.5 |
| 22 | Florida | 38.2 | 47 | Missouri | 30.4 |
| 23 | North Carolina | 38.0 | 48 | North Dakota | 29.7 |
| 24 | Georgia | 37.8 | 49 | South Dakota | 26.9 |
| 25 | Louisiana | 37.2 | 50 | Tennessee | 24.9 |
| | | | | District of Columbia | 47.9 |

Source: Families USA Foundation

"Health Spending: The Growing Threat to the Family Budget" (December 1991) (Reprinted with permission)

*This is a percent paid directly by each family and does not include payments made by business. It is a percent of annual family health payments. See beginning of this chapter for definitions.

# Projected Average Annual Family Health Payments Paid through General Taxes in 2000

## Projected National Average = $4,400 per Family*

| RANK | STATE | GENERAL TAXES | RANK | STATE | GENERAL TAXES |
|---|---|---|---|---|---|
| 1 | New York | $7,149 | 26 | Maine | $3,872 |
| 2 | Massachusetts | 5,968 | 27 | Wisconsin | 3,846 |
| 3 | Connecticut | 5,880 | 28 | South Carolina | 3,819 |
| 4 | New Jersey | 5,582 | 29 | Indiana | 3,815 |
| 5 | Maryland | 5,273 | 30 | Utah | 3,793 |
| 6 | Rhode Island | 5,176 | 31 | Nevada | 3,783 |
| 7 | Virginia | 5,108 | 32 | Iowa | 3,707 |
| 8 | Hawaii | 4,997 | 33 | Missouri | 3,649 |
| 9 | California | 4,659 | 34 | North Carolina | 3,641 |
| 10 | Illinois | 4,505 | 35 | Nebraska | 3,639 |
| 11 | Georgia | 4,414 | 36 | Florida | 3,607 |
| 12 | Ohio | 4,314 | 37 | North Dakota | 3,575 |
| 13 | Washington | 4,296 | 38 | Montana | 3,567 |
| 14 | Minnesota | 4,282 | 39 | Vermont | 3,512 |
| 15 | Oregon | 4,262 | 40 | Kentucky | 3,503 |
| 16 | Delaware | 4,230 | 41 | New Mexico | 3,484 |
| 17 | Michigan | 4,197 | 42 | West Virginia | 3,383 |
| 18 | Wyoming | 4,163 | 43 | Arkansas | 3,332 |
| 19 | Louisiana | 4,145 | 44 | New Hampshire | 3,263 |
| 20 | Colorado | 4,113 | 45 | Arizona | 3,191 |
| 21 | Pennsylvania | 4,039 | 46 | Idaho | 3,110 |
| 22 | Alabama | 4,015 | 47 | Mississippi | 3,019 |
| 23 | Oklahoma | 3,966 | 48 | South Dakota | 2,947 |
| 24 | Kansas | 3,965 | 49 | Alaska | 2,697 |
| 25 | Texas | 3,913 | 50 | Tennessee | 2,615 |
| | | | | District of Columbia | 5,508 |

Source: Families USA Foundation

"Health Spending: The Growing Threat to the Family Budget" (December 1991) (Reprinted with permission)

*This is an average paid directly by each family and does not include payments made by business. It is a subset of average annual family health payments. See beginning of this chapter for definitions.

# Projected Percent of Average Annual Family Health Payments Paid through General Taxes in 2000

## Projected National Average = 46.8% Paid through General Taxes*

| RANK | STATE | PERCENT | | RANK | STATE | PERCENT |
|---|---|---|---|---|---|---|
| 1 | New York | 56.3 | | 26 | Alabama | 45.1 |
| 2 | Maryland | 53.4 | | 26 | Nevada | 45.1 |
| 3 | Virginia | 53.0 | | 28 | Maine | 44.8 |
| 4 | Wyoming | 52.4 | | 29 | Texas | 44.5 |
| 5 | New Jersey | 51.9 | | 30 | Arizona | 44.2 |
| 6 | Washington | 51.4 | | 31 | Arkansas | 44.0 |
| 7 | South Carolina | 51.1 | | 31 | Vermont | 44.0 |
| 8 | Hawaii | 50.0 | | 33 | West Virginia | 43.9 |
| 8 | Massachusetts | 50.0 | | 34 | Florida | 43.8 |
| 10 | Montana | 49.9 | | 35 | Ohio | 43.6 |
| 11 | Georgia | 49.7 | | 36 | Indiana | 43.5 |
| 12 | New Mexico | 49.0 | | 37 | Minnesota | 43.4 |
| 13 | Kentucky | 48.8 | | 38 | Illinois | 43.2 |
| 14 | Louisiana | 48.7 | | 39 | Pennsylvania | 42.2 |
| 15 | Connecticut | 48.6 | | 40 | Michigan | 41.7 |
| 15 | Oregon | 48.6 | | 41 | Wisconsin | 41.2 |
| 17 | Colorado | 47.9 | | 42 | Iowa | 41.1 |
| 18 | California | 47.7 | | 43 | New Hampshire | 40.5 |
| 18 | Rhode Island | 47.7 | | 44 | Kansas | 40.3 |
| 20 | Oklahoma | 47.4 | | 45 | Nebraska | 38.9 |
| 21 | Delaware | 46.7 | | 46 | Missouri | 38.7 |
| 21 | North Carolina | 46.7 | | 46 | North Dakota | 38.7 |
| 23 | Utah | 46.3 | | 48 | Alaska | 37.1 |
| 24 | Idaho | 46.2 | | 49 | Tennessee | 35.3 |
| 25 | Mississippi | 45.8 | | 50 | South Dakota | 35.2 |

District of Columbia     58.3

Source: Families USA Foundation

*"Health Spending: The Growing Threat to the Family Budget"* (December 1991) (Reprinted with permission)

*This is a percent paid directly by each family and does not include payments made by business.  It is a percent of annual family health payments.  See beginning of this chapter for definitions.

# Health Care Payments Paid by Business in 1991

## National Total = $237,641,000,000*

| RANK | STATE | PAYMENTS | % | RANK | STATE | PAYMENTS | % |
|------|-------|----------|---|------|-------|----------|---|
| 1 | California | $35,109,000,000 | 14.77% | 26 | Kansas | $2,619,000,000 | 1.10% |
| 2 | New York | 20,117,000,000 | 8.47% | 27 | Iowa | 2,613,000,000 | 1.10% |
| 3 | Illinois | 13,248,000,000 | 5.57% | 28 | Alabama | 2,580,000,000 | 1.09% |
| 4 | Pennsylvania | 12,700,000,000 | 5.34% | 29 | Kentucky | 2,106,000,000 | 0.89% |
| 5 | Texas | 12,619,000,000 | 5.31% | 30 | Oklahoma | 1,875,000,000 | 0.79% |
| 6 | Ohio | 11,412,000,000 | 4.80% | 31 | South Carolina | 1,844,000,000 | 0.78% |
| 7 | Michigan | 10,609,000,000 | 4.46% | 32 | Nebraska | 1,589,000,000 | 0.67% |
| 8 | Florida | 9,506,000,000 | 4.00% | 33 | Nevada | 1,327,000,000 | 0.56% |
| 9 | New Jersey | 8,777,000,000 | 3.69% | 34 | Arkansas | 1,313,000,000 | 0.55% |
| 10 | Massachusetts | 8,236,000,000 | 3.47% | 35 | New Hampshire | 1,285,000,000 | 0.54% |
| 11 | Connecticut | 5,327,000,000 | 2.24% | 36 | West Virginia | 1,236,000,000 | 0.52% |
| 12 | Missouri | 5,172,000,000 | 2.18% | 37 | Utah | 1,234,000,000 | 0.52% |
| 13 | Minnesota | 5,144,000,000 | 2.16% | 38 | Mississippi | 1,228,000,000 | 0.52% |
| 14 | Wisconsin | 5,002,000,000 | 2.10% | 39 | Maine | 1,176,000,000 | 0.49% |
| 15 | Indiana | 4,705,000,000 | 1.98% | 40 | Hawaii | 1,173,000,000 | 0.49% |
| 16 | Washington | 4,619,000,000 | 1.94% | 41 | Rhode Island | 1,157,000,000 | 0.49% |
| 17 | Tennessee | 4,402,000,000 | 1.85% | 42 | New Mexico | 949,000,000 | 0.40% |
| 18 | Georgia | 4,361,000,000 | 1.84% | 43 | Alaska | 854,000,000 | 0.36% |
| 19 | North Carolina | 4,104,000,000 | 1.73% | 44 | Delaware | 667,000,000 | 0.28% |
| 20 | Virginia | 3,999,000,000 | 1.68% | 45 | Idaho | 664,000,000 | 0.28% |
| 21 | Maryland | 3,607,000,000 | 1.52% | 46 | North Dakota | 640,000,000 | 0.27% |
| 22 | Colorado | 3,284,000,000 | 1.38% | 47 | Montana | 617,000,000 | 0.26% |
| 23 | Louisiana | 3,206,000,000 | 1.35% | 48 | South Dakota | 596,000,000 | 0.25% |
| 24 | Arizona | 3,002,000,000 | 1.26% | 49 | Vermont | 483,000,000 | 0.20% |
| 25 | Oregon | 2,664,000,000 | 1.12% | 50 | Wyoming | 344,000,000 | 0.14% |
| | | | | | District of Columbia | 541,000,000 | 0.23% |

Source: Families USA Foundation

*"Health Spending: The Growing Threat to the Family Budget" (December 1991) (Reprinted with permission)*

*Reflects payments made directly by business and does not inlcude payments made by families. See beginning of this chapter for definitions.

# Percent of Health Care Payments Paid by Business in 1991

## National Rate = 34.3% Paid by Business*

| RANK | STATE | PERCENT | RANK | STATE | PERCENT |
|------|-------|---------|------|-------|---------|
| 1 | Alaska | 50.4 | 26 | Missouri | 35.0 |
| 2 | Connecticut | 41.8 | 27 | Nebraska | 34.9 |
| 3 | New Hampshire | 41.2 | 28 | Vermont | 34.8 |
| 4 | Tennessee | 38.2 | 29 | Idaho | 34.7 |
| 5 | Nevada | 38.0 | 29 | South Dakota | 34.7 |
| 6 | California | 37.9 | 31 | Iowa | 34.5 |
| 7 | Michigan | 37.7 | 32 | Wyoming | 34.3 |
| 8 | Massachusetts | 37.3 | 33 | Delaware | 33.2 |
| 9 | Maine | 37.0 | 34 | Indiana | 33.0 |
| 9 | Minnesota | 37.0 | 35 | Louisiana | 32.9 |
| 9 | Pennsylvania | 37.0 | 36 | West Virginia | 32.4 |
| 12 | Illinois | 36.6 | 37 | New York | 32.0 |
| 13 | Washington | 36.3 | 38 | New Mexico | 31.5 |
| 14 | Wisconsin | 36.2 | 39 | Texas | 30.5 |
| 15 | Hawaii | 36.1 | 40 | Kentucky | 29.3 |
| 15 | Ohio | 36.1 | 41 | Florida | 29.2 |
| 17 | New Jersey | 35.9 | 42 | North Carolina | 28.8 |
| 18 | Montana | 35.8 | 43 | Georgia | 28.2 |
| 18 | North Dakota | 35.8 | 44 | South Carolina | 27.7 |
| 20 | Rhode Island | 35.7 | 45 | Mississippi | 27.6 |
| 21 | Kansas | 35.6 | 46 | Alabama | 27.5 |
| 22 | Oregon | 35.5 | 46 | Maryland | 27.5 |
| 23 | Arizona | 35.4 | 48 | Arkansas | 27.2 |
| 23 | Utah | 35.4 | 49 | Oklahoma | 26.9 |
| 25 | Colorado | 35.2 | 50 | Virginia | 26.2 |

District of Columbia          29.0

Source: Families USA Foundation

"Health Spending: The Growing Threat to the Family Budget" (December 1991) (Reprinted with permission)

*As a percent of total health care payments by business and families. See beginning of this chapter for definitions.

# Total Business Health Care Payments per Employee in 1991

## National per Employee = $1,897*

| RANK | STATE | PER EMPLOYEE | | RANK | STATE | PER EMPLOYEE |
|---|---|---|---|---|---|---|
| 1 | Alaska | $3,310 | | 26 | Oregon | $1,767 |
| 2 | Connecticut | 2,958 | | 27 | Arizona | 1,762 |
| 3 | Massachusetts | 2,634 | | 28 | Iowa | 1,724 |
| 4 | California | 2,367 | | 29 | Indiana | 1,682 |
| 5 | New York | 2,344 | | 30 | Louisiana | 1,659 |
| 6 | Michigan | 2,335 | | 31 | South Dakota | 1,651 |
| 7 | Rhode Island | 2,255 | | 32 | West Virginia | 1,579 |
| 8 | Illinois | 2,197 | | 33 | Vermont | 1,553 |
| 9 | New Jersey | 2,184 | | 34 | Utah | 1,533 |
| 10 | Pennsylvania | 2,141 | | 35 | Montana | 1,531 |
| 11 | Minnesota | 2,116 | | 36 | Florida | 1,478 |
| 12 | Ohio | 2,098 | | 37 | Texas | 1,475 |
| 13 | Hawaii | 2,091 | | 38 | Wyoming | 1,433 |
| 14 | Nevada | 2,045 | | 39 | Maryland | 1,412 |
| 15 | New Hampshire | 2,027 | | 40 | Georgia | 1,377 |
| 16 | Kansas | 2,022 | | 41 | Alabama | 1,362 |
| 17 | North Dakota | 2,019 | | 42 | New Mexico | 1,327 |
| 18 | Wisconsin | 1,930 | | 43 | Idaho | 1,317 |
| 19 | Missouri | 1,923 | | 44 | Oklahoma | 1,236 |
| 20 | Colorado | 1,871 | | 45 | Virginia | 1,210 |
| 21 | Nebraska | 1,854 | | 46 | Kentucky | 1,208 |
| 22 | Washington | 1,849 | | 47 | North Carolina | 1,191 |
| 23 | Delaware | 1,832 | | 48 | Arkansas | 1,174 |
| 24 | Tennessee | 1,822 | | 49 | South Carolina | 1,057 |
| 25 | Maine | 1,818 | | 50 | Mississippi | 1,038 |

District of Columbia          1,918

*Source: Morgan Quitno Corporation*

*Calculated by the editors using total business health care payments data from Families USA Foundation and dividing by U.S. Department of Labor annual average civilian labor force for 1991.  See beginning of this chapter for definitions.*

# Average Business Annual Health Care Payment per Family in 1991

## National Average = $2,239 per Family*

| RANK | STATE | AVERAGE PAYMENT | | RANK | STATE | AVERAGE PAYMENT |
|------|-------|-----------------|--|------|-------|-----------------|
| 1 | Alaska | $3,910 | | 26 | Iowa | $2,122 |
| 2 | Connecticut | 3,890 | | 27 | Washington | 2,117 |
| 3 | Massachusetts | 3,164 | | 28 | South Dakota | 2,056 |
| 4 | Michigan | 2,768 | | 29 | Utah | 2,017 |
| 5 | Rhode Island | 2,733 | | 30 | Indiana | 1,957 |
| 6 | New Jersey | 2,722 | | 31 | Vermont | 1,949 |
| 7 | California | 2,708 | | 32 | Arizona | 1,882 |
| 8 | New Hampshire | 2,701 | | 33 | Louisiana | 1,868 |
| 9 | Illinois | 2,700 | | 34 | Wyoming | 1,810 |
| 10 | Minnesota | 2,684 | | 35 | Texas | 1,796 |
| 11 | New York | 2,625 | | 36 | Montana | 1,755 |
| 12 | Hawaii | 2,594 | | 37 | Maryland | 1,697 |
| 13 | Ohio | 2,531 | | 38 | West Virginia | 1,653 |
| 14 | Pennsylvania | 2,524 | | 39 | Georgia | 1,633 |
| 15 | Kansas | 2,477 | | 40 | Florida | 1,623 |
| 16 | Wisconsin | 2,406 | | 41 | Idaho | 1,594 |
| 17 | Nevada | 2,393 | | 42 | Virginia | 1,547 |
| 18 | Missouri | 2,353 | | 43 | Alabama | 1,541 |
| 19 | North Dakota | 2,335 | | 44 | New Mexico | 1,518 |
| 20 | Maine | 2,322 | | 45 | North Carolina | 1,471 |
| 21 | Nebraska | 2,286 | | 46 | Oklahoma | 1,393 |
| 22 | Delaware | 2,181 | | 47 | Kentucky | 1,329 |
| 23 | Tennessee | 2,152 | | 48 | South Carolina | 1,308 |
| 24 | Oregon | 2,146 | | 49 | Arkansas | 1,301 |
| 25 | Colorado | 2,141 | | 50 | Mississippi | 1,149 |
| | | | | | District of Columbia | 1,754 |

Source: Families USA Foundation

"Health Spending: The Growing Threat to the Family Budget" (December 1991) (Reprinted with permission)

*This is an average paid directly by business and does not include payments made directly by families. See beginning of this chapter for definitions.

# Health Care Payments Paid by Business in 1980

## National Total = $74,083,000,000*

| RANK | STATE | PAYMENTS | % | RANK | STATE | PAYMENTS | % |
|------|-------|----------|---|------|-------|----------|---|
| 1 | California | $8,971,000,000 | 12.11% | 26 | Kansas | $830,000,000 | 1.12% |
| 2 | New York | 6,717,000,000 | 9.07% | 27 | Kentucky | 827,000,000 | 1.12% |
| 3 | Illinois | 4,563,000,000 | 6.16% | 28 | Alabama | 826,000,000 | 1.11% |
| 4 | Ohio | 4,315,000,000 | 5.82% | 29 | Arizona | 800,000,000 | 1.08% |
| 5 | Pennsylvania | 4,291,000,000 | 5.79% | 30 | Oklahoma | 700,000,000 | 0.94% |
| 6 | Michigan | 3,832,000,000 | 5.17% | 31 | South Carolina | 550,000,000 | 0.74% |
| 7 | Texas | 3,810,000,000 | 5.14% | 32 | Nebraska | 525,000,000 | 0.71% |
| 8 | New Jersey | 2,623,000,000 | 3.54% | 33 | West Virginia | 458,000,000 | 0.62% |
| 9 | Massachusetts | 2,326,000,000 | 3.14% | 34 | Mississippi | 455,000,000 | 0.61% |
| 10 | Florida | 2,227,000,000 | 3.01% | 35 | Arkansas | 440,000,000 | 0.59% |
| 11 | Indiana | 1,787,000,000 | 2.41% | 36 | Rhode Island | 385,000,000 | 0.52% |
| 12 | Wisconsin | 1,764,000,000 | 2.38% | 37 | New Mexico | 329,000,000 | 0.44% |
| 13 | Minnesota | 1,640,000,000 | 2.21% | 38 | Utah | 324,000,000 | 0.44% |
| 14 | Missouri | 1,601,000,000 | 2.16% | 39 | New Hampshire | 319,000,000 | 0.43% |
| 15 | Connecticut | 1,519,000,000 | 2.05% | 40 | Maine | 310,000,000 | 0.42% |
| 16 | Tennessee | 1,472,000,000 | 1.99% | 41 | Nevada | 306,000,000 | 0.41% |
| 17 | Washington | 1,346,000,000 | 1.82% | 42 | Hawaii | 305,000,000 | 0.41% |
| 18 | Louisiana | 1,310,000,000 | 1.77% | 43 | North Dakota | 230,000,000 | 0.31% |
| 19 | Georgia | 1,245,000,000 | 1.68% | 44 | Idaho | 220,000,000 | 0.30% |
| 20 | North Carolina | 1,237,000,000 | 1.67% | 45 | Montana | 211,000,000 | 0.28% |
| 21 | Maryland | 1,180,000,000 | 1.59% | 46 | South Dakota | 193,000,000 | 0.26% |
| 22 | Virginia | 1,175,000,000 | 1.59% | 47 | Alaska | 185,000,000 | 0.25% |
| 23 | Iowa | 976,000,000 | 1.32% | 48 | Delaware | 164,000,000 | 0.22% |
| 24 | Colorado | 969,000,000 | 1.31% | 49 | Vermont | 136,000,000 | 0.18% |
| 25 | Oregon | 860,000,000 | 1.16% | 50 | Wyoming | 119,000,000 | 0.16% |
|  |  |  |  |  | District of Columbia | 180,000,000 | 0.24% |

Source: Families USA Foundation

*"Health Spending: The Growing Threat to the Family Budget"* (December 1991) (Reprinted with permission)

*Reflects payments made directly by business and does not inlcude payments made by families. See beginning of this chapter for definitions.

# Percent of Health Care Payments Paid by Business in 1980

## National Rate = 32.3%*

| RANK | STATE | PERCENT | RANK | STATE | PERCENT |
|------|-------|---------|------|-------|---------|
| 1 | Alaska | 43.2 | 25 | Montana | 33.0 |
| 2 | New Hampshire | 38.1 | 27 | Maine | 32.8 |
| 3 | Connecticut | 38.0 | 28 | Iowa | 32.6 |
| 4 | Michigan | 36.4 | 29 | Vermont | 32.5 |
| 5 | Tennessee | 36.3 | 30 | Hawaii | 32.3 |
| 6 | Ohio | 36.0 | 31 | Nebraska | 32.1 |
| 7 | New Mexico | 35.6 | 32 | Missouri | 31.8 |
| 8 | Rhode Island | 35.5 | 33 | New York | 31.1 |
| 9 | Nevada | 35.4 | 34 | South Dakota | 31.0 |
| 10 | California | 34.8 | 35 | Utah | 30.8 |
| 10 | Illinois | 34.8 | 35 | Wyoming | 30.8 |
| 10 | Oregon | 34.8 | 37 | Kentucky | 29.0 |
| 13 | Minnesota | 34.6 | 38 | West Virginia | 28.2 |
| 13 | Pennsylvania | 34.6 | 39 | Mississippi | 27.9 |
| 15 | Wisconsin | 34.5 | 40 | Texas | 27.8 |
| 16 | Arizona | 34.4 | 41 | Delaware | 27.6 |
| 17 | North Dakota | 33.8 | 42 | Maryland | 27.1 |
| 18 | New Jersey | 33.7 | 42 | North Carolina | 27.1 |
| 18 | Washington | 33.7 | 44 | Georgia | 27.0 |
| 20 | Idaho | 33.4 | 45 | Oklahoma | 26.1 |
| 21 | Colorado | 33.2 | 46 | Arkansas | 26.0 |
| 21 | Kansas | 33.2 | 47 | Florida | 25.9 |
| 21 | Massachusetts | 33.2 | 48 | South Carolina | 25.5 |
| 24 | Indiana | 33.1 | 49 | Alabama | 25.4 |
| 25 | Louisiana | 33.0 | 50 | Virginia | 24.8 |
| | | | | District of Columbia | 25.4 |

Source: Families USA Foundation

"Health Spending: The Growing Threat to the Family Budget" (December 1991) (Reprinted with permission)

*As a percent of total health care payments by business and families. See beginning of this chapter for definitions.

# Projected Health Care Payments Paid by Business in 2000

## Projected National Total = $511,439,000,000*

| RANK | STATE | PAYMENTS | % | RANK | STATE | PAYMENTS | % |
|---|---|---|---|---|---|---|---|
| 1 | California | $81,334,000,000 | 15.90% | 26 | Oregon | $5,571,000,000 | 1.09% |
| 2 | New York | 40,006,000,000 | 7.82% | 27 | Kansas | 5,259,000,000 | 1.03% |
| 3 | Texas | 29,838,000,000 | 5.83% | 28 | Iowa | 4,718,000,000 | 0.92% |
| 4 | Illinois | 26,082,000,000 | 5.10% | 29 | Kentucky | 4,346,000,000 | 0.85% |
| 5 | Pennsylvania | 24,576,000,000 | 4.81% | 30 | South Carolina | 4,130,000,000 | 0.81% |
| 6 | Florida | 23,760,000,000 | 4.65% | 31 | Oklahoma | 3,942,000,000 | 0.77% |
| 7 | Ohio | 22,292,000,000 | 4.36% | 32 | Nevada | 3,235,000,000 | 0.63% |
| 8 | Michigan | 21,219,000,000 | 4.15% | 33 | New Hampshire | 3,193,000,000 | 0.62% |
| 9 | New Jersey | 19,275,000,000 | 3.77% | 34 | Nebraska | 3,047,000,000 | 0.60% |
| 10 | Massachusetts | 17,070,000,000 | 3.34% | 35 | Utah | 2,802,000,000 | 0.55% |
| 11 | Connecticut | 11,604,000,000 | 2.27% | 36 | Mississippi | 2,774,000,000 | 0.54% |
| 12 | Georgia | 10,753,000,000 | 2.10% | 37 | Arkansas | 2,770,000,000 | 0.54% |
| 13 | Missouri | 10,682,000,000 | 2.09% | 38 | Hawaii | 2,716,000,000 | 0.53% |
| 14 | Minnesota | 10,308,000,000 | 2.02% | 39 | Maine | 2,516,000,000 | 0.49% |
| 15 | Tennessee | 10,085,000,000 | 1.97% | 40 | Rhode Island | 2,452,000,000 | 0.48% |
| 16 | Washington | 9,994,000,000 | 1.95% | 41 | New Mexico | 2,445,000,000 | 0.48% |
| 17 | Wisconsin | 9,741,000,000 | 1.90% | 42 | West Virginia | 2,432,000,000 | 0.48% |
| 18 | North Carolina | 9,346,000,000 | 1.83% | 43 | Alaska | 2,163,000,000 | 0.42% |
| 19 | Indiana | 9,219,000,000 | 1.80% | 44 | Idaho | 1,376,000,000 | 0.27% |
| 20 | Virginia | 8,989,000,000 | 1.76% | 45 | Delaware | 1,325,000,000 | 0.26% |
| 21 | Maryland | 8,090,000,000 | 1.58% | 46 | Montana | 1,257,000,000 | 0.25% |
| 22 | Arizona | 7,662,000,000 | 1.50% | 47 | North Dakota | 1,225,000,000 | 0.24% |
| 23 | Colorado | 7,414,000,000 | 1.45% | 48 | South Dakota | 1,185,000,000 | 0.23% |
| 24 | Louisiana | 6,907,000,000 | 1.35% | 49 | Vermont | 1,012,000,000 | 0.20% |
| 25 | Alabama | 5,587,000,000 | 1.09% | 50 | Wyoming | 708,000,000 | 0.14% |
| | | | | | District of Columbia | 1,007,000,000 | 0.20% |

Source: Families USA Foundation

*"Health Spending: The Growing Threat to the Family Budget"* (December 1991) (Reprinted with permission)

*Reflects payments made directly by business and does not inlcude payments made by families. See beginning of this chapter for definitions.

# Projected Percent of Health Care Payments Paid by Business in 2000

## Projected National Rate = 32.4%*

| RANK | STATE | PERCENT | | RANK | STATE | PERCENT |
|------|-------|---------|---|------|-------|---------|
| 1 | Alaska | 51.9 | | 26 | Colorado | 33.2 |
| 2 | New Hampshire | 40.9 | | 26 | Hawaii | 33.2 |
| 3 | Connecticut | 40.0 | | 28 | Nebraska | 33.0 |
| 4 | Tennessee | 38.5 | | 28 | Vermont | 33.0 |
| 5 | Nevada | 36.7 | | 30 | Idaho | 32.8 |
| 6 | California | 36.2 | | 31 | Iowa | 32.4 |
| 7 | Michigan | 35.9 | | 32 | Wyoming | 32.3 |
| 8 | Maine | 35.6 | | 33 | Louisiana | 32.1 |
| 9 | Massachusetts | 35.1 | | 34 | West Virginia | 31.7 |
| 10 | Minnesota | 34.9 | | 35 | Indiana | 30.9 |
| 10 | Pennsylvania | 34.9 | | 36 | Delaware | 30.5 |
| 12 | Illinois | 34.4 | | 37 | New Mexico | 30.3 |
| 12 | North Dakota | 34.4 | | 38 | New York | 29.5 |
| 12 | Washington | 34.4 | | 39 | Texas | 29.4 |
| 15 | Wisconsin | 34.1 | | 40 | Florida | 28.5 |
| 16 | Montana | 34.0 | | 41 | Kentucky | 27.9 |
| 16 | Ohio | 34.0 | | 42 | North Carolina | 27.3 |
| 16 | Rhode Island | 34.0 | | 43 | Georgia | 27.0 |
| 19 | Arizona | 33.9 | | 44 | Mississippi | 26.9 |
| 20 | Kansas | 33.8 | | 45 | Alabama | 26.1 |
| 20 | New Jersey | 33.8 | | 45 | South Carolina | 26.1 |
| 22 | Utah | 33.6 | | 47 | Arkansas | 25.8 |
| 23 | Oregon | 33.5 | | 48 | Maryland | 25.6 |
| 24 | Missouri | 33.3 | | 49 | Oklahoma | 25.5 |
| 24 | South Dakota | 33.3 | | 50 | Virginia | 24.4 |

District of Columbia        25.5

Source: Families USA Foundation

"Health Spending: The Growing Threat to the Family Budget" (December 1991) (Reprinted with permission)

*As a percent of total health care payments by business and families. See beginning of this chapter for definitions.

# Health Care Payments Paid by Business for Insurance in 1991

## National Total = $131,360,000,000*

| RANK | STATE | PAYMENTS | % | RANK | STATE | PAYMENTS | % |
|---|---|---|---|---|---|---|---|
| 1 | California | $20,382,000,000 | 15.52% | 26 | Oregon | $1,487,000,000 | 1.13% |
| 2 | New York | 10,918,000,000 | 8.31% | 27 | Alabama | 1,332,000,000 | 1.01% |
| 3 | Illinois | 8,221,000,000 | 6.26% | 28 | Louisiana | 1,200,000,000 | 0.91% |
| 4 | Pennsylvania | 7,527,000,000 | 5.73% | 29 | Nebraska | 1,045,000,000 | 0.80% |
| 5 | Ohio | 6,762,000,000 | 5.15% | 30 | Kentucky | 940,000,000 | 0.72% |
| 6 | Michigan | 6,203,000,000 | 4.72% | 31 | South Carolina | 863,000,000 | 0.66% |
| 7 | Texas | 5,994,000,000 | 4.56% | 32 | Oklahoma | 861,000,000 | 0.66% |
| 8 | Massachusetts | 5,039,000,000 | 3.84% | 33 | Nevada | 843,000,000 | 0.64% |
| 9 | New Jersey | 4,656,000,000 | 3.54% | 34 | Hawaii | 744,000,000 | 0.57% |
| 10 | Florida | 4,630,000,000 | 3.52% | 35 | Utah | 735,000,000 | 0.56% |
| 11 | Missouri | 3,435,000,000 | 2.61% | 36 | Rhode Island | 691,000,000 | 0.53% |
| 12 | Minnesota | 3,205,000,000 | 2.44% | 37 | Maine | 655,000,000 | 0.50% |
| 13 | Wisconsin | 3,180,000,000 | 2.42% | 38 | New Hampshire | 632,000,000 | 0.48% |
| 14 | Indiana | 3,058,000,000 | 2.33% | 39 | Arkansas | 580,000,000 | 0.44% |
| 15 | Connecticut | 2,699,000,000 | 2.05% | 40 | Mississippi | 491,000,000 | 0.37% |
| 16 | Washington | 2,483,000,000 | 1.89% | 41 | West Virginia | 453,000,000 | 0.34% |
| 17 | Georgia | 2,016,000,000 | 1.53% | 42 | New Mexico | 445,000,000 | 0.34% |
| 18 | Colorado | 1,986,000,000 | 1.51% | 43 | South Dakota | 392,000,000 | 0.30% |
| 19 | North Carolina | 1,976,000,000 | 1.50% | 44 | North Dakota | 391,000,000 | 0.30% |
| 20 | Virginia | 1,957,000,000 | 1.49% | 45 | Idaho | 363,000,000 | 0.28% |
| 21 | Arizona | 1,830,000,000 | 1.39% | 46 | Montana | 294,000,000 | 0.22% |
| 22 | Maryland | 1,720,000,000 | 1.31% | 47 | Vermont | 293,000,000 | 0.22% |
| 23 | Kansas | 1,706,000,000 | 1.30% | 48 | Alaska | 283,000,000 | 0.22% |
| 24 | Iowa | 1,683,000,000 | 1.28% | 49 | Delaware | 264,000,000 | 0.20% |
| 25 | Tennessee | 1,596,000,000 | 1.21% | 50 | Wyoming | 171,000,000 | 0.13% |
| | | | | | District of Columbia | 49,000,000 | 0.04% |

*Source: Families USA Foundation*

*"Health Spending: The Growing Threat to the Family Budget" (December 1991) (Reprinted with permission)*

*This is a total paid directly by business and does not include payments made by families. It is a subset of annual business health care payments. See beginning of this chapter for definitions.*

# Percent of Health Care Payments Paid by Business for Insurance in 1991

## National Rate = 55.3% *

| RANK | STATE | PERCENT | RANK | STATE | PERCENT |
|------|-------|---------|------|-------|---------|
| 1 | Missouri | 66.4 | 26 | New York | 54.3 |
| 2 | South Dakota | 65.9 | 27 | Washington | 53.8 |
| 3 | Nebraska | 65.8 | 28 | New Jersey | 53.0 |
| 4 | Kansas | 65.1 | 29 | Alabama | 51.6 |
| 5 | Indiana | 65.0 | 30 | Connecticut | 50.7 |
| 6 | Iowa | 64.4 | 31 | Wyoming | 49.6 |
| 7 | Wisconsin | 63.6 | 32 | New Hampshire | 49.2 |
| 8 | Nevada | 63.5 | 33 | Virginia | 48.9 |
| 9 | Hawaii | 63.4 | 34 | Florida | 48.7 |
| 10 | Minnesota | 62.3 | 35 | North Carolina | 48.2 |
| 11 | Illinois | 62.1 | 36 | Maryland | 47.7 |
| 12 | Massachusetts | 61.2 | 36 | Montana | 47.7 |
| 12 | North Dakota | 61.2 | 38 | Texas | 47.5 |
| 14 | Arizona | 61.0 | 39 | New Mexico | 46.9 |
| 15 | Vermont | 60.7 | 40 | South Carolina | 46.8 |
| 16 | Colorado | 60.5 | 41 | Georgia | 46.2 |
| 17 | Rhode Island | 59.8 | 42 | Oklahoma | 45.9 |
| 18 | Utah | 59.6 | 43 | Kentucky | 44.6 |
| 19 | Ohio | 59.3 | 44 | Arkansas | 44.2 |
| 19 | Pennsylvania | 59.3 | 45 | Mississippi | 40.0 |
| 21 | Michigan | 58.5 | 46 | Delaware | 39.7 |
| 22 | California | 58.1 | 47 | Louisiana | 37.4 |
| 23 | Oregon | 55.8 | 48 | West Virginia | 36.6 |
| 24 | Maine | 55.7 | 49 | Tennessee | 36.3 |
| 25 | Idaho | 54.6 | 50 | Alaska | 33.1 |
| | | | | District of Columbia | 9.1 |

Source: Families USA Foundation

"Health Spending: The Growing Threat to the Family Budget" (December 1991) (Reprinted with permission)

*This is a percent paid directly by business and does not include payments made by families. It is a percent of annual business health care payments.
See beginning of this chapter for definitions.

# Health Care Payments Paid by Business for Insurance in 1980

## National Total = $43,268,000,000*

| RANK | STATE | PAYMENTS | % | RANK | STATE | PAYMENTS | % |
|------|-------|----------|---|------|-------|----------|---|
| 1 | California | $4,887,000,000 | 11.29% | 26 | Kentucky | $467,000,000 | 1.08% |
| 2 | New York | 4,084,000,000 | 9.44% | 27 | Arizona | 455,000,000 | 1.05% |
| 3 | Illinois | 2,911,000,000 | 6.73% | 28 | Oregon | 451,000,000 | 1.04% |
| 4 | Ohio | 2,747,000,000 | 6.35% | 29 | Alabama | 438,000,000 | 1.01% |
| 5 | Pennsylvania | 2,715,000,000 | 6.27% | 30 | Nebraska | 358,000,000 | 0.83% |
| 6 | Michigan | 2,353,000,000 | 5.44% | 31 | Oklahoma | 341,000,000 | 0.79% |
| 7 | Texas | 1,930,000,000 | 4.46% | 32 | Rhode Island | 254,000,000 | 0.59% |
| 8 | New Jersey | 1,604,000,000 | 3.71% | 33 | West Virginia | 239,000,000 | 0.55% |
| 9 | Massachusetts | 1,537,000,000 | 3.55% | 34 | South Carolina | 238,000,000 | 0.55% |
| 10 | Indiana | 1,233,000,000 | 2.85% | 35 | Mississippi | 234,000,000 | 0.54% |
| 11 | Wisconsin | 1,222,000,000 | 2.82% | 36 | Arkansas | 217,000,000 | 0.50% |
| 12 | Missouri | 1,115,000,000 | 2.58% | 37 | Utah | 204,000,000 | 0.47% |
| 13 | Florida | 1,108,000,000 | 2.56% | 38 | Maine | 185,000,000 | 0.43% |
| 14 | Minnesota | 1,035,000,000 | 2.39% | 39 | Hawaii | 181,000,000 | 0.42% |
| 15 | Connecticut | 866,000,000 | 2.00% | 40 | Nevada | 177,000,000 | 0.41% |
| 16 | Maryland | 704,000,000 | 1.63% | 41 | New Hampshire | 172,000,000 | 0.40% |
| 17 | Washington | 682,000,000 | 1.58% | 42 | North Dakota | 149,000,000 | 0.34% |
| 18 | North Carolina | 680,000,000 | 1.57% | 43 | New Mexico | 132,000,000 | 0.31% |
| 19 | Georgia | 669,000,000 | 1.55% | 44 | South Dakota | 131,000,000 | 0.30% |
| 20 | Iowa | 657,000,000 | 1.52% | 45 | Idaho | 117,000,000 | 0.27% |
| 21 | Virginia | 641,000,000 | 1.48% | 46 | Montana | 111,000,000 | 0.26% |
| 22 | Tennessee | 626,000,000 | 1.45% | 47 | Vermont | 89,000,000 | 0.21% |
| 23 | Colorado | 610,000,000 | 1.41% | 48 | Delaware | 88,000,000 | 0.20% |
| 24 | Louisiana | 539,000,000 | 1.25% | 49 | Alaska | 66,000,000 | 0.15% |
| 25 | Kansas | 532,000,000 | 1.23% | 50 | Wyoming | 64,000,000 | 0.15% |
|  |  |  |  |  | District of Columbia | 20,000,000 | 0.05% |

Source: Families USA Foundation

"Health Spending: The Growing Threat to the Family Budget" (December 1991) (Reprinted with permission)

*This is a total paid directly by business and does not include payments made by families. It is a subset of annual business health care payments. See beginning of this chapter for definitions.

# Percent of Health Care Payments Paid by Business for Insurance in 1980

## National Rate = 58.4%*

| RANK | STATE | PERCENT | | RANK | STATE | PERCENT |
|------|-------|---------|---|------|-------|---------|
| 1 | Missouri | 69.6 | | 26 | Arizona | 56.9 |
| 2 | Wisconsin | 69.3 | | 27 | Kentucky | 56.5 |
| 3 | Indiana | 69.0 | | 28 | North Carolina | 55.0 |
| 4 | Nebraska | 68.3 | | 29 | California | 54.5 |
| 5 | South Dakota | 67.8 | | 29 | Virginia | 54.5 |
| 6 | Iowa | 67.3 | | 31 | New Hampshire | 54.0 |
| 7 | Massachusetts | 66.0 | | 31 | Wyoming | 54.0 |
| 8 | Rhode Island | 65.9 | | 33 | Georgia | 53.8 |
| 9 | Vermont | 65.7 | | 34 | Delaware | 53.4 |
| 10 | North Dakota | 65.0 | | 35 | Idaho | 53.2 |
| 11 | Kansas | 64.1 | | 36 | Alabama | 53.0 |
| 12 | Illinois | 63.8 | | 37 | Montana | 52.7 |
| 13 | Ohio | 63.7 | | 38 | Oregon | 52.5 |
| 14 | Pennsylvania | 63.3 | | 39 | West Virginia | 52.2 |
| 15 | Minnesota | 63.1 | | 40 | Mississippi | 51.4 |
| 15 | Utah | 63.1 | | 41 | Washington | 50.7 |
| 17 | Colorado | 62.9 | | 42 | Texas | 50.6 |
| 18 | Michigan | 61.4 | | 43 | Florida | 49.7 |
| 19 | New Jersey | 61.1 | | 44 | Arkansas | 49.5 |
| 20 | New York | 60.8 | | 45 | Oklahoma | 48.7 |
| 21 | Maine | 59.7 | | 46 | South Carolina | 43.3 |
| 21 | Maryland | 59.7 | | 47 | Tennessee | 42.5 |
| 23 | Hawaii | 59.2 | | 48 | Louisiana | 41.2 |
| 24 | Nevada | 57.9 | | 49 | New Mexico | 40.0 |
| 25 | Connecticut | 57.0 | | 50 | Alaska | 36.0 |

District of Columbia     11.2

Source: Families USA Foundation

"Health Spending: The Growing Threat to the Family Budget" (December 1991) (Reprinted with permission)

*This is a percent paid directly by business and does not include payments made by families. It is a percent of annual business health care payments.
See beginning of this chapter for definitions.

# Projected Health Care Payments Paid by Business for Insurance in 2000

## Projected National Total = $271,613,000,000*

| RANK | STATE | PAYMENTS | % | RANK | STATE | PAYMENTS | % |
|---|---|---|---|---|---|---|---|
| 1 | California | $45,634,000,000 | 16.80% | 26 | Iowa | $2,910,000,000 | 1.07% |
| 2 | New York | 21,076,000,000 | 7.76% | 27 | Alabama | 2,737,000,000 | 1.01% |
| 3 | Illinois | 15,732,000,000 | 5.79% | 28 | Louisiana | 2,333,000,000 | 0.86% |
| 4 | Pennsylvania | 13,976,000,000 | 5.15% | 29 | Nevada | 1,999,000,000 | 0.74% |
| 5 | Texas | 13,598,000,000 | 5.01% | 30 | Nebraska | 1,946,000,000 | 0.72% |
| 6 | Ohio | 12,743,000,000 | 4.69% | 31 | South Carolina | 1,854,000,000 | 0.68% |
| 7 | Michigan | 11,960,000,000 | 4.40% | 32 | Kentucky | 1,802,000,000 | 0.66% |
| 8 | Florida | 11,090,000,000 | 4.08% | 33 | Hawaii | 1,720,000,000 | 0.63% |
| 9 | Massachusetts | 10,107,000,000 | 3.72% | 34 | Oklahoma | 1,718,000,000 | 0.63% |
| 10 | New Jersey | 9,940,000,000 | 3.66% | 35 | Utah | 1,613,000,000 | 0.59% |
| 11 | Missouri | 6,942,000,000 | 2.56% | 36 | New Hampshire | 1,508,000,000 | 0.56% |
| 12 | Minnesota | 6,425,000,000 | 2.37% | 37 | Rhode Island | 1,422,000,000 | 0.52% |
| 13 | Wisconsin | 6,039,000,000 | 2.22% | 38 | Maine | 1,339,000,000 | 0.49% |
| 14 | Indiana | 5,820,000,000 | 2.14% | 39 | Arkansas | 1,179,000,000 | 0.43% |
| 15 | Connecticut | 5,564,000,000 | 2.05% | 40 | New Mexico | 1,108,000,000 | 0.41% |
| 16 | Washington | 5,122,000,000 | 1.89% | 41 | Mississippi | 1,030,000,000 | 0.38% |
| 17 | Georgia | 4,845,000,000 | 1.78% | 42 | West Virginia | 802,000,000 | 0.30% |
| 18 | Arizona | 4,609,000,000 | 1.70% | 43 | South Dakota | 757,000,000 | 0.28% |
| 19 | North Carolina | 4,362,000,000 | 1.61% | 44 | Idaho | 722,000,000 | 0.27% |
| 20 | Colorado | 4,360,000,000 | 1.61% | 45 | North Dakota | 708,000,000 | 0.26% |
| 21 | Virginia | 4,257,000,000 | 1.57% | 46 | Alaska | 698,000,000 | 0.26% |
| 22 | Maryland | 3,748,000,000 | 1.38% | 47 | Vermont | 601,000,000 | 0.22% |
| 23 | Kansas | 3,323,000,000 | 1.22% | 48 | Delaware | 562,000,000 | 0.21% |
| 24 | Tennessee | 3,288,000,000 | 1.21% | 49 | Montana | 559,000,000 | 0.21% |
| 25 | Oregon | 2,998,000,000 | 1.10% | 50 | Wyoming | 331,000,000 | 0.12% |
| | | | | | District of Columbia | 99,000,000 | 0.04% |

*Source: Families USA Foundation*

*"Health Spending: The Growing Threat to the Family Budget" (December 1991) (Reprinted with permission)*

*This is a total paid directly by business and does not include payments made by families. It is a subset of annual business health care payments. See beginning of this chapter for definitions.*

# Projected Percent of Health Care Payments Paid by Business for Insurance in 2000

## Projected National Percent = 53.1%*

| RANK | STATE | PERCENT | RANK | STATE | PERCENT |
|------|-------|---------|------|-------|---------|
| 1 | Missouri | 65.0 | 26 | Idaho | 52.5 |
| 2 | Nebraska | 63.9 | 27 | New Jersey | 51.6 |
| 2 | South Dakota | 63.9 | 28 | Washington | 51.2 |
| 4 | Hawaii | 63.3 | 29 | Alabama | 49.0 |
| 5 | Kansas | 63.2 | 30 | Connecticut | 48.0 |
| 6 | Indiana | 63.1 | 31 | Virginia | 47.4 |
| 7 | Minnesota | 62.3 | 32 | New Hampshire | 47.2 |
| 8 | Wisconsin | 62.0 | 33 | Wyoming | 46.8 |
| 9 | Nevada | 61.8 | 34 | Florida | 46.7 |
| 10 | Iowa | 61.7 | 34 | North Carolina | 46.7 |
| 11 | Illinois | 60.3 | 36 | Maryland | 46.3 |
| 12 | Arizona | 60.2 | 37 | Texas | 45.6 |
| 13 | Vermont | 59.3 | 38 | New Mexico | 45.3 |
| 14 | Massachusetts | 59.2 | 39 | Georgia | 45.1 |
| 15 | Colorado | 58.8 | 40 | South Carolina | 44.9 |
| 16 | Rhode Island | 58.0 | 41 | Montana | 44.4 |
| 17 | North Dakota | 57.8 | 42 | Oklahoma | 43.6 |
| 18 | Utah | 57.6 | 43 | Arkansas | 42.6 |
| 19 | Ohio | 57.2 | 44 | Delaware | 42.4 |
| 20 | Pennsylvania | 56.9 | 45 | Kentucky | 41.5 |
| 21 | Michigan | 56.4 | 46 | Mississippi | 37.1 |
| 22 | California | 56.1 | 47 | Louisiana | 33.8 |
| 23 | Oregon | 53.8 | 48 | West Virginia | 33.0 |
| 24 | Maine | 53.2 | 49 | Tennessee | 32.6 |
| 25 | New York | 52.7 | 50 | Alaska | 32.3 |
| | | | | District of Columbia | 9.8 |

Source: Families USA Foundation

"Health Spending: The Growing Threat to the Family Budget" (December 1991) (Reprinted with permission)

*This is a percent paid directly by business and does not include payments made by families. It is a percent of annual business health care payments. See beginning of this chapter for definitions.

# Health Care Payments Paid by Business for Medicare Payroll Tax in 1991

## National Total = $39,204,000,000*

| RANK | STATE | PAYMENTS | % | RANK | STATE | PAYMENTS | % |
|------|-------|----------|---|------|-------|----------|---|
| 1 | California | $4,621,000,000 | 11.79% | 26 | Oregon | $410,000,000 | 1.05% |
| 2 | New York | 4,329,000,000 | 11.04% | 27 | Iowa | 394,000,000 | 1.00% |
| 3 | Texas | 2,215,000,000 | 5.65% | 28 | Oklahoma | 384,000,000 | 0.98% |
| 4 | Illinois | 2,066,000,000 | 5.27% | 29 | South Carolina | 383,000,000 | 0.98% |
| 5 | Pennsylvania | 1,967,000,000 | 5.02% | 30 | Kentucky | 380,000,000 | 0.97% |
| 6 | Ohio | 1,789,000,000 | 4.56% | 31 | Kansas | 359,000,000 | 0.92% |
| 7 | Michigan | 1,768,000,000 | 4.51% | 32 | Arkansas | 313,000,000 | 0.80% |
| 8 | New Jersey | 1,627,000,000 | 4.15% | 33 | Nebraska | 245,000,000 | 0.62% |
| 9 | Florida | 1,522,000,000 | 3.88% | 34 | Mississippi | 222,000,000 | 0.57% |
| 10 | Massachusetts | 1,169,000,000 | 2.98% | 35 | Delaware | 216,000,000 | 0.55% |
| 11 | Georgia | 907,000,000 | 2.31% | 36 | Utah | 183,000,000 | 0.47% |
| 12 | North Carolina | 884,000,000 | 2.25% | 37 | West Virginia | 181,000,000 | 0.46% |
| 13 | Virginia | 841,000,000 | 2.15% | 38 | New Hampshire | 172,000,000 | 0.44% |
| 14 | Minnesota | 818,000,000 | 2.09% | 39 | Rhode Island | 171,000,000 | 0.44% |
| 15 | Wisconsin | 817,000,000 | 2.08% | 40 | New Mexico | 163,000,000 | 0.42% |
| 16 | Missouri | 802,000,000 | 2.05% | 41 | Hawaii | 154,000,000 | 0.39% |
| 17 | Maryland | 793,000,000 | 2.02% | 42 | Nevada | 140,000,000 | 0.36% |
| 18 | Indiana | 782,000,000 | 1.99% | 43 | Maine | 136,000,000 | 0.35% |
| 19 | Connecticut | 777,000,000 | 1.98% | 44 | Alaska | 119,000,000 | 0.30% |
| 20 | Washington | 674,000,000 | 1.72% | 45 | Idaho | 115,000,000 | 0.29% |
| 21 | Tennessee | 658,000,000 | 1.68% | 46 | Montana | 87,000,000 | 0.22% |
| 22 | Louisiana | 497,000,000 | 1.27% | 47 | North Dakota | 80,000,000 | 0.20% |
| 23 | Colorado | 479,000,000 | 1.22% | 48 | Vermont | 78,000,000 | 0.20% |
| 24 | Alabama | 459,000,000 | 1.17% | 49 | South Dakota | 74,000,000 | 0.19% |
| 25 | Arizona | 447,000,000 | 1.14% | 50 | Wyoming | 58,000,000 | 0.15% |
| | | | | | District of Columbia | 278,000,000 | 0.71% |

Source: Families USA Foundation

"Health Spending: The Growing Threat to the Family Budget" (December 1991) (Reprinted with permission)

*This is a total paid directly by business and does not include payments made by families. It is a subset of annual business health care payments. See beginning of this chapter for definitions.

# Percent of Health Care Payments Paid by Business for Medicare Payroll Tax in 1991

## National Rate = 16.5%*

| RANK | STATE | PERCENT | | RANK | STATE | PERCENT |
|------|-------|---------|--|------|-------|---------|
| 1 | Delaware | 32.4 | | 26 | Louisiana | 15.5 |
| 2 | Arkansas | 23.8 | | 26 | Missouri | 15.5 |
| 3 | Maryland | 22.0 | | 26 | Pennsylvania | 15.5 |
| 4 | North Carolina | 21.6 | | 29 | Nebraska | 15.4 |
| 5 | New York | 21.5 | | 29 | Oregon | 15.4 |
| 6 | Virginia | 21.0 | | 31 | Iowa | 15.1 |
| 7 | Georgia | 20.8 | | 32 | Tennessee | 15.0 |
| 7 | South Carolina | 20.8 | | 33 | Arizona | 14.9 |
| 9 | Oklahoma | 20.5 | | 34 | Rhode Island | 14.8 |
| 10 | New Jersey | 18.5 | | 34 | Utah | 14.8 |
| 11 | Mississippi | 18.1 | | 36 | Colorado | 14.6 |
| 12 | Kentucky | 18.0 | | 36 | Connecticut | 14.6 |
| 13 | Alabama | 17.8 | | 36 | Washington | 14.6 |
| 14 | Texas | 17.6 | | 36 | West Virginia | 14.6 |
| 15 | Idaho | 17.4 | | 40 | Massachusetts | 14.2 |
| 16 | New Mexico | 17.1 | | 41 | Montana | 14.1 |
| 17 | Wyoming | 16.9 | | 42 | Alaska | 14.0 |
| 18 | Michigan | 16.7 | | 43 | Kansas | 13.7 |
| 19 | Indiana | 16.6 | | 44 | New Hampshire | 13.4 |
| 20 | Wisconsin | 16.3 | | 45 | California | 13.2 |
| 21 | Vermont | 16.2 | | 46 | Hawaii | 13.1 |
| 22 | Florida | 16.0 | | 47 | North Dakota | 12.5 |
| 23 | Minnesota | 15.9 | | 48 | South Dakota | 12.4 |
| 24 | Ohio | 15.7 | | 49 | Maine | 11.5 |
| 25 | Illinois | 15.6 | | 50 | Nevada | 10.5 |

District of Columbia     51.4

Source: Families USA Foundation

*"Health Spending: The Growing Threat to the Family Budget" (December 1991) (Reprinted with permission)*

*This is a percent paid directly by business and does not include payments made by families. It is a percent of annual business health care payments.
See beginning of this chapter for definitions.

268

# Health Care Payments Paid by Business for Medicare Payroll Tax in 1980

## National Total = $11,745,000,000*

| RANK | STATE | PAYMENTS | % | RANK | STATE | PAYMENTS | % |
|------|-------|----------|---|------|-------|----------|---|
| 1 | California | $1,259,000,000 | 10.72% | 26 | Iowa | $142,000,000 | 1.21% |
| 2 | New York | 1,207,000,000 | 10.28% | 27 | Oregon | 134,000,000 | 1.14% |
| 3 | Texas | 735,000,000 | 6.26% | 28 | Kentucky | 132,000,000 | 1.12% |
| 4 | Illinois | 687,000,000 | 5.85% | 29 | South Carolina | 123,000,000 | 1.05% |
| 5 | Pennsylvania | 641,000,000 | 5.46% | 30 | Arizona | 120,000,000 | 1.02% |
| 6 | Ohio | 610,000,000 | 5.19% | 31 | Kansas | 115,000,000 | 0.98% |
| 7 | Michigan | 579,000,000 | 4.93% | 32 | Arkansas | 85,000,000 | 0.72% |
| 8 | New Jersey | 417,000,000 | 3.55% | 33 | Nebraska | 78,000,000 | 0.66% |
| 9 | Florida | 402,000,000 | 3.42% | 34 | Mississippi | 76,000,000 | 0.65% |
| 10 | Massachusetts | 305,000,000 | 2.60% | 35 | West Virginia | 75,000,000 | 0.64% |
| 11 | Indiana | 288,000,000 | 2.45% | 36 | New Mexico | 51,000,000 | 0.43% |
| 12 | Wisconsin | 265,000,000 | 2.26% | 37 | Utah | 50,000,000 | 0.43% |
| 13 | North Carolina | 258,000,000 | 2.20% | 38 | Rhode Island | 49,000,000 | 0.42% |
| 14 | Minnesota | 257,000,000 | 2.19% | 39 | Hawaii | 45,000,000 | 0.38% |
| 15 | Missouri | 254,000,000 | 2.16% | 40 | Idaho | 43,000,000 | 0.37% |
| 16 | Georgia | 232,000,000 | 1.98% | 41 | New Hampshire | 43,000,000 | 0.37% |
| 17 | Virginia | 221,000,000 | 1.88% | 42 | Delaware | 41,000,000 | 0.35% |
| 18 | Tennessee | 216,000,000 | 1.84% | 43 | Maine | 41,000,000 | 0.35% |
| 19 | Maryland | 205,000,000 | 1.75% | 44 | Nevada | 38,000,000 | 0.32% |
| 20 | Washington | 202,000,000 | 1.72% | 45 | Montana | 33,000,000 | 0.28% |
| 21 | Connecticut | 198,000,000 | 1.69% | 46 | North Dakota | 28,000,000 | 0.24% |
| 22 | Louisiana | 185,000,000 | 1.58% | 47 | South Dakota | 28,000,000 | 0.24% |
| 23 | Alabama | 152,000,000 | 1.29% | 48 | Vermont | 21,000,000 | 0.18% |
| 24 | Colorado | 146,000,000 | 1.24% | 49 | Wyoming | 20,000,000 | 0.17% |
| 25 | Oklahoma | 144,000,000 | 1.23% | 50 | Alaska | 9,000,000 | 0.08% |
| | | | | | District of Columbia | 64,000,000 | 0.54% |

Source: Families USA Foundation

"Health Spending: The Growing Threat to the Family Budget" (December 1991) (Reprinted with permission)

*This is a total paid directly by business and does not include payments made by families. It is a subset of annual business health care payments. See beginning of this chapter for definitions.

# Percent of Health Care Payments Paid by Business for Medicare Payroll Tax in 1980

## National Rate = 15.9%*

| RANK | STATE | PERCENT | RANK | STATE | PERCENT |
|------|-------|---------|------|-------|---------|
| 1 | Delaware | 24.7 | 25 | Vermont | 15.3 |
| 2 | South Carolina | 22.4 | 27 | Colorado | 15.1 |
| 3 | North Carolina | 20.9 | 27 | Illinois | 15.1 |
| 4 | Oklahoma | 20.5 | 27 | Michigan | 15.1 |
| 5 | Idaho | 19.6 | 30 | Arizona | 15.0 |
| 6 | Arkansas | 19.3 | 30 | Washington | 15.0 |
| 6 | Texas | 19.3 | 30 | Wisconsin | 15.0 |
| 8 | Virginia | 18.8 | 33 | Nebraska | 14.9 |
| 9 | Georgia | 18.6 | 33 | Pennsylvania | 14.9 |
| 10 | Alabama | 18.3 | 35 | Hawaii | 14.7 |
| 11 | Florida | 18.0 | 35 | Tennessee | 14.7 |
| 11 | New York | 18.0 | 37 | Iowa | 14.5 |
| 13 | Maryland | 17.3 | 38 | South Dakota | 14.3 |
| 14 | Wyoming | 16.8 | 39 | Louisiana | 14.1 |
| 15 | Mississippi | 16.7 | 39 | Ohio | 14.1 |
| 16 | West Virginia | 16.3 | 41 | California | 14.0 |
| 17 | Indiana | 16.1 | 42 | Kansas | 13.8 |
| 18 | Kentucky | 15.9 | 43 | New Hampshire | 13.5 |
| 18 | Missouri | 15.9 | 44 | Maine | 13.1 |
| 18 | New Jersey | 15.9 | 44 | Massachusetts | 13.1 |
| 21 | Minnesota | 15.7 | 46 | Connecticut | 13.0 |
| 22 | Montana | 15.6 | 47 | Rhode Island | 12.6 |
| 22 | Oregon | 15.6 | 48 | Nevada | 12.4 |
| 24 | New Mexico | 15.4 | 49 | North Dakota | 12.3 |
| 25 | Utah | 15.3 | 50 | Alaska | 4.7 |

| | | |
|---|---|---|
| | District of Columbia | 35.8 |

Source: Families USA Foundation

"Health Spending: The Growing Threat to the Family Budget" (December 1991) (Reprinted with permission)

*This is a percent paid directly by business and does not include payments made by families. It is a percent of annual business health care payments. See beginning of this chapter for definitions.

# Projected Health Care Payments Paid by Business for Medicare Payroll Tax in 2000

## Projected National Total = $68,566,000,000*

| RANK | STATE | PAYMENTS | % | RANK | STATE | PAYMENTS | % |
|------|-------|----------|---|------|-------|----------|---|
| 1 | California | $8,814,000,000 | 12.85% | 26 | Oregon | $704,000,000 | 1.03% |
| 2 | New York | 7,115,000,000 | 10.38% | 27 | South Carolina | 703,000,000 | 1.03% |
| 3 | Texas | 4,286,000,000 | 6.25% | 28 | Oklahoma | 656,000,000 | 0.96% |
| 4 | Illinois | 3,366,000,000 | 4.91% | 29 | Kentucky | 622,000,000 | 0.91% |
| 5 | Pennsylvania | 3,112,000,000 | 4.54% | 30 | Kansas | 596,000,000 | 0.87% |
| 6 | Florida | 3,107,000,000 | 4.53% | 31 | Iowa | 580,000,000 | 0.85% |
| 7 | New Jersey | 2,958,000,000 | 4.31% | 32 | Arkansas | 542,000,000 | 0.79% |
| 8 | Michigan | 2,901,000,000 | 4.23% | 33 | Mississippi | 398,000,000 | 0.58% |
| 9 | Ohio | 2,870,000,000 | 4.19% | 34 | Nebraska | 389,000,000 | 0.57% |
| 10 | Massachusetts | 1,997,000,000 | 2.91% | 35 | New Hampshire | 350,000,000 | 0.51% |
| 11 | Georgia | 1,863,000,000 | 2.72% | 36 | New Mexico | 346,000,000 | 0.50% |
| 12 | North Carolina | 1,664,000,000 | 2.43% | 37 | Utah | 343,000,000 | 0.50% |
| 13 | Virginia | 1,570,000,000 | 2.29% | 38 | Rhode Island | 300,000,000 | 0.44% |
| 14 | Maryland | 1,482,000,000 | 2.16% | 39 | Nevada | 282,000,000 | 0.41% |
| 15 | Missouri | 1,381,000,000 | 2.01% | 40 | Delaware | 276,000,000 | 0.40% |
| 16 | Connecticut | 1,363,000,000 | 1.99% | 41 | West Virginia | 273,000,000 | 0.40% |
| 17 | Wisconsin | 1,321,000,000 | 1.93% | 42 | Hawaii | 262,000,000 | 0.38% |
| 18 | Indiana | 1,266,000,000 | 1.85% | 43 | Maine | 236,000,000 | 0.34% |
| 19 | Washington | 1,186,000,000 | 1.73% | 44 | Idaho | 196,000,000 | 0.29% |
| 20 | Tennessee | 1,158,000,000 | 1.69% | 45 | Montana | 141,000,000 | 0.21% |
| 21 | Minnesota | 1,148,000,000 | 1.67% | 46 | Vermont | 137,000,000 | 0.20% |
| 22 | Arizona | 960,000,000 | 1.40% | 47 | North Dakota | 123,000,000 | 0.18% |
| 23 | Colorado | 896,000,000 | 1.31% | 48 | South Dakota | 121,000,000 | 0.18% |
| 24 | Louisiana | 824,000,000 | 1.20% | 49 | Alaska | 104,000,000 | 0.15% |
| 25 | Alabama | 807,000,000 | 1.18% | 50 | Wyoming | 96,000,000 | 0.14% |
| | | | | | District of Columbia | 379,000,000 | 0.55% |

Source: Families USA Foundation

*"Health Spending: The Growing Threat to the Family Budget"* (December 1991) (Reprinted with permission)

*This is a total paid directly by business and does not include payments made by families. It is a subset of annual business health care payments. See beginning of this chapter for definitions.

# Projected Percent of Health Care Payments Paid by Business for Medicare Payroll Tax in 2000

## Projected National Rate = 13.4%*

| RANK | STATE | PERCENT | RANK | STATE | PERCENT |
|---|---|---|---|---|---|
| 1 | Delaware | 20.8 | 26 | Nebraska | 12.8 |
| 2 | Arkansas | 19.6 | 27 | Pennsylvania | 12.7 |
| 3 | Maryland | 18.3 | 28 | Oregon | 12.6 |
| 4 | New York | 17.8 | 29 | Arizona | 12.5 |
| 4 | North Carolina | 17.8 | 30 | Iowa | 12.3 |
| 6 | Virginia | 17.5 | 30 | Rhode Island | 12.3 |
| 7 | Georgia | 17.3 | 32 | Utah | 12.2 |
| 8 | South Carolina | 17.0 | 33 | Colorado | 12.1 |
| 9 | Oklahoma | 16.7 | 34 | Louisiana | 11.9 |
| 10 | New Jersey | 15.3 | 34 | Washington | 11.9 |
| 11 | Alabama | 14.4 | 36 | Connecticut | 11.7 |
| 11 | Mississippi | 14.4 | 36 | Massachusetts | 11.7 |
| 11 | Texas | 14.4 | 38 | Tennessee | 11.5 |
| 14 | Kentucky | 14.3 | 39 | Kansas | 11.3 |
| 15 | Idaho | 14.2 | 40 | Montana | 11.2 |
| 15 | New Mexico | 14.2 | 40 | West Virginia | 11.2 |
| 17 | Indiana | 13.7 | 42 | Minnesota | 11.1 |
| 17 | Michigan | 13.7 | 43 | New Hampshire | 10.9 |
| 19 | Wisconsin | 13.6 | 44 | California | 10.8 |
| 19 | Wyoming | 13.6 | 45 | South Dakota | 10.2 |
| 21 | Vermont | 13.5 | 46 | North Dakota | 10.1 |
| 22 | Florida | 13.1 | 47 | Hawaii | 9.6 |
| 23 | Illinois | 12.9 | 48 | Maine | 9.4 |
| 23 | Missouri | 12.9 | 49 | Nevada | 8.7 |
| 23 | Ohio | 12.9 | 50 | Alaska | 4.8 |
| | | | | District of Columbia | 37.7 |

Source: Families USA Foundation

"Health Spending: The Growing Threat to the Family Budget" (December 1991) (Reprinted with permission)

*This is a percent paid directly by business and does not include payments made by families. It is a percent of annual business health care payments. See beginning of this chapter for definitions.

# Health Care Payments Paid by Business through General Taxes in 1991

## National Total = $47,965,000,000*

| RANK | STATE | PAYMENTS | % | | RANK | STATE | PAYMENTS | % |
|------|-------|----------|---|---|------|-------|----------|---|
| 1 | California | $6,817,000,000 | 14.21% | | 26 | Colorado | $508,000,000 | 1.06% |
| 2 | New York | 3,935,000,000 | 8.20% | | 27 | South Carolina | 454,000,000 | 0.95% |
| 3 | Texas | 2,806,000,000 | 5.85% | | 28 | Iowa | 427,000,000 | 0.89% |
| 4 | Florida | 2,442,000,000 | 5.09% | | 29 | Kansas | 419,000,000 | 0.87% |
| 5 | Pennsylvania | 2,222,000,000 | 4.63% | | 30 | Mississippi | 409,000,000 | 0.85% |
| 6 | Illinois | 2,134,000,000 | 4.45% | | 31 | Oklahoma | 406,000,000 | 0.85% |
| 7 | New Jersey | 2,009,000,000 | 4.19% | | 32 | New Hampshire | 382,000,000 | 0.80% |
| 8 | Michigan | 1,954,000,000 | 4.07% | | 33 | Oregon | 372,000,000 | 0.78% |
| 9 | Tennessee | 1,923,000,000 | 4.01% | | 34 | Alaska | 345,000,000 | 0.72% |
| 10 | Ohio | 1,652,000,000 | 3.44% | | 35 | West Virginia | 328,000,000 | 0.68% |
| 11 | Connecticut | 1,515,000,000 | 3.16% | | 36 | Arkansas | 296,000,000 | 0.62% |
| 12 | Massachusetts | 1,460,000,000 | 3.04% | | 37 | Nebraska | 231,000,000 | 0.48% |
| 13 | Louisiana | 1,088,000,000 | 2.27% | | 38 | New Mexico | 228,000,000 | 0.48% |
| 14 | Georgia | 1,043,000,000 | 2.17% | | 39 | Utah | 219,000,000 | 0.46% |
| 15 | North Carolina | 1,033,000,000 | 2.15% | | 40 | Nevada | 205,000,000 | 0.43% |
| 16 | Washington | 937,000,000 | 1.95% | | 41 | Rhode Island | 183,000,000 | 0.38% |
| 17 | Virginia | 928,000,000 | 1.93% | | 42 | Maine | 171,000,000 | 0.36% |
| 18 | Maryland | 804,000,000 | 1.68% | | 43 | Hawaii | 169,000,000 | 0.35% |
| 19 | Minnesota | 742,000,000 | 1.55% | | 44 | Delaware | 146,000,000 | 0.30% |
| 20 | Wisconsin | 720,000,000 | 1.50% | | 45 | North Dakota | 134,000,000 | 0.28% |
| 21 | Indiana | 709,000,000 | 1.48% | | 46 | Idaho | 132,000,000 | 0.28% |
| 22 | Missouri | 688,000,000 | 1.43% | | 47 | Montana | 128,000,000 | 0.27% |
| 23 | Alabama | 577,000,000 | 1.20% | | 48 | South Dakota | 102,000,000 | 0.21% |
| 24 | Kentucky | 574,000,000 | 1.20% | | 49 | Vermont | 80,000,000 | 0.17% |
| 25 | Arizona | 552,000,000 | 1.15% | | 50 | Wyoming | 80,000,000 | 0.17% |
| | | | | | | District of Columbia | 146,000,000 | 0.30% |

Source: Families USA Foundation

"Health Spending: The Growing Threat to the Family Budget" (December 1991) (Reprinted with permission)

*This is a total paid directly by business and does not include payments made by families. It is a subset of annual business health care payments. See beginning of this chapter for definitions.

# Percent of Health Care Payments Paid by Business through General Taxes in 1991

## National Rate = 20.2%*

| RANK | STATE | PERCENT | | RANK | STATE | PERCENT |
|------|-------|---------|---|------|-------|---------|
| 1 | Tennessee | 43.7 | | 26 | Idaho | 19.8 |
| 2 | Alaska | 40.4 | | 27 | New York | 19.6 |
| 3 | Louisiana | 33.9 | | 28 | California | 19.4 |
| 4 | Mississippi | 33.3 | | 29 | Arizona | 18.4 |
| 5 | New Hampshire | 29.7 | | 29 | Michigan | 18.4 |
| 6 | Connecticut | 28.4 | | 31 | Massachusetts | 17.7 |
| 7 | Kentucky | 27.3 | | 31 | Utah | 17.7 |
| 8 | West Virginia | 26.5 | | 33 | Pennsylvania | 17.5 |
| 9 | Florida | 25.7 | | 34 | South Dakota | 17.1 |
| 10 | North Carolina | 25.2 | | 35 | Vermont | 16.5 |
| 11 | South Carolina | 24.6 | | 36 | Iowa | 16.3 |
| 12 | New Mexico | 24.1 | | 37 | Illinois | 16.1 |
| 13 | Georgia | 23.9 | | 38 | Kansas | 16.0 |
| 14 | Wyoming | 23.4 | | 39 | Rhode Island | 15.8 |
| 15 | Virginia | 23.2 | | 40 | Colorado | 15.5 |
| 16 | New Jersey | 22.9 | | 41 | Nevada | 15.4 |
| 17 | Arkansas | 22.6 | | 42 | Indiana | 15.1 |
| 18 | Alabama | 22.4 | | 43 | Maine | 14.5 |
| 19 | Maryland | 22.3 | | 43 | Nebraska | 14.5 |
| 20 | Texas | 22.2 | | 43 | Ohio | 14.5 |
| 21 | Delaware | 21.9 | | 46 | Hawaii | 14.4 |
| 22 | Oklahoma | 21.7 | | 46 | Minnesota | 14.4 |
| 23 | North Dakota | 21.0 | | 46 | Wisconsin | 14.4 |
| 24 | Montana | 20.8 | | 49 | Oregon | 14.0 |
| 25 | Washington | 20.3 | | 50 | Missouri | 13.3 |

District of Columbia 27.1

Source: Families USA Foundation

"Health Spending: The Growing Threat to the Family Budget" (December 1991) (Reprinted with permission)

*This is a percent paid directly by business and does not include payments made by families. It is a percent of annual business health care payments. See beginning of this chapter for definitions.

# Health Care Payments Paid by Business through General Taxes in 1980

## National Total = $13,070,000,000*

| RANK | STATE | PAYMENTS | % | RANK | STATE | PAYMENTS | % |
|------|-------|----------|---|------|-------|----------|---|
| 1 | California | $1,940,000,000 | 14.84% | 26 | South Carolina | $146,000,000 | 1.12% |
| 2 | New York | 1,080,000,000 | 8.26% | 27 | Oklahoma | 143,000,000 | 1.09% |
| 3 | Texas | 764,000,000 | 5.85% | 28 | Kentucky | 140,000,000 | 1.07% |
| 4 | Pennsylvania | 624,000,000 | 4.77% | 29 | Kansas | 137,000,000 | 1.05% |
| 5 | Illinois | 603,000,000 | 4.61% | 30 | Oregon | 125,000,000 | 0.96% |
| 6 | Michigan | 560,000,000 | 4.28% | 31 | Iowa | 124,000,000 | 0.95% |
| 7 | Tennessee | 559,000,000 | 4.28% | 32 | New Mexico | 117,000,000 | 0.90% |
| 8 | Ohio | 536,000,000 | 4.10% | 33 | Mississippi | 112,000,000 | 0.86% |
| 9 | Florida | 520,000,000 | 3.98% | 34 | Arkansas | 92,000,000 | 0.70% |
| 10 | New Jersey | 430,000,000 | 3.29% | 35 | New Hampshire | 78,000,000 | 0.60% |
| 11 | Louisiana | 422,000,000 | 3.23% | 36 | Alaska | 77,000,000 | 0.59% |
| 12 | Connecticut | 383,000,000 | 2.93% | 37 | Nebraska | 66,000,000 | 0.50% |
| 13 | Massachusetts | 325,000,000 | 2.49% | 38 | Nevada | 54,000,000 | 0.41% |
| 14 | Washington | 286,000,000 | 2.19% | 39 | Rhode Island | 53,000,000 | 0.41% |
| 15 | Georgia | 243,000,000 | 1.86% | 40 | Utah | 49,000,000 | 0.37% |
| 16 | North Carolina | 227,000,000 | 1.74% | 41 | West Virginia | 48,000,000 | 0.37% |
| 17 | Virginia | 219,000,000 | 1.68% | 42 | Hawaii | 47,000,000 | 0.36% |
| 18 | Minnesota | 208,000,000 | 1.59% | 43 | Montana | 45,000,000 | 0.34% |
| 19 | Indiana | 206,000,000 | 1.58% | 44 | North Dakota | 43,000,000 | 0.33% |
| 20 | Wisconsin | 183,000,000 | 1.40% | 45 | Maine | 40,000,000 | 0.31% |
| 21 | Alabama | 176,000,000 | 1.35% | 46 | Idaho | 39,000,000 | 0.30% |
| 22 | Maryland | 170,000,000 | 1.30% | 47 | South Dakota | 28,000,000 | 0.21% |
| 23 | Missouri | 165,000,000 | 1.26% | 48 | Wyoming | 27,000,000 | 0.21% |
| 24 | Arizona | 160,000,000 | 1.22% | 49 | Delaware | 25,000,000 | 0.19% |
| 25 | Colorado | 151,000,000 | 1.16% | 50 | Vermont | 17,000,000 | 0.13% |
| | | | | | District of Columbia | 58,000,000 | 0.44% |

Source: Families USA Foundation

"Health Spending: The Growing Threat to the Family Budget" (December 1991) (Reprinted with permission)

*This is a total paid directly by business and does not include payments made by families. It is a subset of annual business health care payments. See beginning of this chapter for definitions.

# Percent of Health Care Payments Paid by Business through General Taxes in 1980

## National Rate = 17.6%*

| RANK | STATE | PERCENT | | RANK | STATE | PERCENT |
|------|-------|---------|--|------|-------|---------|
| 1 | Alaska | 41.7 | | 26 | Kansas | 16.5 |
| 2 | Tennessee | 38.0 | | 27 | New Jersey | 16.4 |
| 3 | New Mexico | 35.6 | | 28 | New York | 16.1 |
| 4 | Louisiana | 32.2 | | 29 | Colorado | 15.6 |
| 5 | South Carolina | 26.5 | | 30 | Hawaii | 15.4 |
| 6 | Connecticut | 25.2 | | 31 | Utah | 15.0 |
| 7 | Mississippi | 24.7 | | 32 | Delaware | 14.9 |
| 8 | New Hampshire | 24.3 | | 33 | Michigan | 14.6 |
| 9 | Florida | 23.4 | | 34 | Oregon | 14.5 |
| 10 | Wyoming | 22.8 | | 34 | Pennsylvania | 14.5 |
| 11 | California | 21.6 | | 36 | Maryland | 14.4 |
| 12 | Alabama | 21.3 | | 37 | South Dakota | 14.3 |
| 13 | Montana | 21.2 | | 38 | Massachusetts | 14.0 |
| 13 | Washington | 21.2 | | 39 | Rhode Island | 13.7 |
| 15 | Arkansas | 21.0 | | 40 | Illinois | 13.2 |
| 16 | Oklahoma | 20.4 | | 41 | Maine | 13.0 |
| 17 | Texas | 20.1 | | 42 | Vermont | 12.9 |
| 18 | Arizona | 20.0 | | 43 | Iowa | 12.7 |
| 19 | Georgia | 19.5 | | 43 | Minnesota | 12.7 |
| 20 | Virginia | 18.7 | | 45 | Nebraska | 12.5 |
| 21 | North Dakota | 18.6 | | 46 | Ohio | 12.4 |
| 22 | North Carolina | 18.4 | | 47 | Indiana | 11.5 |
| 23 | Idaho | 17.8 | | 48 | West Virginia | 10.6 |
| 24 | Nevada | 17.5 | | 49 | Wisconsin | 10.4 |
| 25 | Kentucky | 16.9 | | 50 | Missouri | 10.3 |

District of Columbia     32.2

Source: Families USA Foundation

"Health Spending: The Growing Threat to the Family Budget" (December 1991) (Reprinted with permission)

*This is a percent paid directly by business and does not include payments made by families. It is a percent of annual business health care payments. See beginning of this chapter for definitions.

# Projected Health Care Payments Paid by Business through General Taxes in 2000

## National Projected Total = $125,061,000,000*

| RANK | STATE | PAYMENTS | % | RANK | STATE | PAYMENTS | % |
|---|---|---|---|---|---|---|---|
| 1 | California | $18,392,000,000 | 14.71% | 26 | Colorado | $1,371,000,000 | 1.10% |
| 2 | New York | 9,736,000,000 | 7.79% | 27 | South Carolina | 1,216,000,000 | 0.97% |
| 3 | Texas | 7,749,000,000 | 6.20% | 28 | Mississippi | 1,089,000,000 | 0.87% |
| 4 | Florida | 7,043,000,000 | 5.63% | 29 | New Hampshire | 1,064,000,000 | 0.85% |
| 5 | Pennsylvania | 5,379,000,000 | 4.30% | 30 | Alaska | 1,054,000,000 | 0.84% |
| 6 | New Jersey | 5,182,000,000 | 4.14% | 31 | Oklahoma | 1,050,000,000 | 0.84% |
| 7 | Illinois | 5,161,000,000 | 4.13% | 32 | Kansas | 1,037,000,000 | 0.83% |
| 8 | Tennessee | 5,106,000,000 | 4.08% | 33 | Iowa | 1,010,000,000 | 0.81% |
| 9 | Michigan | 4,837,000,000 | 3.87% | 34 | Oregon | 951,000,000 | 0.76% |
| 10 | Ohio | 4,053,000,000 | 3.24% | 35 | West Virginia | 795,000,000 | 0.64% |
| 11 | Connecticut | 3,879,000,000 | 3.10% | 36 | Arkansas | 759,000,000 | 0.61% |
| 12 | Massachusetts | 3,654,000,000 | 2.92% | 37 | New Mexico | 666,000,000 | 0.53% |
| 13 | Georgia | 2,948,000,000 | 2.36% | 38 | Utah | 599,000,000 | 0.48% |
| 14 | Louisiana | 2,806,000,000 | 2.24% | 39 | Nevada | 574,000,000 | 0.46% |
| 15 | North Carolina | 2,785,000,000 | 2.23% | 40 | Nebraska | 566,000,000 | 0.45% |
| 16 | Virginia | 2,469,000,000 | 1.97% | 41 | Rhode Island | 466,000,000 | 0.37% |
| 17 | Washington | 2,437,000,000 | 1.95% | 42 | Hawaii | 451,000,000 | 0.36% |
| 18 | Maryland | 2,127,000,000 | 1.70% | 43 | Maine | 435,000,000 | 0.35% |
| 19 | Minnesota | 1,861,000,000 | 1.49% | 44 | Delaware | 390,000,000 | 0.31% |
| 20 | Indiana | 1,790,000,000 | 1.43% | 45 | Idaho | 334,000,000 | 0.27% |
| 21 | Missouri | 1,782,000,000 | 1.42% | 46 | Montana | 323,000,000 | 0.26% |
| 22 | Wisconsin | 1,756,000,000 | 1.40% | 47 | North Dakota | 322,000,000 | 0.26% |
| 23 | Arizona | 1,593,000,000 | 1.27% | 48 | South Dakota | 245,000,000 | 0.20% |
| 24 | Alabama | 1,538,000,000 | 1.23% | 49 | Wyoming | 203,000,000 | 0.16% |
| 25 | Kentucky | 1,452,000,000 | 1.16% | 50 | Vermont | 200,000,000 | 0.16% |
| | | | | | District of Columbia | 375,000,000 | 0.30% |

Source: Families USA Foundation

"Health Spending: The Growing Threat to the Family Budget" (December 1991) (Reprinted with permission)

*This is a total paid directly by business and does not include payments made by families. It is a subset of annual business health care payments. See beginning of this chapter for definitions.

# Projected Percent of Health Care Payments Paid by Business through General Taxes in 2000

## Projected National Rate = 24.5%*

| RANK | STATE | PERCENT | | RANK | STATE | PERCENT |
|------|-------|---------|---|------|-------|---------|
| 1 | Tennessee | 50.6 | | 26 | Idaho | 24.3 |
| 2 | Alaska | 48.7 | | 26 | New York | 24.3 |
| 3 | Louisiana | 40.6 | | 28 | Michigan | 22.8 |
| 4 | Mississippi | 39.3 | | 29 | California | 22.6 |
| 5 | Connecticut | 33.4 | | 30 | Pennsylvania | 21.9 |
| 5 | Kentucky | 33.4 | | 31 | Iowa | 21.4 |
| 7 | New Hampshire | 33.3 | | 31 | Massachusetts | 21.4 |
| 8 | West Virginia | 32.7 | | 31 | Utah | 21.4 |
| 9 | North Carolina | 29.8 | | 34 | Arizona | 20.8 |
| 10 | Florida | 29.6 | | 35 | South Dakota | 20.7 |
| 11 | Delaware | 29.5 | | 36 | Illinois | 19.8 |
| 12 | South Carolina | 29.4 | | 37 | Kansas | 19.7 |
| 13 | Wyoming | 28.7 | | 37 | Vermont | 19.7 |
| 14 | Alabama | 27.5 | | 39 | Indiana | 19.4 |
| 14 | Virginia | 27.5 | | 40 | Rhode Island | 19.0 |
| 16 | Arkansas | 27.4 | | 41 | Nebraska | 18.6 |
| 16 | Georgia | 27.4 | | 42 | Colorado | 18.5 |
| 18 | New Mexico | 27.2 | | 43 | Ohio | 18.2 |
| 19 | New Jersey | 26.9 | | 44 | Minnesota | 18.1 |
| 20 | Oklahoma | 26.6 | | 45 | Wisconsin | 18.0 |
| 21 | Maryland | 26.3 | | 46 | Nevada | 17.7 |
| 21 | North Dakota | 26.3 | | 47 | Maine | 17.3 |
| 23 | Texas | 26.0 | | 48 | Oregon | 17.1 |
| 24 | Montana | 25.7 | | 49 | Missouri | 16.7 |
| 25 | Washington | 24.4 | | 50 | Hawaii | 16.6 |

District of Columbia                 37.2

Source: Families USA Foundation

    "Health Spending: The Growing Threat to the Family Budget" (December 1991) (Reprinted with permission)

*This is a percent paid directly by business and does not include payments made by families. It is a percent of annual business health care payments. See beginning of this chapter for definitions.

# Health Care Payments Paid by Business for Other Costs in 1991

## National Total = $19,112,000,000*

| RANK | STATE | PAYMENTS | % | RANK | STATE | PAYMENTS | % |
|---|---|---|---|---|---|---|---|
| 1 | California | $3,290,000,000 | 17.21% | 26 | Alabama | $212,000,000 | 1.11% |
| 2 | Texas | 1,605,000,000 | 8.40% | 26 | Kentucky | 212,000,000 | 1.11% |
| 3 | Ohio | 1,209,000,000 | 6.33% | 28 | North Carolina | 211,000,000 | 1.10% |
| 4 | Pennsylvania | 984,000,000 | 5.15% | 29 | Arizona | 172,000,000 | 0.90% |
| 5 | New York | 934,000,000 | 4.89% | 30 | Indiana | 156,000,000 | 0.82% |
| 6 | Florida | 912,000,000 | 4.77% | 31 | South Carolina | 144,000,000 | 0.75% |
| 7 | Illinois | 827,000,000 | 4.33% | 32 | Nevada | 139,000,000 | 0.73% |
| 8 | Michigan | 685,000,000 | 3.58% | 33 | Kansas | 135,000,000 | 0.71% |
| 9 | Massachusetts | 568,000,000 | 2.97% | 34 | Arkansas | 124,000,000 | 0.65% |
| 10 | Washington | 525,000,000 | 2.75% | 35 | New Mexico | 113,000,000 | 0.59% |
| 11 | New Jersey | 485,000,000 | 2.54% | 36 | Rhode Island | 111,000,000 | 0.58% |
| 12 | Louisiana | 421,000,000 | 2.20% | 37 | Iowa | 109,000,000 | 0.57% |
| 13 | Georgia | 395,000,000 | 2.07% | 38 | Alaska | 108,000,000 | 0.57% |
| 13 | Oregon | 395,000,000 | 2.07% | 39 | Montana | 107,000,000 | 0.56% |
| 15 | Minnesota | 379,000,000 | 1.98% | 40 | Hawaii | 106,000,000 | 0.55% |
| 16 | Connecticut | 336,000,000 | 1.76% | 40 | Mississippi | 106,000,000 | 0.55% |
| 17 | Colorado | 311,000,000 | 1.63% | 42 | New Hampshire | 99,000,000 | 0.52% |
| 18 | Maryland | 289,000,000 | 1.51% | 43 | Utah | 98,000,000 | 0.51% |
| 19 | Wisconsin | 286,000,000 | 1.50% | 44 | Nebraska | 68,000,000 | 0.36% |
| 20 | West Virginia | 275,000,000 | 1.44% | 45 | Idaho | 54,000,000 | 0.28% |
| 21 | Virginia | 274,000,000 | 1.43% | 46 | Delaware | 39,000,000 | 0.20% |
| 22 | Missouri | 248,000,000 | 1.30% | 47 | Wyoming | 35,000,000 | 0.18% |
| 23 | Oklahoma | 224,000,000 | 1.17% | 48 | North Dakota | 34,000,000 | 0.18% |
| 23 | Tennessee | 224,000,000 | 1.17% | 49 | Vermont | 32,000,000 | 0.17% |
| 25 | Maine | 214,000,000 | 1.12% | 50 | South Dakota | 28,000,000 | 0.15% |
| | | | | | District of Columbia | 67,000,000 | 0.35% |

Source: Families USA Foundation

"Health Spending: The Growing Threat to the Family Budget" (December 1991) (Reprinted with permission)

*This is a total paid directly by business and does not include payments made by families. It is a subset of annual business health care payments. See beginning of this chapter for definitions.

# Percent of Health Care Payments Paid by Business for Other Costs in 1991

## National Rate = 8.0%*

| RANK | STATE | PERCENT | | RANK | STATE | PERCENT |
|------|-------|---------|---|------|-------|---------|
| 1 | West Virginia | 22.2 | | 26 | Utah | 7.9 |
| 2 | Maine | 18.2 | | 27 | Pennsylvania | 7.8 |
| 3 | Montana | 17.3 | | 27 | South Carolina | 7.8 |
| 4 | Oregon | 14.8 | | 29 | New Hampshire | 7.7 |
| 5 | Louisiana | 13.1 | | 30 | Minnesota | 7.4 |
| 6 | Texas | 12.7 | | 31 | Massachusetts | 6.9 |
| 7 | Alaska | 12.6 | | 31 | Virginia | 6.9 |
| 8 | New Mexico | 11.9 | | 33 | Vermont | 6.6 |
| 8 | Oklahoma | 11.9 | | 34 | Michigan | 6.5 |
| 10 | Washington | 11.4 | | 35 | Connecticut | 6.3 |
| 11 | Ohio | 10.6 | | 36 | Illinois | 6.2 |
| 12 | Nevada | 10.5 | | 37 | Delaware | 5.9 |
| 13 | Kentucky | 10.1 | | 38 | Arizona | 5.7 |
| 13 | Wyoming | 10.1 | | 38 | Wisconsin | 5.7 |
| 15 | Florida | 9.6 | | 40 | New Jersey | 5.5 |
| 15 | Rhode Island | 9.6 | | 41 | North Dakota | 5.3 |
| 17 | Colorado | 9.5 | | 42 | Kansas | 5.2 |
| 18 | Arkansas | 9.4 | | 43 | North Carolina | 5.1 |
| 18 | California | 9.4 | | 43 | Tennessee | 5.1 |
| 20 | Georgia | 9.1 | | 45 | Missouri | 4.8 |
| 21 | Hawaii | 9.0 | | 46 | South Dakota | 4.7 |
| 22 | Mississippi | 8.6 | | 47 | New York | 4.6 |
| 23 | Alabama | 8.2 | | 48 | Nebraska | 4.3 |
| 23 | Idaho | 8.2 | | 49 | Iowa | 4.2 |
| 25 | Maryland | 8.0 | | 50 | Indiana | 3.3 |

District of Columbia     12.4

Source: Families USA Foundation

"Health Spending: The Growing Threat to the Family Budget" (December 1991) (Reprinted with permission)

*This is a percent paid directly by business and does not include payments made by families. It is a percent of annual business health care payments. See beginning of this chapter for definitions.

# Health Care Payments Paid by Business for Other Costs in 1980

## National Total = $6,000,000,000*

| RANK | STATE | PAYMENTS | % | RANK | STATE | PAYMENTS | % |
|------|-------|----------|---|------|-------|----------|---|
| 1 | California | $885,000,000 | 14.75% | 26 | Arizona | $65,000,000 | 1.08% |
| 2 | Ohio | 422,000,000 | 7.03% | 27 | Colorado | 62,000,000 | 1.03% |
| 3 | Texas | 381,000,000 | 6.35% | 28 | Alabama | 61,000,000 | 1.02% |
| 4 | Illinois | 362,000,000 | 6.03% | 29 | Indiana | 60,000,000 | 1.00% |
| 5 | New York | 346,000,000 | 5.77% | 30 | Iowa | 54,000,000 | 0.90% |
| 6 | Michigan | 340,000,000 | 5.67% | 31 | Kansas | 46,000,000 | 0.77% |
| 7 | Pennsylvania | 311,000,000 | 5.18% | 32 | Arkansas | 45,000,000 | 0.75% |
| 8 | Florida | 197,000,000 | 3.28% | 33 | Maine | 44,000,000 | 0.73% |
| 9 | Washington | 176,000,000 | 2.93% | 34 | South Carolina | 43,000,000 | 0.72% |
| 10 | New Jersey | 172,000,000 | 2.87% | 35 | Nevada | 38,000,000 | 0.63% |
| 11 | Louisiana | 164,000,000 | 2.73% | 36 | Alaska | 33,000,000 | 0.55% |
| 12 | Massachusetts | 161,000,000 | 2.68% | 36 | Hawaii | 33,000,000 | 0.55% |
| 13 | Oregon | 149,000,000 | 2.48% | 36 | Mississippi | 33,000,000 | 0.55% |
| 14 | Minnesota | 140,000,000 | 2.33% | 39 | Rhode Island | 30,000,000 | 0.50% |
| 15 | Maryland | 102,000,000 | 1.70% | 40 | New Mexico | 29,000,000 | 0.48% |
| 16 | Georgia | 101,000,000 | 1.68% | 41 | New Hampshire | 26,000,000 | 0.43% |
| 17 | West Virginia | 96,000,000 | 1.60% | 42 | Nebraska | 23,000,000 | 0.38% |
| 18 | Virginia | 94,000,000 | 1.57% | 43 | Montana | 22,000,000 | 0.37% |
| 18 | Wisconsin | 94,000,000 | 1.57% | 44 | Idaho | 21,000,000 | 0.35% |
| 20 | Kentucky | 88,000,000 | 1.47% | 44 | Utah | 21,000,000 | 0.35% |
| 21 | Oklahoma | 73,000,000 | 1.22% | 46 | Delaware | 11,000,000 | 0.18% |
| 22 | Connecticut | 72,000,000 | 1.20% | 47 | North Dakota | 9,000,000 | 0.15% |
| 23 | North Carolina | 71,000,000 | 1.18% | 48 | Vermont | 8,000,000 | 0.13% |
| 24 | Tennessee | 70,000,000 | 1.17% | 48 | Wyoming | 8,000,000 | 0.13% |
| 25 | Missouri | 67,000,000 | 1.12% | 50 | South Dakota | 7,000,000 | 0.12% |
| | | | | | District of Columbia | 38,000,000 | 0.63% |

Source: Families USA Foundation

*"Health Spending: The Growing Threat to the Family Budget"* (December 1991) (Reprinted with permission)

*This is a total paid directly by business and does not include payments made by families. It is a subset of annual business health care payments. See beginning of this chapter for definitions.

## Percent of Health Care Payments Paid by Business for Other Costs in 1980

## National Rate = 8.1%*

| RANK | STATE | PERCENT | RANK | STATE | PERCENT |
|------|-------|---------|------|-------|---------|
| 1 | West Virginia | 20.9 | 26 | Illinois | 7.9 |
| 2 | Alaska | 17.7 | 27 | Rhode Island | 7.8 |
| 3 | Oregon | 17.4 | 27 | South Carolina | 7.8 |
| 4 | Maine | 14.2 | 29 | Alabama | 7.4 |
| 5 | Washington | 13.1 | 30 | Mississippi | 7.2 |
| 6 | Louisiana | 12.5 | 30 | Pennsylvania | 7.2 |
| 7 | Nevada | 12.3 | 32 | Delaware | 6.9 |
| 8 | Hawaii | 10.7 | 32 | Massachusetts | 6.9 |
| 9 | Kentucky | 10.6 | 34 | New Jersey | 6.6 |
| 9 | Montana | 10.6 | 35 | Utah | 6.5 |
| 11 | Oklahoma | 10.4 | 36 | Colorado | 6.4 |
| 12 | Arkansas | 10.3 | 36 | Wyoming | 6.4 |
| 13 | Texas | 10.0 | 38 | Vermont | 6.0 |
| 14 | California | 9.9 | 39 | North Carolina | 5.8 |
| 15 | Ohio | 9.8 | 40 | Iowa | 5.5 |
| 16 | Idaho | 9.4 | 40 | Kansas | 5.5 |
| 17 | Michigan | 8.9 | 42 | Wisconsin | 5.3 |
| 17 | New Mexico | 8.9 | 43 | New York | 5.2 |
| 19 | Florida | 8.8 | 44 | Tennessee | 4.8 |
| 20 | Maryland | 8.6 | 45 | Connecticut | 4.7 |
| 21 | Minnesota | 8.5 | 46 | Nebraska | 4.3 |
| 22 | Arizona | 8.2 | 47 | Missouri | 4.2 |
| 22 | New Hampshire | 8.2 | 48 | North Dakota | 4.0 |
| 24 | Georgia | 8.1 | 49 | South Dakota | 3.7 |
| 25 | Virginia | 8.0 | 50 | Indiana | 3.3 |

District of Columbia     20.8

Source: Families USA Foundation

"Health Spending: The Growing Threat to the Family Budget" (December 1991) (Reprinted with permission)

*This is a percent paid directly by business and does not include payments made by families. It is a percent of annual business health care payments. See beginning of this chapter for definitions.

# Projected Health Care Payments Paid by Business for Other Costs in 2000

## Projected National Total = $46,200,000,000*

| RANK | STATE | PAYMENTS | % | RANK | STATE | PAYMENTS | % |
|------|-------|----------|---|------|-------|----------|---|
| 1 | California | $8,494,000,000 | 18.39% | 26 | Maine | $506,000,000 | 1.10% |
| 2 | Texas | 4,205,000,000 | 9.10% | 27 | Alabama | 504,000,000 | 1.09% |
| 3 | Ohio | 2,626,000,000 | 5.68% | 28 | Arizona | 499,000,000 | 1.08% |
| 4 | Florida | 2,520,000,000 | 5.45% | 29 | Kentucky | 470,000,000 | 1.02% |
| 5 | Pennsylvania | 2,108,000,000 | 4.56% | 30 | Nevada | 381,000,000 | 0.82% |
| 6 | New York | 2,079,000,000 | 4.50% | 31 | South Carolina | 357,000,000 | 0.77% |
| 7 | Illinois | 1,823,000,000 | 3.95% | 32 | Indiana | 343,000,000 | 0.74% |
| 8 | Michigan | 1,522,000,000 | 3.29% | 33 | New Mexico | 326,000,000 | 0.71% |
| 9 | Massachusetts | 1,313,000,000 | 2.84% | 34 | Alaska | 308,000,000 | 0.67% |
| 10 | Washington | 1,249,000,000 | 2.70% | 35 | Kansas | 304,000,000 | 0.66% |
| 11 | New Jersey | 1,195,000,000 | 2.59% | 36 | Arkansas | 291,000,000 | 0.63% |
| 12 | Georgia | 1,097,000,000 | 2.37% | 37 | Hawaii | 283,000,000 | 0.61% |
| 13 | Louisiana | 945,000,000 | 2.05% | 38 | New Hampshire | 272,000,000 | 0.59% |
| 14 | Oregon | 918,000,000 | 1.99% | 39 | Rhode Island | 263,000,000 | 0.57% |
| 15 | Minnesota | 876,000,000 | 1.90% | 40 | Mississippi | 257,000,000 | 0.56% |
| 16 | Connecticut | 798,000,000 | 1.73% | 41 | Utah | 248,000,000 | 0.54% |
| 17 | Colorado | 788,000,000 | 1.71% | 42 | Montana | 234,000,000 | 0.51% |
| 18 | Maryland | 733,000,000 | 1.59% | 43 | Iowa | 217,000,000 | 0.47% |
| 19 | Virginia | 693,000,000 | 1.50% | 44 | Nebraska | 146,000,000 | 0.32% |
| 20 | Wisconsin | 625,000,000 | 1.35% | 45 | Idaho | 124,000,000 | 0.27% |
| 21 | Missouri | 577,000,000 | 1.25% | 46 | Delaware | 97,000,000 | 0.21% |
| 22 | West Virginia | 562,000,000 | 1.22% | 47 | Wyoming | 78,000,000 | 0.17% |
| 23 | North Carolina | 536,000,000 | 1.16% | 48 | Vermont | 75,000,000 | 0.16% |
| 24 | Tennessee | 532,000,000 | 1.15% | 49 | North Dakota | 71,000,000 | 0.15% |
| 25 | Oklahoma | 517,000,000 | 1.12% | 50 | South Dakota | 62,000,000 | 0.13% |
| | | | | | District of Columbia | 154,000,000 | 0.33% |

Source: Families USA Foundation

"Health Spending: The Growing Threat to the Family Budget" (December 1991) (Reprinted with permission)

*This is a total paid directly by business and does not include payments made by families. It is a subset of annual business health care payments. See beginning of this chapter for definitions.

# Projected Percent of Health Care Payments Paid by Business for Other Costs in 2000

## Projected National Rate = 9.0%*

| RANK | STATE | PERCENT | RANK | STATE | PERCENT |
|------|-------|---------|------|-------|---------|
| 1 | West Virginia | 23.1 | 26 | Utah | 8.8 |
| 2 | Maine | 20.1 | 27 | South Carolina | 8.7 |
| 3 | Montana | 18.6 | 28 | Pennsylvania | 8.6 |
| 4 | Oregon | 16.5 | 29 | Minnesota | 8.5 |
| 5 | Alaska | 14.2 | 29 | New Hampshire | 8.5 |
| 6 | Texas | 14.1 | 31 | Massachusetts | 7.7 |
| 7 | Louisiana | 13.7 | 31 | Virginia | 7.7 |
| 8 | New Mexico | 13.3 | 33 | Vermont | 7.4 |
| 9 | Oklahoma | 13.1 | 34 | Delaware | 7.3 |
| 10 | Washington | 12.5 | 35 | Michigan | 7.2 |
| 11 | Nevada | 11.8 | 36 | Illinois | 7.0 |
| 11 | Ohio | 11.8 | 37 | Connecticut | 6.9 |
| 13 | Wyoming | 11.0 | 38 | Arizona | 6.5 |
| 14 | Kentucky | 10.8 | 39 | Wisconsin | 6.4 |
| 15 | Rhode Island | 10.7 | 40 | New Jersey | 6.2 |
| 16 | Colorado | 10.6 | 41 | Kansas | 5.8 |
| 16 | Florida | 10.6 | 41 | North Dakota | 5.8 |
| 18 | Arkansas | 10.5 | 43 | North Carolina | 5.7 |
| 19 | California | 10.4 | 44 | Missouri | 5.4 |
| 19 | Hawaii | 10.4 | 45 | Tennessee | 5.3 |
| 21 | Georgia | 10.2 | 46 | New York | 5.2 |
| 22 | Mississippi | 9.3 | 46 | South Dakota | 5.2 |
| 23 | Maryland | 9.1 | 48 | Nebraska | 4.8 |
| 24 | Alabama | 9.0 | 49 | Iowa | 4.6 |
| 24 | Idaho | 9.0 | 50 | Indiana | 3.7 |

District of Columbia      15.3

Source: Families USA Foundation

"Health Spending: The Growing Threat to the Family Budget" (December 1991) (Reprinted with permission)

*This is a percent paid directly by business and does not include payments made by families. It is a percent of annual business health care payments. See beginning of this chapter for definitions.

# Medicaid Expenditures in 1991

## National Total = $77,048,353,128*

| RANK | STATE | EXPENDITURES | % | | RANK | STATE | EXPENDITURES | % |
|---|---|---|---|---|---|---|---|---|
| 1 | New York | $13,728,452,104 | 17.82% | | 26 | Alabama | $805,455,097 | 1.05% |
| 2 | California | 7,578,546,773 | 9.84% | | 27 | Iowa | 765,942,643 | 0.99% |
| 3 | Ohio | 3,653,431,706 | 4.74% | | 28 | Mississippi | 754,917,219 | 0.98% |
| 4 | Texas | 3,532,103,915 | 4.58% | | 29 | Arkansas | 687,966,888 | 0.89% |
| 5 | Pennsylvania | 3,436,164,827 | 4.46% | | 30 | Colorado | 672,796,175 | 0.87% |
| 6 | Florida | 2,944,357,129 | 3.82% | | 31 | Oregon | 666,526,383 | 0.87% |
| 7 | Massachusetts | 2,828,315,291 | 3.67% | | 32 | Rhode Island | 657,057,749 | 0.85% |
| 8 | Illinois | 2,731,167,804 | 3.54% | | 33 | Kansas | 552,987,169 | 0.72% |
| 9 | New Jersey | 2,724,720,584 | 3.54% | | 34 | West Virginia | 542,490,046 | 0.70% |
| 10 | Michigan | 2,540,086,697 | 3.30% | | 35 | Maine | 536,347,763 | 0.70% |
| 11 | Georgia | 1,799,296,327 | 2.34% | | 36 | Nebraska | 389,846,429 | 0.51% |
| 12 | North Carolina | 1,787,569,509 | 2.32% | | 37 | New Mexico | 342,245,846 | 0.44% |
| 13 | Louisiana | 1,723,278,206 | 2.24% | | 38 | Utah | 311,339,546 | 0.40% |
| 14 | Indiana | 1,661,776,563 | 2.16% | | 39 | New Hampshire | 292,351,687 | 0.38% |
| 15 | Connecticut | 1,629,898,556 | 2.12% | | 40 | Hawaii | 237,529,281 | 0.31% |
| 16 | Minnesota | 1,561,303,611 | 2.03% | | 41 | North Dakota | 226,937,494 | 0.29% |
| 17 | Tennessee | 1,485,247,776 | 1.93% | | 42 | Idaho | 223,048,358 | 0.29% |
| 18 | Wisconsin | 1,471,011,102 | 1.91% | | 43 | Vermont | 196,715,470 | 0.26% |
| 19 | Maryland | 1,292,245,064 | 1.68% | | 44 | South Dakota | 196,305,653 | 0.25% |
| 20 | Virginia | 1,218,430,424 | 1.58% | | 45 | Montana | 193,229,100 | 0.25% |
| 21 | Kentucky | 1,200,294,186 | 1.56% | | 46 | Delaware | 186,056,982 | 0.24% |
| 22 | Washington | 1,131,408,143 | 1.47% | | 47 | Nevada | 178,169,850 | 0.23% |
| 23 | Missouri | 1,117,882,322 | 1.45% | | 48 | Alaska | 160,194,502 | 0.21% |
| 24 | South Carolina | 910,287,195 | 1.18% | | 49 | Wyoming | 90,177,377 | 0.12% |
| 25 | Oklahoma | 814,372,251 | 1.06% | | 50 | Arizona | 83,871,151 | 0.11% |
| | | | | | | District of Columbia | 445,856,191 | 0.58% |
| | | | | | | Puerto Rico | 146,135,200 | 0.19% |

Source: U.S. Department of Health and Human Services, Health Care Financing Administration

Unpublished data

*For fiscal year ending September 30, 1991.

# Medicaid Recipients in 1991

## National Total = 28,279,781 Recipients*

| RANK | STATE | RECIPIENTS | % | RANK | STATE | RECIPIENTS | % |
|---|---|---|---|---|---|---|---|
| 1 | California | 4,019,084 | 14.21% | 26 | Arizona | 313,142 | 1.11% |
| 2 | New York | 2,461,537 | 8.70% | 27 | Oklahoma | 304,659 | 1.08% |
| 3 | Texas | 1,728,629 | 6.11% | 28 | Arkansas | 284,674 | 1.01% |
| 4 | Ohio | 1,299,285 | 4.59% | 29 | West Virginia | 283,708 | 1.00% |
| 5 | Pennsylvania | 1,277,428 | 4.52% | 30 | Connecticut | 271,903 | 0.96% |
| 6 | Florida | 1,248,883 | 4.42% | 31 | Oregon | 263,303 | 0.93% |
| 7 | Illinois | 1,144,272 | 4.05% | 32 | Iowa | 261,419 | 0.92% |
| 8 | Michigan | 1,112,533 | 3.93% | 33 | Colorado | 223,444 | 0.79% |
| 9 | Georgia | 746,241 | 2.64% | 34 | Kansas | 209,329 | 0.74% |
| 10 | Tennessee | 697,411 | 2.47% | 35 | Rhode Island | 163,704 | 0.58% |
| 11 | North Carolina | 667,203 | 2.36% | 36 | New Mexico | 161,995 | 0.57% |
| 12 | Massachusetts | 651,056 | 2.30% | 37 | Maine | 150,623 | 0.53% |
| 13 | Louisiana | 640,562 | 2.27% | 38 | Nebraska | 133,751 | 0.47% |
| 14 | New Jersey | 614,073 | 2.17% | 39 | Utah | 129,274 | 0.46% |
| 15 | Kentucky | 525,497 | 1.86% | 40 | Hawaii | 91,162 | 0.32% |
| 16 | Washington | 506,279 | 1.79% | 41 | Vermont | 70,699 | 0.25% |
| 17 | Missouri | 503,310 | 1.78% | 42 | Idaho | 70,060 | 0.25% |
| 18 | Mississippi | 469,684 | 1.66% | 43 | Montana | 63,615 | 0.22% |
| 19 | Virginia | 442,073 | 1.56% | 44 | New Hampshire | 59,684 | 0.21% |
| 20 | Minnesota | 421,738 | 1.49% | 45 | Nevada | 59,296 | 0.21% |
| 21 | Wisconsin | 415,942 | 1.47% | 46 | South Dakota | 57,145 | 0.20% |
| 22 | Indiana | 415,167 | 1.47% | 47 | North Dakota | 52,539 | 0.19% |
| 23 | Alabama | 403,255 | 1.43% | 48 | Alaska | 51,288 | 0.18% |
| 24 | South Carolina | 375,233 | 1.33% | 49 | Delaware | 50,680 | 0.18% |
| 25 | Maryland | 362,520 | 1.28% | 50 | Wyoming | 36,804 | 0.13% |
| | | | | | District of Columbia | 100,065 | 0.35% |
| | | | | | Puerto Rico | 1,201,199 | 4.25% |

Source: U.S. Department of Health and Human Services, Health Care Financing Administration
Unpublished data

*For fiscal year ending September 30, 1991.

# Medicaid Cost per Recipient in 1991

## National Per Capita = $2,725 per Recipient*

| RANK | STATE | PER CAPITA | RANK | STATE | PER CAPITA |
|------|-------|-----------|------|-------|-----------|
| 1 | Connecticut | $5,994 | 25 | Pennsylvania | $2,690 |
| 2 | New York | 5,577 | 27 | North Carolina | 2,679 |
| 3 | New Hampshire | 4,898 | 28 | Oklahoma | 2,673 |
| 4 | New Jersey | 4,437 | 29 | Kansas | 2,642 |
| 5 | Massachusetts | 4,344 | 30 | Hawaii | 2,606 |
| 6 | North Dakota | 4,319 | 31 | Oregon | 2,531 |
| 7 | Rhode Island | 4,014 | 32 | Wyoming | 2,450 |
| 8 | Indiana | 4,003 | 33 | South Carolina | 2,426 |
| 9 | Minnesota | 3,702 | 34 | Arkansas | 2,417 |
| 10 | Delaware | 3,671 | 35 | Georgia | 2,411 |
| 11 | Maryland | 3,565 | 36 | Utah | 2,408 |
| 12 | Maine | 3,561 | 37 | Illinois | 2,387 |
| 13 | Wisconsin | 3,537 | 38 | Florida | 2,358 |
| 14 | South Dakota | 3,435 | 39 | Kentucky | 2,284 |
| 15 | Idaho | 3,184 | 40 | Michigan | 2,283 |
| 16 | Alaska | 3,123 | 41 | Washington | 2,235 |
| 17 | Montana | 3,037 | 42 | Missouri | 2,221 |
| 18 | Colorado | 3,011 | 43 | Tennessee | 2,130 |
| 19 | Nevada | 3,005 | 44 | New Mexico | 2,113 |
| 20 | Iowa | 2,930 | 45 | Texas | 2,043 |
| 21 | Nebraska | 2,915 | 46 | Alabama | 1,997 |
| 22 | Ohio | 2,812 | 47 | West Virginia | 1,912 |
| 23 | Vermont | 2,782 | 48 | California | 1,886 |
| 24 | Virginia | 2,756 | 49 | Mississippi | 1,607 |
| 25 | Louisiana | 2,690 | 50 | Arizona | 268 |
| | | | | District of Columbia | 4,456 |
| | | | | Puerto Rico | 122 |

Source: U.S. Department of Health and Human Services, Health Care Financing Administration
   Unpublished data

*For fiscal year ending September 30, 1991.

# Medicare Benefit Payments in 1991

## National Total = $113,991,000,000*

| RANK | STATE | BENEFITS | % | RANK | STATE | BENEFITS | % |
|---|---|---|---|---|---|---|---|
| 1 | California | $11,416,000,000 | 10.01% | 26 | Oklahoma | $1,431,000,000 | 1.26% |
| 2 | New York | 9,947,000,000 | 8.73% | 27 | Iowa | 1,245,000,000 | 1.09% |
| 3 | Florida | 8,122,000,000 | 7.13% | 28 | Arkansas | 1,209,000,000 | 1.06% |
| 4 | Pennsylvania | 7,548,000,000 | 6.62% | 29 | South Carolina | 1,166,000,000 | 1.02% |
| 5 | Texas | 6,312,000,000 | 5.54% | 30 | Kansas | 1,124,000,000 | 0.99% |
| 6 | Ohio | 5,730,000,000 | 5.03% | 31 | Mississippi | 1,109,000,000 | 0.97% |
| 7 | Illinois | 5,318,000,000 | 4.67% | 32 | Colorado | 1,001,000,000 | 0.88% |
| 8 | Michigan | 4,624,000,000 | 4.06% | 33 | Oregon | 995,000,000 | 0.87% |
| 9 | New Jersey | 3,687,000,000 | 3.23% | 34 | West Virginia | 912,000,000 | 0.80% |
| 10 | Massachusetts | 3,286,000,000 | 2.88% | 35 | Nebraska | 611,000,000 | 0.54% |
| 11 | Missouri | 2,594,000,000 | 2.28% | 36 | Rhode Island | 506,000,000 | 0.44% |
| 12 | North Carolina | 2,506,000,000 | 2.20% | 37 | Maine | 500,000,000 | 0.44% |
| 13 | Georgia | 2,488,000,000 | 2.18% | 38 | New Mexico | 489,000,000 | 0.43% |
| 14 | Indiana | 2,392,000,000 | 2.10% | 39 | Nevada | 459,000,000 | 0.40% |
| 15 | Tennessee | 2,312,000,000 | 2.03% | 40 | Utah | 419,000,000 | 0.37% |
| 16 | Virginia | 2,251,000,000 | 1.97% | 41 | New Hampshire | 385,000,000 | 0.34% |
| 17 | Maryland | 2,236,000,000 | 1.96% | 42 | Montana | 332,000,000 | 0.29% |
| 18 | Louisiana | 2,195,000,000 | 1.93% | 43 | Idaho | 331,000,000 | 0.29% |
| 19 | Alabama | 2,042,000,000 | 1.79% | 44 | Delaware | 303,000,000 | 0.27% |
| 20 | Wisconsin | 2,001,000,000 | 1.76% | 45 | Hawaii | 282,000,000 | 0.25% |
| 21 | Washington | 1,757,000,000 | 1.54% | 45 | North Dakota | 282,000,000 | 0.25% |
| 22 | Kentucky | 1,731,000,000 | 1.52% | 45 | South Dakota | 282,000,000 | 0.25% |
| 23 | Arizona | 1,651,000,000 | 1.45% | 48 | Vermont | 192,000,000 | 0.17% |
| 24 | Connecticut | 1,612,000,000 | 1.41% | 49 | Wyoming | 152,000,000 | 0.13% |
| 25 | Minnesota | 1,451,000,000 | 1.27% | 50 | Alaska | 90,000,000 | 0.08% |
| | | | | | District of Columbia | 366,000,000 | 0.32% |

Source: U.S. Department of Health and Human Services, Health Care Financing Administration
    unpublished data

*For fiscal year 1991. Includes payments to aged and disabled enrollees. Total includes $624,000,000 in payments to addresses in territories, foreign addresses and "residence unknown."

# Medicare Enrollees in 1991

## National Total = 34,870,240 Enrollees*

| RANK | STATE | ENROLLEES | % | RANK | STATE | ENROLLEES | % |
|---|---|---|---|---|---|---|---|
| 1 | California | 3,351,755 | 9.61% | 26 | Iowa | 460,901 | 1.32% |
| 2 | New York | 2,529,403 | 7.25% | 27 | Oklahoma | 458,312 | 1.31% |
| 3 | Florida | 2,402,039 | 6.89% | 28 | South Carolina | 454,216 | 1.30% |
| 4 | Pennsylvania | 1,984,781 | 5.69% | 29 | Oregon | 433,577 | 1.24% |
| 5 | Texas | 1,872,659 | 5.37% | 30 | Arkansas | 397,233 | 1.14% |
| 6 | Ohio | 1,571,301 | 4.51% | 31 | Mississippi | 371,052 | 1.06% |
| 7 | Illinois | 1,553,086 | 4.45% | 32 | Colorado | 369,493 | 1.06% |
| 8 | Michigan | 1,256,925 | 3.60% | 33 | Kansas | 367,885 | 1.06% |
| 9 | New Jersey | 1,108,627 | 3.18% | 34 | West Virginia | 312,299 | 0.90% |
| 10 | North Carolina | 917,034 | 2.63% | 35 | Nebraska | 239,894 | 0.69% |
| 11 | Massachusetts | 879,175 | 2.52% | 36 | Maine | 186,059 | 0.53% |
| 12 | Missouri | 791,893 | 2.27% | 37 | New Mexico | 185,533 | 0.53% |
| 13 | Indiana | 774,887 | 2.22% | 38 | Utah | 165,520 | 0.47% |
| 14 | Georgia | 749,919 | 2.15% | 39 | Rhode Island | 160,637 | 0.46% |
| 15 | Virginia | 740,511 | 2.12% | 40 | Nevada | 150,622 | 0.43% |
| 16 | Wisconsin | 722,976 | 2.07% | 41 | New Hampshire | 140,798 | 0.40% |
| 17 | Tennessee | 706,476 | 2.03% | 42 | Idaho | 135,407 | 0.39% |
| 18 | Washington | 629,630 | 1.81% | 43 | Hawaii | 131,091 | 0.38% |
| 19 | Minnesota | 596,834 | 1.71% | 44 | Montana | 120,054 | 0.34% |
| 20 | Alabama | 593,107 | 1.70% | 45 | South Dakota | 111,493 | 0.32% |
| 21 | Maryland | 553,623 | 1.59% | 46 | North Dakota | 99,661 | 0.29% |
| 22 | Kentucky | 542,794 | 1.56% | 47 | Delaware | 90,588 | 0.26% |
| 23 | Louisiana | 540,501 | 1.55% | 48 | Vermont | 75,789 | 0.22% |
| 24 | Arizona | 517,186 | 1.48% | 49 | Wyoming | 53,427 | 0.15% |
| 25 | Connecticut | 475,926 | 1.36% | 50 | Alaska | 26,516 | 0.08% |
| | | | | | District of Columbia | 77,882 | 0.22% |

Source: U.S. Department of Health and Human Services, Health Care Financing Administration
   unpublished data

*As of July 1, 1991. Includes aged and disabled enrollees. Total includes 731,253 enrollees in territories, foreign countries and whose residences are unknown.

# Medicare Payments per Enrollee in 1991

## National Rate = $3,269 per Enrollee*

| RANK | STATE | PER ENROLLEE | | RANK | STATE | PER ENROLLEE |
|---|---|---|---|---|---|---|
| 1 | Louisiana | $4,061 | | 26 | Nevada | $3,045 |
| 2 | Maryland | 4,040 | | 27 | Arkansas | 3,043 |
| 3 | New York | 3,932 | | 28 | Virginia | 3,039 |
| 4 | Pennsylvania | 3,803 | | 29 | Mississippi | 2,989 |
| 5 | Massachusetts | 3,738 | | 30 | West Virginia | 2,921 |
| 6 | Michigan | 3,679 | | 31 | Wyoming | 2,839 |
| 7 | Ohio | 3,646 | | 32 | North Dakota | 2,831 |
| 8 | Alabama | 3,443 | | 33 | Washington | 2,790 |
| 9 | Illinois | 3,424 | | 34 | Wisconsin | 2,768 |
| 10 | California | 3,406 | | 35 | Montana | 2,762 |
| 11 | Connecticut | 3,387 | | 36 | New Hampshire | 2,733 |
| 12 | Florida | 3,381 | | 36 | North Carolina | 2,733 |
| 13 | Alaska | 3,375 | | 38 | Colorado | 2,710 |
| 14 | Texas | 3,371 | | 39 | Iowa | 2,700 |
| 15 | Delaware | 3,344 | | 40 | Maine | 2,686 |
| 16 | New Jersey | 3,326 | | 41 | New Mexico | 2,636 |
| 17 | Georgia | 3,318 | | 42 | South Carolina | 2,566 |
| 18 | Missouri | 3,276 | | 43 | Nebraska | 2,546 |
| 19 | Tennessee | 3,272 | | 44 | Utah | 2,533 |
| 20 | Arizona | 3,193 | | 44 | Vermont | 2,533 |
| 21 | Kentucky | 3,189 | | 46 | South Dakota | 2,529 |
| 22 | Rhode Island | 3,147 | | 47 | Idaho | 2,446 |
| 23 | Oklahoma | 3,122 | | 48 | Minnesota | 2,430 |
| 24 | Indiana | 3,087 | | 49 | Oregon | 2,295 |
| 25 | Kansas | 3,055 | | 50 | Hawaii | 2,152 |

District of Columbia          4,698

Source: U.S. Department of Health and Human Services, Health Care Financing Administration
    unpublished data

*For fiscal year 1991. Includes payments to aged and disabled enrollees. National rate includes payments to addresses in territories, foreign addresses and "residence unknown."

# Percent of Population Enrolled in Medicare in 1991

## National Rate = 13.54%*

| RANK | STATE | PERCENT |
|---|---|---|
| 1 | Florida | 18.09 |
| 2 | West Virginia | 17.34 |
| 3 | Arkansas | 16.75 |
| 4 | Pennsylvania | 16.59 |
| 5 | Iowa | 16.49 |
| 6 | Rhode Island | 16.00 |
| 7 | South Dakota | 15.86 |
| 8 | North Dakota | 15.69 |
| 9 | Missouri | 15.35 |
| 10 | Maine | 15.07 |
| 11 | Nebraska | 15.06 |
| 12 | Montana | 14.86 |
| 13 | Oregon | 14.84 |
| 14 | Kansas | 14.74 |
| 15 | Massachusetts | 14.66 |
| 16 | Kentucky | 14.62 |
| 17 | Wisconsin | 14.59 |
| 18 | Alabama | 14.50 |
| 19 | Connecticut | 14.46 |
| 20 | Oklahoma | 14.44 |
| 21 | Ohio | 14.36 |
| 22 | Mississippi | 14.32 |
| 23 | New Jersey | 14.29 |
| 24 | Tennessee | 14.26 |
| 25 | New York | 14.01 |

| RANK | STATE | PERCENT |
|---|---|---|
| 26 | Indiana | 13.81 |
| 27 | Arizona | 13.79 |
| 28 | North Carolina | 13.61 |
| 29 | Minnesota | 13.47 |
| 30 | Illinois | 13.45 |
| 31 | Michigan | 13.42 |
| 32 | Vermont | 13.37 |
| 33 | Delaware | 13.32 |
| 34 | Idaho | 13.03 |
| 35 | South Carolina | 12.76 |
| 36 | New Hampshire | 12.74 |
| 37 | Louisiana | 12.71 |
| 38 | Washington | 12.55 |
| 39 | New Mexico | 11.99 |
| 40 | Virginia | 11.78 |
| 41 | Nevada | 11.73 |
| 42 | Wyoming | 11.61 |
| 43 | Hawaii | 11.55 |
| 44 | Maryland | 11.39 |
| 45 | Georgia | 11.32 |
| 46 | California | 11.03 |
| 47 | Colorado | 10.94 |
| 48 | Texas | 10.79 |
| 49 | Utah | 9.35 |
| 50 | Alaska | 4.65 |

| | District of Columbia | 13.02 |
|---|---|---|

Source: U.S. Department of Health and Human Services, Health Care Financing Administration
  unpublished data

*Rates calculated by the editors using 1991 Census resident population figures. As of July 1, 1991. Includes aged and disabled enrollees. Total percent is only for residents of the 50 states, the District of Columbia and those whose address is unknown (34,152,964 enrollees).

# Medicare Aged Program Benefit Payments in 1991

## National Total = $101,319,000,000*

| RANK | STATE | BENEFITS | % | | RANK | STATE | BENEFITS | % |
|------|-------|----------|---|---|------|-------|----------|---|
| 1 | California | $10,038,000,000 | 9.91% | | 26 | Oklahoma | $1,290,000,000 | 1.27% |
| 2 | New York | 8,893,000,000 | 8.78% | | 27 | Iowa | 1,128,000,000 | 1.11% |
| 3 | Florida | 7,440,000,000 | 7.34% | | 28 | Arkansas | 1,065,000,000 | 1.05% |
| 4 | Pennsylvania | 6,839,000,000 | 6.75% | | 29 | Kansas | 1,030,000,000 | 1.02% |
| 5 | Texas | 5,589,000,000 | 5.52% | | 30 | South Carolina | 979,000,000 | 0.97% |
| 6 | Ohio | 5,119,000,000 | 5.05% | | 31 | Mississippi | 940,000,000 | 0.93% |
| 7 | Illinois | 4,735,000,000 | 4.67% | | 32 | Oregon | 892,000,000 | 0.88% |
| 8 | Michigan | 4,107,000,000 | 4.05% | | 33 | Colorado | 881,000,000 | 0.87% |
| 9 | New Jersey | 3,309,000,000 | 3.27% | | 34 | West Virginia | 798,000,000 | 0.79% |
| 10 | Massachusetts | 2,972,000,000 | 2.93% | | 35 | Nebraska | 555,000,000 | 0.55% |
| 11 | Missouri | 2,310,000,000 | 2.28% | | 36 | Rhode Island | 456,000,000 | 0.45% |
| 12 | North Carolina | 2,140,000,000 | 2.11% | | 37 | Maine | 447,000,000 | 0.44% |
| 13 | Georgia | 2,117,000,000 | 2.09% | | 38 | New Mexico | 425,000,000 | 0.42% |
| 14 | Indiana | 2,114,000,000 | 2.09% | | 39 | Nevada | 413,000,000 | 0.41% |
| 15 | Tennessee | 2,009,000,000 | 1.98% | | 40 | Utah | 379,000,000 | 0.37% |
| 16 | Maryland | 1,987,000,000 | 1.96% | | 41 | New Hampshire | 347,000,000 | 0.34% |
| 17 | Virginia | 1,953,000,000 | 1.93% | | 42 | Idaho | 306,000,000 | 0.30% |
| 18 | Louisiana | 1,882,000,000 | 1.86% | | 43 | Montana | 298,000,000 | 0.29% |
| 19 | Wisconsin | 1,797,000,000 | 1.77% | | 44 | Delaware | 271,000,000 | 0.27% |
| 20 | Alabama | 1,768,000,000 | 1.74% | | 45 | North Dakota | 262,000,000 | 0.26% |
| 21 | Washington | 1,571,000,000 | 1.55% | | 46 | South Dakota | 257,000,000 | 0.25% |
| 22 | Kentucky | 1,500,000,000 | 1.48% | | 47 | Hawaii | 246,000,000 | 0.24% |
| 23 | Arizona | 1,489,000,000 | 1.47% | | 48 | Vermont | 172,000,000 | 0.17% |
| 24 | Connecticut | 1,464,000,000 | 1.44% | | 49 | Wyoming | 135,000,000 | 0.13% |
| 25 | Minnesota | 1,311,000,000 | 1.29% | | 50 | Alaska | 76,000,000 | 0.08% |
| | | | | | | District of Columbia | 314,000,000 | 0.31% |

Source: U.S. Department of Health and Human Services, Health Care Financing Administration
   unpublished data

*For fiscal year 1991.  Total includes $517,000,000 in payments to addresses in territories, foreign addresses and "residence unknown."

# Medicare Aged Program Enrollees in 1991

## National Total = 31,484,779 Aged Enrollees*

| RANK | STATE | ENROLLEES | % | RANK | STATE | ENROLLEES | % |
|---|---|---|---|---|---|---|---|
| 1 | California | 3,048,494 | 9.68% | 26 | Iowa | 425,488 | 1.35% |
| 2 | New York | 2,294,259 | 7.29% | 27 | Oklahoma | 417,051 | 1.32% |
| 3 | Florida | 2,229,882 | 7.08% | 28 | Oregon | 398,492 | 1.27% |
| 4 | Pennsylvania | 1,824,329 | 5.79% | 29 | South Carolina | 393,145 | 1.25% |
| 5 | Texas | 1,703,982 | 5.41% | 30 | Arkansas | 347,195 | 1.10% |
| 6 | Illinois | 1,416,452 | 4.50% | 31 | Kansas | 340,786 | 1.08% |
| 7 | Ohio | 1,410,956 | 4.48% | 32 | Colorado | 332,636 | 1.06% |
| 8 | Michigan | 1,121,440 | 3.56% | 33 | Mississippi | 315,669 | 1.00% |
| 9 | New Jersey | 1,020,175 | 3.24% | 34 | West Virginia | 267,279 | 0.85% |
| 10 | North Carolina | 806,437 | 2.56% | 35 | Nebraska | 222,954 | 0.71% |
| 11 | Massachusetts | 803,420 | 2.55% | 36 | Maine | 166,878 | 0.53% |
| 12 | Missouri | 713,885 | 2.27% | 37 | New Mexico | 165,103 | 0.52% |
| 13 | Indiana | 695,548 | 2.21% | 38 | Utah | 151,828 | 0.48% |
| 14 | Virginia | 660,553 | 2.10% | 39 | Rhode Island | 146,162 | 0.46% |
| 15 | Wisconsin | 657,325 | 2.09% | 40 | Nevada | 136,734 | 0.43% |
| 16 | Georgia | 649,564 | 2.06% | 41 | New Hampshire | 129,085 | 0.41% |
| 17 | Tennessee | 617,837 | 1.96% | 42 | Idaho | 124,198 | 0.39% |
| 18 | Washington | 573,789 | 1.82% | 43 | Hawaii | 121,946 | 0.39% |
| 19 | Minnesota | 551,000 | 1.75% | 44 | Montana | 107,765 | 0.34% |
| 20 | Alabama | 515,488 | 1.64% | 45 | South Dakota | 102,752 | 0.33% |
| 21 | Maryland | 506,332 | 1.61% | 46 | North Dakota | 92,104 | 0.29% |
| 22 | Arizona | 471,814 | 1.50% | 47 | Delaware | 81,877 | 0.26% |
| 23 | Louisiana | 466,461 | 1.48% | 48 | Vermont | 68,556 | 0.22% |
| 24 | Kentucky | 464,085 | 1.47% | 49 | Wyoming | 48,779 | 0.15% |
| 25 | Connecticut | 441,386 | 1.40% | 50 | Alaska | 23,157 | 0.07% |
| | | | | | District of Columbia | 70,938 | 0.23% |

Source: U.S. Department of Health and Human Services, Health Care Financing Administration
   unpublished data

*As of July 1, 1991. Total includes 621,329 enrollees in territories, foreign countries and whose residences are unknown.

# Medicare Aged Program Benefit Payments per Aged Enrollee in 1991

## National Rate = $3,218 per Aged Enrollee*

| RANK | STATE | PER ENROLLEE | | RANK | STATE | PER ENROLLEE |
|------|-------|--------------|---|------|-------|--------------|
| 1 | Louisiana | $4,035 | | 26 | Kansas | $3,021 |
| 2 | Maryland | 3,924 | | 27 | Nevada | 3,017 |
| 3 | New York | 3,876 | | 28 | West Virginia | 2,985 |
| 4 | Pennsylvania | 3,749 | | 29 | Mississippi | 2,979 |
| 5 | Massachusetts | 3,699 | | 30 | Virginia | 2,956 |
| 6 | Michigan | 3,663 | | 31 | North Dakota | 2,841 |
| 7 | Ohio | 3,628 | | 32 | Montana | 2,763 |
| 8 | Alabama | 3,429 | | 33 | Wyoming | 2,761 |
| 9 | Illinois | 3,343 | | 34 | Washington | 2,738 |
| 10 | Florida | 3,337 | | 35 | Wisconsin | 2,733 |
| 11 | Connecticut | 3,317 | | 36 | New Hampshire | 2,686 |
| 12 | Delaware | 3,308 | | 37 | Maine | 2,679 |
| 13 | California | 3,293 | | 38 | North Carolina | 2,654 |
| 14 | Texas | 3,280 | | 39 | Iowa | 2,652 |
| 15 | Alaska | 3,271 | | 40 | Colorado | 2,649 |
| 16 | Georgia | 3,258 | | 41 | New Mexico | 2,575 |
| 17 | Tennessee | 3,252 | | 42 | Vermont | 2,511 |
| 18 | New Jersey | 3,243 | | 43 | Utah | 2,499 |
| 19 | Missouri | 3,236 | | 44 | South Dakota | 2,498 |
| 20 | Kentucky | 3,232 | | 45 | South Carolina | 2,491 |
| 21 | Arizona | 3,155 | | 46 | Nebraska | 2,489 |
| 22 | Rhode Island | 3,121 | | 47 | Idaho | 2,460 |
| 23 | Oklahoma | 3,093 | | 48 | Minnesota | 2,379 |
| 24 | Arkansas | 3,069 | | 49 | Oregon | 2,238 |
| 25 | Indiana | 3,039 | | 50 | Hawaii | 2,019 |
| | | | | | District of Columbia | 4,429 |

Source: U.S. Department of Health and Human Services, Health Care Financing Administration
     unpublished data

*For fiscal year 1991.  National rate includes payments to addresses in territories, foreign addresses and "residence unknown."

# Percent of Population Enrolled in Medicare Aged Program in 1991

## National Rate = 12.24%*

| RANK | STATE | PERCENT | RANK | STATE | PERCENT |
|------|-------|---------|------|-------|---------|
| 1 | Florida | 16.80 | 26 | Minnesota | 12.43 |
| 2 | Pennsylvania | 15.25 | 27 | Indiana | 12.40 |
| 3 | Iowa | 15.22 | 28 | Illinois | 12.27 |
| 4 | West Virginia | 14.84 | 29 | Mississippi | 12.18 |
| 5 | Arkansas | 14.64 | 30 | Vermont | 12.09 |
| 6 | South Dakota | 14.62 | 31 | Delaware | 12.04 |
| 7 | Rhode Island | 14.56 | 32 | Michigan | 11.97 |
| 8 | North Dakota | 14.50 | 33 | North Carolina | 11.97 |
| 9 | Nebraska | 14.00 | 34 | Idaho | 11.95 |
| 10 | Missouri | 13.84 | 35 | New Hampshire | 11.68 |
| 11 | Kansas | 13.66 | 36 | Washington | 11.43 |
| 12 | Oregon | 13.64 | 37 | South Carolina | 11.04 |
| 13 | Maine | 13.51 | 38 | Louisiana | 10.97 |
| 14 | Connecticut | 13.41 | 39 | Hawaii | 10.74 |
| 15 | Massachusetts | 13.40 | 40 | New Mexico | 10.67 |
| 16 | Montana | 13.34 | 41 | Nevada | 10.65 |
| 17 | Wisconsin | 13.27 | 42 | Wyoming | 10.60 |
| 18 | New Jersey | 13.15 | 43 | Virginia | 10.51 |
| 19 | Oklahoma | 13.14 | 44 | Maryland | 10.42 |
| 20 | Ohio | 12.90 | 45 | California | 10.03 |
| 21 | New York | 12.70 | 46 | Colorado | 9.85 |
| 22 | Alabama | 12.61 | 47 | Texas | 9.82 |
| 23 | Arizona | 12.58 | 48 | Georgia | 9.81 |
| 24 | Kentucky | 12.50 | 49 | Utah | 8.58 |
| 25 | Tennessee | 12.47 | 50 | Alaska | 4.06 |
| | | | | District of Columbia | 11.86 |

Source: U.S. Department of Health and Human Services, Health Care Financing Administration
    unpublished data

*Rates calculated by the editors using 1991 Census resident population figures. As of July 1, 1991. Includes aged and disabled enrollees. National rate is only for residents of the 50 states, the District of Columbia and those whose address is unknown (30,875,211 enrollees).

# Medicare Disabled Program Benefit Payments in 1991

## National Total = $12,672,000,000*

| RANK | STATE | BENEFITS | % | RANK | STATE | BENEFITS | % |
|---|---|---|---|---|---|---|---|
| 1 | California | $1,378,000,000 | 10.87% | 26 | Connecticut | $148,000,000 | 1.17% |
| 2 | New York | 1,054,000,000 | 8.32% | 27 | Arkansas | 143,000,000 | 1.13% |
| 3 | Texas | 723,000,000 | 5.71% | 28 | Oklahoma | 141,000,000 | 1.11% |
| 4 | Pennsylvania | 709,000,000 | 5.60% | 29 | Minnesota | 140,000,000 | 1.10% |
| 5 | Florida | 682,000,000 | 5.38% | 30 | Colorado | 120,000,000 | 0.95% |
| 6 | Ohio | 611,000,000 | 4.82% | 31 | Iowa | 116,000,000 | 0.92% |
| 7 | Illinois | 583,000,000 | 4.60% | 32 | West Virginia | 114,000,000 | 0.90% |
| 8 | Michigan | 516,000,000 | 4.07% | 33 | Oregon | 103,000,000 | 0.81% |
| 9 | New Jersey | 378,000,000 | 2.98% | 34 | Kansas | 94,000,000 | 0.74% |
| 10 | Georgia | 371,000,000 | 2.93% | 35 | New Mexico | 64,000,000 | 0.51% |
| 11 | North Carolina | 366,000,000 | 2.89% | 36 | Nebraska | 56,000,000 | 0.44% |
| 12 | Massachusetts | 314,000,000 | 2.48% | 37 | Maine | 53,000,000 | 0.42% |
| 13 | Louisiana | 313,000,000 | 2.47% | 38 | Rhode Island | 49,000,000 | 0.39% |
| 14 | Tennessee | 303,000,000 | 2.39% | 39 | Nevada | 46,000,000 | 0.36% |
| 15 | Virginia | 298,000,000 | 2.35% | 40 | Utah | 40,000,000 | 0.32% |
| 16 | Missouri | 284,000,000 | 2.24% | 41 | New Hampshire | 38,000,000 | 0.30% |
| 17 | Indiana | 278,000,000 | 2.19% | 42 | Hawaii | 36,000,000 | 0.28% |
| 18 | Alabama | 274,000,000 | 2.16% | 43 | Montana | 34,000,000 | 0.27% |
| 19 | Maryland | 250,000,000 | 1.97% | 44 | Delaware | 32,000,000 | 0.25% |
| 20 | Kentucky | 231,000,000 | 1.82% | 45 | Idaho | 26,000,000 | 0.21% |
| 21 | Wisconsin | 204,000,000 | 1.61% | 46 | South Dakota | 25,000,000 | 0.20% |
| 22 | South Carolina | 186,000,000 | 1.47% | 47 | North Dakota | 21,000,000 | 0.17% |
| 22 | Washington | 186,000,000 | 1.47% | 48 | Vermont | 20,000,000 | 0.16% |
| 24 | Mississippi | 169,000,000 | 1.33% | 49 | Wyoming | 17,000,000 | 0.13% |
| 25 | Arizona | 163,000,000 | 1.29% | 50 | Alaska | 14,000,000 | 0.11% |
| | | | | | District of Columbia | 52,000,000 | 0.41% |

Source: U.S. Department of Health and Human Services, Health Care Financing Administration
   unpublished data

*For fiscal year 1991. Total includes $108,000,000 in payments to addresses in territories, foreign addresses and "residence unknown."

# Medicare Disabled Program Enrollees in 1991

## National Total = 3,385,461 Disabled Enrollees*

| RANK | STATE | ENROLLEES | % | RANK | STATE | ENROLLEES | % |
|---|---|---|---|---|---|---|---|
| 1 | California | 303,261 | 8.96% | 26 | Minnesota | 45,834 | 1.35% |
| 2 | New York | 235,144 | 6.95% | 27 | Arizona | 45,372 | 1.34% |
| 3 | Florida | 172,157 | 5.09% | 28 | West Virginia | 45,020 | 1.33% |
| 4 | Texas | 168,677 | 4.98% | 29 | Oklahoma | 41,261 | 1.22% |
| 5 | Pennsylvania | 160,452 | 4.74% | 30 | Colorado | 36,857 | 1.09% |
| 6 | Ohio | 160,345 | 4.74% | 31 | Iowa | 35,413 | 1.05% |
| 7 | Illinois | 136,634 | 4.04% | 32 | Oregon | 35,085 | 1.04% |
| 8 | Michigan | 135,485 | 4.00% | 33 | Connecticut | 34,540 | 1.02% |
| 9 | North Carolina | 110,597 | 3.27% | 34 | Kansas | 27,099 | 0.80% |
| 10 | Georgia | 100,355 | 2.96% | 35 | New Mexico | 20,430 | 0.60% |
| 11 | Tennessee | 88,639 | 2.62% | 36 | Maine | 19,181 | 0.57% |
| 12 | New Jersey | 88,452 | 2.61% | 37 | Nebraska | 16,940 | 0.50% |
| 13 | Virginia | 79,958 | 2.36% | 38 | Rhode Island | 14,475 | 0.43% |
| 14 | Indiana | 79,339 | 2.34% | 39 | Nevada | 13,888 | 0.41% |
| 15 | Kentucky | 78,709 | 2.32% | 40 | Utah | 13,692 | 0.40% |
| 16 | Missouri | 78,008 | 2.30% | 41 | Montana | 12,289 | 0.36% |
| 17 | Alabama | 77,619 | 2.29% | 42 | New Hampshire | 11,713 | 0.35% |
| 18 | Massachusetts | 75,755 | 2.24% | 43 | Idaho | 11,209 | 0.33% |
| 19 | Louisiana | 74,040 | 2.19% | 44 | Hawaii | 9,145 | 0.27% |
| 20 | Wisconsin | 65,651 | 1.94% | 45 | South Dakota | 8,741 | 0.26% |
| 21 | South Carolina | 61,071 | 1.80% | 46 | Delaware | 8,711 | 0.26% |
| 22 | Washington | 55,841 | 1.65% | 47 | North Dakota | 7,557 | 0.22% |
| 23 | Mississippi | 55,383 | 1.64% | 48 | Vermont | 7,233 | 0.21% |
| 24 | Arkansas | 50,038 | 1.48% | 49 | Wyoming | 4,648 | 0.14% |
| 25 | Maryland | 47,291 | 1.40% | 50 | Alaska | 3,359 | 0.10% |
| | | | | | District of Columbia | 6,944 | 0.21% |

Source: U.S. Department of Health and Human Services, Health Care Financing Administration
unpublished data

*As of July 1, 1991. Total includes 109,924 enrollees in territories, foreign countries and whose residences are unknown.

# Medicare Disabled Program Benefit Payments per Enrollee in 1991

## National Rate = $3,743 per Disabled Enrollee*

| RANK | STATE | PER ENROLLEE | | RANK | STATE | PER ENROLLEE |
|------|-------|--------------|---|------|-------|--------------|
| 1 | Maryland | $5,277 | | 25 | Tennessee | $3,415 |
| 2 | California | 4,545 | | 27 | Oklahoma | 3,412 |
| 3 | New York | 4,481 | | 28 | Washington | 3,329 |
| 4 | Pennsylvania | 4,421 | | 29 | Nevada | 3,315 |
| 5 | Texas | 4,286 | | 30 | North Carolina | 3,310 |
| 6 | New Jersey | 4,277 | | 31 | Nebraska | 3,297 |
| 7 | Connecticut | 4,275 | | 32 | Iowa | 3,286 |
| 8 | Illinois | 4,264 | | 33 | Colorado | 3,255 |
| 9 | Louisiana | 4,223 | | 34 | New Hampshire | 3,250 |
| 10 | Massachusetts | 4,148 | | 35 | New Mexico | 3,132 |
| 11 | Alaska | 4,095 | | 36 | Wisconsin | 3,112 |
| 12 | Florida | 3,959 | | 37 | Minnesota | 3,055 |
| 13 | Hawaii | 3,919 | | 38 | South Carolina | 3,052 |
| 14 | Michigan | 3,812 | | 39 | Mississippi | 3,048 |
| 15 | Ohio | 3,811 | | 40 | Oregon | 2,942 |
| 16 | Virginia | 3,724 | | 41 | Kentucky | 2,940 |
| 17 | Georgia | 3,701 | | 42 | Utah | 2,910 |
| 18 | Delaware | 3,678 | | 43 | South Dakota | 2,901 |
| 19 | Wyoming | 3,663 | | 44 | Arkansas | 2,863 |
| 20 | Missouri | 3,644 | | 45 | Montana | 2,754 |
| 21 | Arizona | 3,586 | | 46 | Maine | 2,752 |
| 22 | Alabama | 3,533 | | 47 | Vermont | 2,746 |
| 23 | Indiana | 3,499 | | 48 | North Dakota | 2,718 |
| 24 | Kansas | 3,476 | | 49 | West Virginia | 2,539 |
| 25 | Rhode Island | 3,415 | | 50 | Idaho | 2,294 |
| | | | | | District of Columbia | 7,447 |

*Source: U.S. Department of Health and Human Services, Health Care Financing Administration*
      *unpublished data*

*For fiscal year 1991. National figure includes payments to addresses in territories, foreign addresses and "residence unknown."*

# Percent of Population Enrolled in Medicare Disabled Program in 1991

## National Rate = 1.30%*

| RANK | STATE | PERCENT | RANK | STATE | PERCENT |
|---|---|---|---|---|---|
| 1 | West Virginia | 2.50 | 26 | Iowa | 1.27 |
| 2 | Mississippi | 2.14 | 26 | Virginia | 1.27 |
| 3 | Kentucky | 2.12 | 28 | Massachusetts | 1.26 |
| 4 | Arkansas | 2.11 | 29 | South Dakota | 1.24 |
| 5 | Alabama | 1.90 | 30 | Arizona | 1.21 |
| 6 | Tennessee | 1.79 | 31 | Oregon | 1.20 |
| 7 | Louisiana | 1.74 | 32 | North Dakota | 1.19 |
| 8 | South Carolina | 1.72 | 33 | Illinois | 1.18 |
| 9 | North Carolina | 1.64 | 34 | New Jersey | 1.14 |
| 10 | Maine | 1.55 | 35 | Washington | 1.11 |
| 11 | Georgia | 1.52 | 36 | Colorado | 1.09 |
| 11 | Montana | 1.52 | 36 | Kansas | 1.09 |
| 13 | Missouri | 1.51 | 38 | Idaho | 1.08 |
| 14 | Ohio | 1.47 | 38 | Nevada | 1.08 |
| 15 | Michigan | 1.45 | 40 | Nebraska | 1.06 |
| 16 | Rhode Island | 1.44 | 40 | New Hampshire | 1.06 |
| 17 | Indiana | 1.41 | 42 | Connecticut | 1.05 |
| 18 | Pennsylvania | 1.34 | 43 | Minnesota | 1.03 |
| 19 | New Mexico | 1.32 | 44 | Wyoming | 1.01 |
| 19 | Wisconsin | 1.32 | 45 | California | 1.00 |
| 21 | Florida | 1.30 | 46 | Maryland | 0.97 |
| 21 | New York | 1.30 | 46 | Texas | 0.97 |
| 21 | Oklahoma | 1.30 | 48 | Hawaii | 0.81 |
| 24 | Delaware | 1.28 | 49 | Utah | 0.77 |
| 24 | Vermont | 1.28 | 50 | Alaska | 0.59 |

District of Columbia            1.16

*Source: U.S. Department of Health and Human Services, Health Care Financing Administration*
*unpublished data*

*Calculated by the editors using 1991 Census resident population figures. As of July 1, 1991. National rate is only for residents of the 50 states, the District of Columbia and those whose address is unknown.*

# State and Local Government Expenditures for Health Programs in 1990

## National Total = $25,195,512,000*

| RANK | STATE | EXPENDITURES | % | RANK | STATE | EXPENDITURES | % |
|------|-------|--------------|---|------|-------|--------------|---|
| 1 | California | $3,494,936,000 | 13.87% | 26 | Louisiana | $275,962,000 | 1.10% |
| 2 | New York | 2,602,929,000 | 10.33% | 27 | Oregon | 261,333,000 | 1.04% |
| 3 | Michigan | 1,602,873,000 | 6.36% | 28 | Kentucky | 224,869,000 | 0.89% |
| 4 | Florida | 1,602,836,000 | 6.36% | 29 | Iowa | 190,697,000 | 0.76% |
| 5 | Ohio | 1,179,668,000 | 4.68% | 30 | Oklahoma | 174,549,000 | 0.69% |
| 6 | Illinois | 983,314,000 | 3.90% | 31 | Hawaii | 162,026,000 | 0.64% |
| 7 | Pennsylvania | 942,725,000 | 3.74% | 32 | Kansas | 158,714,000 | 0.63% |
| 8 | Texas | 920,884,000 | 3.65% | 33 | Mississippi | 157,547,000 | 0.63% |
| 9 | Massachusetts | 869,296,000 | 3.45% | 34 | Alaska | 148,357,000 | 0.59% |
| 10 | North Carolina | 778,168,000 | 3.09% | 35 | Rhode Island | 147,823,000 | 0.59% |
| 11 | Washington | 683,428,000 | 2.71% | 36 | Utah | 147,276,000 | 0.58% |
| 12 | Virginia | 669,877,000 | 2.66% | 37 | New Mexico | 144,509,000 | 0.57% |
| 13 | New Jersey | 566,467,000 | 2.25% | 38 | Arkansas | 144,244,000 | 0.57% |
| 14 | Maryland | 505,038,000 | 2.00% | 39 | West Virginia | 127,526,000 | 0.51% |
| 15 | Georgia | 488,733,000 | 1.94% | 40 | New Hampshire | 110,884,000 | 0.44% |
| 16 | Wisconsin | 454,735,000 | 1.80% | 41 | Delaware | 110,575,000 | 0.44% |
| 17 | South Carolina | 431,483,000 | 1.71% | 42 | Maine | 97,299,000 | 0.39% |
| 18 | Minnesota | 423,202,000 | 1.68% | 43 | Nevada | 92,731,000 | 0.37% |
| 19 | Missouri | 418,155,000 | 1.66% | 44 | Montana | 85,450,000 | 0.34% |
| 20 | Alabama | 409,093,000 | 1.62% | 45 | Idaho | 74,620,000 | 0.30% |
| 21 | Tennessee | 391,639,000 | 1.55% | 46 | Nebraska | 63,498,000 | 0.25% |
| 22 | Connecticut | 362,395,000 | 1.44% | 47 | South Dakota | 62,478,000 | 0.25% |
| 23 | Indiana | 341,054,000 | 1.35% | 48 | Wyoming | 52,172,000 | 0.21% |
| 24 | Arizona | 319,395,000 | 1.27% | 49 | Vermont | 46,615,000 | 0.19% |
| 25 | Colorado | 307,678,000 | 1.22% | 50 | North Dakota | 25,304,000 | 0.10% |
| | | | | | District of Columbia | 158,453,000 | 0.63% |

Source: U.S. Bureau of the Census

"Government Finances: 1989-90" (series GF/90-5, December 1991)

*Includes outpatient health services other than hospital care, research and education, categorical health programs, treatment and immunization clinics, nursing and environmental health activities. Includes capital expenditures.

# Per Capita State and Local Government Expenditures for Health Programs in 1990

## National Per Capita = $101.30*

| RANK | STATE | PER CAPITA | RANK | STATE | PER CAPITA |
|---|---|---|---|---|---|
| 1 | Alaska | $269.72 | 26 | South Dakota | $89.77 |
| 2 | Michigan | 172.44 | 27 | Arizona | 87.14 |
| 3 | Delaware | 165.99 | 28 | Illinois | 86.02 |
| 4 | Rhode Island | 147.31 | 29 | Utah | 85.48 |
| 5 | Hawaii | 146.20 | 30 | Vermont | 82.83 |
| 6 | New York | 144.68 | 31 | Missouri | 81.72 |
| 7 | Massachusetts | 144.49 | 32 | Tennessee | 80.30 |
| 8 | Washington | 140.43 | 33 | Pennsylvania | 79.34 |
| 9 | Florida | 123.89 | 34 | Maine | 79.24 |
| 10 | South Carolina | 123.75 | 35 | Nevada | 77.16 |
| 11 | California | 117.44 | 36 | Georgia | 75.44 |
| 12 | North Carolina | 117.39 | 37 | Idaho | 74.12 |
| 13 | Wyoming | 115.02 | 38 | New Jersey | 73.28 |
| 14 | Connecticut | 110.25 | 39 | West Virginia | 71.11 |
| 15 | Ohio | 108.75 | 40 | Iowa | 68.68 |
| 16 | Virginia | 108.27 | 41 | Louisiana | 65.39 |
| 17 | Montana | 106.94 | 42 | Kansas | 64.06 |
| 18 | Maryland | 105.62 | 43 | Indiana | 61.52 |
| 19 | Alabama | 101.25 | 44 | Arkansas | 61.36 |
| 20 | New Hampshire | 99.96 | 45 | Mississippi | 61.23 |
| 21 | Minnesota | 96.73 | 46 | Kentucky | 61.02 |
| 22 | New Mexico | 95.38 | 47 | Oklahoma | 55.49 |
| 23 | Colorado | 93.39 | 48 | Texas | 54.21 |
| 24 | Wisconsin | 92.96 | 49 | Nebraska | 40.23 |
| 25 | Oregon | 91.94 | 50 | North Dakota | 39.61 |
| | | | | District of Columbia | 261.09 |

Source: U.S. Bureau of the Census
    "Government Finances: 1989-90" (series GF/90-5, December 1991)
*Calculated by the editors using 1990 Census resident population figures. Includes outpatient health services other than hospital care, research and education, categorical health programs, treatment and immunization clinics, nursing, environmental health activities and capital expenditures.

# State and Local Government Expenditures for Hospitals in 1990

## National Total = $53,287,092,000*

| RANK | STATE | EXPENDITURES | % | RANK | STATE | EXPENDITURES | % |
|------|-------|--------------|---|------|-------|--------------|---|
| 1 | New York | $7,187,732,000 | 13.49% | 26 | Wisconsin | $632,064,000 | 1.19% |
| 2 | California | 6,939,192,000 | 13.02% | 27 | Kentucky | 531,837,000 | 1.00% |
| 3 | Texas | 3,482,359,000 | 6.54% | 28 | Kansas | 509,634,000 | 0.96% |
| 4 | Georgia | 2,740,531,000 | 5.14% | 29 | Colorado | 480,753,000 | 0.90% |
| 5 | Florida | 2,564,106,000 | 4.81% | 30 | Nebraska | 478,346,000 | 0.90% |
| 6 | Michigan | 1,819,229,000 | 3.41% | 31 | Oregon | 447,686,000 | 0.84% |
| 7 | North Carolina | 1,647,655,000 | 3.09% | 32 | Arkansas | 410,425,000 | 0.77% |
| 8 | Ohio | 1,642,913,000 | 3.08% | 33 | Maryland | 334,448,000 | 0.63% |
| 9 | Alabama | 1,525,304,000 | 2.86% | 34 | Arizona | 327,668,000 | 0.61% |
| 10 | Massachusetts | 1,420,864,000 | 2.67% | 35 | New Mexico | 297,895,000 | 0.56% |
| 11 | Louisiana | 1,352,007,000 | 2.54% | 36 | Nevada | 250,658,000 | 0.47% |
| 12 | Indiana | 1,350,319,000 | 2.53% | 37 | Utah | 250,436,000 | 0.47% |
| 13 | Illinois | 1,343,914,000 | 2.52% | 38 | West Virginia | 233,128,000 | 0.44% |
| 14 | Tennessee | 1,271,659,000 | 2.39% | 39 | Wyoming | 197,454,000 | 0.37% |
| 15 | Virginia | 1,207,732,000 | 2.27% | 40 | Hawaii | 179,248,000 | 0.34% |
| 16 | South Carolina | 1,151,002,000 | 2.16% | 41 | Idaho | 172,607,000 | 0.32% |
| 17 | Minnesota | 1,124,249,000 | 2.11% | 42 | Rhode Island | 124,567,000 | 0.23% |
| 18 | Pennsylvania | 1,044,747,000 | 1.96% | 43 | Maine | 103,893,000 | 0.19% |
| 19 | New Jersey | 1,038,102,000 | 1.95% | 44 | North Dakota | 62,776,000 | 0.12% |
| 20 | Mississippi | 940,374,000 | 1.76% | 45 | Alaska | 62,055,000 | 0.12% |
| 21 | Washington | 838,497,000 | 1.57% | 46 | Montana | 60,974,000 | 0.11% |
| 22 | Iowa | 819,831,000 | 1.54% | 47 | South Dakota | 52,624,000 | 0.10% |
| 23 | Missouri | 806,511,000 | 1.51% | 48 | New Hampshire | 47,319,000 | 0.09% |
| 24 | Oklahoma | 729,173,000 | 1.37% | 49 | Delaware | 46,716,000 | 0.09% |
| 25 | Connecticut | 675,367,000 | 1.27% | 50 | Vermont | 22,690,000 | 0.04% |
| | | | | | District of Columbia | 305,822,000 | 0.57% |

Source: U.S. Bureau of the Census

   "Government Finances: 1989-90" (series GF/90-5, December 1991)

*Financing, construction acquisition, maintenance or operation of hospital facilities, provision of hospital care and support of public or private hospitals.

# Per Capita State and Local Government Expenditures for Hospitals in 1990

## National Per Capita = $214.25*

| RANK | STATE | PER CAPITA | | RANK | STATE | PER CAPITA |
|------|-------|------------|---|------|-------|------------|
| 1 | Wyoming | $435.32 | | 26 | Washington | $172.29 |
| 2 | Georgia | 423.04 | | 27 | Idaho | 171.45 |
| 3 | New York | 399.53 | | 28 | Hawaii | 161.74 |
| 4 | Alabama | 377.50 | | 29 | Missouri | 157.61 |
| 5 | Mississippi | 365.45 | | 30 | Oregon | 157.51 |
| 6 | South Carolina | 330.11 | | 31 | Ohio | 151.46 |
| 7 | Louisiana | 320.38 | | 32 | Colorado | 145.93 |
| 8 | Nebraska | 303.06 | | 33 | Utah | 145.36 |
| 9 | Iowa | 295.25 | | 34 | Kentucky | 144.31 |
| 10 | Tennessee | 260.74 | | 35 | New Jersey | 134.29 |
| 11 | Minnesota | 256.97 | | 36 | West Virginia | 129.99 |
| 12 | North Carolina | 248.57 | | 37 | Wisconsin | 129.21 |
| 13 | Indiana | 243.56 | | 38 | Rhode Island | 124.14 |
| 14 | Massachusetts | 236.16 | | 39 | Illinois | 117.57 |
| 15 | California | 233.17 | | 40 | Alaska | 112.82 |
| 16 | Oklahoma | 231.81 | | 41 | North Dakota | 98.27 |
| 17 | Nevada | 208.56 | | 42 | Arizona | 89.40 |
| 18 | Kansas | 205.70 | | 43 | Pennsylvania | 87.93 |
| 19 | Connecticut | 205.46 | | 44 | Maine | 84.61 |
| 20 | Texas | 205.01 | | 45 | Montana | 76.31 |
| 21 | Florida | 198.19 | | 46 | South Dakota | 75.61 |
| 22 | New Mexico | 196.62 | | 47 | Delaware | 70.13 |
| 23 | Michigan | 195.71 | | 48 | Maryland | 69.95 |
| 24 | Virginia | 195.19 | | 49 | New Hampshire | 42.66 |
| 25 | Arkansas | 174.60 | | 50 | Vermont | 40.32 |

District of Columbia          503.91

Source: U.S. Bureau of the Census

   "Government Finances: 1989-90" (series GF/90-5, December 1991)

*Calculated by the editors using 1990 Census resident population figures. Financing, construction acquisition, maintenance or operation of hospital facilities, provision of hospital care and support of public or private hospitals.

# Hospital Semiprivate Room Charges in 1990

## National Average = $297 per Day for Hospital Semiprivate Room*

| RANK | STATE | AVERAGE CHARGE | RANK | STATE | AVERAGE CHARGE |
|---|---|---|---|---|---|
| 1 | Connecticut | $456 | 26 | Maryland | $266 |
| 2 | California | 453 | 27 | Idaho | 259 |
| 3 | Alaska | 407 | 28 | Indiana | 258 |
| 4 | Delaware | 385 | 29 | Kansas | 256 |
| 5 | Vermont | 378 | 30 | New Mexico | 254 |
| 6 | Pennsylvania | 375 | 31 | Nevada | 251 |
| 7 | Utah | 353 | 32 | Kentucky | 242 |
| 8 | Massachusetts | 351 | 33 | Wyoming | 234 |
| 9 | Hawaii | 348 | 34 | North Dakota | 230 |
| 10 | Rhode Island | 342 | 35 | Texas | 223 |
| 11 | New York | 339 | 35 | West Virginia | 223 |
| 12 | Oregon | 338 | 37 | Wisconsin | 222 |
| 13 | Michigan | 337 | 38 | Iowa | 221 |
| 14 | Maine | 335 | 39 | North Carolina | 220 |
| 15 | Washington | 334 | 39 | Oklahoma | 220 |
| 16 | Colorado | 321 | 39 | Virginia | 220 |
| 17 | Montana | 318 | 42 | South Carolina | 212 |
| 18 | Ohio | 308 | 43 | Alabama | 210 |
| 19 | New Hampshire | 304 | 44 | Nebraska | 209 |
| 20 | Arizona | 300 | 44 | South Dakota | 209 |
| 20 | Illinois | 300 | 46 | Louisiana | 203 |
| 22 | Minnesota | 282 | 47 | Georgia | 198 |
| 23 | New Jersey | 273 | 48 | Tennessee | 183 |
| 24 | Florida | 271 | 49 | Arkansas | 170 |
| 25 | Missouri | 268 | 50 | Mississippi | 167 |
| | | | | District of Columbia | 325 |

Source: Health Insurance Association of America

"Hospital Semiprivate Room Charges Survey, 1989" (Reprinted with permission from the H.I.A.A.)

*As of January 1990.

304

## Percent Change in Hospital Semiprivate Room Charges, 1989 to 1990

## National Percent Change = 12.5% Increase

| RANK | STATE | PERCENT CHANGE | RANK | STATE | PERCENT CHANGE |
|------|-------|----------------|------|-------|----------------|
| 1 | Vermont | 24.8 | 26 | Kentucky | 11.5 |
| 2 | New Jersey | 20.8 | 27 | Idaho | 11.2 |
| 3 | Maine | 20.1 | 28 | Texas | 10.4 |
| 4 | North Carolina | 18.9 | 29 | Delaware | 10.0 |
| 5 | Pennsylvania | 17.9 | 29 | Georgia | 10.0 |
| 6 | Mississippi | 17.6 | 31 | Hawaii | 9.8 |
| 7 | Colorado | 17.5 | 32 | Ohio | 9.6 |
| 8 | Arizona | 17.2 | 33 | Illinois | 9.1 |
| 9 | California | 15.9 | 34 | Missouri | 8.9 |
| 10 | Minnesota | 15.6 | 35 | North Dakota | 7.9 |
| 11 | Rhode Island | 15.5 | 36 | Alaska | 7.7 |
| 12 | Connecticut | 15.2 | 36 | Michigan | 7.7 |
| 13 | Indiana | 14.7 | 38 | Utah | 7.6 |
| 14 | Maryland | 14.2 | 39 | Massachusetts | 7.3 |
| 15 | Florida | 13.4 | 39 | Oklahoma | 7.3 |
| 15 | Virginia | 13.4 | 41 | Kansas | 7.1 |
| 17 | Nebraska | 13.0 | 42 | Wyoming | 6.9 |
| 18 | New York | 12.6 | 43 | South Carolina | 6.5 |
| 19 | Alabama | 12.3 | 44 | New Mexico | 5.8 |
| 19 | Oregon | 12.3 | 44 | Tennessee | 5.8 |
| 21 | Louisiana | 12.2 | 46 | Arkansas | 5.6 |
| 22 | Washington | 12.1 | 47 | Iowa | 5.2 |
| 23 | Montana | 12.0 | 48 | Nevada | 5.0 |
| 24 | New Hampshire | 11.8 | 49 | West Virginia | 4.7 |
| 24 | South Dakota | 11.8 | 50 | Wisconsin | 3.7 |

District of Columbia          0.0

Source: Health Insurance Association of America

"Hospital Semiprivate Room Charges Survey, 1989" (Reprinted with permission from the H.I.A.A.)

# Gross Median Practice Income for Physicians in 1990

## National Median = $249,580*

| RANK | STATE | GROSS INCOME | | RANK | STATE | GROSS INCOME |
|------|-------|--------------|---|------|-------|--------------|
| 1 | Texas | $340,280 | | | | |
| 2 | Florida | 270,830 | | | | |
| 3 | Virginia | 261,110 | | | | |
| 4 | Illinois | 257,500 | | | | |
| 5 | California | 256,250 | | | | |
| 6 | New Jersey | 250,000 | | | | |
| 6 | New York | 250,000 | | | | |
| 8 | Ohio | 233,330 | | | | |
| 9 | Pennsylvania | 228,570 | | | | |
| 10 | Massachusetts | 221,150 | | | | |

Source: Medical Economics Publishing Company (Copyright 1991, reprinted with permission)
    "The Medical Economics Continuing Survey 1991"
*Data available for selected states only.  National median is for all states, not just those shown separately.

# Net Median Practice Income for Physicians in 1990

## National Median = $141,720*

| RANK | STATE | NET INCOME | | RANK | STATE | NET INCOME |
|------|-------|-----------|---|------|-------|-----------|
| 1 | Texas | $165,630 | | | | |
| 2 | Florida | 155,560 | | | | |
| 3 | Massachusetts | 150,000 | | | | |
| 3 | New Jersey | 150,000 | | | | |
| 5 | New York | 144,500 | | | | |
| 6 | Ohio | 143,330 | | | | |
| 7 | Illinois | 142,500 | | | | |
| 8 | California | 140,830 | | | | |
| 9 | Virginia | 140,630 | | | | |
| 10 | Pennsylvania | 131,000 | | | | |

*Source: Medical Economics Publishing Company (Copyright 1991, reprinted with permission)*
*"The Medical Economics Continuing Survey 1991"*
*Data available for selected states only. National median is for all states, not just those shown separately. Using a different methodology, the 1992 survey shows a 1991 national net median of $140,090. No state breakdowns were compiled in 1992.*

# V. INCIDENCE OF DISEASE

# V. INCIDENCE OF DISEASE (continued)

# Estimated New Cancer Cases in 1992

## National Total = 1,130,000 New Cancer Cases*

| RANK | STATE | CASES | % | RANK | STATE | CASES | % |
|------|-------|-------|-----|------|-------|-------|-----|
| 1 | California | 116,000 | 10.27% | 26 | Oklahoma | 14,800 | 1.31% |
| 2 | New York | 87,000 | 7.70% | 27 | South Carolina | 14,500 | 1.28% |
| 3 | Florida | 76,000 | 6.73% | 28 | Oregon | 13,700 | 1.21% |
| 4 | Pennsylvania | 66,000 | 5.84% | 29 | Iowa | 13,500 | 1.19% |
| 5 | Texas | 60,000 | 5.31% | 30 | Arkansas | 12,600 | 1.12% |
| 6 | Illinois | 53,000 | 4.69% | 31 | Mississippi | 12,500 | 1.11% |
| 7 | Ohio | 52,500 | 4.65% | 32 | Kansas | 11,000 | 0.97% |
| 8 | Michigan | 40,600 | 3.59% | 33 | Colorado | 10,600 | 0.94% |
| 9 | New Jersey | 39,400 | 3.49% | 34 | West Virginia | 10,200 | 0.90% |
| 10 | North Carolina | 30,000 | 2.65% | 35 | Nebraska | 7,100 | 0.63% |
| 11 | Massachusetts | 29,600 | 2.62% | 36 | Maine | 6,400 | 0.57% |
| 12 | Georgia | 26,500 | 2.35% | 37 | Nevada | 5,300 | 0.47% |
| 12 | Indiana | 26,500 | 2.35% | 37 | Rhode Island | 5,300 | 0.47% |
| 14 | Virginia | 26,400 | 2.34% | 39 | New Mexico | 5,200 | 0.46% |
| 15 | Missouri | 24,900 | 2.20% | 40 | New Hampshire | 5,100 | 0.45% |
| 16 | Tennessee | 23,500 | 2.08% | 41 | Utah | 4,000 | 0.35% |
| 17 | Wisconsin | 22,000 | 1.95% | 42 | Idaho | 3,800 | 0.34% |
| 18 | Maryland | 21,600 | 1.91% | 43 | Hawaii | 3,600 | 0.32% |
| 19 | Alabama | 20,200 | 1.79% | 44 | Montana | 3,500 | 0.31% |
| 20 | Louisiana | 19,500 | 1.73% | 45 | Delaware | 3,300 | 0.29% |
| 20 | Washington | 19,500 | 1.73% | 46 | South Dakota | 3,200 | 0.28% |
| 22 | Minnesota | 18,400 | 1.63% | 47 | North Dakota | 2,900 | 0.26% |
| 23 | Kentucky | 18,000 | 1.59% | 48 | Vermont | 2,400 | 0.21% |
| 24 | Arizona | 16,000 | 1.42% | 49 | Wyoming | 1,600 | 0.14% |
| 25 | Connecticut | 15,800 | 1.40% | 50 | Alaska | 1,200 | 0.11% |
| | | | | | District of Columbia | 3,800 | 0.34% |

Source: American Cancer Society

*"Cancer Facts & Figures – 1992" (Copyright 1992, Reprinted with permission from the American Cancer Society)*

*These estimates are offered as a rough guide and should not be regarded as definitive. They are calculated according to the distribution of estimated 1992 cancer deaths by state. Totals do not include carcinoma in situ or basal and squamous cell skin cancers.*

# Estimated New Cancer Cases per 100,000 Population in 1992

## National Estimated Rate = 448.10 New Cancer Cases per 100,000 Population*

| RANK | STATE | RATE | | RANK | STATE | RATE |
|---|---|---|---|---|---|---|
| 1 | Florida | 572.42 | | 26 | South Dakota | 455.19 |
| 2 | West Virginia | 566.35 | | 27 | Nebraska | 445.70 |
| 3 | Pennsylvania | 551.79 | | 28 | North Carolina | 445.30 |
| 4 | Arkansas | 531.20 | | 29 | Maryland | 444.44 |
| 5 | Rhode Island | 527.89 | | 30 | Wisconsin | 444.00 |
| 6 | Maine | 518.22 | | 31 | Kansas | 440.88 |
| 7 | New Jersey | 507.73 | | 32 | Michigan | 433.39 |
| 8 | Alabama | 494.01 | | 33 | Montana | 433.17 |
| 9 | Massachusetts | 493.66 | | 34 | Arizona | 426.67 |
| 10 | Delaware | 485.29 | | 35 | Vermont | 423.28 |
| 11 | Kentucky | 484.78 | | 36 | Virginia | 419.98 |
| 12 | Iowa | 483.01 | | 37 | Minnesota | 415.16 |
| 13 | Missouri | 482.75 | | 38 | Nevada | 412.77 |
| 14 | Mississippi | 482.25 | | 39 | South Carolina | 407.30 |
| 15 | New York | 481.78 | | 40 | Georgia | 400.12 |
| 16 | Connecticut | 480.10 | | 41 | Washington | 388.60 |
| 17 | Ohio | 479.93 | | 42 | California | 381.83 |
| 18 | Tennessee | 474.46 | | 43 | Idaho | 365.74 |
| 19 | Indiana | 472.37 | | 44 | Wyoming | 347.83 |
| 20 | Oregon | 468.86 | | 45 | Texas | 345.84 |
| 21 | Oklahoma | 466.14 | | 46 | New Mexico | 335.92 |
| 22 | New Hampshire | 461.54 | | 47 | Hawaii | 317.18 |
| 23 | Illinois | 459.15 | | 48 | Colorado | 313.89 |
| 24 | Louisiana | 458.61 | | 49 | Utah | 225.99 |
| 25 | North Dakota | 456.69 | | 50 | Alaska | 210.53 |

District of Columbia     635.45

Source: American Cancer Society

"Cancer Facts & Figures – 1992" (Copyright 1992, Reprinted with permission from the American Cancer Society)

*Calculated by the editors using 1991 Census resident population figures. These estimates are offered as a rough guide and should not be regarded as definitive. They are calculated according to the distribution of estimated 1992 cancer deaths by state.

# Estimated New Female Breast Cancer Cases in 1992

## National Total = 180,000 New Female Breast Cancer Cases*

| RANK | STATE | CASES | % | RANK | STATE | CASES | % |
|------|-------|-------|---|------|-------|-------|---|
| 1 | California | 18,000 | 10.00% | 26 | Iowa | 2,300 | 1.28% |
| 2 | New York | 15,900 | 8.83% | 26 | South Carolina | 2,300 | 1.28% |
| 3 | Florida | 11,200 | 6.22% | 28 | Oklahoma | 2,100 | 1.17% |
| 4 | Pennsylvania | 10,700 | 5.94% | 28 | Oregon | 2,100 | 1.17% |
| 5 | Texas | 8,700 | 4.83% | 30 | Colorado | 1,800 | 1.00% |
| 6 | Illinois | 8,600 | 4.78% | 30 | Kansas | 1,800 | 1.00% |
| 6 | Ohio | 8,600 | 4.78% | 32 | Arkansas | 1,700 | 0.94% |
| 8 | New Jersey | 6,700 | 3.72% | 32 | Mississippi | 1,700 | 0.94% |
| 9 | Michigan | 6,600 | 3.67% | 34 | West Virginia | 1,400 | 0.78% |
| 10 | Massachusetts | 5,400 | 3.00% | 35 | Nebraska | 1,200 | 0.67% |
| 11 | North Carolina | 5,100 | 2.83% | 36 | Rhode Island | 1,000 | 0.56% |
| 12 | Georgia | 4,400 | 2.44% | 37 | New Hampshire | 900 | 0.50% |
| 13 | Virginia | 4,300 | 2.39% | 37 | New Mexico | 900 | 0.50% |
| 14 | Indiana | 4,100 | 2.28% | 39 | Maine | 850 | 0.47% |
| 15 | Missouri | 3,900 | 2.17% | 40 | Nevada | 750 | 0.42% |
| 16 | Tennessee | 3,600 | 2.00% | 41 | Utah | 700 | 0.39% |
| 17 | Maryland | 3,500 | 1.94% | 42 | Delaware | 600 | 0.33% |
| 17 | Wisconsin | 3,500 | 1.94% | 43 | South Dakota | 550 | 0.31% |
| 19 | Minnesota | 3,200 | 1.78% | 44 | Idaho | 500 | 0.28% |
| 19 | Washington | 3,200 | 1.78% | 45 | Vermont | 475 | 0.26% |
| 21 | Alabama | 2,700 | 1.50% | 46 | Montana | 450 | 0.25% |
| 21 | Connecticut | 2,700 | 1.50% | 47 | Hawaii | 425 | 0.24% |
| 23 | Louisiana | 2,600 | 1.44% | 47 | North Dakota | 425 | 0.24% |
| 24 | Arizona | 2,400 | 1.33% | 49 | Wyoming | 300 | 0.17% |
| 24 | Kentucky | 2,400 | 1.33% | 50 | Alaska | 175 | 0.10% |
| | | | | | District of Columbia | 600 | 0.33% |

Source: American Cancer Society

"Cancer Facts & Figures – 1992" (Copyright 1992, Reprinted with permission from the American Cancer Society)

*These estimates are offered as a rough guide and should not be regarded as definitive. They are calculated according to the distribution of estimated 1992 cancer deaths by state.

# Estimated New Female Breast Cancer Cases per 100,000 Female Population in 1992

## National Estimated Rate = 141.21 New Breast Cancer Cases per 100,000 Female Population*

| RANK | STATE | RATE | RANK | STATE | RATE |
|---|---|---|---|---|---|
| 1 | Rhode Island | 191.58 | 26 | Arkansas | 139.61 |
| 2 | Delaware | 174.83 | 27 | Michigan | 138.00 |
| 3 | Pennsylvania | 172.93 | 28 | Virginia | 136.36 |
| 4 | Massachusetts | 172.65 | 29 | Maine | 134.90 |
| 5 | New York | 169.79 | 30 | North Dakota | 132.56 |
| 6 | Florida | 167.76 | 31 | Wyoming | 132.40 |
| 7 | New Jersey | 167.73 | 32 | Georgia | 131.98 |
| 8 | Vermont | 165.35 | 33 | Washington | 130.46 |
| 9 | Iowa | 160.62 | 34 | Oklahoma | 130.05 |
| 10 | Connecticut | 159.36 | 35 | Arizona | 129.41 |
| 11 | New Hampshire | 159.09 | 36 | Alabama | 128.30 |
| 12 | South Dakota | 155.58 | 37 | South Carolina | 127.91 |
| 13 | Ohio | 153.00 | 38 | Nevada | 127.13 |
| 14 | West Virginia | 150.22 | 39 | Mississippi | 126.62 |
| 15 | North Carolina | 149.37 | 40 | Kentucky | 126.31 |
| 16 | Nebraska | 148.34 | 41 | California | 121.11 |
| 17 | Missouri | 147.02 | 42 | Louisiana | 118.80 |
| 18 | Illinois | 146.30 | 43 | New Mexico | 116.91 |
| 19 | Oregon | 145.30 | 44 | Montana | 111.58 |
| 20 | Indiana | 143.56 | 45 | Colorado | 108.23 |
| 21 | Minnesota | 143.50 | 46 | Texas | 100.92 |
| 22 | Kansas | 142.53 | 47 | Idaho | 98.85 |
| 23 | Tennessee | 142.39 | 48 | Utah | 80.73 |
| 24 | Maryland | 142.11 | 49 | Hawaii | 78.08 |
| 25 | Wisconsin | 140.07 | 50 | Alaska | 67.26 |

District of Columbia    185.23

Source: American Cancer Society

"Cancer Facts & Figures – 1992" (Copyright 1992, Reprinted with permission from the American Cancer Society)

*Calculated by the editors using 1990 Census resident population figures. These estimates are offered as a rough guide and should not be regarded as definitive. They are calculated according to the distribution of estimated 1992 cancer deaths by state.

# Percentage of Women 40 and Older Who Reported Ever Having a Mammogram in 1989

## National Percent = 62.6% of Women 40 and Older

| RANK | STATE | PERCENT | RANK | STATE | PERCENT |
|------|-------|---------|------|-------|---------|
| 1 | Minnesota | 73.0 | 26 | Kentucky | 58.0 |
| 2 | Massachusetts | 71.4 | 27 | Indiana | 57.2 |
| 3 | Rhode Island | 70.9 | 28 | West Virginia | 56.3 |
| 4 | Hawaii | 69.2 | 29 | Tennessee | 56.2 |
| 5 | New Hampshire | 68.3 | 30 | Alabama | 54.6 |
| 6 | California | 68.0 | 31 | Missouri | 53.3 |
| 7 | Wisconsin | 67.4 | 32 | Nebraska | 52.0 |
| 8 | Maryland | 67.2 | – | Alaska* | N/A |
| 9 | Texas | 67.0 | – | Arkansas* | N/A |
| 10 | Washington | 66.5 | – | Colorado* | N/A |
| 11 | North Dakota | 65.3 | – | Connecticut* | N/A |
| 12 | Ohio | 64.0 | – | Delaware* | N/A |
| 12 | Utah | 64.0 | – | Iowa* | N/A |
| 14 | Maine | 63.2 | – | Kansas* | N/A |
| 15 | Georgia | 63.0 | – | Louisiana* | N/A |
| 16 | New Mexico | 62.2 | – | Michigan* | N/A |
| 17 | New York | 62.1 | – | Mississippi* | N/A |
| 18 | Illinois | 61.8 | – | Nevada* | N/A |
| 19 | Florida | 61.6 | – | New Jersey* | N/A |
| 20 | Arizona | 61.4 | – | Oklahoma* | N/A |
| 21 | North Carolina | 61.2 | – | Oregon* | N/A |
| 22 | South Dakota | 60.8 | – | Pennsylvania* | N/A |
| 23 | Montana | 60.1 | – | Vermont* | N/A |
| 24 | Idaho | 59.4 | – | Virginia* | N/A |
| 25 | South Carolina | 58.2 | – | Wyoming* | N/A |

District of Columbia                79.0

*Source: U.S. Department of Health and Human Services, Centers for Disease Control*

*"Cancer Screening Behaviors Among U.S. Women" (Morbidity and Mortality Weekly Report, Vol. 41, No. SS-2, April 24, 1992)*

*\*Not available.*

# Estimated New Colon and Rectum Cancer Cases in 1992

## National Total = 156,000 New Colon and Rectum Cancer Cases*

| RANK | STATE | CASES | % | RANK | STATE | CASES | % |
|------|-------|-------|---|------|-------|-------|---|
| 1 | California | 15,000 | 9.62% | 26 | Arizona | 2,000 | 1.28% |
| 2 | New York | 13,700 | 8.78% | 27 | Oklahoma | 1,800 | 1.15% |
| 3 | Florida | 10,600 | 6.79% | 28 | South Carolina | 1,800 | 1.15% |
| 4 | Pennsylvania | 10,000 | 6.41% | 29 | Arkansas | 1,700 | 1.09% |
| 5 | Illinois | 8,100 | 5.19% | 30 | Kansas | 1,700 | 1.09% |
| 6 | Ohio | 7,600 | 4.87% | 31 | Oregon | 1,700 | 1.09% |
| 7 | Texas | 7,100 | 4.55% | 32 | Mississippi | 1,600 | 1.03% |
| 8 | New Jersey | 6,100 | 3.91% | 33 | Colorado | 1,500 | 0.96% |
| 9 | Michigan | 5,200 | 3.33% | 34 | West Virginia | 1,400 | 0.90% |
| 10 | Massachusetts | 4,500 | 2.88% | 35 | Nebraska | 1,000 | 0.64% |
| 11 | North Carolina | 4,000 | 2.56% | 36 | Maine | 950 | 0.61% |
| 12 | Indiana | 3,600 | 2.31% | 37 | Rhode Island | 800 | 0.51% |
| 13 | Virginia | 3,400 | 2.18% | 37 | New Hampshire | 750 | 0.48% |
| 13 | Missouri | 3,300 | 2.12% | 39 | New Mexico | 750 | 0.48% |
| 15 | Tennessee | 3,200 | 2.05% | 40 | Hawaii | 600 | 0.38% |
| 16 | Wisconsin | 3,200 | 2.05% | 41 | Nevada | 600 | 0.38% |
| 17 | Georgia | 3,100 | 1.99% | 42 | Idaho | 550 | 0.35% |
| 18 | Maryland | 2,900 | 1.86% | 43 | Montana | 550 | 0.35% |
| 19 | Minnesota | 2,600 | 1.67% | 44 | Utah | 550 | 0.35% |
| 20 | Connecticut | 2,400 | 1.54% | 45 | South Dakota | 500 | 0.32% |
| 20 | Louisiana | 2,400 | 1.54% | 46 | Delaware | 475 | 0.30% |
| 22 | Washington | 2,400 | 1.54% | 47 | North Dakota | 425 | 0.27% |
| 23 | Alabama | 2,300 | 1.47% | 48 | Vermont | 325 | 0.21% |
| 24 | Kentucky | 2,300 | 1.47% | 49 | Wyoming | 200 | 0.13% |
| 25 | Iowa | 2,100 | 1.35% | 50 | Alaska | 125 | 0.08% |
| | | | | | District of Columbia | 550 | 0.35% |

Source: American Cancer Society

*"Cancer Facts & Figures – 1992"* (Copyright 1992, Reprinted with permission from the American Cancer Society)

*These estimates are offered as a rough guide and should not be regarded as definitive. They are calculated according to the distribution of estimated 1992 cancer deaths by state.

# Estimated New Colon and Rectum Cancer Cases per 100,000 Population in 1992

## National Estimated Rate = 61.86 New Colon and Rectum Cancer Cases per 100,000 Population*

| RANK | STATE | RATE | RANK | STATE | RATE |
|------|-------|------|------|-------|------|
| 1 | Pennsylvania | 83.61 | 26 | Mississippi | 61.73 |
| 2 | Florida | 79.84 | 27 | Maryland | 59.67 |
| 3 | Rhode Island | 79.68 | 28 | North Carolina | 59.37 |
| 4 | New Jersey | 78.61 | 29 | Minnesota | 58.66 |
| 5 | West Virginia | 77.73 | 30 | Oregon | 58.18 |
| 6 | Maine | 76.92 | 31 | Vermont | 57.32 |
| 7 | New York | 75.87 | 32 | Oklahoma | 56.69 |
| 8 | Iowa | 75.13 | 33 | Louisiana | 56.44 |
| 9 | Massachusetts | 75.05 | 34 | Alabama | 56.25 |
| 10 | Connecticut | 72.93 | 35 | Michigan | 55.51 |
| 11 | Arkansas | 71.67 | 36 | Virginia | 54.09 |
| 12 | South Dakota | 71.12 | 37 | Arizona | 53.33 |
| 13 | Illinois | 70.17 | 37 | Idaho | 52.94 |
| 13 | Delaware | 69.85 | 39 | Hawaii | 52.86 |
| 15 | Ohio | 69.48 | 40 | South Carolina | 50.56 |
| 16 | Kansas | 68.14 | 41 | California | 49.37 |
| 17 | Montana | 68.07 | 42 | New Mexico | 48.45 |
| 18 | New Hampshire | 67.87 | 43 | Washington | 47.83 |
| 19 | North Dakota | 66.93 | 44 | Georgia | 46.81 |
| 20 | Tennessee | 64.61 | 45 | Nevada | 46.73 |
| 20 | Wisconsin | 64.58 | 46 | Colorado | 44.42 |
| 22 | Indiana | 64.17 | 47 | Wyoming | 43.48 |
| 23 | Missouri | 63.98 | 48 | Texas | 40.92 |
| 24 | Nebraska | 62.77 | 49 | Utah | 31.07 |
| 25 | Kentucky | 61.94 | 50 | Alaska | 21.93 |

District of Columbia 91.97

Source: American Cancer Society

*"Cancer Facts & Figures – 1992" (Copyright 1992, Reprinted with permission from the American Cancer Society)*

*Calculated by the editors using 1991 Census resident population figures. These estimates are offered as a rough guide and should not be regarded as definitive. They are calculated according to the distribution of estimated 1992 cancer deaths by state.*

# Estimated New Cases of Leukemia in 1992

## National Total = 28,200 New Cases of Leukemia*

| RANK | STATE | CASES | % | RANK | STATE | CASES | % |
|------|-------|-------|---|------|-------|-------|---|
| 1 | California | 3,100 | 10.99% | 26 | Connecticut | 375 | 1.33% |
| 2 | New York | 1,900 | 6.74% | 27 | Arkansas | 350 | 1.24% |
| 3 | Florida | 1,800 | 6.38% | 27 | Kentucky | 350 | 1.24% |
| 3 | Pennsylvania | 1,800 | 6.38% | 27 | Oregon | 350 | 1.24% |
| 5 | Texas | 1,700 | 6.03% | 30 | Iowa | 325 | 1.15% |
| 6 | Illinois | 1,300 | 4.61% | 30 | Kansas | 325 | 1.15% |
| 6 | Ohio | 1,300 | 4.61% | 32 | Colorado | 300 | 1.06% |
| 8 | Michigan | 1,000 | 3.55% | 33 | Mississippi | 275 | 0.98% |
| 9 | New Jersey | 900 | 3.19% | 34 | West Virginia | 250 | 0.89% |
| 10 | Massachusetts | 700 | 2.48% | 35 | Nebraska | 175 | 0.62% |
| 10 | North Carolina | 700 | 2.48% | 35 | New Mexico | 175 | 0.62% |
| 12 | Indiana | 650 | 2.30% | 37 | Maine | 150 | 0.53% |
| 13 | Georgia | 600 | 2.13% | 38 | Nevada | 125 | 0.44% |
| 13 | Missouri | 600 | 2.13% | 38 | Utah | 125 | 0.44% |
| 13 | Tennessee | 600 | 2.13% | 40 | Idaho | 100 | 0.35% |
| 13 | Virginia | 600 | 2.13% | 40 | New Hampshire | 100 | 0.35% |
| 13 | Wisconsin | 600 | 2.13% | 40 | North Dakota | 100 | 0.35% |
| 18 | Minnesota | 550 | 1.95% | 40 | Rhode Island | 100 | 0.35% |
| 19 | Maryland | 500 | 1.77% | 40 | South Dakota | 100 | 0.35% |
| 19 | Washington | 500 | 1.77% | 45 | Delaware | 80 | 0.28% |
| 21 | Alabama | 450 | 1.60% | 45 | Montana | 80 | 0.28% |
| 21 | Arizona | 450 | 1.60% | 45 | Vermont | 80 | 0.28% |
| 23 | Louisiana | 425 | 1.51% | 45 | Wyoming | 80 | 0.28% |
| 24 | Oklahoma | 400 | 1.42% | 49 | Hawaii | 75 | 0.27% |
| 24 | South Carolina | 400 | 1.42% | 50 | Alaska | 40 | 0.14% |
| | | | | | District of Columbia | 90 | 0.32% |

Source: American Cancer Society

"Cancer Facts & Figures – 1992" (Copyright 1992, Reprinted with permission from the American Cancer Society)

*These estimates are offered as a rough guide and should not be regarded as definitive. They are calculated according to the distribution of estimated 1992 cancer deaths by state.

# Estimated New Cases of Leukemia per 100,000 Population in 1992

## National Estimated Rate = 11.18 New Cases of Leukemia per 100,000 Population*

| RANK | STATE | RATE | RANK | STATE | RATE |
|------|-------|------|------|-------|------|
| 1 | Wyoming | 17.39 | 26 | Illinois | 11.26 |
| 2 | North Dakota | 15.75 | 27 | South Carolina | 11.24 |
| 3 | Pennsylvania | 15.05 | 28 | Alabama | 11.01 |
| 4 | Arkansas | 14.76 | 29 | Nebraska | 10.99 |
| 5 | South Dakota | 14.22 | 30 | Michigan | 10.67 |
| 6 | Vermont | 14.11 | 31 | Mississippi | 10.61 |
| 7 | West Virginia | 13.88 | 32 | New York | 10.52 |
| 8 | Florida | 13.56 | 33 | North Carolina | 10.39 |
| 9 | Kansas | 13.03 | 34 | Maryland | 10.29 |
| 10 | Oklahoma | 12.60 | 35 | California | 10.20 |
| 11 | Minnesota | 12.41 | 36 | Louisiana | 10.00 |
| 12 | Maine | 12.15 | 37 | Rhode Island | 9.96 |
| 13 | Tennessee | 12.11 | 37 | Washington | 9.96 |
| 13 | Wisconsin | 12.11 | 39 | Montana | 9.90 |
| 15 | Arizona | 12.00 | 40 | Texas | 9.80 |
| 16 | Oregon | 11.98 | 41 | Nevada | 9.74 |
| 17 | Ohio | 11.88 | 42 | Idaho | 9.62 |
| 18 | Delaware | 11.76 | 43 | Virginia | 9.55 |
| 19 | Massachusetts | 11.67 | 44 | Kentucky | 9.43 |
| 20 | Iowa | 11.63 | 45 | Georgia | 9.06 |
| 20 | Missouri | 11.63 | 46 | New Hampshire | 9.05 |
| 22 | New Jersey | 11.60 | 47 | Colorado | 8.88 |
| 23 | Indiana | 11.59 | 48 | Utah | 7.06 |
| 24 | Connecticut | 11.39 | 49 | Alaska | 7.02 |
| 25 | New Mexico | 11.30 | 50 | Hawaii | 6.61 |

District of Columbia          15.05

Source: American Cancer Society

*"Cancer Facts & Figures – 1992"* (Copyright 1992, Reprinted with permission from the American Cancer Society)

*Calculated by the editors using 1991 Census resident population figures. These estimates are offered as a rough guide and should not be regarded as definitive. They are calculated according to the distribution of estimated 1992 cancer deaths by state.

# Estimated New Lung Cancer Cases in 1992

## National Total = 168,000 New Lung Cancer Cases*

| RANK | STATE | CASES | % | RANK | STATE | CASES | % |
|---|---|---|---|---|---|---|---|
| 1 | California | 17,000 | 10.12% | 25 | Minnesota | 2,300 | 1.37% |
| 2 | Florida | 12,000 | 7.14% | 25 | South Carolina | 2,300 | 1.37% |
| 3 | New York | 11,400 | 6.79% | 28 | Connecticut | 2,200 | 1.31% |
| 4 | Pennsylvania | 9,300 | 5.54% | 29 | Oregon | 2,100 | 1.25% |
| 5 | Texas | 9,000 | 5.36% | 30 | Iowa | 2,000 | 1.19% |
| 6 | Ohio | 8,000 | 4.76% | 30 | Mississippi | 2,000 | 1.19% |
| 7 | Illinois | 7,600 | 4.52% | 32 | West Virginia | 1,800 | 1.07% |
| 8 | Michigan | 6,000 | 3.57% | 33 | Kansas | 1,600 | 0.95% |
| 9 | New Jersey | 5,400 | 3.21% | 34 | Colorado | 1,400 | 0.83% |
| 10 | North Carolina | 4,700 | 2.80% | 35 | Nebraska | 1,100 | 0.65% |
| 11 | Virginia | 4,200 | 2.50% | 36 | Nevada | 950 | 0.57% |
| 12 | Georgia | 4,100 | 2.44% | 37 | Maine | 900 | 0.54% |
| 12 | Indiana | 4,100 | 2.44% | 38 | Rhode Island | 750 | 0.45% |
| 14 | Massachusetts | 4,000 | 2.38% | 39 | New Hampshire | 700 | 0.42% |
| 14 | Missouri | 4,000 | 2.38% | 40 | New Mexico | 600 | 0.36% |
| 14 | Tennessee | 4,000 | 2.38% | 41 | Delaware | 500 | 0.30% |
| 17 | Kentucky | 3,300 | 1.96% | 41 | Hawaii | 500 | 0.30% |
| 17 | Maryland | 3,300 | 1.96% | 41 | Idaho | 500 | 0.30% |
| 19 | Alabama | 3,200 | 1.90% | 41 | Montana | 500 | 0.30% |
| 19 | Louisiana | 3,200 | 1.90% | 45 | South Dakota | 450 | 0.27% |
| 21 | Washington | 3,000 | 1.79% | 46 | North Dakota | 375 | 0.22% |
| 22 | Wisconsin | 2,800 | 1.67% | 47 | Utah | 350 | 0.21% |
| 23 | Arizona | 2,500 | 1.49% | 47 | Vermont | 350 | 0.21% |
| 24 | Oklahoma | 2,400 | 1.43% | 49 | Alaska | 250 | 0.15% |
| 25 | Arkansas | 2,300 | 1.37% | 50 | Wyoming | 225 | 0.13% |
| | | | | | District of Columbia | 500 | 0.30% |

Source: American Cancer Society

"Cancer Facts & Figures – 1992" (Copyright 1992, Reprinted with permission from the American Cancer Society)

*These estimates are offered as a rough guide and should not be regarded as definitive. They are calculated according to the distribution of estimated 1992 cancer deaths by state.

## Estimated New Lung Cancer Cases per 100,000 Population in 1992

### National Estimated Rate = 66.62 New Lung Cancer Cases per 100,000 Population*

| RANK | STATE | RATE | RANK | STATE | RATE |
|------|-------|------|------|-------|------|
| 1 | West Virginia | 99.94 | 26 | Massachusetts | 66.71 |
| 2 | Arkansas | 96.96 | 27 | Arizona | 66.67 |
| 3 | Florida | 90.38 | 28 | Illinois | 65.84 |
| 4 | Kentucky | 88.88 | 29 | South Carolina | 64.61 |
| 5 | Tennessee | 80.76 | 30 | Kansas | 64.13 |
| 6 | Alabama | 78.26 | 31 | Michigan | 64.05 |
| 7 | Pennsylvania | 77.75 | 32 | South Dakota | 64.01 |
| 8 | Missouri | 77.55 | 33 | New Hampshire | 63.35 |
| 9 | Mississippi | 77.16 | 34 | New York | 63.13 |
| 10 | Oklahoma | 75.59 | 35 | Georgia | 61.91 |
| 11 | Louisiana | 75.26 | 36 | Montana | 61.88 |
| 12 | Rhode Island | 74.70 | 37 | Vermont | 61.73 |
| 13 | Nevada | 73.99 | 38 | Washington | 59.78 |
| 14 | Delaware | 73.53 | 39 | North Dakota | 59.06 |
| 15 | Ohio | 73.13 | 40 | Wisconsin | 56.51 |
| 16 | Indiana | 73.08 | 41 | California | 55.96 |
| 17 | Maine | 72.87 | 42 | Minnesota | 51.90 |
| 18 | Oregon | 71.87 | 43 | Texas | 51.88 |
| 19 | Iowa | 71.56 | 44 | Wyoming | 48.91 |
| 20 | North Carolina | 69.76 | 45 | Idaho | 48.12 |
| 21 | New Jersey | 69.59 | 46 | Hawaii | 44.05 |
| 22 | Nebraska | 69.05 | 47 | Alaska | 43.86 |
| 23 | Maryland | 67.90 | 48 | Colorado | 41.46 |
| 24 | Connecticut | 66.85 | 49 | New Mexico | 38.76 |
| 25 | Virginia | 66.82 | 50 | Utah | 19.77 |

District of Columbia        83.61

Source: American Cancer Society

"Cancer Facts & Figures – 1992" (Copyright 1992, Reprinted with permission from the American Cancer Society)

*Calculated by the editors using 1991 Census resident population figures. These estimates are offered as a rough guide and should not be regarded as definitive. They are calculated according to the distribution of estimated 1992 cancer deaths by state.

# Estimated New Oral Cancer Cases in 1992

## National Total = 30,300 New Oral Cancer Cases*

| RANK | STATE | CASES | % | RANK | STATE | CASES | % |
|------|-------|-------|------|------|-------|-------|------|
| 1 | California | 3,200 | 10.56% | 26 | Iowa | 400 | 1.32% |
| 2 | New York | 2,600 | 8.58% | 26 | Kentucky | 400 | 1.32% |
| 3 | Florida | 2,500 | 8.25% | 28 | Oregon | 350 | 1.16% |
| 4 | Texas | 1,500 | 4.95% | 29 | Mississippi | 325 | 1.07% |
| 5 | Pennsylvania | 1,400 | 4.62% | 30 | Arizona | 300 | 0.99% |
| 6 | Ohio | 1,300 | 4.29% | 31 | Colorado | 275 | 0.91% |
| 7 | Illinois | 1,200 | 3.96% | 32 | Arkansas | 250 | 0.83% |
| 8 | Michigan | 1,100 | 3.63% | 33 | Kansas | 225 | 0.74% |
| 8 | New Jersey | 1,100 | 3.63% | 33 | Rhode Island | 225 | 0.74% |
| 10 | Georgia | 1,000 | 3.30% | 33 | West Virginia | 225 | 0.74% |
| 11 | Massachusetts | 900 | 2.97% | 36 | Maine | 200 | 0.66% |
| 11 | North Carolina | 900 | 2.97% | 37 | New Hampshire | 150 | 0.50% |
| 13 | Virginia | 700 | 2.31% | 38 | Hawaii | 125 | 0.41% |
| 14 | Alabama | 600 | 1.98% | 38 | Montana | 125 | 0.41% |
| 14 | Indiana | 600 | 1.98% | 38 | Nevada | 125 | 0.41% |
| 14 | Louisiana | 600 | 1.98% | 41 | Delaware | 100 | 0.33% |
| 14 | South Carolina | 600 | 1.98% | 41 | Idaho | 100 | 0.33% |
| 18 | Maryland | 550 | 1.82% | 41 | Nebraska | 100 | 0.33% |
| 18 | Tennessee | 550 | 1.82% | 41 | New Mexico | 100 | 0.33% |
| 18 | Wisconsin | 550 | 1.82% | 45 | Utah | 90 | 0.30% |
| 21 | Missouri | 500 | 1.65% | 46 | North Dakota | 80 | 0.26% |
| 22 | Connecticut | 450 | 1.49% | 47 | Alaska | 50 | 0.17% |
| 22 | Oklahoma | 450 | 1.49% | 47 | South Dakota | 50 | 0.17% |
| 22 | Washington | 450 | 1.49% | 47 | Vermont | 50 | 0.17% |
| 25 | Minnesota | 425 | 1.40% | 50 | Wyoming | 30 | 0.10% |
| | | | | | District of Columbia | 125 | 0.41% |

Source: American Cancer Society

"Cancer Facts & Figures – 1992" (Copyright 1992, Reprinted with permission from the American Cancer Society)

*These estimates are offered as a rough guide and should not be regarded as definitive. They are calculated according to the distribution of estimated 1992 cancer deaths by state.

# Estimated New Oral Cancer Cases per 100,000 Population in 1992

## National Estimated Rate = 12.02 New Oral Cancer Cases per 100,000 Population*

| RANK | STATE | RATE | RANK | STATE | RATE |
|---|---|---|---|---|---|
| 1 | Rhode Island | 22.41 | 26 | Virginia | 11.14 |
| 2 | Florida | 18.83 | 27 | Tennessee | 11.10 |
| 3 | South Carolina | 16.85 | 27 | Wisconsin | 11.10 |
| 4 | Maine | 16.19 | 29 | Hawaii | 11.01 |
| 5 | Montana | 15.47 | 30 | Kentucky | 10.77 |
| 6 | Georgia | 15.10 | 31 | Indiana | 10.70 |
| 7 | Massachusetts | 15.01 | 32 | Arkansas | 10.54 |
| 8 | Delaware | 14.71 | 33 | California | 10.53 |
| 9 | Alabama | 14.67 | 34 | Illinois | 10.40 |
| 10 | New York | 14.40 | 35 | Nevada | 9.74 |
| 11 | Iowa | 14.31 | 36 | Missouri | 9.69 |
| 12 | New Jersey | 14.18 | 37 | Idaho | 9.62 |
| 13 | Oklahoma | 14.17 | 38 | Minnesota | 9.59 |
| 14 | Louisiana | 14.11 | 39 | Kansas | 9.02 |
| 15 | Connecticut | 13.67 | 40 | Washington | 8.97 |
| 16 | New Hampshire | 13.57 | 41 | Vermont | 8.82 |
| 17 | North Carolina | 13.36 | 42 | Alaska | 8.77 |
| 18 | North Dakota | 12.60 | 43 | Texas | 8.65 |
| 19 | Mississippi | 12.54 | 44 | Colorado | 8.14 |
| 20 | West Virginia | 12.49 | 45 | Arizona | 8.00 |
| 21 | Oregon | 11.98 | 46 | South Dakota | 7.11 |
| 22 | Ohio | 11.88 | 47 | Wyoming | 6.52 |
| 23 | Michigan | 11.74 | 48 | New Mexico | 6.46 |
| 24 | Pennsylvania | 11.70 | 49 | Nebraska | 6.28 |
| 25 | Maryland | 11.32 | 50 | Utah | 5.08 |
| | | | | District of Columbia | 20.90 |

*Source: American Cancer Society*

*"Cancer Facts & Figures – 1992" (Copyright 1992, Reprinted with permission from the American Cancer Society)*

*Calculated by the editors using 1991 Census resident population figures. These estimates are offered as a rough guide and should not be regarded as definitive. They are calculated according to the distribution of estimated 1992 cancer deaths by state.*

# Estimated New Cancer of the Pancreas Cases in 1992

## National Total = 28,300 New Cancer of the Pancreas Cases*

| RANK | STATE | CASES | % | RANK | STATE | CASES | % |
|---|---|---|---|---|---|---|---|
| 1 | California | 3,000 | 10.60% | 26 | Arizona | 350 | 1.24% |
| 2 | New York | 2,300 | 8.13% | 26 | Mississippi | 350 | 1.24% |
| 3 | Florida | 2,000 | 7.07% | 26 | Oklahoma | 350 | 1.24% |
| 4 | Pennsylvania | 1,500 | 5.30% | 26 | Oregon | 350 | 1.24% |
| 4 | Texas | 1,500 | 5.30% | 30 | Arkansas | 325 | 1.15% |
| 6 | Illinois | 1,400 | 4.95% | 30 | Iowa | 325 | 1.15% |
| 7 | Ohio | 1,200 | 4.24% | 32 | Colorado | 300 | 1.06% |
| 8 | Michigan | 1,000 | 3.53% | 33 | Kansas | 275 | 0.97% |
| 9 | New Jersey | 900 | 3.18% | 34 | West Virginia | 250 | 0.88% |
| 10 | North Carolina | 800 | 2.83% | 35 | Nebraska | 175 | 0.62% |
| 11 | Massachusetts | 700 | 2.47% | 36 | Maine | 150 | 0.53% |
| 12 | Georgia | 650 | 2.30% | 36 | Nevada | 150 | 0.53% |
| 13 | Indiana | 600 | 2.12% | 36 | New Mexico | 150 | 0.53% |
| 13 | Missouri | 600 | 2.12% | 39 | Idaho | 125 | 0.44% |
| 13 | Virginia | 600 | 2.12% | 39 | New Hampshire | 125 | 0.44% |
| 16 | Louisiana | 550 | 1.94% | 39 | Rhode Island | 125 | 0.44% |
| 16 | Maryland | 550 | 1.94% | 39 | Utah | 125 | 0.44% |
| 16 | Minnesota | 550 | 1.94% | 43 | Hawaii | 100 | 0.35% |
| 16 | Tennessee | 550 | 1.94% | 44 | Montana | 90 | 0.32% |
| 16 | Wisconsin | 550 | 1.94% | 44 | South Dakota | 90 | 0.32% |
| 21 | Alabama | 500 | 1.77% | 46 | North Dakota | 80 | 0.28% |
| 22 | Washington | 475 | 1.68% | 47 | Delaware | 70 | 0.25% |
| 23 | Connecticut | 425 | 1.50% | 48 | Vermont | 60 | 0.21% |
| 24 | Kentucky | 375 | 1.33% | 49 | Alaska | 40 | 0.14% |
| 24 | South Carolina | 375 | 1.33% | 49 | Wyoming | 40 | 0.14% |
| | | | | | District of Columbia | 80 | 0.28% |

Source: American Cancer Society

*"Cancer Facts & Figures – 1992" (Copyright 1992, Reprinted with permission from the American Cancer Society)*

*These estimates are offered as a rough guide and should not be regarded as definitive. They are calculated according to the distribution of estimated 1992 cancer deaths by state.*

# Estimated New Cases of Cancer of the Pancreas per 100,000 Population in 1992

## National Estimated Rate = 11.22 New Cases of Cancer of the Pancreas per 100,000 Population*

| RANK | STATE | RATE |
|------|-------|------|
| 1 | Florida | 15.06 |
| 2 | West Virginia | 13.88 |
| 3 | Arkansas | 13.70 |
| 4 | Mississippi | 13.50 |
| 5 | Louisiana | 12.94 |
| 6 | Connecticut | 12.91 |
| 7 | South Dakota | 12.80 |
| 8 | New York | 12.74 |
| 9 | North Dakota | 12.60 |
| 10 | Pennsylvania | 12.54 |
| 11 | Rhode Island | 12.45 |
| 12 | Minnesota | 12.41 |
| 13 | Alabama | 12.23 |
| 14 | Maine | 12.15 |
| 15 | Illinois | 12.13 |
| 16 | Idaho | 12.03 |
| 17 | Oregon | 11.98 |
| 18 | North Carolina | 11.87 |
| 19 | Nevada | 11.68 |
| 20 | Massachusetts | 11.67 |
| 21 | Iowa | 11.63 |
| 21 | Missouri | 11.63 |
| 23 | New Jersey | 11.60 |
| 24 | Maryland | 11.32 |
| 25 | New Hampshire | 11.31 |

| RANK | STATE | RATE |
|------|-------|------|
| 26 | Montana | 11.14 |
| 27 | Tennessee | 11.10 |
| 27 | Wisconsin | 11.10 |
| 29 | Kansas | 11.02 |
| 29 | Oklahoma | 11.02 |
| 31 | Nebraska | 10.99 |
| 32 | Ohio | 10.97 |
| 33 | Indiana | 10.70 |
| 34 | Michigan | 10.67 |
| 35 | Vermont | 10.58 |
| 36 | South Carolina | 10.53 |
| 37 | Delaware | 10.29 |
| 38 | Kentucky | 10.10 |
| 39 | California | 9.87 |
| 40 | Georgia | 9.81 |
| 41 | New Mexico | 9.69 |
| 42 | Virginia | 9.55 |
| 43 | Washington | 9.47 |
| 44 | Arizona | 9.33 |
| 45 | Colorado | 8.88 |
| 46 | Hawaii | 8.81 |
| 47 | Wyoming | 8.70 |
| 48 | Texas | 8.65 |
| 49 | Utah | 7.06 |
| 50 | Alaska | 7.02 |

| | District of Columbia | 13.38 |

Source: American Cancer Society

"Cancer Facts & Figures – 1992" (Copyright 1992, Reprinted with permission from the American Cancer Society)

*Calculated by the editors using 1991 Census resident population figures. These estimates are offered as a rough guide and should not be regarded as definitive. They are calculated according to the distribution of estimated 1992 cancer deaths by state.

# Estimated New Prostate Cancer Cases in 1992

## National Total = 132,000 New Prostate Cancer Cases*

| RANK | STATE | CASES | % | RANK | STATE | CASES | % |
|---|---|---|---|---|---|---|---|
| 1 | California | 13,000 | 9.85% | 25 | Oregon | 1,800 | 1.36% |
| 2 | Florida | 9,600 | 7.27% | 27 | Kentucky | 1,700 | 1.29% |
| 3 | New York | 9,500 | 7.20% | 28 | Connecticut | 1,600 | 1.21% |
| 4 | Pennsylvania | 7,700 | 5.83% | 28 | Oklahoma | 1,600 | 1.21% |
| 5 | Texas | 6,100 | 4.62% | 30 | Arkansas | 1,500 | 1.14% |
| 6 | Illinois | 5,800 | 4.39% | 30 | Mississippi | 1,500 | 1.14% |
| 7 | Ohio | 5,700 | 4.32% | 32 | Colorado | 1,400 | 1.06% |
| 8 | Michigan | 4,900 | 3.71% | 32 | Kansas | 1,400 | 1.06% |
| 9 | New Jersey | 4,100 | 3.11% | 34 | West Virginia | 1,100 | 0.83% |
| 10 | North Carolina | 4,000 | 3.03% | 35 | Nebraska | 850 | 0.64% |
| 11 | Virginia | 3,400 | 2.58% | 36 | New Mexico | 700 | 0.53% |
| 12 | Georgia | 3,300 | 2.50% | 37 | Maine | 650 | 0.49% |
| 13 | Massachusetts | 3,200 | 2.42% | 37 | New Hampshire | 650 | 0.49% |
| 14 | Indiana | 3,000 | 2.27% | 39 | Rhode Island | 600 | 0.45% |
| 14 | Wisconsin | 3,000 | 2.27% | 39 | Utah | 600 | 0.45% |
| 16 | Missouri | 2,900 | 2.20% | 41 | Idaho | 550 | 0.42% |
| 17 | Tennessee | 2,700 | 2.05% | 42 | Montana | 500 | 0.38% |
| 17 | Washington | 2,700 | 2.05% | 42 | North Dakota | 500 | 0.38% |
| 19 | Minnesota | 2,600 | 1.97% | 42 | South Dakota | 500 | 0.38% |
| 20 | Alabama | 2,400 | 1.82% | 45 | Nevada | 425 | 0.32% |
| 20 | Maryland | 2,400 | 1.82% | 46 | Delaware | 400 | 0.30% |
| 22 | Louisiana | 2,200 | 1.67% | 46 | Vermont | 400 | 0.30% |
| 23 | Arizona | 1,900 | 1.44% | 48 | Hawaii | 375 | 0.28% |
| 23 | South Carolina | 1,900 | 1.44% | 49 | Wyoming | 200 | 0.15% |
| 25 | Iowa | 1,800 | 1.36% | 50 | Alaska | 100 | 0.08% |
| | | | | | District of Columbia | 600 | 0.45% |

Source: American Cancer Society

*"Cancer Facts & Figures – 1992"* (Copyright 1992, Reprinted with permission from the American Cancer Society)

*These estimates are offered as a rough guide and should not be regarded as definitive. They are calculated according to the distribution of estimated 1992 cancer deaths by state.

# Estimated New Prostate Cancer Cases per 100,000 Male Population in 1992

## National Estimated Rate = 108.88 New Prostate Cancer Cases per 100,000 Male Population*

| RANK | STATE | RATE | | RANK | STATE | RATE |
|---|---|---|---|---|---|---|
| 1 | North Dakota | 157.13 | | 26 | Massachusetts | 110.77 |
| 2 | Florida | 153.31 | | 27 | Nebraska | 110.47 |
| 3 | South Dakota | 145.99 | | 28 | New York | 110.14 |
| 4 | Vermont | 145.19 | | 29 | Idaho | 109.79 |
| 5 | Pennsylvania | 135.22 | | 30 | New Jersey | 109.75 |
| 6 | Iowa | 133.85 | | 31 | Ohio | 109.06 |
| 7 | Arkansas | 132.38 | | 32 | Maine | 108.72 |
| 8 | Oregon | 128.84 | | 33 | Michigan | 108.58 |
| 9 | West Virginia | 127.68 | | 34 | Louisiana | 108.30 |
| 10 | Montana | 126.34 | | 35 | Georgia | 104.95 |
| 11 | Wisconsin | 125.37 | | 36 | Arizona | 104.93 |
| 12 | Rhode Island | 124.61 | | 37 | Oklahoma | 104.52 |
| 13 | North Carolina | 124.44 | | 38 | Illinois | 104.46 |
| 14 | Alabama | 123.96 | | 39 | Maryland | 103.51 |
| 15 | Delaware | 123.85 | | 40 | Connecticut | 100.45 |
| 16 | Mississippi | 121.89 | | 41 | Kentucky | 95.23 |
| 17 | Minnesota | 121.20 | | 42 | New Mexico | 93.93 |
| 18 | New Hampshire | 119.59 | | 43 | Wyoming | 88.10 |
| 19 | Missouri | 117.68 | | 44 | California | 87.26 |
| 20 | Kansas | 115.26 | | 45 | Colorado | 85.82 |
| 21 | Tennessee | 114.95 | | 46 | Texas | 72.91 |
| 22 | South Carolina | 112.53 | | 47 | Utah | 70.11 |
| 23 | Virginia | 112.06 | | 48 | Nevada | 69.46 |
| 24 | Washington | 111.86 | | 49 | Hawaii | 66.50 |
| 25 | Indiana | 111.60 | | 50 | Alaska | 34.50 |

District of Columbia        212.04

Source: American Cancer Society

*"Cancer Facts & Figures – 1992"* (Copyright 1992, Reprinted with permission from the American Cancer Society)

*Calculated by the editors using 1990 Census resident population figures. These estimates are offered as a rough guide and should not be regarded as definitive. They are calculated according to the distribution of estimated 1992 cancer deaths by state.*

# Estimated New Skin Melanoma Cases in 1992

## National Total = 32,000 New Skin Melanoma Cases*

| RANK | STATE | CASES | % | RANK | STATE | CASES | % |
|---|---|---|---|---|---|---|---|
| 1 | California | 3,700 | 11.56% | 24 | South Carolina | 450 | 1.41% |
| 2 | New York | 2,600 | 8.13% | 27 | Connecticut | 425 | 1.33% |
| 3 | Florida | 2,200 | 6.88% | 27 | Iowa | 425 | 1.33% |
| 4 | Pennsylvania | 1,800 | 5.63% | 29 | Colorado | 400 | 1.25% |
| 5 | Texas | 1,700 | 5.31% | 29 | Louisiana | 400 | 1.25% |
| 6 | Illinois | 1,300 | 4.06% | 31 | Arkansas | 325 | 1.02% |
| 7 | New Jersey | 1,200 | 3.75% | 31 | Kansas | 325 | 1.02% |
| 7 | Ohio | 1,200 | 3.75% | 33 | Nebraska | 300 | 0.94% |
| 9 | North Carolina | 1,000 | 3.13% | 33 | West Virginia | 300 | 0.94% |
| 10 | Massachusetts | 900 | 2.81% | 35 | Mississippi | 275 | 0.86% |
| 11 | Georgia | 850 | 2.66% | 36 | Maine | 175 | 0.55% |
| 12 | Michigan | 800 | 2.50% | 36 | New Mexico | 175 | 0.55% |
| 13 | Virginia | 750 | 2.34% | 38 | Nevada | 150 | 0.47% |
| 14 | Tennessee | 700 | 2.19% | 38 | Utah | 150 | 0.47% |
| 15 | Indiana | 650 | 2.03% | 40 | Idaho | 125 | 0.39% |
| 15 | Missouri | 650 | 2.03% | 40 | Montana | 125 | 0.39% |
| 15 | Washington | 650 | 2.03% | 40 | New Hampshire | 125 | 0.39% |
| 18 | Maryland | 550 | 1.72% | 40 | Rhode Island | 125 | 0.39% |
| 18 | Wisconsin | 550 | 1.72% | 44 | Delaware | 100 | 0.31% |
| 20 | Alabama | 500 | 1.56% | 44 | South Dakota | 100 | 0.31% |
| 20 | Arizona | 500 | 1.56% | 46 | Hawaii | 80 | 0.25% |
| 22 | Kentucky | 475 | 1.48% | 46 | North Dakota | 80 | 0.25% |
| 22 | Minnesota | 475 | 1.48% | 48 | Vermont | 75 | 0.23% |
| 24 | Oklahoma | 450 | 1.41% | 49 | Wyoming | 60 | 0.19% |
| 24 | Oregon | 450 | 1.41% | 50 | Alaska | 50 | 0.16% |
| | | | | | District of Columbia | 80 | 0.25% |

Source: American Cancer Society

"Cancer Facts & Figures – 1992" (Copyright 1992, Reprinted with permission from the American Cancer Society)

*These estimates are offered as a rough guide and should not be regarded as definitive. They are calculated according to the distribution of estimated 1992 cancer deaths by state.

# Estimated New Skin Melanoma Cases per 100,000 Population in 1992

## National Estimated Rate = 12.69 New Skin Melanoma Cases per 100,000 Population*

| RANK | STATE | RATE | RANK | STATE | RATE |
|------|-------|------|------|-------|------|
| 1 | Nebraska | 18.83 | 26 | South Carolina | 12.64 |
| 2 | West Virginia | 16.66 | 27 | Missouri | 12.60 |
| 3 | Florida | 16.57 | 27 | North Dakota | 12.60 |
| 4 | Montana | 15.47 | 29 | Rhode Island | 12.45 |
| 5 | New Jersey | 15.46 | 30 | Alabama | 12.23 |
| 6 | Oregon | 15.40 | 31 | California | 12.18 |
| 7 | Iowa | 15.21 | 32 | Idaho | 12.03 |
| 8 | Pennsylvania | 15.05 | 33 | Virginia | 11.93 |
| 9 | Massachusetts | 15.01 | 34 | Colorado | 11.84 |
| 10 | North Carolina | 14.84 | 35 | Nevada | 11.68 |
| 11 | Delaware | 14.71 | 36 | Indiana | 11.59 |
| 12 | New York | 14.40 | 37 | Maryland | 11.32 |
| 13 | South Dakota | 14.22 | 38 | New Hampshire | 11.31 |
| 14 | Maine | 14.17 | 39 | New Mexico | 11.30 |
| 14 | Oklahoma | 14.17 | 40 | Illinois | 11.26 |
| 16 | Tennessee | 14.13 | 41 | Wisconsin | 11.10 |
| 17 | Arkansas | 13.70 | 42 | Ohio | 10.97 |
| 18 | Arizona | 13.33 | 43 | Minnesota | 10.72 |
| 19 | Vermont | 13.23 | 44 | Mississippi | 10.61 |
| 20 | Wyoming | 13.04 | 45 | Texas | 9.80 |
| 21 | Kansas | 13.03 | 46 | Louisiana | 9.41 |
| 22 | Washington | 12.95 | 47 | Alaska | 8.77 |
| 23 | Connecticut | 12.91 | 48 | Michigan | 8.54 |
| 24 | Georgia | 12.83 | 49 | Utah | 8.47 |
| 25 | Kentucky | 12.79 | 50 | Hawaii | 7.05 |
| | | | | District of Columbia | 13.38 |

Source: American Cancer Society

"Cancer Facts & Figures - 1992" (Copyright 1992, Reprinted with permission from the American Cancer Society)

*Calculated by the editors using 1991 Census resident population figures. These estimates are offered as a rough guide and should not be regarded as definitive. They are calculated according to the distribution of estimated 1992 cancer deaths by state.

# Estimated New Cancer of the Uterus Cases in 1992

## National Total = 45,500 New Cancer of the Uterus Cases*

| RANK | STATE | CASES | % | RANK | STATE | CASES | % |
|------|-------|-------|-----|------|-------|-------|-----|
| 1 | California | 4,600 | 10.11% | 25 | Oregon | 600 | 1.32% |
| 2 | New York | 3,600 | 7.91% | 25 | Washington | 600 | 1.32% |
| 3 | Pennsylvania | 2,800 | 6.15% | 28 | Connecticut | 550 | 1.21% |
| 4 | Florida | 2,600 | 5.71% | 28 | Mississippi | 550 | 1.21% |
| 5 | Illinois | 2,400 | 5.27% | 30 | Kansas | 475 | 1.04% |
| 5 | Texas | 2,400 | 5.27% | 31 | Iowa | 450 | 0.99% |
| 7 | Ohio | 2,300 | 5.05% | 32 | Arkansas | 425 | 0.93% |
| 8 | Michigan | 1,700 | 3.74% | 32 | West Virginia | 425 | 0.93% |
| 8 | New Jersey | 1,700 | 3.74% | 34 | Colorado | 350 | 0.77% |
| 10 | North Carolina | 1,300 | 2.86% | 35 | Maine | 275 | 0.60% |
| 11 | Massachusetts | 1,100 | 2.42% | 36 | Nebraska | 225 | 0.49% |
| 11 | Tennessee | 1,100 | 2.42% | 36 | Utah | 225 | 0.49% |
| 13 | Georgia | 1,000 | 2.20% | 38 | Idaho | 200 | 0.44% |
| 13 | Indiana | 1,000 | 2.20% | 38 | New Hampshire | 200 | 0.44% |
| 13 | Virginia | 1,000 | 2.20% | 38 | New Mexico | 200 | 0.44% |
| 16 | Alabama | 900 | 1.98% | 38 | Rhode Island | 200 | 0.44% |
| 16 | Louisiana | 900 | 1.98% | 42 | Nevada | 175 | 0.38% |
| 16 | Missouri | 900 | 1.98% | 43 | Delaware | 125 | 0.27% |
| 19 | Wisconsin | 850 | 1.87% | 43 | Hawaii | 125 | 0.27% |
| 20 | Kentucky | 750 | 1.65% | 43 | Montana | 125 | 0.27% |
| 20 | Maryland | 750 | 1.65% | 43 | North Dakota | 125 | 0.27% |
| 22 | Minnesota | 700 | 1.54% | 47 | South Dakota | 100 | 0.22% |
| 22 | Oklahoma | 700 | 1.54% | 48 | Vermont | 90 | 0.20% |
| 22 | South Carolina | 700 | 1.54% | 49 | Wyoming | 60 | 0.13% |
| 25 | Arizona | 600 | 1.32% | 50 | Alaska | 50 | 0.11% |
| | | | | | District of Columbia | 225 | 0.49% |

Source: American Cancer Society

*"Cancer Facts & Figures – 1992" (Copyright 1992, Reprinted with permission from the American Cancer Society)*

*These estimates are offered as a rough guide and should not be regarded as definitive. They are calculated according to the distribution of estimated 1992 cancer deaths by state.*

# Estimated New Cancer of the Uterus Cases per 100,000 Female Population in 1992

## National Estimated Rate = 35.69 New Cancer of the Uterus Cases per 100,000 Female Population*

| RANK | STATE | RATE | RANK | STATE | RATE |
|------|-------|------|------|-------|------|
| 1 | West Virginia | 45.60 | 26 | Indiana | 35.02 |
| 2 | Pennsylvania | 45.25 | 27 | Arkansas | 34.90 |
| 3 | Maine | 43.65 | 28 | Wisconsin | 34.02 |
| 4 | Tennessee | 43.51 | 29 | Missouri | 33.93 |
| 5 | Oklahoma | 43.35 | 30 | Connecticut | 32.46 |
| 6 | Alabama | 42.77 | 31 | Arizona | 32.35 |
| 7 | New Jersey | 42.56 | 32 | Virginia | 31.71 |
| 8 | Oregon | 41.52 | 33 | Iowa | 31.43 |
| 9 | Louisiana | 41.12 | 34 | Minnesota | 31.39 |
| 10 | Mississippi | 40.97 | 35 | Vermont | 31.33 |
| 11 | Ohio | 40.92 | 36 | Montana | 30.99 |
| 12 | Illinois | 40.83 | 37 | California | 30.95 |
| 13 | Idaho | 39.54 | 38 | Maryland | 30.45 |
| 14 | Kentucky | 39.47 | 39 | Georgia | 30.00 |
| 15 | North Dakota | 38.99 | 40 | Nevada | 29.66 |
| 16 | Florida | 38.94 | 41 | South Dakota | 28.29 |
| 17 | South Carolina | 38.93 | 42 | Texas | 27.84 |
| 18 | New York | 38.44 | 43 | Nebraska | 27.81 |
| 19 | Rhode Island | 38.32 | 44 | Wyoming | 26.48 |
| 20 | North Carolina | 38.07 | 45 | New Mexico | 25.98 |
| 21 | Kansas | 37.61 | 46 | Utah | 25.95 |
| 22 | Delaware | 36.42 | 47 | Washington | 24.46 |
| 23 | Michigan | 35.55 | 48 | Hawaii | 22.96 |
| 24 | New Hampshire | 35.35 | 49 | Colorado | 21.05 |
| 25 | Massachusetts | 35.17 | 50 | Alaska | 19.22 |
| | | | | District of Columbia | 69.46 |

Source: American Cancer Society

"Cancer Facts & Figures – 1992" (Copyright 1992, Reprinted with permission from the American Cancer Society)

*Calculated by the editors using 1990 Census resident population figures. These estimates are offered as a rough guide and should not be regarded as definitive. They are calculated according to the distribution of estimated 1992 cancer deaths by state.

# AIDS Cases Reported in 1991

## National Total = 43,389 New AIDS Cases Reported in 1991

| RANK | STATE | CASES | % | RANK | STATE | CASES | % |
|---|---|---|---|---|---|---|---|
| 1 | New York | 8,162 | 18.81% | 26 | Oregon | 258 | 0.59% |
| 2 | California | 7,822 | 18.03% | 27 | Minnesota | 229 | 0.53% |
| 3 | Florida | 5,367 | 12.37% | 28 | Mississippi | 207 | 0.48% |
| 4 | Texas | 3,108 | 7.16% | 29 | Wisconsin | 206 | 0.47% |
| 5 | New Jersey | 2,307 | 5.32% | 30 | Oklahoma | 192 | 0.44% |
| 6 | Illinois | 1,550 | 3.57% | 31 | Hawaii | 190 | 0.44% |
| 7 | Georgia | 1,441 | 3.32% | 32 | Arkansas | 184 | 0.42% |
| 8 | Pennsylvania | 1,194 | 2.75% | 33 | Kentucky | 165 | 0.38% |
| 9 | Massachusetts | 975 | 2.25% | 34 | Utah | 135 | 0.31% |
| 10 | Maryland | 881 | 2.03% | 35 | Kansas | 109 | 0.25% |
| 11 | Louisiana | 753 | 1.74% | 36 | New Mexico | 103 | 0.24% |
| 12 | Virginia | 701 | 1.62% | 37 | Rhode Island | 99 | 0.23% |
| 13 | Missouri | 655 | 1.51% | 38 | Iowa | 97 | 0.22% |
| 14 | Michigan | 573 | 1.32% | 39 | Delaware | 89 | 0.21% |
| 15 | Ohio | 568 | 1.31% | 40 | West Virginia | 65 | 0.15% |
| 16 | Connecticut | 563 | 1.30% | 41 | Nebraska | 63 | 0.15% |
| 17 | Washington | 557 | 1.28% | 42 | Maine | 61 | 0.14% |
| 18 | North Carolina | 543 | 1.25% | 43 | New Hampshire | 45 | 0.10% |
| 19 | Colorado | 436 | 1.00% | 44 | Idaho | 32 | 0.07% |
| 20 | Tennessee | 349 | 0.80% | 45 | Montana | 29 | 0.07% |
| 21 | South Carolina | 337 | 0.78% | 46 | Alaska | 20 | 0.05% |
| 22 | Alabama | 326 | 0.75% | 46 | Vermont | 20 | 0.05% |
| 23 | Indiana | 314 | 0.72% | 48 | Wyoming | 17 | 0.04% |
| 24 | Arizona | 284 | 0.65% | 49 | North Dakota | 4 | 0.01% |
| 25 | Nevada | 264 | 0.61% | 50 | South Dakota | 3 | 0.01% |
| | | | | | District of Columbia | 737 | 1.70% |

Source: U.S. Department of Health and Human Services, Public Health Service
"Morbidity and Mortality Weekly Report" (January 3, 1992, Vol. 40, Nos. 51 & 52)

# AIDS Rate in 1991

## National Rate = 17.21 New AIDS Cases Reported per 100,000 Population*

| RANK | STATE | RATE | RANK | STATE | RATE |
|------|-------|------|------|-------|------|
| 1 | New York | 45.20 | 26 | Arkansas | 7.76 |
| 2 | Florida | 40.42 | 27 | Utah | 7.63 |
| 3 | New Jersey | 29.73 | 28 | Arizona | 7.57 |
| 4 | California | 25.75 | 29 | Tennessee | 7.05 |
| 5 | Georgia | 21.76 | 30 | New Mexico | 6.65 |
| 6 | Nevada | 20.56 | 31 | Michigan | 6.12 |
| 7 | Maryland | 18.13 | 32 | Oklahoma | 6.05 |
| 8 | Texas | 17.91 | 33 | Indiana | 5.60 |
| 9 | Louisiana | 17.71 | 34 | Ohio | 5.19 |
| 10 | Connecticut | 17.11 | 35 | Minnesota | 5.17 |
| 11 | Hawaii | 16.74 | 36 | Maine | 4.94 |
| 12 | Massachusetts | 16.26 | 37 | Kentucky | 4.44 |
| 13 | Illinois | 13.43 | 38 | Kansas | 4.37 |
| 14 | Delaware | 13.09 | 39 | Wisconsin | 4.16 |
| 15 | Colorado | 12.91 | 40 | New Hampshire | 4.07 |
| 16 | Missouri | 12.70 | 41 | Nebraska | 3.95 |
| 17 | Virginia | 11.15 | 42 | Wyoming | 3.70 |
| 18 | Washington | 11.10 | 43 | West Virginia | 3.61 |
| 19 | Pennsylvania | 9.98 | 44 | Montana | 3.59 |
| 20 | Rhode Island | 9.86 | 45 | Vermont | 3.53 |
| 21 | South Carolina | 9.47 | 46 | Alaska | 3.51 |
| 22 | Oregon | 8.83 | 47 | Iowa | 3.47 |
| 23 | North Carolina | 8.06 | 48 | Idaho | 3.08 |
| 24 | Mississippi | 7.99 | 49 | North Dakota | 0.63 |
| 25 | Alabama | 7.97 | 50 | South Dakota | 0.43 |

District of Columbia  123.24

*Source: U.S. Department of Health and Human Services, Public Health Service*

  *"Morbidity and Mortality Weekly Report" (January 3, 1992, Vol. 40, Nos. 51 & 52)*

*Rates calculated by the editors using 1991 Census population estimates.*

# AIDS Cases to 1992

## National Total = 202,730 AIDS Cases*

| RANK | STATE | AIDS CASES | % | RANK | STATE | AIDS CASES | % |
|---|---|---|---|---|---|---|---|
| 1 | New York | 43,066 | 21.24% | 26 | Minnesota | 1,057 | 0.52% |
| 2 | California | 39,065 | 19.27% | 27 | Oklahoma | 945 | 0.47% |
| 3 | Florida | 19,858 | 9.80% | 28 | Nevada | 917 | 0.45% |
| 4 | Texas | 14,691 | 7.25% | 29 | Mississippi | 886 | 0.44% |
| 5 | New Jersey | 12,860 | 6.34% | 30 | Wisconsin | 841 | 0.41% |
| 6 | Illinois | 6,427 | 3.17% | 31 | Hawaii | 832 | 0.41% |
| 7 | Georgia | 5,811 | 2.87% | 32 | Kentucky | 692 | 0.34% |
| 8 | Pennsylvania | 5,715 | 2.82% | 33 | Arkansas | 668 | 0.33% |
| 9 | Massachusetts | 4,309 | 2.13% | 34 | Kansas | 599 | 0.30% |
| 10 | Maryland | 4,185 | 2.06% | 35 | Utah | 485 | 0.24% |
| 11 | Louisiana | 3,128 | 1.54% | 36 | Rhode Island | 484 | 0.24% |
| 12 | Ohio | 2,982 | 1.47% | 37 | New Mexico | 462 | 0.23% |
| 13 | Washington | 2,822 | 1.39% | 38 | Delaware | 406 | 0.20% |
| 14 | Virginia | 2,747 | 1.36% | 39 | Iowa | 326 | 0.16% |
| 15 | Michigan | 2,592 | 1.28% | 40 | Maine | 275 | 0.14% |
| 16 | Missouri | 2,567 | 1.27% | 41 | Nebraska | 252 | 0.12% |
| 17 | Connecticut | 2,474 | 1.22% | 42 | West Virginia | 250 | 0.12% |
| 18 | North Carolina | 2,273 | 1.12% | 43 | New Hampshire | 245 | 0.12% |
| 19 | Colorado | 2,064 | 1.02% | 44 | Alaska | 122 | 0.06% |
| 20 | Arizona | 1,585 | 0.78% | 45 | Idaho | 111 | 0.05% |
| 21 | Tennessee | 1,502 | 0.74% | 46 | Vermont | 95 | 0.05% |
| 22 | South Carolina | 1,409 | 0.70% | 47 | Montana | 85 | 0.04% |
| 23 | Indiana | 1,372 | 0.68% | 48 | Wyoming | 53 | 0.03% |
| 24 | Oregon | 1,324 | 0.65% | 49 | South Dakota | 28 | 0.01% |
| 25 | Alabama | 1,303 | 0.64% | 50 | North Dakota | 24 | 0.01% |
| | | | | | District of Columbia | 3,459 | 1.71% |

Source: U.S. Department of Health and Human Services, Centers for Disease Control
    "HIV/AIDS Surveillance Report" (February 1992)
*Cumulative through January 1992.  AIDS is Acquired Immunodeficiency Syndrome.

# AIDS Cases in Children 12 Years and Younger: To 1992

## National Total = 3,330 AIDS Cases*

| RANK | STATE | AIDS CASES | % | RANK | STATE | AIDS CASES | % |
|------|-------|-----------|-----|------|-------|-----------|-----|
| 1 | New York | 961 | 28.86% | 26 | Indiana | 11 | 0.33% |
| 2 | Florida | 520 | 15.62% | 27 | Arizona | 10 | 0.30% |
| 3 | New Jersey | 358 | 10.75% | 27 | Nevada | 10 | 0.30% |
| 4 | California | 256 | 7.69% | 27 | Utah | 10 | 0.30% |
| 5 | Texas | 161 | 4.83% | 30 | Kentucky | 9 | 0.27% |
| 6 | Illinois | 98 | 2.94% | 30 | Minnesota | 9 | 0.27% |
| 7 | Massachusetts | 92 | 2.76% | 30 | Rhode Island | 9 | 0.27% |
| 8 | Pennsylvania | 91 | 2.73% | 30 | Wisconsin | 9 | 0.27% |
| 9 | Maryland | 90 | 2.70% | 34 | Hawaii | 7 | 0.21% |
| 10 | Connecticut | 69 | 2.07% | 34 | Oregon | 7 | 0.21% |
| 11 | Georgia | 57 | 1.71% | 36 | New Hampshire | 5 | 0.15% |
| 12 | Virginia | 54 | 1.62% | 37 | Delaware | 4 | 0.12% |
| 13 | Louisiana | 51 | 1.53% | 37 | Kansas | 4 | 0.12% |
| 14 | Ohio | 50 | 1.50% | 37 | West Virginia | 4 | 0.12% |
| 15 | Michigan | 42 | 1.26% | 40 | Alaska | 3 | 0.09% |
| 16 | North Carolina | 38 | 1.14% | 40 | Iowa | 3 | 0.09% |
| 17 | Alabama | 29 | 0.87% | 42 | Idaho | 2 | 0.06% |
| 18 | Missouri | 27 | 0.81% | 42 | Maine | 2 | 0.06% |
| 18 | South Carolina | 27 | 0.81% | 42 | Nebraska | 2 | 0.06% |
| 20 | Mississippi | 18 | 0.54% | 42 | New Mexico | 2 | 0.06% |
| 21 | Tennessee | 17 | 0.51% | 42 | Vermont | 2 | 0.06% |
| 22 | Washington | 16 | 0.48% | 47 | Montana | 1 | 0.03% |
| 23 | Arkansas | 14 | 0.42% | 48 | North Dakota | 0 | 0.00% |
| 24 | Colorado | 12 | 0.36% | 48 | South Dakota | 0 | 0.00% |
| 24 | Oklahoma | 12 | 0.36% | 48 | Wyoming | 0 | 0.00% |
| | | | | | District of Columbia | 45 | 1.35% |

Source: U.S. Department of Health and Human Services, Centers for Disease Control
    "HIV/AIDS Surveillance Report" (February 1992)
*Cumulative through January 1992.  AIDS is Acquired Immunodeficiency Syndrome.

# Aseptic Meningitis Cases Reported in 1991

## National Total = 14,102 Aseptic Meningitis Cases*

| RANK | STATE | CASES | % | RANK | STATE | CASES | % |
|---|---|---|---|---|---|---|---|
| 1 | New York | 1,714 | 12.15% | 26 | Wisconsin | 123 | 0.87% |
| 2 | California | 1,288 | 9.13% | 27 | Colorado | 113 | 0.80% |
| 3 | Texas | 1,149 | 8.15% | 28 | Mississippi | 83 | 0.59% |
| 4 | Ohio | 1,001 | 7.10% | 29 | Delaware | 73 | 0.52% |
| 5 | Pennsylvania | 958 | 6.79% | 30 | Arizona | 72 | 0.51% |
| 6 | Florida | 866 | 6.14% | 30 | Kansas | 72 | 0.51% |
| 7 | Michigan | 851 | 6.03% | 32 | Arkansas | 61 | 0.43% |
| 8 | Illinois | 540 | 3.83% | 33 | Hawaii | 57 | 0.40% |
| 9 | Massachusetts | 528 | 3.74% | 33 | West Virginia | 57 | 0.40% |
| 10 | Rhode Island | 484 | 3.43% | 35 | Alaska | 48 | 0.34% |
| 11 | Virginia | 463 | 3.28% | 36 | South Carolina | 40 | 0.28% |
| 12 | North Carolina | 341 | 2.42% | 37 | Nevada | 36 | 0.26% |
| 13 | Georgia | 336 | 2.38% | 38 | Nebraska | 30 | 0.21% |
| 14 | Maryland | 329 | 2.33% | 39 | New Mexico | 21 | 0.15% |
| 15 | Alabama | 293 | 2.08% | 40 | Montana | 18 | 0.13% |
| 16 | Missouri | 262 | 1.86% | 41 | Utah | 17 | 0.12% |
| 17 | Tennessee | 254 | 1.80% | 42 | South Dakota | 13 | 0.09% |
| 18 | Vermont | 230 | 1.63% | 43 | North Dakota | 12 | 0.09% |
| 19 | Indiana | 203 | 1.44% | 44 | Oklahoma | 10 | 0.07% |
| 20 | Kentucky | 200 | 1.42% | 45 | Connecticut | 7 | 0.05% |
| 21 | Iowa | 172 | 1.22% | 46 | Idaho | 0 | 0.00% |
| 22 | New Hampshire | 171 | 1.21% | 46 | New Jersey | 0 | 0.00% |
| 23 | Maine | 155 | 1.10% | 46 | Oregon | 0 | 0.00% |
| 24 | Louisiana | 137 | 0.97% | 46 | Washington | 0 | 0.00% |
| 25 | Minnesota | 136 | 0.96% | 46 | Wyoming | 0 | 0.00% |
| | | | | | District of Columbia | 78 | 0.55% |

*Source: U.S. Department of Health and Human Services, Public Health Service*
*"Morbidity and Mortality Weekly Report" (January 3, 1992, Vol. 40, Nos. 51 & 52)*
*An inflammation of the membranes that envelope the brain and spinal cord.*

# Aseptic Meningitis Rate in 1991

## National Rate = 5.59 Aseptic Meningitis Cases Reported per 100,000 Population*

| RANK | STATE | RATE | RANK | STATE | RATE |
|------|-------|------|------|-------|------|
| 1 | Rhode Island | 48.21 | 26 | Indiana | 3.62 |
| 2 | Vermont | 40.56 | 27 | Colorado | 3.35 |
| 3 | New Hampshire | 15.48 | 28 | Louisiana | 3.22 |
| 4 | Maine | 12.55 | 29 | Mississippi | 3.20 |
| 5 | Delaware | 10.74 | 30 | West Virginia | 3.16 |
| 6 | New York | 9.49 | 31 | Minnesota | 3.07 |
| 7 | Ohio | 9.15 | 32 | Kansas | 2.89 |
| 8 | Michigan | 9.08 | 33 | Nevada | 2.80 |
| 9 | Massachusetts | 8.81 | 34 | Arkansas | 2.57 |
| 10 | Alaska | 8.42 | 35 | Wisconsin | 2.48 |
| 11 | Pennsylvania | 8.01 | 36 | Montana | 2.23 |
| 12 | Virginia | 7.37 | 37 | Arizona | 1.92 |
| 13 | Alabama | 7.17 | 38 | North Dakota | 1.89 |
| 14 | Maryland | 6.77 | 39 | Nebraska | 1.88 |
| 15 | Texas | 6.62 | 40 | South Dakota | 1.85 |
| 16 | Florida | 6.52 | 41 | New Mexico | 1.36 |
| 17 | Iowa | 6.15 | 42 | South Carolina | 1.12 |
| 18 | Kentucky | 5.39 | 43 | Utah | 0.96 |
| 19 | Tennessee | 5.13 | 44 | Oklahoma | 0.31 |
| 20 | Missouri | 5.08 | 45 | Connecticut | 0.21 |
| 21 | Georgia | 5.07 | 46 | Idaho | 0.00 |
| 22 | North Carolina | 5.06 | 46 | New Jersey | 0.00 |
| 23 | Hawaii | 5.02 | 46 | Oregon | 0.00 |
| 24 | Illinois | 4.68 | 46 | Washington | 0.00 |
| 25 | California | 4.24 | 46 | Wyoming | 0.00 |
| | | | | District of Columbia | 13.04 |

Source: U.S. Department of Health and Human Services, Public Health Service
  "Morbidity and Mortality Weekly Report" (January 3, 1992, Vol. 40, Nos. 51 & 52)
*Calculated by the editors using 1991 Census resident population figures.  An inflammation of the membranes that envelope the brain and spinal cord.

# Chickenpox (Varicella) Cases Reported in 1990

## National Total = 173,099 Cases*

| RANK | STATE | CASES | % | RANK | STATE | CASES | % |
|------|-------|-------|---|------|-------|-------|---|
| 1 | Michigan | 38,024 | 21.97% | 26 | Nebraska | 122 | 0.07% |
| 2 | Illinois | 31,189 | 18.02% | 27 | Wyoming | 40 | 0.02% |
| 3 | Texas | 26,636 | 15.39% | 28 | Arkansas | 28 | 0.02% |
| 4 | Arizona | 11,771 | 6.80% | 28 | Delaware | 28 | 0.02% |
| 5 | Missouri | 10,591 | 6.12% | 30 | Nevada | 19 | 0.01% |
| 6 | Ohio | 9,711 | 5.61% | – | Alabama* | N/A | N/A |
| 7 | West Virginia | 6,365 | 3.68% | – | Alaska* | N/A | N/A |
| 8 | Iowa | 5,924 | 3.42% | – | Colorado* | N/A | N/A |
| 9 | Massachusetts | 5,897 | 3.41% | – | Florida* | N/A | N/A |
| 10 | New York | 4,738 | 2.74% | – | Georgia* | N/A | N/A |
| 11 | Kansas | 3,253 | 1.88% | – | Idaho* | N/A | N/A |
| 12 | Kentucky | 2,989 | 1.73% | – | Indiana* | N/A | N/A |
| 13 | Rhode Island | 2,834 | 1.64% | – | Louisiana* | N/A | N/A |
| 14 | Virginia | 2,677 | 1.55% | – | Maryland* | N/A | N/A |
| 15 | Tennessee | 2,363 | 1.37% | – | Minnesota* | N/A | N/A |
| 16 | New Hampshire | 2,299 | 1.33% | – | Mississippi* | N/A | N/A |
| 17 | Hawaii | 2,007 | 1.16% | – | New Jersey* | N/A | N/A |
| 18 | California | 904 | 0.52% | – | New Mexico* | N/A | N/A |
| 19 | South Carolina | 675 | 0.39% | – | North Carolina* | N/A | N/A |
| 20 | North Dakota | 642 | 0.37% | – | Oklahoma* | N/A | N/A |
| 21 | South Dakota | 367 | 0.21% | – | Oregon* | N/A | N/A |
| 22 | Maine | 283 | 0.16% | – | Pennsylvania* | N/A | N/A |
| 23 | Connecticut | 218 | 0.13% | – | Vermont* | N/A | N/A |
| 24 | Utah | 214 | 0.12% | – | Washington* | N/A | N/A |
| 25 | Montana | 196 | 0.11% | – | Wisconsin* | N/A | N/A |
| | | | | | District of Columbia | 95 | 0.05% |

Source: U.S. Department of Health and Human Services, Centers for Disease Control
    "Summary of Notifiable Diseases, United States 1990" (Morbidity and Mortality Weekly, October 4, 1991, Vol. 39, No. 53)
*Chickenpox is not reportable in states marked "N/A" except Wisconsin is not available. Connecticut is for persons age 16 and older only. National total does not include cases for states not reporting.

# Chickenpox (Varicella) Rate in 1990

## National Rate = 111.79 Chickenpox (Varicella) Cases Reported per 100,000 Population*

| RANK | STATE | RATE | RANK | STATE | RATE |
|------|-------|------|------|-------|------|
| 1 | Michigan | 409.07 | 26 | Connecticut | 6.63 |
| 2 | West Virginia | 354.90 | 27 | Delaware | 4.20 |
| 3 | Arizona | 321.15 | 28 | California | 3.04 |
| 4 | Rhode Island | 282.42 | 29 | Nevada | 1.58 |
| 5 | Illinois | 272.86 | 30 | Arkansas | 1.19 |
| 6 | Iowa | 213.34 | – | Alabama* | N/A |
| 7 | New Hampshire | 207.26 | – | Alaska* | N/A |
| 8 | Missouri | 206.97 | – | Colorado* | N/A |
| 9 | Hawaii | 181.10 | – | Florida* | N/A |
| 10 | Texas | 156.81 | – | Georgia* | N/A |
| 11 | Kansas | 131.30 | – | Idaho* | N/A |
| 12 | North Dakota | 100.50 | – | Indiana* | N/A |
| 13 | Massachusetts | 98.02 | – | Louisiana* | N/A |
| 14 | Ohio | 89.53 | – | Maryland* | N/A |
| 15 | Kentucky | 81.11 | – | Minnesota* | N/A |
| 16 | South Dakota | 52.73 | – | Mississippi* | N/A |
| 17 | Tennessee | 48.45 | – | New Jersey* | N/A |
| 18 | Virginia | 43.27 | – | New Mexico* | N/A |
| 19 | New York | 26.34 | – | North Carolina* | N/A |
| 20 | Montana | 24.53 | – | Oklahoma* | N/A |
| 21 | Maine | 23.05 | – | Oregon* | N/A |
| 22 | South Carolina | 19.36 | – | Pennsylvania* | N/A |
| 23 | Utah | 12.42 | – | Vermont* | N/A |
| 24 | Wyoming | 8.82 | – | Washington* | N/A |
| 25 | Nebraska | 7.73 | – | Wisconsin* | N/A |

District of Columbia          15.65

Source: U.S. Department of Health and Human Services, Centers for Disease Control
     "Summary of Notifiable Diseases, United States 1990" (Morbidity and Mortality Weekly, October 4, 1991, Vol. 39, No. 53)
*Calculated by the editors using 1990 Census resident population figures.  Chickenpox is not reportable in states marked "N/A" except Wisconsin is not available.  Connecticut is for persons age 16 and older only.  National rate does not include cases or population for states not reporting.

# Encephalitis Cases Reported in 1991

## National Total = 999 Encephalitis Cases*

| RANK | STATE | CASES | % | RANK | STATE | CASES | % |
|------|-------|-------|---|------|-------|-------|---|
| 1 | California | 114 | 11.41% | 26 | Oklahoma | 8 | 0.80% |
| 2 | Illinois | 94 | 9.41% | 27 | New Hampshire | 7 | 0.70% |
| 3 | Ohio | 90 | 9.01% | 28 | Wisconsin | 6 | 0.60% |
| 4 | Michigan | 60 | 6.01% | 29 | Delaware | 5 | 0.50% |
| 4 | Texas | 60 | 6.01% | 29 | Kansas | 5 | 0.50% |
| 6 | Florida | 52 | 5.21% | 29 | Vermont | 5 | 0.50% |
| 7 | Virginia | 51 | 5.11% | 32 | Iowa | 4 | 0.40% |
| 8 | New York | 45 | 4.50% | 32 | South Dakota | 4 | 0.40% |
| 9 | Minnesota | 38 | 3.80% | 34 | Maine | 3 | 0.30% |
| 10 | Pennsylvania | 36 | 3.60% | 35 | Alaska | 2 | 0.20% |
| 11 | North Carolina | 35 | 3.50% | 35 | Connecticut | 2 | 0.20% |
| 12 | West Virginia | 34 | 3.40% | 35 | Nebraska | 2 | 0.20% |
| 13 | Arkansas | 33 | 3.30% | 35 | North Dakota | 2 | 0.20% |
| 14 | Maryland | 26 | 2.60% | 39 | Hawaii | 1 | 0.10% |
| 15 | Indiana | 25 | 2.50% | 39 | Mississippi | 1 | 0.10% |
| 16 | Tennessee | 21 | 2.10% | 39 | Montana | 1 | 0.10% |
| 17 | Missouri | 18 | 1.80% | 39 | New Mexico | 1 | 0.10% |
| 18 | Louisiana | 17 | 1.70% | 39 | Rhode Island | 1 | 0.10% |
| 19 | Kentucky | 16 | 1.60% | 44 | Idaho | 0 | 0.00% |
| 19 | Massachusetts | 16 | 1.60% | 44 | Nevada | 0 | 0.00% |
| 21 | Arizona | 13 | 1.30% | 44 | New Jersey | 0 | 0.00% |
| 22 | Georgia | 12 | 1.20% | 44 | Oregon | 0 | 0.00% |
| 23 | Alabama | 11 | 1.10% | 44 | South Carolina | 0 | 0.00% |
| 23 | Washington | 11 | 1.10% | 44 | Utah | 0 | 0.00% |
| 25 | Colorado | 9 | 0.90% | 44 | Wyoming | 0 | 0.00% |

District of Columbia    2    0.20%

Source: U.S. Department of Health and Human Services, Public Health Service
   "Morbidity and Mortality Weekly Report" (January 3, 1992, Vol. 40, Nos. 51 & 52)
*Inflammation of the brain.  Includes Primary and Post-infectious cases.

# Encephalitis Rate in 1991

## National Rate = 0.40 Encephalitis Cases Reported per 100,000 Population*

| RANK | STATE | RATE | | RANK | STATE | RATE |
|------|-------|------|---|------|-------|------|
| 1 | West Virginia | 1.89 | | 26 | Alabama | 0.27 |
| 2 | Arkansas | 1.39 | | 26 | Colorado | 0.27 |
| 3 | Vermont | 0.88 | | 26 | Massachusetts | 0.27 |
| 4 | Minnesota | 0.86 | | 29 | New York | 0.25 |
| 5 | Ohio | 0.82 | | 29 | Oklahoma | 0.25 |
| 6 | Illinois | 0.81 | | 31 | Maine | 0.24 |
| 6 | Virginia | 0.81 | | 32 | Washington | 0.22 |
| 8 | Delaware | 0.74 | | 33 | Kansas | 0.20 |
| 9 | Michigan | 0.64 | | 34 | Georgia | 0.18 |
| 10 | New Hampshire | 0.63 | | 35 | Iowa | 0.14 |
| 11 | South Dakota | 0.57 | | 36 | Nebraska | 0.13 |
| 12 | Maryland | 0.53 | | 37 | Montana | 0.12 |
| 13 | North Carolina | 0.52 | | 37 | Wisconsin | 0.12 |
| 14 | Indiana | 0.45 | | 39 | Rhode Island | 0.10 |
| 15 | Kentucky | 0.43 | | 40 | Hawaii | 0.09 |
| 16 | Tennessee | 0.42 | | 41 | Connecticut | 0.06 |
| 17 | Louisiana | 0.40 | | 41 | New Mexico | 0.06 |
| 18 | Florida | 0.39 | | 43 | Mississippi | 0.04 |
| 19 | California | 0.38 | | 44 | Idaho | 0.00 |
| 20 | Alaska | 0.35 | | 44 | Nevada | 0.00 |
| 20 | Arizona | 0.35 | | 44 | New Jersey | 0.00 |
| 20 | Missouri | 0.35 | | 44 | Oregon | 0.00 |
| 20 | Texas | 0.35 | | 44 | South Carolina | 0.00 |
| 24 | North Dakota | 0.31 | | 44 | Utah | 0.00 |
| 25 | Pennsylvania | 0.30 | | 44 | Wyoming | 0.00 |
| | | | | | District of Columbia | 0.33 |

Source: U.S. Department of Health and Human Services, Public Health Service
"Morbidity and Mortality Weekly Report" (January 3, 1992, Vol. 40, Nos. 51 & 52)
*Calculated by the editors using 1991 Census resident population figures. Inflammation of the brain. Includes Primary and Post-infectious cases.

# German Measles (Rubella) Cases Reported in 1991

## National Total = 1,372 German Measles (Rubella) Cases

| RANK | STATE | CASES | % | RANK | STATE | CASES | % |
|---|---|---|---|---|---|---|---|
| 1 | New York | 541 | 39.43% | 26 | Alaska | 1 | 0.07% |
| 2 | Ohio | 283 | 20.63% | 26 | Arkansas | 1 | 0.07% |
| 3 | California | 267 | 19.46% | 26 | Connecticut | 1 | 0.07% |
| 4 | Tennessee | 100 | 7.29% | 26 | Kansas | 1 | 0.07% |
| 5 | Pennsylvania | 43 | 3.13% | 26 | Louisiana | 1 | 0.07% |
| 6 | Michigan | 25 | 1.82% | 26 | Maryland | 1 | 0.07% |
| 7 | Montana | 11 | 0.80% | 26 | New Hampshire | 1 | 0.07% |
| 7 | Utah | 11 | 0.80% | 26 | New Jersey | 1 | 0.07% |
| 9 | Illinois | 8 | 0.58% | 26 | North Dakota | 1 | 0.07% |
| 9 | Washington | 8 | 0.58% | 26 | Wisconsin | 1 | 0.07% |
| 11 | Florida | 7 | 0.51% | 36 | Alabama | 0 | 0.00% |
| 11 | Nevada | 7 | 0.51% | 36 | Delaware | 0 | 0.00% |
| 13 | Hawaii | 6 | 0.44% | 36 | Georgia | 0 | 0.00% |
| 13 | Iowa | 6 | 0.44% | 36 | Idaho | 0 | 0.00% |
| 13 | Minnesota | 6 | 0.44% | 36 | Kentucky | 0 | 0.00% |
| 16 | Missouri | 5 | 0.36% | 36 | Maine | 0 | 0.00% |
| 16 | Oregon | 5 | 0.36% | 36 | Mississippi | 0 | 0.00% |
| 16 | Texas | 5 | 0.36% | 36 | Nebraska | 0 | 0.00% |
| 19 | New Mexico | 4 | 0.29% | 36 | Rhode Island | 0 | 0.00% |
| 20 | Colorado | 3 | 0.22% | 36 | South Carolina | 0 | 0.00% |
| 21 | Arizona | 2 | 0.15% | 36 | South Dakota | 0 | 0.00% |
| 21 | Indiana | 2 | 0.15% | 36 | Vermont | 0 | 0.00% |
| 21 | Massachusetts | 2 | 0.15% | 36 | Virginia | 0 | 0.00% |
| 21 | North Carolina | 2 | 0.15% | 36 | West Virginia | 0 | 0.00% |
| 21 | Oklahoma | 2 | 0.15% | 36 | Wyoming | 0 | 0.00% |

District of Columbia     1     0.07%

Source: U.S. Department of Health and Human Services, Public Health Service
  "Morbidity and Mortality Weekly Report" (January 3, 1992, Vol. 40, Nos. 51 & 52)

# German Measles (Rubella) Rate in 1991

## National Rate = 0.54 German Measles (Rubella) Cases Reported per 100,000 Population*

| RANK | STATE | RATE | RANK | STATE | RATE |
|------|-------|------|------|-------|------|
| 1 | New York | 3.00 | 25 | Indiana | 0.04 |
| 2 | Ohio | 2.59 | 25 | Kansas | 0.04 |
| 3 | Tennessee | 2.02 | 28 | Connecticut | 0.03 |
| 4 | Montana | 1.36 | 28 | Massachusetts | 0.03 |
| 5 | California | 0.88 | 28 | North Carolina | 0.03 |
| 6 | Utah | 0.62 | 28 | Texas | 0.03 |
| 7 | Nevada | 0.55 | 32 | Louisiana | 0.02 |
| 8 | Hawaii | 0.53 | 32 | Maryland | 0.02 |
| 9 | Pennsylvania | 0.36 | 32 | Wisconsin | 0.02 |
| 10 | Michigan | 0.27 | 35 | New Jersey | 0.01 |
| 11 | New Mexico | 0.26 | 36 | Alabama | 0.00 |
| 12 | Iowa | 0.21 | 36 | Delaware | 0.00 |
| 13 | Alaska | 0.18 | 36 | Georgia | 0.00 |
| 14 | Oregon | 0.17 | 36 | Idaho | 0.00 |
| 15 | North Dakota | 0.16 | 36 | Kentucky | 0.00 |
| 15 | Washington | 0.16 | 36 | Maine | 0.00 |
| 17 | Minnesota | 0.14 | 36 | Mississippi | 0.00 |
| 18 | Missouri | 0.10 | 36 | Nebraska | 0.00 |
| 19 | Colorado | 0.09 | 36 | Rhode Island | 0.00 |
| 19 | New Hampshire | 0.09 | 36 | South Carolina | 0.00 |
| 21 | Illinois | 0.07 | 36 | South Dakota | 0.00 |
| 22 | Oklahoma | 0.06 | 36 | Vermont | 0.00 |
| 23 | Arizona | 0.05 | 36 | Virginia | 0.00 |
| 23 | Florida | 0.05 | 36 | West Virginia | 0.00 |
| 25 | Arkansas | 0.04 | 36 | Wyoming | 0.00 |

| | | |
|---|---|---|
| | District of Columbia | 0.17 |

Source: U.S. Department of Health and Human Services, Public Health Service
   "Morbidity and Mortality Weekly Report" (January 3, 1992, Vol. 40, Nos. 51 & 52)
*Calculated by the editors using 1991 Census resident population figures.

# Gonorrhea Cases Reported in 1991

## National Total = 602,577 Gonorrhea Cases

| RANK | STATE | CASES | % | | RANK | STATE | CASES | % |
|---|---|---|---|---|---|---|---|---|
| 1 | Georgia | 44,915 | 7.45% | | 26 | Kentucky | 5,913 | 0.98% |
| 2 | California | 44,679 | 7.41% | | 27 | Washington | 4,566 | 0.76% |
| 3 | New York | 39,163 | 6.50% | | 28 | Kansas | 4,527 | 0.75% |
| 4 | Texas | 36,790 | 6.11% | | 29 | Arizona | 4,457 | 0.74% |
| 5 | Ohio | 36,303 | 6.02% | | 30 | Colorado | 3,809 | 0.63% |
| 6 | Florida | 35,317 | 5.86% | | 31 | Minnesota | 3,083 | 0.51% |
| 7 | Illinois | 34,566 | 5.74% | | 32 | Delaware | 2,961 | 0.49% |
| 8 | North Carolina | 33,695 | 5.59% | | 33 | Nevada | 2,433 | 0.40% |
| 9 | Michigan | 27,015 | 4.48% | | 34 | Oregon | 2,029 | 0.34% |
| 10 | Pennsylvania | 24,244 | 4.02% | | 35 | Iowa | 1,974 | 0.33% |
| 11 | Maryland | 19,656 | 3.26% | | 36 | Nebraska | 1,817 | 0.30% |
| 12 | Tennessee | 19,343 | 3.21% | | 37 | West Virginia | 1,265 | 0.21% |
| 13 | Alabama | 18,212 | 3.02% | | 38 | Rhode Island | 1,196 | 0.20% |
| 14 | Virginia | 18,172 | 3.02% | | 39 | New Mexico | 973 | 0.16% |
| 15 | Missouri | 17,551 | 2.91% | | 40 | Alaska | 891 | 0.15% |
| 16 | Louisiana | 14,934 | 2.48% | | 41 | Hawaii | 671 | 0.11% |
| 17 | South Carolina | 14,055 | 2.33% | | 42 | South Dakota | 348 | 0.06% |
| 18 | Mississippi | 14,006 | 2.32% | | 43 | Utah | 338 | 0.06% |
| 19 | Indiana | 11,840 | 1.96% | | 44 | New Hampshire | 183 | 0.03% |
| 20 | New Jersey | 11,318 | 1.88% | | 45 | Idaho | 161 | 0.03% |
| 21 | Arkansas | 8,009 | 1.33% | | 46 | Maine | 158 | 0.03% |
| 22 | Oklahoma | 6,862 | 1.14% | | 47 | Montana | 100 | 0.02% |
| 23 | Wisconsin | 6,429 | 1.07% | | 48 | Wyoming | 95 | 0.02% |
| 24 | Connecticut | 6,357 | 1.05% | | 49 | North Dakota | 83 | 0.01% |
| 25 | Massachusetts | 6,002 | 1.00% | | 50 | Vermont | 54 | 0.01% |
| | | | | | | District of Columbia | 9,059 | 1.50% |

*Source: U.S. Department of Health and Human Services, Public Health Service*
*"Morbidity and Mortality Weekly Report" (January 3, 1992, Vol. 40, Nos. 51 & 52)*

# Gonorrhea Rate in 1991

## National Rate = Gonorrhea Cases Reported per 100,000 Population*

| RANK | STATE | RATE | RANK | STATE | RATE |
|------|-------|------|------|-------|------|
| 1 | Georgia | 678.17 | 26 | Alaska | 156.32 |
| 2 | Mississippi | 540.35 | 27 | California | 147.07 |
| 3 | North Carolina | 500.15 | 28 | New Jersey | 145.85 |
| 4 | Alabama | 445.39 | 29 | Wisconsin | 129.75 |
| 5 | Delaware | 435.44 | 30 | Rhode Island | 119.12 |
| 6 | Maryland | 404.44 | 31 | Arizona | 118.85 |
| 7 | South Carolina | 394.80 | 32 | Nebraska | 114.06 |
| 8 | Tennessee | 390.53 | 33 | Colorado | 112.79 |
| 9 | Louisiana | 351.22 | 34 | Massachusetts | 100.10 |
| 10 | Missouri | 340.27 | 35 | Washington | 90.99 |
| 11 | Arkansas | 337.65 | 36 | Iowa | 70.63 |
| 12 | Ohio | 331.87 | 37 | West Virginia | 70.24 |
| 13 | Illinois | 299.45 | 38 | Minnesota | 69.56 |
| 14 | Virginia | 289.09 | 39 | Oregon | 69.44 |
| 15 | Michigan | 288.38 | 40 | New Mexico | 62.86 |
| 16 | Florida | 266.00 | 41 | Hawaii | 59.12 |
| 17 | New York | 216.87 | 42 | South Dakota | 49.50 |
| 18 | Oklahoma | 216.13 | 43 | Wyoming | 20.65 |
| 19 | Texas | 212.06 | 44 | Utah | 19.10 |
| 20 | Indiana | 211.05 | 45 | New Hampshire | 16.56 |
| 21 | Pennsylvania | 202.69 | 46 | Idaho | 15.50 |
| 22 | Connecticut | 193.16 | 47 | North Dakota | 13.07 |
| 23 | Nevada | 189.49 | 48 | Maine | 12.79 |
| 24 | Kansas | 181.44 | 49 | Montana | 12.38 |
| 25 | Kentucky | 159.25 | 50 | Vermont | 9.52 |

District of Columbia     1,514.88

Source: U.S. Department of Health and Human Services, Public Health Service
   "Morbidity and Mortality Weekly Report" (January 3, 1992, Vol. 40, Nos. 51 & 52)
*Calculated by the editors using 1991 Census resident population figures.

# Hepatitis (Viral) Cases Reported in 1991

## National Total = 44,086 Hepatitis (Viral) Cases*

| RANK | STATE | CASES | % | RANK | STATE | CASES | % |
|---|---|---|---|---|---|---|---|
| 1 | California | 8,469 | 19.21% | 26 | Oklahoma | 567 | 1.29% |
| 2 | Texas | 4,031 | 9.14% | 27 | Minnesota | 536 | 1.22% |
| 3 | New York | 2,943 | 6.68% | 28 | Nevada | 535 | 1.21% |
| 4 | Florida | 1,742 | 3.95% | 29 | Louisiana | 508 | 1.15% |
| 5 | Illinois | 1,698 | 3.85% | 30 | Utah | 399 | 0.91% |
| 6 | Tennessee | 1,558 | 3.53% | 31 | Arkansas | 385 | 0.87% |
| 7 | Missouri | 1,428 | 3.24% | 32 | Connecticut | 262 | 0.59% |
| 8 | Arizona | 1,359 | 3.08% | 33 | Kentucky | 258 | 0.59% |
| 9 | Washington | 1,155 | 2.62% | 34 | Nebraska | 243 | 0.55% |
| 10 | Wisconsin | 1,120 | 2.54% | 35 | Alabama | 236 | 0.54% |
| 11 | Michigan | 1,106 | 2.51% | 36 | Idaho | 179 | 0.41% |
| 12 | New Mexico | 1,055 | 2.39% | 37 | Montana | 167 | 0.38% |
| 13 | Ohio | 959 | 2.18% | 38 | Wyoming | 158 | 0.36% |
| 14 | Pennsylvania | 942 | 2.14% | 39 | Rhode Island | 156 | 0.35% |
| 15 | Colorado | 920 | 2.09% | 40 | Kansas | 155 | 0.35% |
| 16 | Massachusetts | 908 | 2.06% | 41 | Alaska | 144 | 0.33% |
| 17 | North Carolina | 873 | 1.98% | 42 | Hawaii | 130 | 0.29% |
| 18 | Oregon | 868 | 1.97% | 43 | West Virginia | 109 | 0.25% |
| 19 | Georgia | 865 | 1.96% | 44 | Iowa | 104 | 0.24% |
| 20 | South Dakota | 844 | 1.91% | 45 | New Hampshire | 72 | 0.16% |
| 21 | New Jersey | 750 | 1.70% | 46 | Delaware | 71 | 0.16% |
| 22 | South Carolina | 723 | 1.64% | 46 | North Dakota | 71 | 0.16% |
| 23 | Maryland | 722 | 1.64% | 48 | Maine | 56 | 0.13% |
| 24 | Indiana | 622 | 1.41% | 49 | Mississippi | 53 | 0.12% |
| 25 | Virginia | 589 | 1.34% | 50 | Vermont | 47 | 0.11% |
| | | | | | District of Columbia | 236 | 0.54% |

Source: U.S. Department of Health and Human Services, Public Health Service
   "Morbidity and Mortality Weekly Report" (January 3, 1992, Vol. 40, Nos. 51 & 52)
*An inflammation of the liver. Includes types A, B, NA, NB and unspecified.

# Hepatitis (Viral) Rate in 1991

## National Rate = 17.48 Hepatitis (Viral) Cases Reported per 100,000 Population*

| RANK | STATE | RATE | RANK | STATE | RATE |
|---|---|---|---|---|---|
| 1 | South Dakota | 120.06 | 26 | Illinois | 14.71 |
| 2 | New Mexico | 68.15 | 27 | Florida | 13.12 |
| 3 | Nevada | 41.67 | 28 | Georgia | 13.06 |
| 4 | Arizona | 36.24 | 29 | North Carolina | 12.96 |
| 5 | Wyoming | 34.35 | 30 | Minnesota | 12.09 |
| 6 | Tennessee | 31.46 | 31 | Louisiana | 11.95 |
| 7 | Oregon | 29.71 | 32 | Michigan | 11.81 |
| 8 | California | 27.88 | 33 | Hawaii | 11.45 |
| 9 | Missouri | 27.69 | 34 | North Dakota | 11.18 |
| 10 | Colorado | 27.24 | 35 | Indiana | 11.09 |
| 11 | Alaska | 25.26 | 36 | Delaware | 10.44 |
| 12 | Texas | 23.23 | 37 | New Jersey | 9.66 |
| 13 | Washington | 23.02 | 38 | Virginia | 9.37 |
| 14 | Wisconsin | 22.60 | 39 | Ohio | 8.77 |
| 15 | Utah | 22.54 | 40 | Vermont | 8.29 |
| 16 | Montana | 20.67 | 41 | Connecticut | 7.96 |
| 17 | South Carolina | 20.31 | 42 | Pennsylvania | 7.88 |
| 18 | Oklahoma | 17.86 | 43 | Kentucky | 6.95 |
| 19 | Idaho | 17.23 | 44 | New Hampshire | 6.52 |
| 20 | New York | 16.30 | 45 | Kansas | 6.21 |
| 21 | Arkansas | 16.23 | 46 | West Virginia | 6.05 |
| 22 | Rhode Island | 15.54 | 47 | Alabama | 5.77 |
| 23 | Nebraska | 15.25 | 48 | Maine | 4.53 |
| 24 | Massachusetts | 15.14 | 49 | Iowa | 3.72 |
| 25 | Maryland | 14.86 | 50 | Mississippi | 2.04 |
| | | | | District of Columbia | 39.46 |

Source: U.S. Department of Health and Human Services, Public Health Service
   "Morbidity and Mortality Weekly Report" (January 3, 1992, Vol. 40, Nos. 51 & 52)
*Calculated by the editors using 1991 Census resident population figures. An inflammation of the liver. Includes types A, B, NA, NB and unspecified.
Rates calculated by the editors using 1991 Census population estimates.

# Legionellosis Cases Reported in 1991

## National Total = 1,222 Legionellosis Cases*

| RANK | STATE | CASES | % |
|---|---|---|---|
| 1 | New York | 187 | 15.30% |
| 2 | Ohio | 136 | 11.13% |
| 3 | Pennsylvania | 121 | 9.90% |
| 4 | California | 76 | 6.22% |
| 5 | Massachusetts | 60 | 4.91% |
| 6 | Michigan | 52 | 4.26% |
| 7 | South Carolina | 39 | 3.19% |
| 8 | Florida | 37 | 3.03% |
| 8 | Maryland | 37 | 3.03% |
| 10 | Arizona | 33 | 2.70% |
| 11 | New Jersey | 32 | 2.62% |
| 12 | Wisconsin | 31 | 2.54% |
| 13 | North Carolina | 27 | 2.21% |
| 14 | Georgia | 22 | 1.80% |
| 14 | Illinois | 22 | 1.80% |
| 14 | Oklahoma | 22 | 1.80% |
| 17 | Indiana | 18 | 1.47% |
| 17 | Kentucky | 18 | 1.47% |
| 17 | Tennessee | 18 | 1.47% |
| 20 | Missouri | 17 | 1.39% |
| 20 | Virginia | 17 | 1.39% |
| 22 | Alabama | 16 | 1.31% |
| 23 | Colorado | 15 | 1.23% |
| 24 | Minnesota | 13 | 1.06% |
| 24 | Texas | 13 | 1.06% |

| RANK | STATE | CASES | % |
|---|---|---|---|
| 24 | Washington | 13 | 1.06% |
| 27 | Iowa | 12 | 0.98% |
| 28 | Nevada | 11 | 0.90% |
| 29 | Louisiana | 10 | 0.82% |
| 29 | Nebraska | 10 | 0.82% |
| 31 | New Hampshire | 9 | 0.74% |
| 31 | Utah | 9 | 0.74% |
| 33 | Arkansas | 7 | 0.57% |
| 33 | Montana | 7 | 0.57% |
| 35 | Maine | 6 | 0.49% |
| 35 | Rhode Island | 6 | 0.49% |
| 37 | Idaho | 5 | 0.41% |
| 38 | Kansas | 4 | 0.33% |
| 38 | Vermont | 4 | 0.33% |
| 38 | West Virginia | 4 | 0.33% |
| 41 | Delaware | 3 | 0.25% |
| 41 | New Mexico | 3 | 0.25% |
| 41 | Oregon | 3 | 0.25% |
| 41 | South Dakota | 3 | 0.25% |
| 45 | Hawaii | 2 | 0.16% |
| 46 | Mississippi | 1 | 0.08% |
| 46 | North Dakota | 1 | 0.08% |
| 48 | Alaska | 0 | 0.00% |
| 48 | Connecticut | 0 | 0.00% |
| 48 | Wyoming | 0 | 0.00% |
| | District of Columbia | 10 | 0.82% |

Source: U.S. Department of Health and Human Services, Public Health Service
   "Morbidity and Mortality Weekly Report" (January 3, 1992, Vol. 40, Nos. 51 & 52)
*A pneumonia-like disease (Legionnaire's Disease).

# Legionellosis Rate in 1991

## National Rate = 0.48 Legionellosis Cases Reported per 100,000 Population*

| RANK | STATE | RATE | RANK | STATE | RATE |
|------|-------|------|------|-------|------|
| 1 | Ohio | 1.24 | 26 | North Carolina | 0.40 |
| 2 | South Carolina | 1.10 | 27 | Alabama | 0.39 |
| 3 | New York | 1.04 | 28 | Tennessee | 0.36 |
| 4 | Pennsylvania | 1.01 | 29 | Georgia | 0.33 |
| 5 | Massachusetts | 1.00 | 29 | Missouri | 0.33 |
| 6 | Arizona | 0.88 | 31 | Indiana | 0.32 |
| 7 | Montana | 0.87 | 32 | Arkansas | 0.30 |
| 8 | Nevada | 0.86 | 33 | Minnesota | 0.29 |
| 9 | New Hampshire | 0.81 | 34 | Florida | 0.28 |
| 10 | Maryland | 0.76 | 35 | Virginia | 0.27 |
| 11 | Vermont | 0.71 | 36 | Washington | 0.26 |
| 12 | Oklahoma | 0.69 | 37 | California | 0.25 |
| 13 | Nebraska | 0.63 | 38 | Louisiana | 0.24 |
| 13 | Wisconsin | 0.63 | 39 | West Virginia | 0.22 |
| 15 | Rhode Island | 0.60 | 40 | Illinois | 0.19 |
| 16 | Michigan | 0.56 | 40 | New Mexico | 0.19 |
| 17 | Utah | 0.51 | 42 | Hawaii | 0.18 |
| 18 | Maine | 0.49 | 43 | Kansas | 0.16 |
| 19 | Idaho | 0.48 | 43 | North Dakota | 0.16 |
| 19 | Kentucky | 0.48 | 45 | Oregon | 0.10 |
| 21 | Colorado | 0.44 | 46 | Texas | 0.07 |
| 21 | Delaware | 0.44 | 47 | Mississippi | 0.04 |
| 23 | Iowa | 0.43 | 48 | Alaska | 0.00 |
| 23 | South Dakota | 0.43 | 48 | Connecticut | 0.00 |
| 25 | New Jersey | 0.41 | 48 | Wyoming | 0.00 |

District of Columbia          1.67

Source: U.S. Department of Health and Human Services, Public Health Service
    "Morbidity and Mortality Weekly Report" (January 3, 1992, Vol. 40, Nos. 51 & 52)
*Calculated by the editors using 1991 Census resident population figures. A pneumonia-like disease (Legionnaire's Disease).

# Lyme Disease Cases Reported in 1991

## National Total = 8,884 Lyme Disease Cases*

| RANK | STATE | CASES | % | RANK | STATE | CASES | % |
|---|---|---|---|---|---|---|---|
| 1 | New York | 3,357 | 37.79% | 25 | Kansas | 22 | 0.25% |
| 2 | Connecticut | 1,221 | 13.74% | 27 | Alabama | 18 | 0.20% |
| 3 | Pennsylvania | 1,022 | 11.50% | 28 | Texas | 15 | 0.17% |
| 4 | New Jersey | 852 | 9.59% | 29 | Indiana | 13 | 0.15% |
| 5 | California | 323 | 3.64% | 30 | South Carolina | 10 | 0.11% |
| 6 | Massachusetts | 290 | 3.26% | 31 | Wyoming | 9 | 0.10% |
| 7 | Maryland | 274 | 3.08% | 32 | Nevada | 7 | 0.08% |
| 8 | Virginia | 202 | 2.27% | 32 | Vermont | 7 | 0.08% |
| 9 | Missouri | 193 | 2.17% | 34 | Louisiana | 6 | 0.07% |
| 10 | Rhode Island | 177 | 1.99% | 35 | Utah | 3 | 0.03% |
| 11 | Ohio | 173 | 1.95% | 35 | Washington | 3 | 0.03% |
| 12 | Michigan | 110 | 1.24% | 37 | Idaho | 2 | 0.02% |
| 13 | Minnesota | 85 | 0.96% | 37 | North Dakota | 2 | 0.02% |
| 14 | North Carolina | 81 | 0.91% | 39 | Arizona | 1 | 0.01% |
| 15 | Delaware | 72 | 0.81% | 39 | South Dakota | 1 | 0.01% |
| 16 | Tennessee | 45 | 0.51% | 41 | Alaska | 0 | 0.00% |
| 17 | West Virginia | 44 | 0.50% | 41 | Colorado | 0 | 0.00% |
| 18 | Kentucky | 43 | 0.48% | 41 | Hawaii | 0 | 0.00% |
| 19 | New Hampshire | 35 | 0.39% | 41 | Maine | 0 | 0.00% |
| 20 | Georgia | 31 | 0.35% | 41 | Mississippi | 0 | 0.00% |
| 20 | Oklahoma | 31 | 0.35% | 41 | Montana | 0 | 0.00% |
| 22 | Arkansas | 29 | 0.33% | 41 | Nebraska | 0 | 0.00% |
| 23 | Illinois | 25 | 0.28% | 41 | New Mexico | 0 | 0.00% |
| 24 | Florida | 23 | 0.26% | 41 | Oregon | 0 | 0.00% |
| 25 | Iowa | 22 | 0.25% | 41 | Wisconsin | 0 | 0.00% |
| | | | | | District of Columbia | 5 | 0.06% |

Source: U.S. Department of Health and Human Services, Public Health Service

"Morbidity and Mortality Weekly Report" (January 3, 1992, Vol. 40, Nos. 51 & 52)

*Caused by ticks--lesions followed by arthritis of large joints, myalgia, malaise and neurologic and cardiac manifestations. Named after Old Lyme, CT, where the disease was first reported.

# Lyme Disease Rate in 1991

## National Rate = 3.52 Lyme Disease Cases Reported per 100,000 Population*

| RANK | STATE | RATE | RANK | STATE | RATE |
|---|---|---|---|---|---|
| 1 | Connecticut | 37.10 | 26 | Nevada | 0.55 |
| 2 | New York | 18.59 | 27 | Georgia | 0.47 |
| 3 | Rhode Island | 17.63 | 28 | Alabama | 0.44 |
| 4 | New Jersey | 10.98 | 29 | North Dakota | 0.31 |
| 5 | Delaware | 10.59 | 30 | South Carolina | 0.28 |
| 6 | Pennsylvania | 8.54 | 31 | Indiana | 0.23 |
| 7 | Maryland | 5.64 | 32 | Illinois | 0.22 |
| 8 | Massachusetts | 4.84 | 33 | Idaho | 0.19 |
| 9 | Missouri | 3.74 | 34 | Florida | 0.17 |
| 10 | Virginia | 3.21 | 34 | Utah | 0.17 |
| 11 | New Hampshire | 3.17 | 36 | Louisiana | 0.14 |
| 12 | West Virginia | 2.44 | 36 | South Dakota | 0.14 |
| 13 | Wyoming | 1.96 | 38 | Texas | 0.09 |
| 14 | Minnesota | 1.92 | 39 | Washington | 0.06 |
| 15 | Ohio | 1.58 | 40 | Arizona | 0.03 |
| 16 | Vermont | 1.23 | 41 | Alaska | 0.00 |
| 17 | Arkansas | 1.22 | 41 | Colorado | 0.00 |
| 18 | North Carolina | 1.20 | 41 | Hawaii | 0.00 |
| 19 | Michigan | 1.17 | 41 | Maine | 0.00 |
| 20 | Kentucky | 1.16 | 41 | Mississippi | 0.00 |
| 21 | California | 1.06 | 41 | Montana | 0.00 |
| 22 | Oklahoma | 0.98 | 41 | Nebraska | 0.00 |
| 23 | Tennessee | 0.91 | 41 | New Mexico | 0.00 |
| 24 | Kansas | 0.88 | 41 | Oregon | 0.00 |
| 25 | Iowa | 0.79 | 41 | Wisconsin | 0.00 |
| | | | | District of Columbia | 0.84 |

Source: U.S. Department of Health and Human Services, Public Health Service

"Morbidity and Mortality Weekly Report" (January 3, 1992, Vol. 40, Nos. 51 & 52)

*Calculated by the editors using 1991 Census resident population figures. Caused by ticks--lesions followed by arthritis of large joints, myalgia, malaise and neurologic and cardiac manifestations. Named after Old Lyme, CT, where the disease was first reported.

# Malaria Cases Reported in 1991

## National Total = 1,173 Malaria Cases*

| RANK | STATE | CASES | % | RANK | STATE | CASES | % |
|---|---|---|---|---|---|---|---|
| 1 | California | 321 | 27.37% | 26 | Missouri | 9 | 0.77% |
| 2 | New York | 161 | 13.73% | 27 | Kansas | 8 | 0.68% |
| 3 | Maryland | 61 | 5.20% | 27 | Oklahoma | 8 | 0.68% |
| 4 | New Jersey | 55 | 4.69% | 29 | Alabama | 7 | 0.60% |
| 5 | Virginia | 52 | 4.43% | 29 | Iowa | 7 | 0.60% |
| 6 | Florida | 51 | 4.35% | 31 | New Mexico | 6 | 0.51% |
| 7 | Illinois | 39 | 3.32% | 32 | Hawaii | 5 | 0.43% |
| 8 | Texas | 37 | 3.15% | 32 | Utah | 5 | 0.43% |
| 9 | Massachusetts | 32 | 2.73% | 34 | Vermont | 4 | 0.34% |
| 10 | Michigan | 29 | 2.47% | 35 | Delaware | 3 | 0.26% |
| 11 | Washington | 26 | 2.22% | 35 | Idaho | 3 | 0.26% |
| 12 | Connecticut | 23 | 1.96% | 35 | Indiana | 3 | 0.26% |
| 13 | Georgia | 22 | 1.88% | 35 | West Virginia | 3 | 0.26% |
| 14 | Ohio | 20 | 1.71% | 35 | Wisconsin | 3 | 0.26% |
| 15 | Pennsylvania | 18 | 1.53% | 40 | Kentucky | 2 | 0.17% |
| 16 | Louisiana | 17 | 1.45% | 40 | Nevada | 2 | 0.17% |
| 17 | Arizona | 16 | 1.36% | 40 | New Hampshire | 2 | 0.17% |
| 18 | North Carolina | 15 | 1.28% | 40 | North Dakota | 2 | 0.17% |
| 19 | Colorado | 13 | 1.11% | 40 | South Dakota | 2 | 0.17% |
| 20 | Oregon | 12 | 1.02% | 45 | Maine | 1 | 0.09% |
| 21 | Minnesota | 11 | 0.94% | 45 | Montana | 1 | 0.09% |
| 21 | Tennessee | 11 | 0.94% | 45 | Nebraska | 1 | 0.09% |
| 23 | Arkansas | 10 | 0.85% | 48 | Alaska | 0 | 0.00% |
| 23 | Rhode Island | 10 | 0.85% | 48 | Mississippi | 0 | 0.00% |
| 23 | South Carolina | 10 | 0.85% | 48 | Wyoming | 0 | 0.00% |
| | | | | | District of Columbia | 14 | 1.19% |

Source: U.S. Department of Health and Human Services, Public Health Service
    "Morbidity and Mortality Weekly Report" (January 3, 1992, Vol. 40, Nos. 51 & 52)
*Infectious disease usually transmitted by bites of infected mosquitoes. High fever, shaking chills, sweating, anemia and spenomegaly.

# Malaria Rate in 1991

## National Rate = 0.47 Malaria Cases Reported per 100,000 Population*

| RANK | STATE | RATE | RANK | STATE | RATE |
|---|---|---|---|---|---|
| 1 | Maryland | 1.26 | 26 | South Carolina | 0.28 |
| 2 | California | 1.06 | 26 | South Dakota | 0.28 |
| 3 | Rhode Island | 1.00 | 26 | Utah | 0.28 |
| 4 | New York | 0.89 | 29 | Iowa | 0.25 |
| 5 | Virginia | 0.83 | 29 | Minnesota | 0.25 |
| 6 | New Jersey | 0.71 | 29 | Oklahoma | 0.25 |
| 6 | Vermont | 0.71 | 32 | North Carolina | 0.22 |
| 8 | Connecticut | 0.70 | 32 | Tennessee | 0.22 |
| 9 | Massachusetts | 0.53 | 34 | Texas | 0.21 |
| 10 | Washington | 0.52 | 35 | New Hampshire | 0.18 |
| 11 | Delaware | 0.44 | 35 | Ohio | 0.18 |
| 11 | Hawaii | 0.44 | 37 | Alabama | 0.17 |
| 13 | Arizona | 0.43 | 37 | Missouri | 0.17 |
| 14 | Arkansas | 0.42 | 37 | West Virginia | 0.17 |
| 15 | Oregon | 0.41 | 40 | Nevada | 0.16 |
| 16 | Louisiana | 0.40 | 41 | Pennsylvania | 0.15 |
| 17 | New Mexico | 0.39 | 42 | Montana | 0.12 |
| 18 | Colorado | 0.38 | 43 | Maine | 0.08 |
| 18 | Florida | 0.38 | 44 | Nebraska | 0.06 |
| 20 | Illinois | 0.34 | 44 | Wisconsin | 0.06 |
| 21 | Georgia | 0.33 | 46 | Indiana | 0.05 |
| 22 | Kansas | 0.32 | 46 | Kentucky | 0.05 |
| 23 | Michigan | 0.31 | 48 | Alaska | 0.00 |
| 23 | North Dakota | 0.31 | 48 | Mississippi | 0.00 |
| 25 | Idaho | 0.29 | 48 | Wyoming | 0.00 |

District of Columbia     2.34

Source: U.S. Department of Health and Human Services, Public Health Service
   *"Morbidity and Mortality Weekly Report"* (January 3, 1992, Vol. 40, Nos. 51 & 52)
*Calculated by the editors using 1991 Census resident population figures. Infectious disease usually transmitted by bites of infected mosquitoes. High fever, shaking chills, sweating, anemia and spenomegaly.

# Measles (Rubeola) Cases Reported in 1991

## National Total = 9,488 Measles (Rubeola) Cases*

| RANK | STATE | CASES | % | RANK | STATE | CASES | % |
|------|-------|-------|---|------|-------|-------|---|
| 1 | New York | 2,313 | 24.38% | 26 | Georgia | 15 | 0.16% |
| 2 | California | 1,990 | 20.97% | 27 | Kansas | 13 | 0.14% |
| 3 | Pennsylvania | 1,545 | 16.28% | 27 | South Carolina | 13 | 0.14% |
| 4 | New Jersey | 1,028 | 10.83% | 29 | Colorado | 12 | 0.13% |
| 5 | Arizona | 453 | 4.77% | 30 | Ohio | 11 | 0.12% |
| 6 | Idaho | 452 | 4.76% | 31 | Wisconsin | 9 | 0.09% |
| 7 | Florida | 356 | 3.75% | 32 | Maine | 7 | 0.07% |
| 8 | Utah | 224 | 2.36% | 32 | Tennessee | 7 | 0.07% |
| 9 | Texas | 214 | 2.26% | 34 | Indiana | 6 | 0.06% |
| 10 | Maryland | 178 | 1.88% | 35 | Alaska | 5 | 0.05% |
| 11 | New Mexico | 122 | 1.29% | 35 | Arkansas | 5 | 0.05% |
| 12 | Oregon | 93 | 0.98% | 35 | Vermont | 5 | 0.05% |
| 13 | Washington | 61 | 0.64% | 38 | Rhode Island | 4 | 0.04% |
| 14 | North Carolina | 44 | 0.46% | 39 | Wyoming | 3 | 0.03% |
| 15 | Massachusetts | 43 | 0.45% | 40 | Alabama | 2 | 0.02% |
| 15 | Michigan | 43 | 0.45% | 41 | Missouri | 1 | 0.01% |
| 17 | Virginia | 31 | 0.33% | 41 | Nebraska | 1 | 0.01% |
| 18 | Minnesota | 27 | 0.28% | 43 | Louisiana | 0 | 0.00% |
| 19 | Connecticut | 26 | 0.27% | 43 | Mississippi | 0 | 0.00% |
| 19 | Illinois | 26 | 0.27% | 43 | Montana | 0 | 0.00% |
| 21 | Kentucky | 24 | 0.25% | 43 | New Hampshire | 0 | 0.00% |
| 22 | Delaware | 21 | 0.22% | 43 | North Dakota | 0 | 0.00% |
| 23 | Hawaii | 19 | 0.20% | 43 | Oklahoma | 0 | 0.00% |
| 23 | Nevada | 19 | 0.20% | 43 | South Dakota | 0 | 0.00% |
| 25 | Iowa | 17 | 0.18% | 43 | West Virginia | 0 | 0.00% |
|  |  |  |  |  | District of Columbia | 0 | 0.00% |

Source: U.S. Department of Health and Human Services, Public Health Service
   "Morbidity and Mortality Weekly Report" (January 3, 1992, Vol. 40, Nos. 51 & 52)
*Includes indigenous and imported cases.

# Measles (Rubeola) Rate in 1991

## National Rate = 3.76 Measles (Rubeola) Cases Reported per 100,000 Population*

| RANK | STATE | RATE | RANK | STATE | RATE |
|------|-------|------|------|-------|------|
| 1 | Idaho | 43.50 | 26 | Maine | 0.57 |
| 2 | New Jersey | 13.25 | 27 | Kansas | 0.52 |
| 3 | Pennsylvania | 12.92 | 28 | Virginia | 0.49 |
| 4 | New York | 12.81 | 29 | Michigan | 0.46 |
| 5 | Utah | 12.66 | 30 | Rhode Island | 0.40 |
| 6 | Arizona | 12.08 | 31 | South Carolina | 0.37 |
| 7 | New Mexico | 7.88 | 32 | Colorado | 0.36 |
| 8 | California | 6.55 | 33 | Georgia | 0.23 |
| 9 | Maryland | 3.66 | 33 | Illinois | 0.23 |
| 10 | Oregon | 3.18 | 35 | Arkansas | 0.21 |
| 11 | Delaware | 3.09 | 36 | Wisconsin | 0.18 |
| 12 | Florida | 2.68 | 37 | Tennessee | 0.14 |
| 13 | Hawaii | 1.67 | 38 | Indiana | 0.11 |
| 14 | Nevada | 1.48 | 39 | Ohio | 0.10 |
| 15 | Texas | 1.23 | 40 | Nebraska | 0.06 |
| 16 | Washington | 1.22 | 41 | Alabama | 0.05 |
| 17 | Alaska | 0.88 | 42 | Missouri | 0.02 |
| 17 | Vermont | 0.88 | 43 | Louisiana | 0.00 |
| 19 | Connecticut | 0.79 | 43 | Mississippi | 0.00 |
| 20 | Massachusetts | 0.72 | 43 | Montana | 0.00 |
| 21 | Kentucky | 0.65 | 43 | New Hampshire | 0.00 |
| 21 | North Carolina | 0.65 | 43 | North Dakota | 0.00 |
| 21 | Wyoming | 0.65 | 43 | Oklahoma | 0.00 |
| 24 | Iowa | 0.61 | 43 | South Dakota | 0.00 |
| 24 | Minnesota | 0.61 | 43 | West Virginia | 0.00 |
| | | | | District of Columbia | 0.00 |

Source: U.S. Department of Health and Human Services, Public Health Service
"Morbidity and Mortality Weekly Report" (January 3, 1992, Vol. 40, Nos. 51 & 52)
*Calculated by the editors using 1991 Census resident population figures. Includes indigenous and imported cases.

# Mumps Cases Reported in 1991

## National Total = 4,031 Mumps Cases*

| RANK | STATE | CASES | % | RANK | STATE | CASES | % |
|---|---|---|---|---|---|---|---|
| 1 | California | 499 | 12.38% | 26 | Iowa | 24 | 0.60% |
| 2 | Florida | 445 | 11.04% | 27 | Mississippi | 22 | 0.55% |
| 3 | South Carolina | 380 | 9.43% | 27 | Nevada | 22 | 0.55% |
| 4 | North Carolina | 269 | 6.67% | 29 | Minnesota | 21 | 0.52% |
| 5 | Maryland | 251 | 6.23% | 30 | Alaska | 17 | 0.42% |
| 6 | Texas | 240 | 5.95% | 31 | Oklahoma | 16 | 0.40% |
| 7 | Tennessee | 195 | 4.84% | 32 | Alabama | 15 | 0.37% |
| 8 | Washington | 171 | 4.24% | 32 | Utah | 15 | 0.37% |
| 9 | Illinois | 147 | 3.65% | 34 | Connecticut | 12 | 0.30% |
| 10 | Colorado | 135 | 3.35% | 34 | Idaho | 12 | 0.30% |
| 11 | Pennsylvania | 124 | 3.08% | 36 | Indiana | 9 | 0.22% |
| 12 | Arizona | 122 | 3.03% | 37 | Nebraska | 8 | 0.20% |
| 13 | Michigan | 121 | 3.00% | 38 | Delaware | 7 | 0.17% |
| 14 | Ohio | 112 | 2.78% | 39 | New Hampshire | 6 | 0.15% |
| 15 | New York | 107 | 2.65% | 40 | Wyoming | 5 | 0.12% |
| 16 | Georgia | 86 | 2.13% | 41 | Rhode Island | 4 | 0.10% |
| 17 | Virginia | 70 | 1.74% | 41 | Vermont | 4 | 0.10% |
| 18 | New Jersey | 65 | 1.61% | 43 | Massachusetts | 2 | 0.05% |
| 19 | Arkansas | 44 | 1.09% | 43 | North Dakota | 2 | 0.05% |
| 20 | Louisiana | 41 | 1.02% | 43 | South Dakota | 2 | 0.05% |
| 21 | Missouri | 40 | 0.99% | 46 | Kentucky | 0 | 0.00% |
| 22 | Kansas | 31 | 0.77% | 46 | Maine | 0 | 0.00% |
| 23 | Hawaii | 30 | 0.74% | 46 | Montana | 0 | 0.00% |
| 23 | Wisconsin | 30 | 0.74% | – | New Mexico* | N/A | N/A |
| 25 | West Virginia | 27 | 0.67% | – | Oregon* | N/A | N/A |
| | | | | | District of Columbia | 24 | 0.60% |

Source: U.S. Department of Health and Human Services, Public Health Service

*"Morbidity and Mortality Weekly Report" (January 3, 1992, Vol. 40, Nos. 51 & 52)*

*Mumps is not a notifiable disease in these states.

# Mumps Rate in 1991

## National Rate = 1.60 Mumps Cases Reported per 100,000 Population*

| RANK | STATE | RATE | RANK | STATE | RATE |
|------|-------|------|------|-------|------|
| 1 | South Carolina | 10.67 | 26 | Louisiana | 0.96 |
| 2 | Maryland | 5.16 | 27 | Iowa | 0.86 |
| 3 | Colorado | 4.00 | 28 | Mississippi | 0.85 |
| 4 | North Carolina | 3.99 | 28 | Utah | 0.85 |
| 5 | Tennessee | 3.94 | 30 | New Jersey | 0.84 |
| 6 | Washington | 3.41 | 31 | Missouri | 0.78 |
| 7 | Florida | 3.35 | 32 | Vermont | 0.71 |
| 8 | Arizona | 3.25 | 33 | Wisconsin | 0.61 |
| 9 | Alaska | 2.98 | 34 | New York | 0.59 |
| 10 | Hawaii | 2.64 | 35 | New Hampshire | 0.54 |
| 11 | Arkansas | 1.85 | 36 | Nebraska | 0.50 |
| 12 | Nevada | 1.71 | 36 | Oklahoma | 0.50 |
| 13 | California | 1.64 | 38 | Minnesota | 0.47 |
| 14 | West Virginia | 1.50 | 39 | Rhode Island | 0.40 |
| 15 | Texas | 1.38 | 40 | Alabama | 0.37 |
| 16 | Georgia | 1.30 | 41 | Connecticut | 0.36 |
| 17 | Michigan | 1.29 | 42 | North Dakota | 0.31 |
| 18 | Illinois | 1.27 | 43 | South Dakota | 0.28 |
| 19 | Kansas | 1.24 | 44 | Indiana | 0.16 |
| 20 | Idaho | 1.15 | 45 | Massachusetts | 0.03 |
| 21 | Virginia | 1.11 | 46 | Kentucky | 0.00 |
| 22 | Wyoming | 1.09 | 46 | Maine | 0.00 |
| 23 | Pennsylvania | 1.04 | 46 | Montana | 0.00 |
| 24 | Delaware | 1.03 | – | New Mexico* | N/A |
| 25 | Ohio | 1.02 | – | Oregon* | N/A |

District of Columbia      4.01

Source: U.S. Department of Health and Human Services, Public Health Service
    "Morbidity and Mortality Weekly Report" (January 3, 1992, Vol. 40, Nos. 51 & 52)
*Calculated by the editors using 1991 Census resident population figures. Mumps is not a notifiable disease in New Mexico and Oregon.

# Rabies (Animal) Cases Reported in 1991

## National Total = 6,486 Rabies (Animal) Cases*

| RANK | STATE | CASES | % | RANK | STATE | CASES | % |
|---|---|---|---|---|---|---|---|
| 1 | New Jersey | 976 | 15.05% | 26 | Illinois | 35 | 0.54% |
| 2 | New York | 957 | 14.75% | 27 | Michigan | 33 | 0.51% |
| 3 | Maryland | 564 | 8.70% | 28 | Florida | 30 | 0.46% |
| 4 | California | 462 | 7.12% | 29 | Indiana | 29 | 0.45% |
| 5 | Texas | 375 | 5.78% | 29 | Tennessee | 29 | 0.45% |
| 6 | Pennsylvania | 365 | 5.63% | 31 | Colorado | 25 | 0.39% |
| 7 | Minnesota | 306 | 4.72% | 32 | Missouri | 23 | 0.35% |
| 8 | Georgia | 253 | 3.90% | 32 | North Carolina | 23 | 0.35% |
| 8 | Virginia | 253 | 3.90% | 34 | Ohio | 20 | 0.31% |
| 10 | Connecticut | 185 | 2.85% | 35 | Utah | 19 | 0.29% |
| 11 | Delaware | 183 | 2.82% | 36 | Nebraska | 17 | 0.26% |
| 12 | Oklahoma | 174 | 2.68% | 37 | Massachusetts | 14 | 0.22% |
| 12 | South Dakota | 174 | 2.68% | 38 | Nevada | 11 | 0.17% |
| 14 | Iowa | 155 | 2.39% | 39 | Louisiana | 7 | 0.11% |
| 15 | South Carolina | 113 | 1.74% | 40 | Idaho | 6 | 0.09% |
| 16 | North Dakota | 107 | 1.65% | 40 | New Mexico | 6 | 0.09% |
| 17 | Wyoming | 83 | 1.28% | 42 | Oregon | 5 | 0.08% |
| 18 | Alabama | 76 | 1.17% | 43 | Alaska | 3 | 0.05% |
| 19 | Wisconsin | 65 | 1.00% | 44 | New Hampshire | 2 | 0.03% |
| 20 | Kansas | 60 | 0.93% | 45 | Hawaii | 1 | 0.02% |
| 21 | West Virginia | 52 | 0.80% | 45 | Washington | 1 | 0.02% |
| 22 | Arizona | 50 | 0.77% | 47 | Maine | 0 | 0.00% |
| 23 | Arkansas | 48 | 0.74% | 47 | Mississippi | 0 | 0.00% |
| 23 | Kentucky | 48 | 0.74% | 47 | Rhode Island | 0 | 0.00% |
| 25 | Montana | 41 | 0.63% | 47 | Vermont | 0 | 0.00% |
| | | | | | District of Columbia | 22 | 0.34% |

*Source: U.S. Department of Health and Human Services, Public Health Service*
*"Morbidity and Mortality Weekly Report" (January 3, 1992, Vol. 40, Nos. 51 & 52)*
*There were 3 reported cases of humans with rabies in 1991.*

# Rabies (Animal) Rate in 1991

## National Rate = 2.57 Rabies (Animal) Cases Reported per 100,000 Human Population*

| RANK | STATE | RATE | RANK | STATE | RATE |
|------|-------|------|------|-------|------|
| 1 | Delaware | 26.91 | 26 | Nebraska | 1.07 |
| 2 | South Dakota | 24.75 | 26 | Utah | 1.07 |
| 3 | Wyoming | 18.04 | 28 | Nevada | 0.86 |
| 4 | North Dakota | 16.85 | 29 | Colorado | 0.74 |
| 5 | New Jersey | 12.58 | 30 | Tennessee | 0.59 |
| 6 | Maryland | 11.60 | 31 | Idaho | 0.58 |
| 7 | Minnesota | 6.90 | 32 | Alaska | 0.53 |
| 8 | Connecticut | 5.62 | 33 | Indiana | 0.52 |
| 9 | Iowa | 5.55 | 34 | Missouri | 0.45 |
| 10 | Oklahoma | 5.48 | 35 | New Mexico | 0.39 |
| 11 | New York | 5.30 | 36 | Michigan | 0.35 |
| 12 | Montana | 5.07 | 37 | North Carolina | 0.34 |
| 13 | Virginia | 4.02 | 38 | Illinois | 0.30 |
| 14 | Georgia | 3.82 | 39 | Florida | 0.23 |
| 15 | South Carolina | 3.17 | 39 | Massachusetts | 0.23 |
| 16 | Pennsylvania | 3.05 | 41 | New Hampshire | 0.18 |
| 17 | West Virginia | 2.89 | 41 | Ohio | 0.18 |
| 18 | Kansas | 2.40 | 43 | Oregon | 0.17 |
| 19 | Texas | 2.16 | 44 | Louisiana | 0.16 |
| 20 | Arkansas | 2.02 | 45 | Hawaii | 0.09 |
| 21 | Alabama | 1.86 | 46 | Washington | 0.02 |
| 22 | California | 1.52 | 47 | Maine | 0.00 |
| 23 | Arizona | 1.33 | 47 | Mississippi | 0.00 |
| 24 | Wisconsin | 1.31 | 47 | Rhode Island | 0.00 |
| 25 | Kentucky | 1.29 | 47 | Vermont | 0.00 |

District of Columbia     3.68

Source: U.S. Department of Health and Human Services, Public Health Service
"Morbidity and Mortality Weekly Report" (January 3, 1992, Vol. 40, Nos. 51 & 52)
*Calculated by the editors using 1991 Census resident population figures. There were 3 reported cases of humans with rabies in 1991.

# Salmonellosis Cases Reported in 1990

## National Total = 48,603 Cases of Salmonellosis*

| RANK | STATE | CASES | % | RANK | STATE | CASES | % |
|------|-------|-------|---|------|-------|-------|---|
| 1 | California | 5,725 | 11.78% | 26 | Colorado | 632 | 1.30% |
| 2 | New York | 3,716 | 7.65% | 27 | Mississippi | 583 | 1.20% |
| 3 | Illinois | 3,231 | 6.65% | 28 | Kentucky | 503 | 1.03% |
| 4 | Pennsylvania | 2,891 | 5.95% | 29 | Hawaii | 456 | 0.94% |
| 5 | Florida | 2,562 | 5.27% | 30 | New Mexico | 446 | 0.92% |
| 6 | Texas | 2,315 | 4.76% | 31 | Oklahoma | 437 | 0.90% |
| 7 | Massachusetts | 2,079 | 4.28% | 32 | Arkansas | 430 | 0.88% |
| 8 | New Jersey | 1,870 | 3.85% | 33 | Oregon | 359 | 0.74% |
| 9 | Georgia | 1,633 | 3.36% | 34 | Rhode Island | 316 | 0.65% |
| 10 | Virginia | 1,491 | 3.07% | 35 | Iowa | 313 | 0.64% |
| 11 | Ohio | 1,316 | 2.71% | 36 | Kansas | 295 | 0.61% |
| 12 | Michigan | 1,310 | 2.70% | 37 | Delaware | 291 | 0.60% |
| 13 | North Carolina | 1,265 | 2.60% | 38 | New Hampshire | 272 | 0.56% |
| 14 | Maryland | 1,256 | 2.58% | 39 | Maine | 244 | 0.50% |
| 15 | Wisconsin | 1,175 | 2.42% | 40 | Nebraska | 231 | 0.48% |
| 16 | Connecticut | 916 | 1.88% | 41 | Nevada | 189 | 0.39% |
| 17 | Louisiana | 822 | 1.69% | 42 | Vermont | 175 | 0.36% |
| 18 | Minnesota | 771 | 1.59% | 43 | West Virginia | 173 | 0.36% |
| 19 | Indiana | 748 | 1.54% | 44 | Utah | 150 | 0.31% |
| 20 | Alabama | 728 | 1.50% | 45 | Montana | 112 | 0.23% |
| 21 | South Carolina | 727 | 1.50% | 45 | North Dakota | 112 | 0.23% |
| 22 | Missouri | 723 | 1.49% | 47 | Alaska | 107 | 0.22% |
| 23 | Tennessee | 721 | 1.48% | 48 | Idaho | 94 | 0.19% |
| 24 | Arizona | 706 | 1.45% | 49 | South Dakota | 87 | 0.18% |
| 25 | Washington | 634 | 1.30% | 50 | Wyoming | 52 | 0.11% |
| | | | | | District of Columbia | 213 | 0.44% |

Source: U.S. Department of Health and Human Services, Centers for Disease Control

*"Summary of Notifiable Diseases, United States 1990"* (Morbidity and Mortality Weekly Report, October 4, 1991, Vol. 39, No. 53)

*Any disease caused by a salmonellal infection, which may be manifested as food poisoning with acute gastroenteritis, vomiting and diarrhea.

# Salmonellosis Rate in 1990

## National Rate = 19.54 Salmonellosis Cases Reported per 100,000 Population*

| RANK | STATE | RATE | RANK | STATE | RATE |
|---|---|---|---|---|---|
| 1 | Delaware | 43.68 | 26 | North Carolina | 19.08 |
| 2 | Hawaii | 41.15 | 27 | Arkansas | 18.29 |
| 3 | Massachusetts | 34.56 | 28 | Alabama | 18.02 |
| 4 | Rhode Island | 31.49 | 29 | Minnesota | 17.62 |
| 5 | Vermont | 31.10 | 30 | North Dakota | 17.53 |
| 6 | New Mexico | 29.44 | 31 | Nevada | 15.73 |
| 7 | Illinois | 28.27 | 31 | Tennessee | 14.78 |
| 8 | Connecticut | 27.87 | 31 | Nebraska | 14.64 |
| 9 | Maryland | 26.27 | 31 | Missouri | 14.13 |
| 10 | Georgia | 25.21 | 31 | Michigan | 14.09 |
| 11 | New Hampshire | 24.52 | 31 | Montana | 14.02 |
| 12 | Pennsylvania | 24.33 | 31 | Oklahoma | 13.89 |
| 13 | New Jersey | 24.19 | 31 | Kentucky | 13.65 |
| 14 | Virginia | 24.10 | 31 | Texas | 13.63 |
| 15 | Wisconsin | 24.02 | 31 | Indiana | 13.49 |
| 16 | Mississippi | 22.66 | 31 | Washington | 13.03 |
| 17 | South Carolina | 20.85 | 31 | Oregon | 12.63 |
| 18 | New York | 20.66 | 31 | South Dakota | 12.50 |
| 19 | Maine | 19.87 | 31 | Ohio | 12.13 |
| 20 | Florida | 19.80 | 31 | Kansas | 11.91 |
| 21 | Louisiana | 19.48 | 31 | Wyoming | 11.46 |
| 22 | Alaska | 19.45 | 31 | Iowa | 11.27 |
| 23 | Arizona | 19.26 | 31 | West Virginia | 9.65 |
| 24 | California | 19.24 | 31 | Idaho | 9.34 |
| 25 | Colorado | 19.18 | 31 | Utah | 8.71 |

|  |  |  |
|---|---|---|
| | District of Columbia | 35.10 |

Source: U.S. Department of Health and Human Services, Centers for Disease Control

"Summary of Notifiable Diseases, United States 1990" (Morbidity and Mortality Weekly Report, October 4, 1991, Vol. 39, No. 53)

*Calculated by the editors using 1990 Census resident population figures. Any disease caused by a salmonellal infection, which may be manifested as food poisoning with acute gastroenteritis, vomiting and diarrhea.

## Shigellosis Cases Reported in 1990

### National Total = 27,077 Cases of Shigellosis*

| RANK | STATE | CASES | % | RANK | STATE | CASES | % |
|------|-------|-------|---|------|-------|-------|---|
| 1 | California | 5,703 | 21.06% | 26 | Maryland | 238 | 0.88% |
| 2 | Texas | 3,550 | 13.11% | 27 | Tennessee | 237 | 0.88% |
| 3 | Arizona | 1,988 | 7.34% | 28 | Connecticut | 227 | 0.84% |
| 4 | New York | 1,725 | 6.37% | 29 | Oregon | 178 | 0.66% |
| 5 | Florida | 1,630 | 6.02% | 30 | Virginia | 158 | 0.58% |
| 6 | Illinois | 1,126 | 4.16% | 31 | Delaware | 147 | 0.54% |
| 7 | New Mexico | 948 | 3.50% | 31 | North Dakota | 147 | 0.54% |
| 8 | Pennsylvania | 871 | 3.22% | 33 | Kansas | 135 | 0.50% |
| 9 | Georgia | 721 | 2.66% | 34 | Minnesota | 118 | 0.44% |
| 10 | North Carolina | 667 | 2.46% | 35 | Arkansas | 92 | 0.34% |
| 11 | Ohio | 628 | 2.32% | 36 | South Dakota | 81 | 0.30% |
| 12 | Alabama | 566 | 2.09% | 37 | New Hampshire | 65 | 0.24% |
| 13 | Oklahoma | 511 | 1.89% | 38 | Kentucky | 55 | 0.20% |
| 14 | Michigan | 466 | 1.72% | 39 | Hawaii | 54 | 0.20% |
| 15 | Massachusetts | 409 | 1.51% | 40 | Iowa | 51 | 0.19% |
| 16 | Colorado | 389 | 1.44% | 41 | Nebraska | 48 | 0.18% |
| 17 | South Carolina | 360 | 1.33% | 42 | Montana | 45 | 0.17% |
| 18 | Utah | 355 | 1.31% | 43 | Nevada | 40 | 0.15% |
| 19 | Indiana | 351 | 1.30% | 44 | Rhode Island | 34 | 0.13% |
| 20 | New Jersey | 331 | 1.22% | 45 | Idaho | 26 | 0.10% |
| 21 | Louisiana | 303 | 1.12% | 46 | West Virginia | 22 | 0.08% |
| 22 | Mississippi | 287 | 1.06% | 47 | Vermont | 14 | 0.05% |
| 23 | Missouri | 284 | 1.05% | 48 | Maine | 13 | 0.05% |
| 24 | Wisconsin | 280 | 1.03% | 49 | Alaska | 11 | 0.04% |
| 25 | Washington | 279 | 1.03% | 50 | Wyoming | 10 | 0.04% |
| | | | | | District of Columbia | 103 | 0.38% |

*Source: U.S. Department of Health and Human Services, Centers for Disease Control*
   *"Summary of Notifiable Diseases, United States 1990" (Morbidity and Mortality Weekly Report, October 4, 1991, Vol. 39, No. 53)*
*Produced by infection with Shigella organisms. These cause dysentery.*

# Shigellosis Rate in 1990

## National Rate = 10.89 Shigellosis Cases Reported per 100,000 Population*

| RANK | STATE | RATE | RANK | STATE | RATE |
|---|---|---|---|---|---|
| 1 | New Mexico | 62.57 | 26 | Ohio | 5.79 |
| 2 | Arizona | 54.24 | 27 | Washington | 5.73 |
| 3 | North Dakota | 23.01 | 28 | Wisconsin | 5.72 |
| 4 | Delaware | 22.07 | 29 | Montana | 5.63 |
| 5 | Texas | 20.90 | 30 | Missouri | 5.55 |
| 6 | Utah | 20.61 | 31 | Kansas | 5.45 |
| 7 | California | 19.16 | 32 | Michigan | 5.01 |
| 8 | Oklahoma | 16.24 | 33 | Maryland | 4.98 |
| 9 | Alabama | 14.01 | 34 | Hawaii | 4.87 |
| 10 | Florida | 12.60 | 35 | Tennessee | 4.86 |
| 11 | Colorado | 11.81 | 36 | New Jersey | 4.28 |
| 12 | South Dakota | 11.64 | 37 | Arkansas | 3.91 |
| 13 | Mississippi | 11.15 | 38 | Rhode Island | 3.39 |
| 14 | Georgia | 11.13 | 39 | Nevada | 3.33 |
| 15 | South Carolina | 10.32 | 40 | Nebraska | 3.04 |
| 16 | North Carolina | 10.06 | 41 | Minnesota | 2.70 |
| 17 | Illinois | 9.85 | 42 | Idaho | 2.58 |
| 18 | New York | 9.59 | 43 | Virginia | 2.55 |
| 19 | Pennsylvania | 7.33 | 44 | Vermont | 2.49 |
| 20 | Louisiana | 7.18 | 45 | Wyoming | 2.20 |
| 21 | Connecticut | 6.91 | 46 | Alaska | 2.00 |
| 22 | Massachusetts | 6.80 | 47 | Iowa | 1.84 |
| 23 | Indiana | 6.33 | 48 | Kentucky | 1.49 |
| 24 | Oregon | 6.26 | 49 | West Virginia | 1.23 |
| 25 | New Hampshire | 5.86 | 50 | Maine | 1.06 |

District of Columbia    16.97

Source: U.S. Department of Health and Human Services, Centers for Disease Control
"Summary of Notifiable Diseases, United States 1990" (Morbidity and Mortality Weekly Report, October 4, 1991, Vol. 39, No. 53)
*Calculated by the editors using 1990 Census resident population figures. Produced by infection with Shigella organisms. These cause dysentery.

# Syphilis Cases Reported in 1991

## National Total = 41,006 Syphilis Cases*

| RANK | STATE | CASES | % | RANK | STATE | CASES | % |
|------|-------|-------|---|------|-------|-------|---|
| 1 | New York | 4,117 | 10.04% | 26 | Kansas | 193 | 0.47% |
| 2 | Texas | 3,891 | 9.49% | 27 | Delaware | 185 | 0.45% |
| 3 | Georgia | 2,868 | 6.99% | 28 | Indiana | 179 | 0.44% |
| 4 | Florida | 2,756 | 6.72% | 29 | Washington | 178 | 0.43% |
| 5 | Louisiana | 2,692 | 6.56% | 30 | Nevada | 113 | 0.28% |
| 6 | Illinois | 2,373 | 5.79% | 31 | Kentucky | 112 | 0.27% |
| 7 | California | 2,288 | 5.58% | 32 | Colorado | 87 | 0.21% |
| 8 | North Carolina | 1,967 | 4.80% | 33 | Oregon | 84 | 0.20% |
| 9 | Pennsylvania | 1,711 | 4.17% | 34 | Minnesota | 71 | 0.17% |
| 10 | Alabama | 1,573 | 3.84% | 35 | Iowa | 68 | 0.17% |
| 11 | South Carolina | 1,527 | 3.72% | 36 | Rhode Island | 57 | 0.14% |
| 12 | Tennessee | 1,452 | 3.54% | 37 | West Virginia | 33 | 0.08% |
| 13 | Mississippi | 1,285 | 3.13% | 38 | New Mexico | 30 | 0.07% |
| 14 | New Jersey | 1,213 | 2.96% | 39 | Nebraska | 17 | 0.04% |
| 15 | Michigan | 1,136 | 2.77% | 40 | New Hampshire | 12 | 0.03% |
| 16 | Maryland | 972 | 2.37% | 41 | Wyoming | 11 | 0.03% |
| 17 | Virginia | 871 | 2.12% | 42 | Utah | 9 | 0.02% |
| 18 | Arkansas | 743 | 1.81% | 43 | Hawaii | 8 | 0.02% |
| 19 | Ohio | 662 | 1.61% | 44 | Montana | 6 | 0.01% |
| 20 | Wisconsin | 590 | 1.44% | 45 | Alaska | 4 | 0.01% |
| 21 | Missouri | 589 | 1.44% | 45 | Idaho | 4 | 0.01% |
| 22 | Connecticut | 513 | 1.25% | 47 | Maine | 3 | 0.01% |
| 23 | Massachusetts | 498 | 1.21% | 48 | Vermont | 2 | 0.00% |
| 24 | Arizona | 344 | 0.84% | 49 | South Dakota | 1 | 0.00% |
| 25 | Oklahoma | 205 | 0.50% | 50 | North Dakota | 0 | 0.00% |
| | | | | | District of Columbia | 703 | 1.71% |

Source: U.S. Department of Health and Human Services, Public Health Service
    "Morbidity and Mortality Weekly Report" (January 3, 1992, Vol. 40, Nos. 51 & 52)
*Includes primary and secondary cases.

# Syphilis Rate in 1991

## National Rate = 16.26 Syphilis Cases Reported per 100,000 Population*

| RANK | STATE | RATE | | RANK | STATE | RATE |
|---|---|---|---|---|---|---|
| 1 | Louisiana | 63.31 | | 26 | California | 7.53 |
| 2 | Mississippi | 49.58 | | 27 | Oklahoma | 6.46 |
| 3 | Georgia | 43.30 | | 28 | Ohio | 6.05 |
| 4 | South Carolina | 42.89 | | 29 | Rhode Island | 5.68 |
| 5 | Alabama | 38.47 | | 30 | Washington | 3.55 |
| 6 | Arkansas | 31.32 | | 31 | Indiana | 3.19 |
| 7 | Tennessee | 29.32 | | 32 | Kentucky | 3.02 |
| 8 | North Carolina | 29.20 | | 33 | Oregon | 2.87 |
| 9 | Delaware | 27.21 | | 34 | Colorado | 2.58 |
| 10 | New York | 22.80 | | 35 | Iowa | 2.43 |
| 11 | Texas | 22.43 | | 36 | Wyoming | 2.39 |
| 12 | Florida | 20.76 | | 37 | New Mexico | 1.94 |
| 13 | Illinois | 20.56 | | 38 | West Virginia | 1.83 |
| 14 | Maryland | 20.00 | | 39 | Minnesota | 1.60 |
| 15 | New Jersey | 15.63 | | 40 | New Hampshire | 1.09 |
| 16 | Connecticut | 15.59 | | 41 | Nebraska | 1.07 |
| 17 | Pennsylvania | 14.30 | | 42 | Montana | 0.74 |
| 18 | Virginia | 13.86 | | 43 | Alaska | 0.70 |
| 19 | Michigan | 12.13 | | 43 | Hawaii | 0.70 |
| 20 | Wisconsin | 11.91 | | 45 | Utah | 0.51 |
| 21 | Missouri | 11.42 | | 46 | Idaho | 0.38 |
| 22 | Arizona | 9.17 | | 47 | Vermont | 0.35 |
| 23 | Nevada | 8.80 | | 48 | Maine | 0.24 |
| 24 | Massachusetts | 8.31 | | 49 | South Dakota | 0.14 |
| 25 | Kansas | 7.74 | | 50 | North Dakota | 0.00 |

District of Columbia          117.56

*Source: U.S. Department of Health and Human Services, Public Health Service*
*"Morbidity and Mortality Weekly Report" (January 3, 1992, Vol. 40, Nos. 51 & 52)*
*\*Calculated by the editors using 1991 Census resident population figures. Includes primary and secondary cases.*

# Toxic Shock Syndrome Cases Reported in 1991

## National Total = 274 Toxic Shock Syndrome Cases

| RANK | STATE | CASES | % | RANK | STATE | CASES | % |
|------|-------|-------|-----|------|-------|-------|-----|
| 1 | California | 31 | 11.31% | 26 | New Hampshire | 3 | 1.09% |
| 2 | New York | 23 | 8.39% | 27 | Alabama | 2 | 0.73% |
| 3 | Ohio | 22 | 8.03% | 27 | Maryland | 2 | 0.73% |
| 4 | Pennsylvania | 21 | 7.66% | 27 | Nebraska | 2 | 0.73% |
| 5 | Illinois | 15 | 5.47% | 27 | South Carolina | 2 | 0.73% |
| 5 | Utah | 15 | 5.47% | 31 | Delaware | 1 | 0.36% |
| 7 | Missouri | 13 | 4.74% | 31 | Georgia | 1 | 0.36% |
| 8 | Michigan | 12 | 4.38% | 31 | Idaho | 1 | 0.36% |
| 9 | North Carolina | 11 | 4.01% | 31 | Montana | 1 | 0.36% |
| 10 | Kansas | 9 | 3.28% | 31 | South Dakota | 1 | 0.36% |
| 10 | Minnesota | 9 | 3.28% | 36 | Alaska | 0 | 0.00% |
| 12 | Massachusetts | 8 | 2.92% | 36 | Connecticut | 0 | 0.00% |
| 13 | Iowa | 7 | 2.55% | 36 | Hawaii | 0 | 0.00% |
| 13 | New Mexico | 7 | 2.55% | 36 | Indiana | 0 | 0.00% |
| 13 | Texas | 7 | 2.55% | 36 | Louisiana | 0 | 0.00% |
| 16 | Colorado | 6 | 2.19% | 36 | Mississippi | 0 | 0.00% |
| 17 | Arizona | 5 | 1.82% | 36 | Nevada | 0 | 0.00% |
| 17 | Kentucky | 5 | 1.82% | 36 | New Jersey | 0 | 0.00% |
| 17 | Tennessee | 5 | 1.82% | 36 | North Dakota | 0 | 0.00% |
| 17 | Virginia | 5 | 1.82% | 36 | Oregon | 0 | 0.00% |
| 17 | Washington | 5 | 1.82% | 36 | Rhode Island | 0 | 0.00% |
| 22 | Arkansas | 4 | 1.46% | 36 | Vermont | 0 | 0.00% |
| 22 | Florida | 4 | 1.46% | 36 | West Virginia | 0 | 0.00% |
| 22 | Maine | 4 | 1.46% | 36 | Wisconsin | 0 | 0.00% |
| 22 | Oklahoma | 4 | 1.46% | 36 | Wyoming | 0 | 0.00% |
| | | | | | District of Columbia | 1 | 0.36% |

Source: U.S. Department of Health and Human Services, Public Health Service
"Morbidity and Mortality Weekly Report" (January 3, 1992, Vol. 40, Nos. 51 & 52)

# Toxic Shock Syndrome Rate in 1991

## National Rate = 0.108 Toxic Shock Syndrome Cases Reported per 100,000 Population*

| RANK | STATE | RATE | | RANK | STATE | RATE |
|---|---|---|---|---|---|---|
| 1 | Utah | 0.847 | | 26 | Tennessee | 0.101 |
| 2 | New Mexico | 0.452 | | 27 | Washington | 0.100 |
| 3 | Kansas | 0.361 | | 28 | Idaho | 0.096 |
| 4 | Maine | 0.324 | | 29 | Virginia | 0.080 |
| 5 | New Hampshire | 0.271 | | 30 | South Carolina | 0.056 |
| 6 | Missouri | 0.252 | | 31 | Alabama | 0.049 |
| 7 | Iowa | 0.250 | | 32 | Maryland | 0.041 |
| 8 | Minnesota | 0.203 | | 33 | Texas | 0.040 |
| 9 | Ohio | 0.201 | | 34 | Florida | 0.030 |
| 10 | Colorado | 0.178 | | 35 | Georgia | 0.015 |
| 11 | Pennsylvania | 0.176 | | 36 | Alaska | 0.000 |
| 12 | Arkansas | 0.169 | | 36 | Connecticut | 0.000 |
| 13 | North Carolina | 0.163 | | 36 | Hawaii | 0.000 |
| 14 | Delaware | 0.147 | | 36 | Indiana | 0.000 |
| 15 | South Dakota | 0.142 | | 36 | Louisiana | 0.000 |
| 16 | Kentucky | 0.135 | | 36 | Mississippi | 0.000 |
| 17 | Arizona | 0.133 | | 36 | Nevada | 0.000 |
| 17 | Massachusetts | 0.133 | | 36 | New Jersey | 0.000 |
| 19 | Illinois | 0.130 | | 36 | North Dakota | 0.000 |
| 20 | Michigan | 0.128 | | 36 | Oregon | 0.000 |
| 21 | New York | 0.127 | | 36 | Rhode Island | 0.000 |
| 22 | Nebraska | 0.126 | | 36 | Vermont | 0.000 |
| 22 | Oklahoma | 0.126 | | 36 | West Virginia | 0.000 |
| 24 | Montana | 0.124 | | 36 | Wisconsin | 0.000 |
| 25 | California | 0.102 | | 36 | Wyoming | 0.000 |
| | | | | | District of Columbia | 0.167 |

Source: U.S. Department of Health and Human Services, Public Health Service
   "Morbidity and Mortality Weekly Report" (January 3, 1992, Vol. 40, Nos. 51 & 52)
*Calculated by the editors using 1991 Census resident population figures.

# Tuberculosis Cases Reported in 1991

## National Total = 23,543 Tuberculosis Cases*

| RANK | STATE | CASES | % | RANK | STATE | CASES | % |
|------|-------|-------|---|------|-------|-------|---|
| 1 | California | 4,304 | 18.28% | 26 | Hawaii | 202 | 0.86% |
| 2 | New York | 4,018 | 17.07% | 27 | Oklahoma | 179 | 0.76% |
| 3 | Texas | 2,063 | 8.76% | 28 | Connecticut | 158 | 0.67% |
| 4 | Florida | 1,518 | 6.45% | 29 | Oregon | 132 | 0.56% |
| 5 | Illinois | 1,181 | 5.02% | 30 | Wisconsin | 102 | 0.43% |
| 6 | New Jersey | 917 | 3.90% | 31 | Minnesota | 97 | 0.41% |
| 7 | Georgia | 834 | 3.54% | 32 | Nevada | 90 | 0.38% |
| 8 | Pennsylvania | 692 | 2.94% | 33 | Kansas | 83 | 0.35% |
| 9 | North Carolina | 615 | 2.61% | 33 | Rhode Island | 83 | 0.35% |
| 10 | Tennessee | 593 | 2.52% | 35 | New Mexico | 73 | 0.31% |
| 11 | Michigan | 418 | 1.78% | 36 | Colorado | 69 | 0.29% |
| 11 | South Carolina | 418 | 1.78% | 36 | Iowa | 69 | 0.29% |
| 13 | Maryland | 417 | 1.77% | 38 | West Virginia | 65 | 0.28% |
| 14 | Alabama | 396 | 1.68% | 39 | Alaska | 61 | 0.26% |
| 15 | Massachusetts | 373 | 1.58% | 40 | Utah | 54 | 0.23% |
| 16 | Ohio | 370 | 1.57% | 41 | Delaware | 34 | 0.14% |
| 17 | Kentucky | 336 | 1.43% | 42 | Maine | 33 | 0.14% |
| 18 | Arizona | 310 | 1.32% | 43 | South Dakota | 31 | 0.13% |
| 18 | Virginia | 310 | 1.32% | 44 | Nebraska | 20 | 0.08% |
| 20 | Washington | 302 | 1.28% | 45 | Idaho | 15 | 0.06% |
| 21 | Louisiana | 301 | 1.28% | 46 | Vermont | 12 | 0.05% |
| 22 | Mississippi | 286 | 1.21% | 47 | Montana | 10 | 0.04% |
| 23 | Arkansas | 249 | 1.06% | 48 | North Dakota | 8 | 0.03% |
| 24 | Indiana | 230 | 0.98% | 49 | New Hampshire | 5 | 0.02% |
| 25 | Missouri | 221 | 0.94% | 50 | Wyoming | 4 | 0.02% |
| | | | | | District of Columbia | 182 | 0.77% |

Source: U.S. Department of Health and Human Services, Public Health Service
    "Morbidity and Mortality Weekly Report" (January 3, 1992, Vol. 40, Nos. 51 & 52)
*Infectious disease usually centered in the lungs.

# Tuberculosis Rate in 1991

## National Rate = 9.34 Tuberculosis Cases Reported per 100,000 Population*

| RANK | STATE | RATE | | RANK | STATE | RATE |
|---|---|---|---|---|---|---|
| 1 | New York | 22.25 | | 26 | Delaware | 5.00 |
| 2 | Hawaii | 17.80 | | 27 | Virginia | 4.93 |
| 3 | California | 14.17 | | 28 | Connecticut | 4.80 |
| 4 | Georgia | 12.59 | | 29 | New Mexico | 4.72 |
| 5 | Tennessee | 11.97 | | 30 | Oregon | 4.52 |
| 6 | Texas | 11.89 | | 31 | Michigan | 4.46 |
| 7 | New Jersey | 11.82 | | 32 | South Dakota | 4.41 |
| 8 | South Carolina | 11.74 | | 33 | Missouri | 4.28 |
| 9 | Florida | 11.43 | | 34 | Indiana | 4.10 |
| 10 | Mississippi | 11.03 | | 35 | West Virginia | 3.61 |
| 11 | Alaska | 10.70 | | 36 | Ohio | 3.38 |
| 12 | Arkansas | 10.50 | | 37 | Kansas | 3.33 |
| 13 | Illinois | 10.23 | | 38 | Utah | 3.05 |
| 14 | Alabama | 9.68 | | 39 | Maine | 2.67 |
| 15 | North Carolina | 9.13 | | 40 | Iowa | 2.47 |
| 16 | Kentucky | 9.05 | | 41 | Minnesota | 2.19 |
| 17 | Maryland | 8.58 | | 42 | Vermont | 2.12 |
| 18 | Arizona | 8.27 | | 43 | Wisconsin | 2.06 |
| 18 | Rhode Island | 8.27 | | 44 | Colorado | 2.04 |
| 20 | Louisiana | 7.08 | | 45 | Idaho | 1.44 |
| 21 | Nevada | 7.01 | | 46 | Nebraska | 1.26 |
| 22 | Massachusetts | 6.22 | | 46 | North Dakota | 1.26 |
| 23 | Washington | 6.02 | | 48 | Montana | 1.24 |
| 24 | Pennsylvania | 5.79 | | 49 | Wyoming | 0.87 |
| 25 | Oklahoma | 5.64 | | 50 | New Hampshire | 0.45 |

District of Columbia     30.43

Source: U.S. Department of Health and Human Services, Public Health Service

"Morbidity and Mortality Weekly Report" (January 3, 1992, Vol. 40, Nos. 51 & 52)

*Calculated by the editors using 1991 Census resident population figures. Infectious disease usually centered in the lungs.

# Typhoid Fever Cases Reported in 1991

## National Total = 456 Typhoid Fever Cases*

| RANK | STATE | CASES | % | RANK | STATE | CASES | % |
|---|---|---|---|---|---|---|---|
| 1 | California | 126 | 27.63% | 25 | Kentucky | 2 | 0.44% |
| 2 | New York | 79 | 17.32% | 25 | Minnesota | 2 | 0.44% |
| 3 | Florida | 33 | 7.24% | 25 | New Mexico | 2 | 0.44% |
| 4 | Massachusetts | 28 | 6.14% | 29 | Maine | 1 | 0.22% |
| 5 | Texas | 21 | 4.61% | 29 | Missouri | 1 | 0.22% |
| 6 | Illinois | 20 | 4.39% | 29 | Nevada | 1 | 0.22% |
| 7 | New Jersey | 18 | 3.95% | 29 | New Hampshire | 1 | 0.22% |
| 8 | Hawaii | 12 | 2.63% | 29 | Tennessee | 1 | 0.22% |
| 8 | Michigan | 12 | 2.63% | 29 | West Virginia | 1 | 0.22% |
| 10 | Virginia | 11 | 2.41% | 35 | Alabama | 0 | 0.00% |
| 11 | Maryland | 10 | 2.19% | 35 | Alaska | 0 | 0.00% |
| 11 | Washington | 10 | 2.19% | 35 | Arkansas | 0 | 0.00% |
| 13 | Pennsylvania | 8 | 1.75% | 35 | Delaware | 0 | 0.00% |
| 14 | Arizona | 7 | 1.54% | 35 | Idaho | 0 | 0.00% |
| 14 | Oregon | 7 | 1.54% | 35 | Indiana | 0 | 0.00% |
| 16 | Georgia | 6 | 1.32% | 35 | Iowa | 0 | 0.00% |
| 17 | Louisiana | 5 | 1.10% | 35 | Kansas | 0 | 0.00% |
| 17 | Wisconsin | 5 | 1.10% | 35 | Mississippi | 0 | 0.00% |
| 19 | North Carolina | 4 | 0.88% | 35 | Montana | 0 | 0.00% |
| 19 | Ohio | 4 | 0.88% | 35 | North Dakota | 0 | 0.00% |
| 19 | South Carolina | 4 | 0.88% | 35 | Rhode Island | 0 | 0.00% |
| 22 | Connecticut | 3 | 0.66% | 35 | South Dakota | 0 | 0.00% |
| 22 | Nebraska | 3 | 0.66% | 35 | Utah | 0 | 0.00% |
| 22 | Oklahoma | 3 | 0.66% | 35 | Vermont | 0 | 0.00% |
| 25 | Colorado | 2 | 0.44% | 35 | Wyoming | 0 | 0.00% |
| | | | | | District of Columbia | 3 | 0.66% |

Source: U.S. Department of Health and Human Services, Public Health Service
"Morbidity and Mortality Weekly Report" (January 3, 1992, Vol. 40, Nos. 51 & 52)
*An infectious, often fatal, febrile disease, characterized by intestinal inflammation and ulceration.

# Typhoid Fever Rate in 1991

## National Rate = 0.180 Typhoid Fever Cases Reported per 100,000 Population*

| RANK | STATE | RATE | RANK | STATE | RATE |
|---|---|---|---|---|---|
| 1 | Hawaii | 1.057 | 26 | Pennsylvania | 0.067 |
| 2 | Massachusetts | 0.467 | 27 | Colorado | 0.059 |
| 3 | New York | 0.437 | 27 | North Carolina | 0.059 |
| 4 | California | 0.415 | 29 | West Virginia | 0.056 |
| 5 | Florida | 0.249 | 30 | Kentucky | 0.054 |
| 6 | Oregon | 0.240 | 31 | Minnesota | 0.045 |
| 7 | New Jersey | 0.232 | 32 | Ohio | 0.037 |
| 8 | Maryland | 0.206 | 33 | Tennessee | 0.020 |
| 9 | Washington | 0.199 | 34 | Missouri | 0.019 |
| 10 | Nebraska | 0.188 | 35 | Alabama | 0.000 |
| 11 | Arizona | 0.187 | 35 | Alaska | 0.000 |
| 12 | Virginia | 0.175 | 35 | Arkansas | 0.000 |
| 13 | Illinois | 0.173 | 35 | Delaware | 0.000 |
| 14 | New Mexico | 0.129 | 35 | Idaho | 0.000 |
| 15 | Michigan | 0.128 | 35 | Indiana | 0.000 |
| 16 | Texas | 0.121 | 35 | Iowa | 0.000 |
| 17 | Louisiana | 0.118 | 35 | Kansas | 0.000 |
| 18 | South Carolina | 0.112 | 35 | Mississippi | 0.000 |
| 19 | Wisconsin | 0.101 | 35 | Montana | 0.000 |
| 20 | Oklahoma | 0.094 | 35 | North Dakota | 0.000 |
| 21 | Connecticut | 0.091 | 35 | Rhode Island | 0.000 |
| 21 | Georgia | 0.091 | 35 | South Dakota | 0.000 |
| 23 | New Hampshire | 0.090 | 35 | Utah | 0.000 |
| 24 | Maine | 0.081 | 35 | Vermont | 0.000 |
| 25 | Nevada | 0.078 | 35 | Wyoming | 0.000 |

District of Columbia     0.502

Source: U.S. Department of Health and Human Services, Public Health Service
*"Morbidity and Mortality Weekly Report"* (January 3, 1992, Vol. 40, Nos. 51 & 52)
*Calculated by the editors using 1991 Census resident population figures. An infectious, often fatal, febrile disease, characterized by intestinal inflammation and ulceration.

# Typhus Fever Cases Reported in 1991

## National Total = 635 Typhus Fever Cases*

| RANK | STATE | CASES | % | RANK | STATE | CASES | % |
|------|-------|-------|-----|------|-------|-------|-----|
| 1 | North Carolina | 159 | 25.04% | 25 | Mississippi | 2 | 0.31% |
| 2 | Oklahoma | 81 | 12.76% | 25 | Texas | 2 | 0.31% |
| 3 | Tennessee | 58 | 9.13% | 28 | Connecticut | 1 | 0.16% |
| 4 | Georgia | 40 | 6.30% | 28 | Iowa | 1 | 0.16% |
| 5 | South Carolina | 37 | 5.83% | 28 | Oregon | 1 | 0.16% |
| 6 | Kentucky | 31 | 4.88% | 28 | South Dakota | 1 | 0.16% |
| 7 | Arkansas | 30 | 4.72% | 28 | Washington | 1 | 0.16% |
| 8 | Maryland | 26 | 4.09% | 33 | Alaska | 0 | 0.00% |
| 8 | Missouri | 26 | 4.09% | 33 | Arizona | 0 | 0.00% |
| 10 | Ohio | 25 | 3.94% | 33 | California | 0 | 0.00% |
| 11 | Virginia | 19 | 2.99% | 33 | Delaware | 0 | 0.00% |
| 12 | Alabama | 16 | 2.52% | 33 | Hawaii | 0 | 0.00% |
| 13 | New York | 15 | 2.36% | 33 | Idaho | 0 | 0.00% |
| 14 | Indiana | 10 | 1.57% | 33 | Louisiana | 0 | 0.00% |
| 15 | Massachusetts | 8 | 1.26% | 33 | Maine | 0 | 0.00% |
| 16 | Kansas | 6 | 0.94% | 33 | Minnesota | 0 | 0.00% |
| 16 | Montana | 6 | 0.94% | 33 | Nevada | 0 | 0.00% |
| 16 | New Jersey | 6 | 0.94% | 33 | New Hampshire | 0 | 0.00% |
| 19 | Illinois | 5 | 0.79% | 33 | New Mexico | 0 | 0.00% |
| 19 | Nebraska | 5 | 0.79% | 33 | North Dakota | 0 | 0.00% |
| 21 | Florida | 4 | 0.63% | 33 | Rhode Island | 0 | 0.00% |
| 21 | Pennsylvania | 4 | 0.63% | 33 | Utah | 0 | 0.00% |
| 21 | West Virginia | 4 | 0.63% | 33 | Vermont | 0 | 0.00% |
| 24 | Michigan | 3 | 0.47% | 33 | Wisconsin | 0 | 0.00% |
| 25 | Colorado | 2 | 0.31% | 33 | Wyoming | 0 | 0.00% |
| | | | | | District of Columbia | 0 | 0.00% |

Source: U.S. Department of Health and Human Services, Public Health Service
     "Morbidity and Mortality Weekly Report" (January 3, 1992, Vol. 40, Nos. 51 & 52)
*Tick-borne, RMSF. An acute, infectious disease characterized by great prostration, severe nervous symptoms, and a peculiar eruption of reddish spots on the body.

# Typhus Fever Rate in 1991

## National Rate = 0.252 Typhus Fever Cases Reported per 100,000 Population*

| RANK | STATE | RATE | RANK | STATE | RATE |
|------|-------|------|------|-------|------|
| 1 | Oklahoma | 2.551 | 26 | Oregon | 0.034 |
| 2 | North Carolina | 2.360 | 27 | Pennsylvania | 0.033 |
| 3 | Arkansas | 1.265 | 28 | Michigan | 0.032 |
| 4 | Tennessee | 1.171 | 29 | Connecticut | 0.030 |
| 5 | South Carolina | 1.039 | 29 | Florida | 0.030 |
| 6 | Kentucky | 0.835 | 31 | Washington | 0.020 |
| 7 | Montana | 0.743 | 32 | Texas | 0.012 |
| 8 | Georgia | 0.604 | 33 | Alaska | 0.000 |
| 9 | Maryland | 0.535 | 33 | Arizona | 0.000 |
| 10 | Missouri | 0.504 | 33 | California | 0.000 |
| 11 | Alabama | 0.391 | 33 | Delaware | 0.000 |
| 12 | Nebraska | 0.314 | 33 | Hawaii | 0.000 |
| 13 | Virginia | 0.302 | 33 | Idaho | 0.000 |
| 14 | Kansas | 0.240 | 33 | Louisiana | 0.000 |
| 15 | Ohio | 0.229 | 33 | Maine | 0.000 |
| 16 | West Virginia | 0.222 | 33 | Minnesota | 0.000 |
| 17 | Indiana | 0.178 | 33 | Nevada | 0.000 |
| 18 | South Dakota | 0.142 | 33 | New Hampshire | 0.000 |
| 19 | Massachusetts | 0.133 | 33 | New Mexico | 0.000 |
| 20 | New York | 0.083 | 33 | North Dakota | 0.000 |
| 21 | Mississippi | 0.077 | 33 | Rhode Island | 0.000 |
| 21 | New Jersey | 0.077 | 33 | Utah | 0.000 |
| 23 | Colorado | 0.059 | 33 | Vermont | 0.000 |
| 24 | Illinois | 0.043 | 33 | Wisconsin | 0.000 |
| 25 | Iowa | 0.036 | 33 | Wyoming | 0.000 |
|  |  |  |  | District of Columbia | 0.000 |

Source: U.S. Department of Health and Human Services, Public Health Service

"Morbidity and Mortality Weekly Report" (January 3, 1992, Vol. 40, Nos. 51 & 52)

*Calculated by the editors using 1991 Census resident population figures. Tick-borne, RMSF. An acute, infectious disease characterized by great prostration, severe nervous symptoms, and a peculiar eruption of reddish spots on the body.

# Whooping Cough (Pertussis) Cases Reported in 1991

## National Total = 2,575 Whooping Cough (Pertussis) Cases*

| RANK | STATE | CASES | % | RANK | STATE | CASES | % |
|---|---|---|---|---|---|---|---|
| 1 | California | 263 | 10.21% | 26 | Tennessee | 40 | 1.55% |
| 2 | New York | 191 | 7.42% | 27 | Michigan | 37 | 1.44% |
| 3 | Massachusetts | 178 | 6.91% | 28 | Idaho | 29 | 1.13% |
| 4 | Colorado | 145 | 5.63% | 29 | Iowa | 26 | 1.01% |
| 5 | Washington | 136 | 5.28% | 30 | Virginia | 24 | 0.93% |
| 6 | Ohio | 116 | 4.50% | 31 | Connecticut | 23 | 0.89% |
| 7 | Wisconsin | 97 | 3.77% | 32 | New Hampshire | 22 | 0.85% |
| 8 | Texas | 88 | 3.42% | 33 | Louisiana | 17 | 0.66% |
| 9 | Minnesota | 81 | 3.15% | 34 | Arkansas | 14 | 0.54% |
| 10 | Missouri | 77 | 2.99% | 34 | South Carolina | 14 | 0.54% |
| 11 | Indiana | 71 | 2.76% | 36 | Alaska | 13 | 0.50% |
| 11 | Pennsylvania | 71 | 2.76% | 37 | Kansas | 12 | 0.47% |
| 13 | Arizona | 69 | 2.68% | 37 | New Jersey | 12 | 0.47% |
| 14 | Oregon | 67 | 2.60% | 39 | Nebraska | 9 | 0.35% |
| 15 | Hawaii | 66 | 2.56% | 39 | West Virginia | 9 | 0.35% |
| 16 | Maryland | 63 | 2.45% | 41 | Montana | 6 | 0.23% |
| 17 | Illinois | 61 | 2.37% | 42 | South Dakota | 5 | 0.19% |
| 18 | Florida | 60 | 2.33% | 42 | Vermont | 5 | 0.19% |
| 19 | Alabama | 57 | 2.21% | 44 | Mississippi | 4 | 0.16% |
| 20 | New Mexico | 53 | 2.06% | 44 | North Dakota | 4 | 0.16% |
| 21 | Maine | 52 | 2.02% | 46 | Wyoming | 3 | 0.12% |
| 22 | Georgia | 50 | 1.94% | 47 | Nevada | 2 | 0.08% |
| 23 | Oklahoma | 49 | 1.90% | 48 | Delaware | 0 | 0.00% |
| 24 | North Carolina | 41 | 1.59% | 48 | Kentucky | 0 | 0.00% |
| 24 | Utah | 41 | 1.59% | 48 | Rhode Island | 0 | 0.00% |
| | | | | | District of Columbia | 2 | 0.08% |

Source: U.S. Department of Health and Human Services, Public Health Service
   "Morbidity and Mortality Weekly Report" (January 3, 1992, Vol. 40, Nos. 51 & 52)
*Acute, highly contagious infection of respiratory tract.

# Whooping Cough (Pertussis) Rate in 1991

## National Rate = 1.02 Whooping Cough (Pertussis) Cases Reported per 100,000 Population*

| RANK | STATE | RATE | RANK | STATE | RATE |
|------|-------|------|------|-------|------|
| 1 | Hawaii | 5.81 | 26 | Georgia | 0.75 |
| 2 | Colorado | 4.29 | 27 | Montana | 0.74 |
| 3 | Maine | 4.21 | 28 | South Dakota | 0.71 |
| 4 | New Mexico | 3.42 | 29 | Connecticut | 0.70 |
| 5 | Massachusetts | 2.97 | 30 | Wyoming | 0.65 |
| 6 | Idaho | 2.79 | 31 | North Dakota | 0.63 |
| 7 | Washington | 2.71 | 32 | North Carolina | 0.61 |
| 8 | Utah | 2.32 | 33 | Arkansas | 0.59 |
| 9 | Oregon | 2.29 | 33 | Pennsylvania | 0.59 |
| 10 | Alaska | 2.28 | 35 | Nebraska | 0.56 |
| 11 | New Hampshire | 1.99 | 36 | Illinois | 0.53 |
| 12 | Wisconsin | 1.96 | 37 | Texas | 0.51 |
| 13 | Arizona | 1.84 | 38 | West Virginia | 0.50 |
| 14 | Minnesota | 1.83 | 39 | Kansas | 0.48 |
| 15 | Oklahoma | 1.54 | 40 | Florida | 0.45 |
| 16 | Missouri | 1.49 | 41 | Louisiana | 0.40 |
| 17 | Alabama | 1.39 | 42 | Michigan | 0.39 |
| 18 | Maryland | 1.30 | 42 | South Carolina | 0.39 |
| 19 | Indiana | 1.27 | 44 | Virginia | 0.38 |
| 20 | New York | 1.06 | 45 | Nevada | 0.16 |
| 20 | Ohio | 1.06 | 46 | Mississippi | 0.15 |
| 22 | Iowa | 0.93 | 46 | New Jersey | 0.15 |
| 23 | Vermont | 0.88 | 48 | Delaware | 0.00 |
| 24 | California | 0.87 | 48 | Kentucky | 0.00 |
| 25 | Tennessee | 0.81 | 48 | Rhode Island | 0.00 |

District of Columbia          0.33

Source: U.S. Department of Health and Human Services, Public Health Service

"Morbidity and Mortality Weekly Report" (January 3, 1992, Vol. 40, Nos. 51 & 52)

*Calculated by the editors using 1991 Census resident population figures. Acute, highly contagious infection of respiratory tract.

# VI. PERSONNEL

# VI. PERSONNEL (continued)

# Physicians in 1990

## National Total = 615,421 Physicians*

| RANK | STATE | PHYSICIANS | % | RANK | STATE | PHYSICIANS | % |
|------|-------|-----------|------|------|-------|-----------|------|
| 1 | California | 80,874 | 13.14% | 26 | Kentucky | 6,878 | 1.12% |
| 2 | New York | 61,628 | 10.01% | 27 | Oregon | 6,756 | 1.10% |
| 3 | Texas | 33,357 | 5.42% | 28 | South Carolina | 6,415 | 1.04% |
| 4 | Florida | 32,425 | 5.27% | 29 | Oklahoma | 5,310 | 0.86% |
| 5 | Pennsylvania | 31,369 | 5.10% | 30 | Kansas | 5,037 | 0.82% |
| 6 | Illinois | 27,140 | 4.41% | 31 | Iowa | 4,831 | 0.78% |
| 7 | Ohio | 23,729 | 3.86% | 32 | Arkansas | 4,120 | 0.67% |
| 8 | Massachusetts | 21,904 | 3.56% | 33 | Mississippi | 3,956 | 0.64% |
| 9 | New Jersey | 20,882 | 3.39% | 34 | Utah | 3,511 | 0.57% |
| 10 | Michigan | 18,872 | 3.07% | 35 | West Virginia | 3,490 | 0.57% |
| 11 | Maryland | 18,291 | 2.97% | 36 | New Mexico | 3,289 | 0.53% |
| 12 | Virginia | 14,656 | 2.38% | 37 | Hawaii | 3,097 | 0.50% |
| 13 | North Carolina | 13,990 | 2.27% | 38 | Nebraska | 3,063 | 0.50% |
| 14 | Georgia | 12,689 | 2.06% | 39 | Rhode Island | 2,822 | 0.46% |
| 15 | Washington | 11,955 | 1.94% | 40 | Maine | 2,604 | 0.42% |
| 16 | Missouri | 11,057 | 1.80% | 41 | New Hampshire | 2,582 | 0.42% |
| 17 | Connecticut | 10,892 | 1.77% | 42 | Nevada | 2,006 | 0.33% |
| 18 | Minnesota | 10,661 | 1.73% | 43 | Vermont | 1,673 | 0.27% |
| 19 | Tennessee | 10,643 | 1.73% | 44 | Montana | 1,513 | 0.25% |
| 20 | Wisconsin | 10,258 | 1.67% | 45 | Delaware | 1,500 | 0.24% |
| 21 | Indiana | 9,693 | 1.58% | 46 | Idaho | 1,495 | 0.24% |
| 22 | Louisiana | 8,929 | 1.45% | 47 | North Dakota | 1,246 | 0.20% |
| 23 | Arizona | 8,560 | 1.39% | 48 | South Dakota | 1,159 | 0.19% |
| 24 | Colorado | 8,037 | 1.31% | 49 | Alaska | 915 | 0.15% |
| 25 | Alabama | 7,246 | 1.18% | 50 | Wyoming | 766 | 0.12% |
| | | | | | District of Columbia | 4,318 | 0.70% |

Source: American Medical Association

"Physician Characteristics and Distribution in the U.S." 1992 Edition (Copyright, reprinted with permission)

*As of January 1, 1990. Comprised of federal and nonfederal physicians. Total includes 11,332 physicians in the U.S. territories and possessions, at APO's and FPO's and whose addresses are unknown.

# Male Physicians in 1990

## National Total = 511,227 Male Physicians*

| RANK | STATE | PHYSICIANS | % | RANK | STATE | PHYSICIANS | % |
|---|---|---|---|---|---|---|---|
| 1 | California | 67,347 | 13.17% | 26 | Kentucky | 5,832 | 1.14% |
| 2 | New York | 48,519 | 9.49% | 27 | Oregon | 5,768 | 1.13% |
| 3 | Florida | 28,564 | 5.59% | 28 | South Carolina | 5,628 | 1.10% |
| 4 | Texas | 28,238 | 5.52% | 29 | Oklahoma | 4,576 | 0.90% |
| 5 | Pennsylvania | 25,573 | 5.00% | 30 | Kansas | 4,270 | 0.84% |
| 6 | Illinois | 21,553 | 4.22% | 31 | Iowa | 4,226 | 0.83% |
| 7 | Ohio | 19,649 | 3.84% | 32 | Arkansas | 3,642 | 0.71% |
| 8 | Massachusetts | 17,230 | 3.37% | 33 | Mississippi | 3,470 | 0.68% |
| 9 | New Jersey | 16,668 | 3.26% | 34 | Utah | 3,137 | 0.61% |
| 10 | Michigan | 15,582 | 3.05% | 35 | West Virginia | 3,011 | 0.59% |
| 11 | Maryland | 14,454 | 2.83% | 36 | Nebraska | 2,708 | 0.53% |
| 12 | Virginia | 12,156 | 2.38% | 37 | New Mexico | 2,646 | 0.52% |
| 13 | North Carolina | 11,897 | 2.33% | 38 | Hawaii | 2,584 | 0.51% |
| 14 | Georgia | 10,895 | 2.13% | 39 | Rhode Island | 2,276 | 0.45% |
| 15 | Washington | 10,085 | 1.97% | 40 | Maine | 2,228 | 0.44% |
| 16 | Tennessee | 9,265 | 1.81% | 41 | New Hampshire | 2,225 | 0.44% |
| 17 | Missouri | 9,246 | 1.81% | 42 | Nevada | 1,797 | 0.35% |
| 18 | Connecticut | 8,935 | 1.75% | 43 | Vermont | 1,388 | 0.27% |
| 19 | Minnesota | 8,891 | 1.74% | 44 | Idaho | 1,382 | 0.27% |
| 20 | Wisconsin | 8,745 | 1.71% | 45 | Montana | 1,373 | 0.27% |
| 21 | Indiana | 8,338 | 1.63% | 46 | Delaware | 1,212 | 0.24% |
| 22 | Louisiana | 7,648 | 1.50% | 47 | North Dakota | 1,136 | 0.22% |
| 23 | Arizona | 7,364 | 1.44% | 48 | South Dakota | 1,047 | 0.20% |
| 24 | Colorado | 6,705 | 1.31% | 49 | Alaska | 766 | 0.15% |
| 25 | Alabama | 6,374 | 1.25% | 50 | Wyoming | 696 | 0.14% |
| | | | | | District of Columbia | 3,266 | 0.64% |

Source: American Medical Association

"Physician Characteristics and Distribution in the U.S." 1992 Edition (Copyright, reprinted with permission)

*As of January 1, 1990. Comprised of federal and nonfederal physicians. Total includes 9,016 male physicians in the U.S. territories and possessions, at APO's and FPO's and whose addresses are unknown.

# Female Physicians in 1990

## National Total = 104,194 Female Physicians*

| RANK | STATE | PHYSICIANS | % | | RANK | STATE | PHYSICIANS | % |
|------|-------|-----------|---|---|------|-------|-----------|---|
| 1 | California | 13,527 | 12.98% | | 26 | Oregon | 988 | 0.95% |
| 2 | New York | 13,109 | 12.58% | | 27 | Alabama | 872 | 0.84% |
| 3 | Pennsylvania | 5,796 | 5.56% | | 28 | South Carolina | 787 | 0.76% |
| 4 | Illinois | 5,587 | 5.36% | | 29 | Kansas | 767 | 0.74% |
| 5 | Texas | 5,119 | 4.91% | | 30 | Oklahoma | 734 | 0.70% |
| 6 | Massachusetts | 4,674 | 4.49% | | 31 | New Mexico | 643 | 0.62% |
| 7 | New Jersey | 4,214 | 4.04% | | 32 | Iowa | 605 | 0.58% |
| 8 | Ohio | 4,080 | 3.92% | | 33 | Rhode Island | 546 | 0.52% |
| 9 | Florida | 3,861 | 3.71% | | 34 | Hawaii | 513 | 0.49% |
| 10 | Maryland | 3,837 | 3.68% | | 35 | Mississippi | 486 | 0.47% |
| 11 | Michigan | 3,290 | 3.16% | | 36 | West Virginia | 479 | 0.46% |
| 12 | Virginia | 2,500 | 2.40% | | 37 | Arkansas | 478 | 0.46% |
| 13 | North Carolina | 2,093 | 2.01% | | 38 | Maine | 376 | 0.36% |
| 14 | Connecticut | 1,957 | 1.88% | | 39 | Utah | 374 | 0.36% |
| 15 | Washington | 1,870 | 1.79% | | 40 | New Hampshire | 357 | 0.34% |
| 16 | Missouri | 1,811 | 1.74% | | 41 | Nebraska | 355 | 0.34% |
| 17 | Georgia | 1,794 | 1.72% | | 42 | Delaware | 288 | 0.28% |
| 18 | Minnesota | 1,770 | 1.70% | | 43 | Vermont | 285 | 0.27% |
| 19 | Wisconsin | 1,513 | 1.45% | | 44 | Nevada | 209 | 0.20% |
| 20 | Tennessee | 1,378 | 1.32% | | 45 | Alaska | 149 | 0.14% |
| 21 | Indiana | 1,355 | 1.30% | | 46 | Montana | 140 | 0.13% |
| 22 | Colorado | 1,332 | 1.28% | | 47 | Idaho | 113 | 0.11% |
| 23 | Louisiana | 1,281 | 1.23% | | 48 | South Dakota | 112 | 0.11% |
| 24 | Arizona | 1,196 | 1.15% | | 49 | North Dakota | 110 | 0.11% |
| 25 | Kentucky | 1,046 | 1.00% | | 50 | Wyoming | 70 | 0.07% |
| | | | | | | District of Columbia | 1,052 | 1.01% |

Source: American Medical Association

"Physician Characteristics and Distribution in the U.S." 1992 Edition (Copyright, reprinted with permission)

*As of January 1, 1990. Comprised of federal and nonfederal physicians. Total includes 2,316 female physicians in the U.S. territories and possessions, at APO's and FPO's and whose addresses are unknown.

# Percent of Physicians Who Are Female in 1990

## National Rate = 16.9% of Physicians are Female*

| RANK | STATE | PERCENT | RANK | STATE | PERCENT |
|---|---|---|---|---|---|
| 1 | Massachusetts | 21.3 | 26 | Wisconsin | 14.7 |
| 1 | New York | 21.3 | 27 | Oregon | 14.6 |
| 3 | Maryland | 21.0 | 28 | Maine | 14.4 |
| 4 | Illinois | 20.6 | 29 | Louisiana | 14.3 |
| 5 | New Jersey | 20.2 | 30 | Georgia | 14.1 |
| 6 | New Mexico | 19.6 | 31 | Arizona | 14.0 |
| 7 | Rhode Island | 19.3 | 31 | Indiana | 14.0 |
| 8 | Delaware | 19.2 | 33 | New Hampshire | 13.8 |
| 9 | Pennsylvania | 18.5 | 33 | Oklahoma | 13.8 |
| 10 | Connecticut | 18.0 | 35 | West Virginia | 13.7 |
| 11 | Michigan | 17.4 | 36 | Tennessee | 12.9 |
| 12 | Ohio | 17.2 | 37 | Iowa | 12.5 |
| 13 | Virginia | 17.1 | 38 | Mississippi | 12.3 |
| 14 | Vermont | 17.0 | 38 | South Carolina | 12.3 |
| 15 | California | 16.7 | 40 | Alabama | 12.0 |
| 16 | Colorado | 16.6 | 41 | Florida | 11.9 |
| 16 | Hawaii | 16.6 | 42 | Arkansas | 11.6 |
| 16 | Minnesota | 16.6 | 42 | Nebraska | 11.6 |
| 19 | Missouri | 16.4 | 44 | Utah | 10.7 |
| 20 | Alaska | 16.3 | 45 | Nevada | 10.4 |
| 21 | Washington | 15.6 | 46 | South Dakota | 9.7 |
| 22 | Texas | 15.3 | 47 | Montana | 9.3 |
| 23 | Kansas | 15.2 | 48 | Wyoming | 9.1 |
| 23 | Kentucky | 15.2 | 49 | North Dakota | 8.8 |
| 25 | North Carolina | 15.0 | 50 | Idaho | 7.6 |

District of Columbia     24.4

Source: American Medical Association

"Physician Characteristics and Distribution in the U.S." 1992 edition (Copyright, reprinted with permission)

*Calculated by the editors. Comprised of federal and nonfederal physicians. As of January 1, 1990. National rate includes physicians in U.S. territories and possessions, at APO's and FPO's and whose addresses are unknown.

# Physicians Under 35 Years Old in 1990

## National Total = 134,872 Physicians Under 35 Years Old*

| RANK | STATE | PHYSICIANS | % | RANK | STATE | PHYSICIANS | % |
|---|---|---|---|---|---|---|---|
| 1 | New York | 15,029 | 11.14% | 26 | Kentucky | 1,515 | 1.12% |
| 2 | California | 14,461 | 10.72% | 27 | South Carolina | 1,487 | 1.10% |
| 3 | Pennsylvania | 7,977 | 5.91% | 28 | Iowa | 1,178 | 0.87% |
| 4 | Texas | 7,755 | 5.75% | 29 | Kansas | 1,164 | 0.86% |
| 5 | Illinois | 6,710 | 4.98% | 30 | Oklahoma | 1,074 | 0.80% |
| 6 | Ohio | 5,984 | 4.44% | 31 | Oregon | 997 | 0.74% |
| 7 | Massachusetts | 5,858 | 4.34% | 32 | Mississippi | 843 | 0.63% |
| 8 | Florida | 5,017 | 3.72% | 33 | Arkansas | 836 | 0.62% |
| 9 | Maryland | 4,588 | 3.40% | 34 | Utah | 730 | 0.54% |
| 10 | Michigan | 4,534 | 3.36% | 35 | Rhode Island | 708 | 0.52% |
| 11 | New Jersey | 4,048 | 3.00% | 36 | Nebraska | 690 | 0.51% |
| 12 | North Carolina | 3,544 | 2.63% | 37 | West Virginia | 614 | 0.46% |
| 13 | Virginia | 3,463 | 2.57% | 38 | Hawaii | 581 | 0.43% |
| 14 | Missouri | 2,931 | 2.17% | 39 | New Mexico | 543 | 0.40% |
| 15 | Georgia | 2,818 | 2.09% | 40 | New Hampshire | 446 | 0.33% |
| 16 | Minnesota | 2,782 | 2.06% | 41 | Maine | 365 | 0.27% |
| 17 | Tennessee | 2,557 | 1.90% | 42 | Vermont | 341 | 0.25% |
| 18 | Connecticut | 2,546 | 1.89% | 43 | Delaware | 311 | 0.23% |
| 19 | Wisconsin | 2,353 | 1.74% | 44 | Nevada | 265 | 0.20% |
| 20 | Louisiana | 2,127 | 1.58% | 45 | North Dakota | 222 | 0.16% |
| 21 | Indiana | 2,014 | 1.49% | 46 | South Dakota | 204 | 0.15% |
| 22 | Washington | 2,010 | 1.49% | 47 | Idaho | 169 | 0.13% |
| 23 | Alabama | 1,741 | 1.29% | 48 | Montana | 148 | 0.11% |
| 24 | Arizona | 1,638 | 1.21% | 49 | Alaska | 121 | 0.09% |
| 25 | Colorado | 1,598 | 1.18% | 50 | Wyoming | 107 | 0.08% |
| | | | | | District of Columbia | 1,043 | 0.77% |

*Source: American Medical Association*

   *"Physician Characteristics and Distribution in the U.S." 1992 Edition (Copyright, reprinted with permission)*
*As of January 1, 1990. Comprised of federal and nonfederal physicians. Total includes 2,087 physicians in the U.S. territories and possessions, at APO's and FPO's and whose addresses are unknown.*

# Percent of Physicians Under 35 Years Old in 1990

## National Rate = 21.9% of Physicians Under 35 Years Old*

| RANK | STATE | PERCENT | RANK | STATE | PERCENT |
|------|-------|---------|------|-------|---------|
| 1 | Massachusetts | 26.7 | 26 | Indiana | 20.8 |
| 2 | Missouri | 26.5 | 26 | Utah | 20.8 |
| 3 | Minnesota | 26.1 | 28 | Delaware | 20.7 |
| 4 | Pennsylvania | 25.4 | 29 | Vermont | 20.4 |
| 5 | North Carolina | 25.3 | 30 | Arkansas | 20.3 |
| 6 | Ohio | 25.2 | 31 | Oklahoma | 20.2 |
| 7 | Maryland | 25.1 | 32 | Colorado | 19.9 |
| 7 | Rhode Island | 25.1 | 33 | New Jersey | 19.4 |
| 9 | Illinois | 24.7 | 34 | Arizona | 19.1 |
| 10 | Iowa | 24.4 | 35 | Hawaii | 18.8 |
| 10 | New York | 24.4 | 36 | California | 17.9 |
| 12 | Alabama | 24.0 | 37 | North Dakota | 17.8 |
| 12 | Michigan | 24.0 | 38 | South Dakota | 17.6 |
| 12 | Tennessee | 24.0 | 38 | West Virginia | 17.6 |
| 15 | Louisiana | 23.8 | 40 | New Hampshire | 17.3 |
| 16 | Virginia | 23.6 | 41 | Washington | 16.8 |
| 17 | Connecticut | 23.4 | 42 | New Mexico | 16.5 |
| 18 | South Carolina | 23.2 | 43 | Florida | 15.5 |
| 18 | Texas | 23.2 | 44 | Oregon | 14.8 |
| 20 | Kansas | 23.1 | 45 | Maine | 14.0 |
| 21 | Wisconsin | 22.9 | 45 | Wyoming | 14.0 |
| 22 | Nebraska | 22.5 | 47 | Alaska | 13.2 |
| 23 | Georgia | 22.2 | 47 | Nevada | 13.2 |
| 24 | Kentucky | 22.0 | 49 | Idaho | 11.3 |
| 25 | Mississippi | 21.3 | 50 | Montana | 9.8 |
| | | | | District of Columbia | 24.2 |

Source: American Medical Association

"Physician Characteristics and Distribution in the U.S." 1992 edition (Copyright, reprinted with permission)

*Calculated by the editors. Comprised of federal and nonfederal physicians. As of January 1, 1990. National rate includes physicians in U.S. territories and possessions, at APO's and FPO's and whose addresses are unknown.

# Physicians 35 to 44 Years Old in 1990

## National Total = 184,742 Physicians 35 to 44 Years Old*

| RANK | STATE | PHYSICIANS | % | RANK | STATE | PHYSICIANS | % |
|------|-------|-----------:|------:|------|-------|-----------:|------:|
| 1 | California | 24,315 | 13.16% | 26 | Oregon | 2,210 | 1.20% |
| 2 | New York | 17,110 | 9.26% | 27 | Kentucky | 2,166 | 1.17% |
| 3 | Texas | 10,299 | 5.57% | 28 | South Carolina | 1,962 | 1.06% |
| 4 | Florida | 9,147 | 4.95% | 29 | Oklahoma | 1,632 | 0.88% |
| 5 | Pennsylvania | 9,111 | 4.93% | 30 | Kansas | 1,429 | 0.77% |
| 6 | Illinois | 7,956 | 4.31% | 31 | Iowa | 1,423 | 0.77% |
| 7 | Massachusetts | 6,788 | 3.67% | 32 | Arkansas | 1,278 | 0.69% |
| 8 | Ohio | 6,589 | 3.57% | 33 | New Mexico | 1,186 | 0.64% |
| 9 | New Jersey | 6,451 | 3.49% | 34 | Mississippi | 1,181 | 0.64% |
| 10 | Maryland | 5,801 | 3.14% | 35 | Utah | 1,180 | 0.64% |
| 11 | Michigan | 5,479 | 2.97% | 36 | West Virginia | 1,053 | 0.57% |
| 12 | Virginia | 4,424 | 2.39% | 37 | Hawaii | 1,000 | 0.54% |
| 13 | North Carolina | 4,306 | 2.33% | 38 | Nebraska | 984 | 0.53% |
| 14 | Washington | 4,141 | 2.24% | 39 | New Hampshire | 866 | 0.47% |
| 15 | Georgia | 4,068 | 2.20% | 40 | Maine | 835 | 0.45% |
| 16 | Minnesota | 3,390 | 1.83% | 41 | Rhode Island | 761 | 0.41% |
| 17 | Tennessee | 3,378 | 1.83% | 42 | Nevada | 700 | 0.38% |
| 18 | Missouri | 3,292 | 1.78% | 43 | Vermont | 526 | 0.28% |
| 19 | Connecticut | 3,248 | 1.76% | 44 | Montana | 485 | 0.26% |
| 20 | Wisconsin | 3,134 | 1.70% | 45 | Idaho | 481 | 0.26% |
| 21 | Indiana | 2,993 | 1.62% | 46 | North Dakota | 448 | 0.24% |
| 22 | Louisiana | 2,703 | 1.46% | 47 | Delaware | 400 | 0.22% |
| 23 | Colorado | 2,661 | 1.44% | 48 | South Dakota | 383 | 0.21% |
| 24 | Arizona | 2,467 | 1.34% | 49 | Alaska | 373 | 0.20% |
| 25 | Alabama | 2,248 | 1.22% | 50 | Wyoming | 269 | 0.15% |
|  |  |  |  |  | District of Columbia | 1,138 | 0.62% |

Source: American Medical Association

"Physician Characteristics and Distribution in the U.S." 1992 Edition (Copyright, reprinted with permission)

*As of January 1, 1990. Comprised of federal and nonfederal physicians. Total includes 2,895 physicians in the U.S. territories and possessions, at APO's and FPO's and whose addresses are unknown.

# Physicians 45 to 54 Years Old in 1990

## National Total = 116,803 Physicians 45 to 54 Years Old*

| RANK | STATE | PHYSICIANS | % | RANK | STATE | PHYSICIANS | % |
|------|-------|-----------|-----|------|-------|-----------|-----|
| 1 | California | 16,367 | 14.01% | 26 | Alabama | 1,342 | 1.15% |
| 2 | New York | 11,201 | 9.59% | 27 | Kentucky | 1,288 | 1.10% |
| 3 | Texas | 6,361 | 5.45% | 28 | South Carolina | 1,121 | 0.96% |
| 4 | Florida | 6,150 | 5.27% | 29 | Oklahoma | 1,018 | 0.87% |
| 5 | Illinois | 5,398 | 4.62% | 30 | Kansas | 959 | 0.82% |
| 6 | Pennsylvania | 5,389 | 4.61% | 31 | Iowa | 849 | 0.73% |
| 7 | New Jersey | 4,337 | 3.71% | 32 | West Virginia | 836 | 0.72% |
| 8 | Ohio | 4,237 | 3.63% | 33 | Arkansas | 806 | 0.69% |
| 9 | Massachusetts | 3,801 | 3.25% | 34 | Mississippi | 744 | 0.64% |
| 10 | Michigan | 3,624 | 3.10% | 35 | Utah | 680 | 0.58% |
| 11 | Maryland | 3,525 | 3.02% | 36 | New Mexico | 657 | 0.56% |
| 12 | Virginia | 2,797 | 2.39% | 37 | Hawaii | 561 | 0.48% |
| 13 | Georgia | 2,608 | 2.23% | 38 | Nebraska | 526 | 0.45% |
| 14 | North Carolina | 2,368 | 2.03% | 39 | Rhode Island | 509 | 0.44% |
| 15 | Washington | 2,321 | 1.99% | 40 | Maine | 488 | 0.42% |
| 16 | Missouri | 2,019 | 1.73% | 41 | New Hampshire | 466 | 0.40% |
| 17 | Connecticut | 1,949 | 1.67% | 42 | Nevada | 413 | 0.35% |
| 18 | Wisconsin | 1,906 | 1.63% | 43 | Montana | 355 | 0.30% |
| 19 | Tennessee | 1,879 | 1.61% | 44 | Idaho | 330 | 0.28% |
| 20 | Minnesota | 1,769 | 1.51% | 45 | Delaware | 305 | 0.26% |
| 21 | Indiana | 1,726 | 1.48% | 46 | Vermont | 298 | 0.26% |
| 22 | Louisiana | 1,675 | 1.43% | 47 | North Dakota | 247 | 0.21% |
| 23 | Colorado | 1,614 | 1.38% | 48 | Alaska | 229 | 0.20% |
| 24 | Arizona | 1,574 | 1.35% | 49 | South Dakota | 210 | 0.18% |
| 25 | Oregon | 1,460 | 1.25% | 50 | Wyoming | 151 | 0.13% |
| | | | | | District of Columbia | 945 | 0.81% |

Source: American Medical Association

"Physician Characteristics and Distribution in the U.S." 1992 Edition (Copyright, reprinted with permission)

*As of January 1, 1990. Comprised of federal and nonfederal physicians. Total includes 2,415 physicians in the U.S. territories and possessions, at APO's and FPO's and whose addresses are unknown.

# Physicians 55 to 64 Years Old in 1990

## National Total = 83,614 Physicians 55 to 64 Years Old*

| RANK | STATE | PHYSICIANS | % |
|---|---|---|---|
| 1 | California | 11,633 | 13.91% |
| 2 | New York | 8,712 | 10.42% |
| 3 | Texas | 4,640 | 5.55% |
| 4 | Florida | 4,439 | 5.31% |
| 5 | Pennsylvania | 4,072 | 4.87% |
| 6 | Ohio | 3,338 | 3.99% |
| 7 | Illinois | 3,272 | 3.91% |
| 8 | New Jersey | 3,011 | 3.60% |
| 9 | Michigan | 2,704 | 3.23% |
| 10 | Massachusetts | 2,429 | 2.91% |
| 11 | Maryland | 2,245 | 2.68% |
| 12 | Virginia | 1,969 | 2.35% |
| 13 | North Carolina | 1,772 | 2.12% |
| 14 | Georgia | 1,666 | 1.99% |
| 15 | Washington | 1,558 | 1.86% |
| 16 | Connecticut | 1,462 | 1.75% |
| 17 | Wisconsin | 1,443 | 1.73% |
| 18 | Missouri | 1,421 | 1.70% |
| 19 | Tennessee | 1,405 | 1.68% |
| 20 | Indiana | 1,396 | 1.67% |
| 21 | Minnesota | 1,332 | 1.59% |
| 22 | Louisiana | 1,231 | 1.47% |
| 23 | Arizona | 1,199 | 1.43% |
| 24 | Colorado | 1,043 | 1.25% |
| 25 | Kentucky | 946 | 1.13% |

| RANK | STATE | PHYSICIANS | % |
|---|---|---|---|
| 26 | Alabama | 930 | 1.11% |
| 27 | Oregon | 919 | 1.10% |
| 28 | South Carolina | 848 | 1.01% |
| 29 | Oklahoma | 773 | 0.92% |
| 30 | Kansas | 666 | 0.80% |
| 31 | Iowa | 628 | 0.75% |
| 32 | Mississippi | 605 | 0.72% |
| 33 | Arkansas | 552 | 0.66% |
| 34 | Hawaii | 444 | 0.53% |
| 35 | West Virginia | 442 | 0.53% |
| 36 | Utah | 418 | 0.50% |
| 37 | Nebraska | 412 | 0.49% |
| 38 | Rhode Island | 387 | 0.46% |
| 39 | New Mexico | 380 | 0.45% |
| 40 | Maine | 359 | 0.43% |
| 41 | Nevada | 327 | 0.39% |
| 41 | New Hampshire | 327 | 0.39% |
| 43 | Delaware | 248 | 0.30% |
| 44 | Montana | 221 | 0.26% |
| 45 | Idaho | 219 | 0.26% |
| 46 | Vermont | 194 | 0.23% |
| 47 | North Dakota | 188 | 0.22% |
| 48 | South Dakota | 160 | 0.19% |
| 49 | Alaska | 131 | 0.16% |
| 50 | Wyoming | 113 | 0.14% |
| | District of Columbia | 605 | 0.72% |

Source: American Medical Association

"Physician Characteristics and Distribution in the U.S." 1992 Edition (Copyright, reprinted with permission)

*As of January 1, 1990. Comprised of federal and nonfederal physicians. Total includes 1,780 physicians in the U.S. territories and possessions, at APO's and FPO's and whose addresses are unknown.

# Physicians 65 Years Old and Older in 1990

## National Total = 95,389 Physicians 65 Years Old and Older*

| RANK | STATE | PHYSICIANS | % | RANK | STATE | PHYSICIANS | % |
|---|---|---|---|---|---|---|---|
| 1 | California | 14,098 | 14.78% | 26 | South Carolina | 997 | 1.05% |
| 2 | New York | 9,576 | 10.04% | 27 | Alabama | 985 | 1.03% |
| 3 | Florida | 7,672 | 8.04% | 28 | Kentucky | 963 | 1.01% |
| 4 | Pennsylvania | 4,820 | 5.05% | 29 | Kansas | 819 | 0.86% |
| 5 | Texas | 4,302 | 4.51% | 30 | Oklahoma | 813 | 0.85% |
| 6 | Illinois | 3,804 | 3.99% | 31 | Iowa | 753 | 0.79% |
| 7 | Ohio | 3,581 | 3.75% | 32 | Arkansas | 648 | 0.68% |
| 8 | New Jersey | 3,035 | 3.18% | 33 | Mississippi | 583 | 0.61% |
| 9 | Massachusetts | 3,028 | 3.17% | 34 | Maine | 557 | 0.58% |
| 10 | Michigan | 2,531 | 2.65% | 35 | West Virginia | 545 | 0.57% |
| 11 | Maryland | 2,132 | 2.24% | 36 | New Mexico | 523 | 0.55% |
| 12 | Virginia | 2,003 | 2.10% | 37 | Hawaii | 511 | 0.54% |
| 13 | North Carolina | 2,000 | 2.10% | 38 | Utah | 503 | 0.53% |
| 14 | Washington | 1,925 | 2.02% | 39 | New Hampshire | 477 | 0.50% |
| 15 | Connecticut | 1,687 | 1.77% | 40 | Rhode Island | 457 | 0.48% |
| 16 | Arizona | 1,682 | 1.76% | 41 | Nebraska | 451 | 0.47% |
| 17 | Indiana | 1,564 | 1.64% | 42 | Vermont | 314 | 0.33% |
| 18 | Georgia | 1,529 | 1.60% | 43 | Montana | 304 | 0.32% |
| 19 | Tennessee | 1,424 | 1.49% | 44 | Nevada | 301 | 0.32% |
| 20 | Wisconsin | 1,422 | 1.49% | 45 | Idaho | 296 | 0.31% |
| 21 | Missouri | 1,394 | 1.46% | 46 | Delaware | 236 | 0.25% |
| 22 | Minnesota | 1,388 | 1.46% | 47 | South Dakota | 202 | 0.21% |
| 23 | Louisiana | 1,193 | 1.25% | 48 | North Dakota | 141 | 0.15% |
| 24 | Oregon | 1,170 | 1.23% | 49 | Wyoming | 126 | 0.13% |
| 25 | Colorado | 1,121 | 1.18% | 50 | Alaska | 61 | 0.06% |
| | | | | | District of Columbia | 587 | 0.62% |

Source: American Medical Association

"Physician Characteristics and Distribution in the U.S." 1992 Edition (Copyright, reprinted with permission)

*As of January 1, 1990. Comprised of federal and nonfederal physicians. Total includes 2,155 physicians in the U.S. territories and possessions, at APO's and FPO's and whose addresses are unknown.

# Percent of Physicians 65 Years Old and Older in 1990

## National Rate = 15.5% of Physicians are 65 Years Old and Older*

| RANK | STATE | PERCENT | RANK | STATE | PERCENT |
|------|-------|---------|------|-------|---------|
| 1 | Florida | 23.7 | 26 | Oklahoma | 15.3 |
| 2 | Maine | 21.4 | 27 | Ohio | 15.1 |
| 3 | Montana | 20.1 | 28 | Nevada | 15.0 |
| 4 | Idaho | 19.8 | 29 | Mississippi | 14.7 |
| 5 | Arizona | 19.6 | 29 | Nebraska | 14.7 |
| 6 | Vermont | 18.8 | 31 | New Jersey | 14.5 |
| 7 | New Hampshire | 18.5 | 32 | North Carolina | 14.3 |
| 8 | California | 17.4 | 32 | Utah | 14.3 |
| 8 | South Dakota | 17.4 | 34 | Illinois | 14.0 |
| 10 | Oregon | 17.3 | 34 | Kentucky | 14.0 |
| 11 | Hawaii | 16.5 | 36 | Colorado | 13.9 |
| 12 | Wyoming | 16.4 | 36 | Wisconsin | 13.9 |
| 13 | Kansas | 16.3 | 38 | Massachusetts | 13.8 |
| 14 | Rhode Island | 16.2 | 39 | Virginia | 13.7 |
| 15 | Indiana | 16.1 | 40 | Alabama | 13.6 |
| 15 | Washington | 16.1 | 41 | Louisiana | 13.4 |
| 17 | New Mexico | 15.9 | 41 | Michigan | 13.4 |
| 18 | Arkansas | 15.7 | 41 | Tennessee | 13.4 |
| 18 | Delaware | 15.7 | 44 | Minnesota | 13.0 |
| 20 | Iowa | 15.6 | 45 | Texas | 12.9 |
| 20 | West Virginia | 15.6 | 46 | Missouri | 12.6 |
| 22 | Connecticut | 15.5 | 47 | Georgia | 12.0 |
| 22 | New York | 15.5 | 48 | Maryland | 11.7 |
| 22 | South Carolina | 15.5 | 49 | North Dakota | 11.3 |
| 25 | Pennsylvania | 15.4 | 50 | Alaska | 6.7 |

District of Columbia        13.6

Source: American Medical Association

"Physician Characteristics and Distribution in the U.S." 1992 edition (Copyright, reprinted with permission)

*Calculated by the editors. Comprised of federal and nonfederal physicians. As of January 1, 1990. National rate includes physicians in U.S. territories and possessions, at APO's and FPO's and whose addresses are unknown.

# Federal Physicians in 1990

## National Total = 20,475 Federal Physicians*

| RANK | STATE | PHYSICIANS | % | RANK | STATE | PHYSICIANS | % |
|---|---|---|---|---|---|---|---|
| 1 | California | 2,589 | 12.64% | 26 | Minnesota | 203 | 0.99% |
| 2 | Texas | 1,710 | 8.35% | 26 | Mississippi | 203 | 0.99% |
| 3 | Maryland | 1,575 | 7.69% | 28 | Oregon | 194 | 0.95% |
| 4 | Florida | 942 | 4.60% | 29 | Connecticut | 193 | 0.94% |
| 5 | New York | 884 | 4.32% | 30 | Kentucky | 177 | 0.86% |
| 6 | Virginia | 861 | 4.21% | 31 | Kansas | 176 | 0.86% |
| 7 | Georgia | 760 | 3.71% | 32 | New Mexico | 175 | 0.85% |
| 8 | Washington | 630 | 3.08% | 33 | Arkansas | 154 | 0.75% |
| 9 | Pennsylvania | 545 | 2.66% | 34 | Alaska | 138 | 0.67% |
| 10 | Illinois | 537 | 2.62% | 35 | Indiana | 135 | 0.66% |
| 11 | North Carolina | 498 | 2.43% | 36 | Nebraska | 108 | 0.53% |
| 12 | Ohio | 490 | 2.39% | 37 | Utah | 105 | 0.51% |
| 13 | Colorado | 431 | 2.11% | 38 | Iowa | 103 | 0.50% |
| 14 | Massachusetts | 429 | 2.10% | 39 | West Virginia | 102 | 0.50% |
| 15 | Arizona | 334 | 1.63% | 40 | Nevada | 85 | 0.42% |
| 16 | South Carolina | 319 | 1.56% | 41 | Maine | 82 | 0.40% |
| 17 | Tennessee | 309 | 1.51% | 42 | Rhode Island | 78 | 0.38% |
| 18 | New Jersey | 303 | 1.48% | 43 | New Hampshire | 75 | 0.37% |
| 19 | Missouri | 298 | 1.46% | 44 | South Dakota | 66 | 0.32% |
| 20 | Hawaii | 288 | 1.41% | 45 | Montana | 61 | 0.30% |
| 21 | Alabama | 282 | 1.38% | 46 | Idaho | 60 | 0.29% |
| 22 | Michigan | 252 | 1.23% | 47 | Delaware | 51 | 0.25% |
| 23 | Louisiana | 240 | 1.17% | 47 | North Dakota | 51 | 0.25% |
| 24 | Oklahoma | 215 | 1.05% | 49 | Vermont | 42 | 0.21% |
| 25 | Wisconsin | 209 | 1.02% | 50 | Wyoming | 32 | 0.16% |
| | | | | | District of Columbia | 389 | 1.90% |

Source: American Medical Association

   "Physician Characteristics and Distribution in the U.S." 1992 Edition (Copyright, reprinted with permission)

*As of January 1, 1990. Total includes 1,307 physicians in the U.S. territories and possessions, at APO's and FPO's and whose addresses are unknown.

384

# Federal Physicians per 100,000 Population in 1990

## National Rate = 8.23 Federal Physicians per 100,000 Population*

| RANK | STATE | RATE | | RANK | STATE | RATE |
|---|---|---|---|---|---|---|
| 1 | Maryland | 32.94 | | 26 | Alabama | 6.98 |
| 2 | Hawaii | 25.99 | | 27 | Nebraska | 6.84 |
| 3 | Alaska | 25.09 | | 28 | Oklahoma | 6.83 |
| 4 | Virginia | 13.92 | | 28 | Oregon | 6.83 |
| 5 | Colorado | 13.08 | | 30 | New Hampshire | 6.76 |
| 6 | Washington | 12.95 | | 31 | Maine | 6.68 |
| 7 | Georgia | 11.73 | | 32 | Arkansas | 6.55 |
| 8 | New Mexico | 11.55 | | 33 | Tennessee | 6.34 |
| 9 | Texas | 10.07 | | 34 | Utah | 6.09 |
| 10 | South Dakota | 9.48 | | 35 | Idaho | 5.96 |
| 11 | South Carolina | 9.15 | | 36 | Connecticut | 5.87 |
| 12 | Arizona | 9.11 | | 37 | Missouri | 5.82 |
| 13 | California | 8.70 | | 38 | Louisiana | 5.69 |
| 14 | North Dakota | 7.98 | | 38 | West Virginia | 5.69 |
| 15 | Mississippi | 7.89 | | 40 | New York | 4.91 |
| 16 | Rhode Island | 7.77 | | 41 | Kentucky | 4.80 |
| 17 | Delaware | 7.66 | | 42 | Illinois | 4.70 |
| 18 | Montana | 7.63 | | 43 | Minnesota | 4.64 |
| 19 | North Carolina | 7.51 | | 44 | Pennsylvania | 4.59 |
| 20 | Vermont | 7.46 | | 45 | Ohio | 4.52 |
| 21 | Florida | 7.28 | | 46 | Wisconsin | 4.27 |
| 22 | Massachusetts | 7.13 | | 47 | New Jersey | 3.92 |
| 23 | Kansas | 7.10 | | 48 | Iowa | 3.71 |
| 24 | Nevada | 7.07 | | 49 | Michigan | 2.71 |
| 25 | Wyoming | 7.05 | | 50 | Indiana | 2.43 |

District of Columbia                 64.10

Source: American Medical Association
*"Physician Characteristics and Distribution in the U.S." 1992 Edition (Copyright, reprinted with permission)*
*Calculated by the editors using 1990 Census resident population figures. As of January 1, 1990. National rate includes physicians in the U.S. territories and possessions not shown separately.*

# Nonfederal Physicians in 1990

## National Total = 592,166 Physicians*

| RANK | STATE | PHYSICIANS | % | | RANK | STATE | PHYSICIANS | % |
|---|---|---|---|---|---|---|---|---|
| 1 | California | 78,285 | 13.22% | | 26 | Kentucky | 6,701 | 1.13% |
| 2 | New York | 60,744 | 10.26% | | 27 | Oregon | 6,562 | 1.11% |
| 3 | Texas | 31,647 | 5.34% | | 28 | South Carolina | 6,096 | 1.03% |
| 4 | Florida | 31,483 | 5.32% | | 29 | Oklahoma | 5,095 | 0.86% |
| 5 | Pennsylvania | 30,824 | 5.21% | | 30 | Kansas | 4,861 | 0.82% |
| 6 | Illinois | 26,603 | 4.49% | | 31 | Iowa | 4,728 | 0.80% |
| 7 | Ohio | 23,239 | 3.92% | | 32 | Arkansas | 3,966 | 0.67% |
| 8 | Massachusetts | 21,475 | 3.63% | | 33 | Mississippi | 3,753 | 0.63% |
| 9 | New Jersey | 20,579 | 3.48% | | 34 | Utah | 3,406 | 0.58% |
| 10 | Michigan | 18,620 | 3.14% | | 35 | West Virginia | 3,388 | 0.57% |
| 11 | Maryland | 16,716 | 2.82% | | 36 | New Mexico | 3,114 | 0.53% |
| 12 | Virginia | 13,795 | 2.33% | | 37 | Nebraska | 2,955 | 0.50% |
| 13 | North Carolina | 13,492 | 2.28% | | 38 | Hawaii | 2,809 | 0.47% |
| 14 | Georgia | 11,929 | 2.01% | | 39 | Rhode Island | 2,744 | 0.46% |
| 15 | Washington | 11,325 | 1.91% | | 40 | Maine | 2,522 | 0.43% |
| 16 | Missouri | 10,759 | 1.82% | | 41 | New Hampshire | 2,507 | 0.42% |
| 17 | Connecticut | 10,699 | 1.81% | | 42 | Nevada | 1,921 | 0.32% |
| 18 | Minnesota | 10,458 | 1.77% | | 43 | Vermont | 1,631 | 0.28% |
| 19 | Tennessee | 10,334 | 1.75% | | 44 | Montana | 1,452 | 0.25% |
| 20 | Wisconsin | 10,049 | 1.70% | | 45 | Delaware | 1,449 | 0.24% |
| 21 | Indiana | 9,558 | 1.61% | | 46 | Idaho | 1,435 | 0.24% |
| 22 | Louisiana | 8,689 | 1.47% | | 47 | North Dakota | 1,195 | 0.20% |
| 23 | Arizona | 8,226 | 1.39% | | 48 | South Dakota | 1,093 | 0.18% |
| 24 | Colorado | 7,606 | 1.28% | | 49 | Alaska | 777 | 0.13% |
| 25 | Alabama | 6,964 | 1.18% | | 50 | Wyoming | 734 | 0.12% |
| | | | | | | District of Columbia | 3,929 | 0.66% |

*Source: American Medical Association*

*"Physician Characteristics and Distribution in the U.S." 1992 edition (Copyright, reprinted with permission)*

*As of January 1, 1990. Total includes 7,259 physicians in U.S. territories and possessions not shown separately.*

# Nonfederal Physicians per 100,000 Population in 1990

## National Rate = 238.10 Physicians per 100,000 Population*

| RANK | STATE | RATE | | RANK | STATE | RATE |
|---|---|---|---|---|---|---|
| 1 | Massachusetts | 356.94 | | 26 | Wisconsin | 205.43 |
| 2 | Maryland | 349.60 | | 27 | Maine | 205.39 |
| 3 | New York | 337.65 | | 28 | North Carolina | 203.54 |
| 4 | Connecticut | 325.48 | | 29 | Michigan | 200.32 |
| 5 | Vermont | 289.82 | | 30 | Utah | 197.70 |
| 6 | Rhode Island | 273.45 | | 31 | Kansas | 196.20 |
| 7 | New Jersey | 266.22 | | 32 | West Virginia | 188.91 |
| 8 | California | 263.05 | | 33 | Nebraska | 187.22 |
| 9 | Pennsylvania | 259.43 | | 34 | North Dakota | 187.07 |
| 10 | Hawaii | 253.47 | | 35 | Texas | 186.31 |
| 11 | Florida | 243.34 | | 36 | Georgia | 184.14 |
| 12 | Minnesota | 239.03 | | 37 | Kentucky | 181.83 |
| 13 | Illinois | 232.73 | | 38 | Montana | 181.71 |
| 14 | Washington | 232.70 | | 39 | South Carolina | 174.84 |
| 15 | Colorado | 230.88 | | 40 | Indiana | 172.40 |
| 16 | Oregon | 230.87 | | 41 | Alabama | 172.35 |
| 17 | New Hampshire | 226.01 | | 42 | Iowa | 170.27 |
| 18 | Arizona | 224.43 | | 43 | Arkansas | 168.71 |
| 19 | Virginia | 222.95 | | 44 | Oklahoma | 161.97 |
| 20 | Delaware | 217.51 | | 45 | Wyoming | 161.82 |
| 21 | Ohio | 214.24 | | 46 | Nevada | 159.84 |
| 22 | Tennessee | 211.88 | | 47 | South Dakota | 157.04 |
| 23 | Missouri | 210.26 | | 48 | Mississippi | 145.85 |
| 24 | Louisiana | 205.90 | | 49 | Idaho | 142.54 |
| 25 | New Mexico | 205.54 | | 50 | Alaska | 141.26 |

District of Columbia      647.39

Source: American Medical Association

"Physician Characteristics and Distribution in the U.S." 1992 edition (Copyright, reprinted with permission)

*Calculated by the editors using 1990 Census resident population figures. As of January 1, 1990. National rate includes physicians in U.S. territories and possessions not shown separately.

# Active Nonfederal Physicians in 1990

## National Total = 539,513 Active Physicians*

| RANK | STATE | PHYSICIANS | % | RANK | STATE | PHYSICIANS | % |
|---|---|---|---|---|---|---|---|
| 1 | California | 70,062 | 12.99% | 26 | Kentucky | 6,202 | 1.15% |
| 2 | New York | 56,395 | 10.45% | 27 | Oregon | 5,778 | 1.07% |
| 3 | Texas | 29,451 | 5.46% | 28 | South Carolina | 5,541 | 1.03% |
| 4 | Pennsylvania | 28,293 | 5.24% | 29 | Oklahoma | 4,697 | 0.87% |
| 5 | Florida | 26,123 | 4.84% | 30 | Kansas | 4,360 | 0.81% |
| 6 | Illinois | 24,680 | 4.57% | 31 | Iowa | 4,280 | 0.79% |
| 7 | Ohio | 21,379 | 3.96% | 32 | Arkansas | 3,595 | 0.67% |
| 8 | Massachusetts | 19,910 | 3.69% | 33 | Mississippi | 3,455 | 0.64% |
| 9 | New Jersey | 18,971 | 3.52% | 34 | Utah | 3,145 | 0.58% |
| 10 | Michigan | 17,129 | 3.17% | 35 | West Virginia | 3,086 | 0.57% |
| 11 | Maryland | 15,484 | 2.87% | 36 | New Mexico | 2,768 | 0.51% |
| 12 | Virginia | 12,615 | 2.34% | 37 | Nebraska | 2,741 | 0.51% |
| 13 | North Carolina | 12,262 | 2.27% | 38 | Rhode Island | 2,515 | 0.47% |
| 14 | Georgia | 11,144 | 2.07% | 39 | Hawaii | 2,491 | 0.46% |
| 15 | Missouri | 10,100 | 1.87% | 40 | New Hampshire | 2,199 | 0.41% |
| 16 | Washington | 10,006 | 1.85% | 41 | Maine | 2,155 | 0.40% |
| 17 | Connecticut | 9,820 | 1.82% | 42 | Nevada | 1,746 | 0.32% |
| 18 | Tennessee | 9,619 | 1.78% | 43 | Vermont | 1,432 | 0.27% |
| 19 | Minnesota | 9,574 | 1.77% | 44 | Delaware | 1,329 | 0.25% |
| 20 | Wisconsin | 9,172 | 1.70% | 45 | Montana | 1,263 | 0.23% |
| 21 | Indiana | 8,764 | 1.62% | 46 | Idaho | 1,259 | 0.23% |
| 22 | Louisiana | 8,173 | 1.51% | 47 | North Dakota | 1,102 | 0.20% |
| 23 | Arizona | 6,961 | 1.29% | 48 | South Dakota | 992 | 0.18% |
| 24 | Colorado | 6,894 | 1.28% | 49 | Alaska | 734 | 0.14% |
| 25 | Alabama | 6,464 | 1.20% | 50 | Wyoming | 654 | 0.12% |
|  |  |  |  |  | District of Columbia | 3,674 | 0.68% |

*Source: American Medical Association*

*"Physician Characteristics and Distribution in the U.S." 1992 edition (Copyright, reprinted with permission)*

*\*Calculated by the editors by subtracting inactive physicians from total physicians. As of January 1, 1990. Total includes physicians in U.S. territories and possessions not shown separately.*

# Active Nonfederal Physicians per 100,000 Population in 1990

## National Rate = 216.92 Active Physicians per 100,000 Population*

| RANK | STATE | RATE | | RANK | STATE | RATE |
|---|---|---|---|---|---|---|
| 1 | Massachusetts | 330.93 | | 26 | North Carolina | 184.99 |
| 2 | Maryland | 323.83 | | 27 | Michigan | 184.28 |
| 3 | New York | 313.47 | | 28 | New Mexico | 182.70 |
| 4 | Connecticut | 298.74 | | 29 | Utah | 182.55 |
| 5 | Vermont | 254.46 | | 30 | Kansas | 175.98 |
| 6 | Rhode Island | 250.63 | | 31 | Maine | 175.50 |
| 7 | New Jersey | 245.41 | | 32 | Nebraska | 173.66 |
| 8 | Pennsylvania | 238.12 | | 33 | Texas | 173.38 |
| 9 | California | 235.42 | | 34 | North Dakota | 172.51 |
| 10 | Hawaii | 224.77 | | 35 | West Virginia | 172.07 |
| 11 | Minnesota | 218.83 | | 36 | Georgia | 172.02 |
| 12 | Illinois | 215.91 | | 37 | Kentucky | 168.29 |
| 13 | Colorado | 209.26 | | 38 | Alabama | 159.98 |
| 14 | Washington | 205.60 | | 39 | South Carolina | 158.92 |
| 15 | Virginia | 203.88 | | 40 | Indiana | 158.08 |
| 16 | Oregon | 203.28 | | 41 | Montana | 158.06 |
| 17 | Florida | 201.91 | | 42 | Iowa | 154.14 |
| 18 | Delaware | 199.50 | | 43 | Arkansas | 152.93 |
| 19 | New Hampshire | 198.24 | | 44 | Oklahoma | 149.32 |
| 20 | Missouri | 197.38 | | 45 | Nevada | 145.28 |
| 21 | Tennessee | 197.22 | | 46 | Wyoming | 144.18 |
| 22 | Ohio | 197.09 | | 47 | South Dakota | 142.53 |
| 23 | Louisiana | 193.67 | | 48 | Mississippi | 134.27 |
| 24 | Arizona | 189.92 | | 49 | Alaska | 133.44 |
| 25 | Wisconsin | 187.50 | | 50 | Idaho | 125.06 |
| | | | | | District of Columbia | 605.37 |

Source: American Medical Association

"Physician Characteristics and Distribution in the U.S." 1992 edition (Copyright, reprinted with permission)

*Calculated by the editors using 1990 Census resident population figures and by subtracting Inactive Physicians from Total Physicians. As of January 1, 1990. National rate includes physicians in U.S. territories and possessions not shown separately.

# Nonfederal Physicians in Patient Care in 1990

## National Total = 487,796 Physicians*

| RANK | STATE | PHYSICIANS | % | RANK | STATE | PHYSICIANS | % |
|---|---|---|---|---|---|---|---|
| 1 | California | 63,109 | 12.94% | 26 | Kentucky | 5,815 | 1.19% |
| 2 | New York | 49,468 | 10.14% | 27 | Oregon | 5,374 | 1.10% |
| 3 | Texas | 26,992 | 5.53% | 28 | South Carolina | 5,170 | 1.06% |
| 4 | Pennsylvania | 25,610 | 5.25% | 29 | Oklahoma | 4,358 | 0.89% |
| 5 | Florida | 24,092 | 4.94% | 30 | Kansas | 4,050 | 0.83% |
| 6 | Illinois | 22,396 | 4.59% | 31 | Iowa | 3,905 | 0.80% |
| 7 | Ohio | 19,586 | 4.02% | 32 | Arkansas | 3,384 | 0.69% |
| 8 | New Jersey | 17,137 | 3.51% | 33 | Mississippi | 3,283 | 0.67% |
| 9 | Massachusetts | 16,875 | 3.46% | 34 | Utah | 2,869 | 0.59% |
| 10 | Michigan | 15,622 | 3.20% | 35 | West Virginia | 2,855 | 0.59% |
| 11 | Maryland | 12,882 | 2.64% | 36 | Nebraska | 2,534 | 0.52% |
| 12 | Virginia | 11,576 | 2.37% | 37 | New Mexico | 2,521 | 0.52% |
| 13 | North Carolina | 11,105 | 2.28% | 38 | Hawaii | 2,316 | 0.47% |
| 14 | Georgia | 10,337 | 2.12% | 39 | Rhode Island | 2,245 | 0.46% |
| 15 | Missouri | 9,109 | 1.87% | 40 | New Hampshire | 2,052 | 0.42% |
| 16 | Washington | 9,074 | 1.86% | 41 | Maine | 2,010 | 0.41% |
| 17 | Tennessee | 8,907 | 1.83% | 42 | Nevada | 1,639 | 0.34% |
| 18 | Minnesota | 8,755 | 1.79% | 43 | Vermont | 1,269 | 0.26% |
| 19 | Connecticut | 8,653 | 1.77% | 44 | Delaware | 1,222 | 0.25% |
| 20 | Wisconsin | 8,476 | 1.74% | 45 | Montana | 1,216 | 0.25% |
| 21 | Indiana | 8,130 | 1.67% | 46 | Idaho | 1,208 | 0.25% |
| 22 | Louisiana | 7,566 | 1.55% | 47 | North Dakota | 1,041 | 0.21% |
| 23 | Arizona | 6,481 | 1.33% | 48 | South Dakota | 934 | 0.19% |
| 24 | Colorado | 6,276 | 1.29% | 49 | Alaska | 686 | 0.14% |
| 25 | Alabama | 5,999 | 1.23% | 50 | Wyoming | 616 | 0.13% |
| | | | | | District of Columbia | 2,988 | 0.61% |

Source: American Medical Association

"Physician Characteristics and Distribution in the U.S." 1992 edition (Copyright, reprinted with permission)

*As of January 1, 1990. Total includes 6,035 physicians in U.S. territories and possessions not shown separately. Patient Care excludes those physicians in administration, teaching and research.

# Nonfederal Physicians in Patient Care per 100,000 Population in 1990

## National Rate = 196.13 Physicians in Patient Care per 100,000 Population*

| RANK | STATE | RATE | RANK | STATE | RATE |
|------|-------|------|------|-------|------|
| 1 | Massachusetts | 280.48 | 26 | Michigan | 168.06 |
| 2 | New York | 274.97 | 27 | North Carolina | 167.53 |
| 3 | Maryland | 269.42 | 28 | Utah | 166.53 |
| 4 | Connecticut | 263.24 | 29 | New Mexico | 166.40 |
| 5 | Vermont | 225.50 | 30 | Maine | 163.69 |
| 6 | Rhode Island | 223.73 | 31 | Kansas | 163.47 |
| 7 | New Jersey | 221.69 | 32 | North Dakota | 162.96 |
| 8 | Pennsylvania | 215.54 | 33 | Nebraska | 160.54 |
| 9 | California | 212.06 | 34 | Georgia | 159.57 |
| 10 | Hawaii | 208.98 | 35 | West Virginia | 159.19 |
| 11 | Minnesota | 200.11 | 36 | Texas | 158.90 |
| 12 | Illinois | 195.93 | 37 | Kentucky | 157.79 |
| 13 | Colorado | 190.51 | 38 | Montana | 152.18 |
| 14 | Oregon | 189.07 | 39 | Alabama | 148.47 |
| 15 | Virginia | 187.09 | 40 | South Carolina | 148.28 |
| 16 | Washington | 186.45 | 41 | Indiana | 146.64 |
| 17 | Florida | 186.21 | 42 | Arkansas | 143.96 |
| 18 | New Hampshire | 184.99 | 43 | Iowa | 140.63 |
| 19 | Delaware | 183.44 | 44 | Oklahoma | 138.54 |
| 20 | Tennessee | 182.63 | 45 | Nevada | 136.38 |
| 21 | Ohio | 180.56 | 46 | Wyoming | 135.81 |
| 22 | Louisiana | 179.29 | 47 | South Dakota | 134.19 |
| 23 | Missouri | 178.01 | 48 | Mississippi | 127.58 |
| 24 | Arizona | 176.82 | 49 | Alaska | 124.72 |
| 25 | Wisconsin | 173.27 | 50 | Idaho | 119.99 |
|  |  |  |  | District of Columbia | 492.34 |

Source: American Medical Association

"Physician Characteristics and Distribution in the U.S." 1992 edition (Copyright, reprinted with permission)

*Calculated by the editors using 1990 Census resident population figures. As of January 1, 1990. National rate includes physicians in U.S. territories and possessions not shown separately. Patient Care excludes those physicians in administration, teaching and research.

391

# Nonfederal Physicians in General/Family Practice in 1990

## National Total = 68,428 General/Family Practitioners*

| RANK | STATE | PHYSICIANS | % | RANK | STATE | PHYSICIANS | % |
|---|---|---|---|---|---|---|---|
| 1 | California | 8,863 | 12.95% | 26 | Iowa | 977 | 1.43% |
| 2 | Texas | 4,356 | 6.37% | 27 | Massachusetts | 942 | 1.38% |
| 3 | Pennsylvania | 3,520 | 5.14% | 28 | Arkansas | 909 | 1.33% |
| 4 | Florida | 3,494 | 5.11% | 29 | Kansas | 886 | 1.29% |
| 5 | New York | 3,369 | 4.92% | 30 | Oklahoma | 880 | 1.29% |
| 6 | Illinois | 3,127 | 4.57% | 31 | Oregon | 864 | 1.26% |
| 7 | Ohio | 2,777 | 4.06% | 32 | Mississippi | 727 | 1.06% |
| 8 | Indiana | 1,932 | 2.82% | 33 | Nebraska | 634 | 0.93% |
| 9 | Minnesota | 1,918 | 2.80% | 34 | West Virginia | 573 | 0.84% |
| 10 | Washington | 1,912 | 2.79% | 35 | Connecticut | 572 | 0.84% |
| 11 | Michigan | 1,908 | 2.79% | 36 | New Mexico | 463 | 0.68% |
| 12 | North Carolina | 1,769 | 2.59% | 37 | Maine | 422 | 0.62% |
| 13 | Virginia | 1,738 | 2.54% | 38 | Utah | 415 | 0.61% |
| 14 | Wisconsin | 1,653 | 2.42% | 39 | Idaho | 337 | 0.49% |
| 15 | New Jersey | 1,432 | 2.09% | 40 | New Hampshire | 308 | 0.45% |
| 16 | Georgia | 1,367 | 2.00% | 41 | South Dakota | 302 | 0.44% |
| 17 | Tennessee | 1,274 | 1.86% | 42 | Montana | 289 | 0.42% |
| 18 | Kentucky | 1,140 | 1.67% | 43 | North Dakota | 274 | 0.40% |
| 19 | South Carolina | 1,119 | 1.64% | 44 | Hawaii | 272 | 0.40% |
| 20 | Colorado | 1,062 | 1.55% | 45 | Nevada | 262 | 0.38% |
| 21 | Alabama | 1,040 | 1.52% | 46 | Wyoming | 190 | 0.28% |
| 22 | Maryland | 1,016 | 1.48% | 47 | Vermont | 189 | 0.28% |
| 23 | Arizona | 1,008 | 1.47% | 48 | Alaska | 181 | 0.26% |
| 24 | Louisiana | 1,007 | 1.47% | 49 | Delaware | 169 | 0.25% |
| 25 | Missouri | 989 | 1.45% | 49 | Rhode Island | 169 | 0.25% |
| | | | | | District of Columbia | 166 | 0.24% |

Source: American Medical Association

"Physician Characteristics and Distribution in the U.S." 1992 Edition (Copyright, reprinted with permission)

*As of January 1, 1990.  Total includes 1,270 nonfederal physicians in the U.S. territories and possessions not shown separately.

# Nonfederal Physicians in General/Family Practice per 100,000 Population in 1990

## National Rate = 27.51 General/Family Practitioners per 100,000 Population*

| RANK | STATE | RATE | | RANK | STATE | RATE |
|---|---|---|---|---|---|---|
| 1 | Minnesota | 43.84 | | 26 | Virginia | 28.09 |
| 2 | South Dakota | 43.39 | | 27 | Oklahoma | 27.98 |
| 3 | North Dakota | 42.89 | | 28 | New Hampshire | 27.77 |
| 4 | Wyoming | 41.89 | | 29 | Arizona | 27.50 |
| 5 | Nebraska | 40.17 | | 30 | Illinois | 27.36 |
| 6 | Washington | 39.29 | | 31 | Florida | 27.01 |
| 7 | Arkansas | 38.67 | | 32 | North Carolina | 26.69 |
| 8 | Montana | 36.17 | | 33 | Tennessee | 26.12 |
| 9 | Kansas | 35.76 | | 34 | Alabama | 25.74 |
| 10 | Iowa | 35.18 | | 35 | Texas | 25.64 |
| 11 | Indiana | 34.85 | | 36 | Ohio | 25.60 |
| 12 | Maine | 34.37 | | 37 | Delaware | 25.37 |
| 13 | Wisconsin | 33.79 | | 38 | Hawaii | 24.54 |
| 14 | Vermont | 33.58 | | 39 | Utah | 24.09 |
| 15 | Idaho | 33.47 | | 40 | Louisiana | 23.86 |
| 16 | Alaska | 32.91 | | 41 | Nevada | 21.80 |
| 17 | Colorado | 32.24 | | 42 | Maryland | 21.25 |
| 18 | South Carolina | 32.09 | | 43 | Georgia | 21.10 |
| 19 | West Virginia | 31.95 | | 44 | Michigan | 20.53 |
| 20 | Kentucky | 30.93 | | 45 | Missouri | 19.33 |
| 21 | New Mexico | 30.56 | | 46 | New York | 18.73 |
| 22 | Oregon | 30.40 | | 47 | New Jersey | 18.52 |
| 23 | California | 29.78 | | 48 | Connecticut | 17.40 |
| 24 | Pennsylvania | 29.63 | | 49 | Rhode Island | 16.84 |
| 25 | Mississippi | 28.25 | | 50 | Massachusetts | 15.66 |

District of Columbia        27.35

Source: American Medical Association

"Physician Characteristics and Distribution in the U.S." 1992 edition (Copyright, reprinted with permission)

*Calculated by the editors using 1990 Census resident population figures. As of January 1, 1990. National rate includes physicians in U.S. territories and possessions not shown separately.

# Nonfederal Physicians in Medical Specialties in 1990

## National Total = 173,751 Specialists*

| RANK | STATE | SPECIALISTS | % | RANK | STATE | SPECIALISTS | % |
|------|-------|-------------|---|------|-------|-------------|---|
| 1 | California | 22,169 | 12.76% | 26 | Kentucky | 1,693 | 0.97% |
| 2 | New York | 21,586 | 12.42% | 27 | Oregon | 1,669 | 0.96% |
| 3 | Pennsylvania | 9,225 | 5.31% | 28 | South Carolina | 1,397 | 0.80% |
| 4 | Texas | 8,431 | 4.85% | 29 | Oklahoma | 1,292 | 0.74% |
| 5 | Illinois | 8,292 | 4.77% | 30 | Iowa | 1,099 | 0.63% |
| 6 | Florida | 8,076 | 4.65% | 31 | Kansas | 1,074 | 0.62% |
| 7 | Massachusetts | 7,791 | 4.48% | 32 | Rhode Island | 1,070 | 0.62% |
| 8 | New Jersey | 7,314 | 4.21% | 33 | Utah | 921 | 0.53% |
| 9 | Ohio | 6,713 | 3.86% | 34 | Mississippi | 876 | 0.50% |
| 10 | Maryland | 5,728 | 3.30% | 35 | Arkansas | 874 | 0.50% |
| 11 | Michigan | 5,486 | 3.16% | 36 | Hawaii | 840 | 0.48% |
| 12 | North Carolina | 3,861 | 2.22% | 37 | West Virginia | 796 | 0.46% |
| 13 | Virginia | 3,856 | 2.22% | 38 | New Mexico | 784 | 0.45% |
| 14 | Connecticut | 3,715 | 2.14% | 39 | Nebraska | 724 | 0.42% |
| 15 | Missouri | 3,532 | 2.03% | 40 | New Hampshire | 679 | 0.39% |
| 16 | Georgia | 3,318 | 1.91% | 41 | Maine | 593 | 0.34% |
| 17 | Tennessee | 3,022 | 1.74% | 42 | Nevada | 490 | 0.28% |
| 18 | Minnesota | 2,963 | 1.71% | 43 | Vermont | 468 | 0.27% |
| 19 | Washington | 2,768 | 1.59% | 44 | Delaware | 393 | 0.23% |
| 20 | Wisconsin | 2,651 | 1.53% | 45 | Montana | 306 | 0.18% |
| 21 | Louisiana | 2,382 | 1.37% | 46 | Idaho | 268 | 0.15% |
| 22 | Indiana | 2,212 | 1.27% | 46 | North Dakota | 268 | 0.15% |
| 23 | Colorado | 2,078 | 1.20% | 48 | South Dakota | 213 | 0.12% |
| 24 | Arizona | 2,069 | 1.19% | 49 | Alaska | 164 | 0.09% |
| 25 | Alabama | 1,976 | 1.14% | 50 | Wyoming | 124 | 0.07% |
| | | | | | District of Columbia | 1,356 | 0.78% |

Source: American Medical Association

*"Physician Characteristics and Distribution in the U.S."* 1992 edition (Copyright, reprinted with permission)

*As of January 1, 1990. Total includes 2,110 physicians in U.S. territories and possessions not shown separately. Medical Specialties are Allergy/Immunology, Cardiovascular Diseases, Dermatology, Gastroenterology, Internal Medicine, Pediatrics, Pediatric Cardiology and Pulmonary Diseases.

# Nonfederal Physicians in Medical Specialties per 100,000 Population in 1990

## National Rate = 69.86 Medical Specialty Physicians per 100,000 Population*

| RANK | STATE | RATE | | RANK | STATE | RATE |
|---|---|---|---|---|---|---|
| 1 | Massachusetts | 129.50 | | 25 | Louisiana | 56.45 |
| 2 | New York | 119.99 | | 27 | Wisconsin | 54.19 |
| 3 | Maryland | 119.80 | | 28 | Utah | 53.46 |
| 4 | Connecticut | 113.02 | | 29 | New Mexico | 51.75 |
| 5 | Rhode Island | 106.63 | | 30 | Georgia | 51.22 |
| 6 | New Jersey | 94.62 | | 31 | Texas | 49.63 |
| 7 | Vermont | 83.16 | | 32 | Alabama | 48.90 |
| 8 | Pennsylvania | 77.64 | | 33 | Maine | 48.29 |
| 9 | Hawaii | 75.80 | | 34 | Kentucky | 45.94 |
| 10 | California | 74.49 | | 35 | Nebraska | 45.87 |
| 11 | Illinois | 72.54 | | 36 | West Virginia | 44.38 |
| 12 | Missouri | 69.02 | | 37 | Kansas | 43.35 |
| 13 | Minnesota | 67.72 | | 38 | North Dakota | 41.95 |
| 14 | Colorado | 63.08 | | 39 | Oklahoma | 41.07 |
| 15 | Florida | 62.42 | | 40 | Nevada | 40.77 |
| 16 | Virginia | 62.32 | | 41 | South Carolina | 40.07 |
| 17 | Tennessee | 61.96 | | 42 | Indiana | 39.90 |
| 18 | Ohio | 61.89 | | 43 | Iowa | 39.58 |
| 19 | New Hampshire | 61.21 | | 44 | Montana | 38.29 |
| 20 | Michigan | 59.02 | | 45 | Arkansas | 37.18 |
| 21 | Delaware | 58.99 | | 46 | Mississippi | 34.04 |
| 22 | Oregon | 58.72 | | 47 | South Dakota | 30.60 |
| 23 | North Carolina | 58.25 | | 48 | Alaska | 29.82 |
| 24 | Washington | 56.88 | | 49 | Wyoming | 27.34 |
| 25 | Arizona | 56.45 | | 50 | Idaho | 26.62 |

| | | |
|---|---|---|
| | District of Columbia | 223.43 |

Source: American Medical Association
   "Physician Characteristics and Distribution in the U.S." 1992 edition (Copyright, reprinted with permission)
*Calculated by the editors using 1990 Census resident population figures. As of January 1, 1990. National rate includes physicians in the U.S. territories and possessions not shown separately. Medical Specialties are Allergy/Immunology, Cardiovascular Diseases, Dermatology, Gastroenterology, Internal Medicine, Pediatrics, Pediatric Cardiology and Pulmonary Diseases.

# Nonfederal Physicians in Internal Medicine in 1990

## National Total = 94,252 Internal Medicine Physicians*

| RANK | STATE | PHYSICIANS | % | RANK | STATE | PHYSICIANS | % |
|------|-------|-----------|------|------|-------|-----------|------|
| 1 | New York | 12,510 | 13.27% | 26 | Oregon | 993 | 1.05% |
| 2 | California | 11,569 | 12.27% | 27 | Kentucky | 845 | 0.90% |
| 3 | Pennsylvania | 5,267 | 5.59% | 28 | South Carolina | 705 | 0.75% |
| 4 | Illinois | 4,749 | 5.04% | 29 | Oklahoma | 667 | 0.71% |
| 5 | Massachusetts | 4,744 | 5.03% | 30 | Rhode Island | 632 | 0.67% |
| 6 | Texas | 4,121 | 4.37% | 31 | Kansas | 586 | 0.62% |
| 7 | Florida | 3,861 | 4.10% | 32 | Iowa | 556 | 0.59% |
| 8 | New Jersey | 3,852 | 4.09% | 33 | Hawaii | 479 | 0.51% |
| 9 | Ohio | 3,597 | 3.82% | 34 | West Virginia | 442 | 0.47% |
| 10 | Maryland | 3,205 | 3.40% | 35 | Mississippi | 441 | 0.47% |
| 11 | Michigan | 3,145 | 3.34% | 36 | Utah | 430 | 0.46% |
| 12 | Connecticut | 2,136 | 2.27% | 37 | Arkansas | 405 | 0.43% |
| 13 | North Carolina | 2,085 | 2.21% | 38 | New Mexico | 381 | 0.40% |
| 14 | Virginia | 2,053 | 2.18% | 39 | Nebraska | 373 | 0.40% |
| 15 | Missouri | 1,966 | 2.09% | 40 | New Hampshire | 364 | 0.39% |
| 16 | Minnesota | 1,724 | 1.83% | 41 | Maine | 310 | 0.33% |
| 17 | Georgia | 1,716 | 1.82% | 42 | Vermont | 283 | 0.30% |
| 18 | Tennessee | 1,671 | 1.77% | 43 | Nevada | 275 | 0.29% |
| 19 | Wisconsin | 1,492 | 1.58% | 44 | Delaware | 199 | 0.21% |
| 20 | Washington | 1,482 | 1.57% | 45 | Montana | 162 | 0.17% |
| 21 | Louisiana | 1,176 | 1.25% | 46 | North Dakota | 147 | 0.16% |
| 22 | Indiana | 1,132 | 1.20% | 47 | Idaho | 145 | 0.15% |
| 23 | Alabama | 1,106 | 1.17% | 48 | South Dakota | 122 | 0.13% |
| 24 | Colorado | 1,052 | 1.12% | 49 | Alaska | 82 | 0.09% |
| 25 | Arizona | 1,033 | 1.10% | 50 | Wyoming | 71 | 0.08% |
| | | | | | District of Columbia | 770 | 0.82% |

Source: American Medical Association

*"Physician Characteristics and Distribution in the U.S." 1992 edition (Copyright, reprinted with permission)*

*As of January 1, 1990. Total includes 946 physicians in the U.S. territories and possessions not shown separately. Internal Medicine includes Diabetes, Endocrinology, Geriatrics, Hematology, Infectious Diseases, Nephrology, Nutrition, Medical Oncology and Rheumatology.*

# Nonfederal Physicians in Internal Medicine per 100,000 Population in 1990

## National Rate = 37.90 Internal Medicine Physicians per 100,000 Population*

| RANK | STATE | RATE | RANK | STATE | RATE |
|------|-------|------|------|-------|------|
| 1 | Massachusetts | 78.85 | 26 | Arizona | 28.18 |
| 2 | New York | 69.54 | 27 | Louisiana | 27.87 |
| 3 | Maryland | 67.03 | 28 | Alabama | 27.37 |
| 4 | Connecticut | 64.98 | 29 | Georgia | 26.49 |
| 5 | Rhode Island | 62.98 | 30 | Maine | 25.25 |
| 6 | Vermont | 50.29 | 31 | New Mexico | 25.15 |
| 7 | New Jersey | 49.83 | 32 | Utah | 24.96 |
| 8 | Pennsylvania | 44.33 | 33 | West Virginia | 24.64 |
| 9 | Hawaii | 43.22 | 34 | Texas | 24.26 |
| 10 | Illinois | 41.55 | 35 | Kansas | 23.65 |
| 11 | Minnesota | 39.40 | 36 | Nebraska | 23.63 |
| 12 | California | 38.87 | 37 | North Dakota | 23.01 |
| 13 | Missouri | 38.42 | 38 | Kentucky | 22.93 |
| 14 | Oregon | 34.94 | 39 | Nevada | 22.88 |
| 15 | Tennessee | 34.26 | 40 | Oklahoma | 21.20 |
| 16 | Michigan | 33.83 | 41 | Indiana | 20.42 |
| 17 | Virginia | 33.18 | 42 | Montana | 20.27 |
| 18 | Ohio | 33.16 | 43 | South Carolina | 20.22 |
| 19 | New Hampshire | 32.81 | 44 | Iowa | 20.02 |
| 20 | Colorado | 31.93 | 45 | South Dakota | 17.53 |
| 21 | North Carolina | 31.45 | 46 | Arkansas | 17.23 |
| 22 | Wisconsin | 30.50 | 47 | Mississippi | 17.14 |
| 23 | Washington | 30.45 | 48 | Wyoming | 15.65 |
| 24 | Delaware | 29.87 | 49 | Alaska | 14.91 |
| 25 | Florida | 29.84 | 50 | Idaho | 14.40 |

District of Columbia     126.87

Source: American Medical Association

"Physician Characteristics and Distribution in the U.S." 1992 Edition (Copyright, reprinted with permission)

*Calculated by the editors using 1990 Census resident population figures. As of January 1, 1990. National rate includes physicians in the U.S. territories and possessions not shown separately. Internal Medicine includes Diabetes, Endocrinology, Geriatrics, Hematology, Infectious Diseases, Nephrology, Nutrition, Medical Oncology and Rheumatology.

## Nonfederal Physicians in Pediatrics in 1990

## National Total = 39,897 Pediatricians*

| RANK | STATE | PEDIATRICIANS | % | RANK | STATE | PEDIATRICIANS | % |
|------|-------|---------------|---|------|-------|---------------|---|
| 1 | California | 5,235 | 13.12% | 26 | Alabama | 432 | 1.08% |
| 2 | New York | 4,773 | 11.96% | 27 | South Carolina | 363 | 0.91% |
| 3 | Texas | 2,167 | 5.43% | 28 | Oklahoma | 317 | 0.79% |
| 4 | Illinois | 1,826 | 4.58% | 28 | Oregon | 317 | 0.79% |
| 5 | New Jersey | 1,777 | 4.45% | 30 | Utah | 259 | 0.65% |
| 6 | Pennsylvania | 1,738 | 4.36% | 31 | Kansas | 257 | 0.64% |
| 7 | Florida | 1,725 | 4.32% | 32 | Mississippi | 245 | 0.61% |
| 8 | Ohio | 1,646 | 4.13% | 33 | Iowa | 241 | 0.60% |
| 9 | Massachusetts | 1,491 | 3.74% | 34 | Arkansas | 232 | 0.58% |
| 10 | Maryland | 1,351 | 3.39% | 35 | New Mexico | 230 | 0.58% |
| 11 | Michigan | 1,176 | 2.95% | 36 | Hawaii | 221 | 0.55% |
| 12 | Virginia | 948 | 2.38% | 37 | Rhode Island | 216 | 0.54% |
| 13 | North Carolina | 922 | 2.31% | 38 | Nebraska | 173 | 0.43% |
| 14 | Georgia | 817 | 2.05% | 39 | West Virginia | 170 | 0.43% |
| 15 | Connecticut | 777 | 1.95% | 40 | New Hampshire | 165 | 0.41% |
| 16 | Missouri | 758 | 1.90% | 41 | Maine | 144 | 0.36% |
| 17 | Tennessee | 694 | 1.74% | 42 | Delaware | 104 | 0.26% |
| 18 | Washington | 631 | 1.58% | 43 | Vermont | 101 | 0.25% |
| 19 | Louisiana | 622 | 1.56% | 44 | Nevada | 80 | 0.20% |
| 20 | Wisconsin | 584 | 1.46% | 45 | Montana | 64 | 0.16% |
| 21 | Minnesota | 580 | 1.45% | 46 | Idaho | 62 | 0.16% |
| 22 | Indiana | 512 | 1.28% | 47 | North Dakota | 61 | 0.15% |
| 23 | Colorado | 501 | 1.26% | 48 | Alaska | 54 | 0.14% |
| 24 | Arizona | 498 | 1.25% | 49 | South Dakota | 44 | 0.11% |
| 25 | Kentucky | 441 | 1.11% | 50 | Wyoming | 33 | 0.08% |
| | | | | | District of Columbia | 333 | 0.83% |

Source: American Medical Association

"Physician Characteristics and Distribution in the U.S." 1992 Edition (Copyright, reprinted with permission)

*As of January 1, 1990. Total includes 789 physicians in U.S. territories and possessions not shown separately. Pediatrics includes Adolescent Medicine, Neonatal-Perinatal, Pediatric Allergy, Pediatric Endocrinology, Pediatric Pulmonology, Pediatric Hematology-Oncology and Pediatric Nephrology.

# Nonfederal Physicians in Pediatrics per 100,000 Population 17 Years and Younger in 1990

## National Rate = 62.73 Pediatricians per 100,000 Population 17 Years and Younger*

| RANK | STATE | RATE | RANK | STATE | RATE |
|------|-------|------|------|-------|------|
| 1 | Maryland | 116.24 | 26 | Michigan | 47.83 |
| 2 | New York | 112.05 | 27 | Georgia | 47.30 |
| 3 | Massachusetts | 110.19 | 28 | Maine | 46.60 |
| 4 | Connecticut | 103.66 | 29 | Kentucky | 46.22 |
| 5 | New Jersey | 98.75 | 30 | Wisconsin | 45.31 |
| 6 | Rhode Island | 95.71 | 31 | Texas | 44.81 |
| 7 | Hawaii | 78.89 | 32 | Oregon | 43.78 |
| 8 | Vermont | 70.59 | 33 | Utah | 41.28 |
| 9 | California | 67.54 | 34 | Alabama | 40.80 |
| 10 | Delaware | 63.67 | 35 | Nebraska | 40.33 |
| 11 | Virginia | 63.00 | 36 | South Carolina | 39.45 |
| 12 | Pennsylvania | 62.19 | 37 | Kansas | 38.84 |
| 13 | Illinois | 61.97 | 38 | West Virginia | 38.32 |
| 14 | Florida | 60.18 | 39 | Oklahoma | 37.87 |
| 15 | New Hampshire | 59.19 | 40 | Arkansas | 37.35 |
| 16 | Ohio | 58.79 | 41 | Indiana | 35.17 |
| 17 | Colorado | 58.17 | 42 | North Dakota | 34.78 |
| 18 | Missouri | 57.65 | 43 | Iowa | 33.52 |
| 19 | North Carolina | 57.40 | 44 | Mississippi | 32.81 |
| 20 | Tennessee | 57.04 | 45 | Alaska | 31.33 |
| 21 | New Mexico | 51.48 | 46 | Montana | 28.82 |
| 22 | Arizona | 50.76 | 47 | Nevada | 26.94 |
| 23 | Louisiana | 50.68 | 48 | Wyoming | 24.35 |
| 24 | Washington | 50.02 | 49 | South Dakota | 22.17 |
| 25 | Minnesota | 49.71 | 50 | Idaho | 20.10 |

District of Columbia     284.39

Source: American Medical Association

*"Physician Characteristics and Distribution in the U.S." 1992 Edition (Copyright, reprinted with permission)*

*Calculated by the editors using 1990 Census resident population figures. As of January 1, 1990. National rate includes physicians in the U.S. territories and possessions not shown separately. Pediatrics includes Adolescent Medicine, Neonatal-Perinatal, Pediatric Allergy, Pediatric Endocrinology, Pediatric Pulmonology, Pediatric Hematology-Oncology and Pediatric Nephrology.*

# Nonfederal Physicians in Surgical Specialties in 1990

## National Total = 132,604 Surgical Specialty Physicians*

| RANK | STATE | PHYSICIANS | % | RANK | STATE | PHYSICIANS | % |
|------|-------|-----------|-----|------|-------|-----------|-----|
| 1 | California | 16,744 | 12.63% | 26 | Kentucky | 1,592 | 1.20% |
| 2 | New York | 12,993 | 9.80% | 27 | Oregon | 1,518 | 1.14% |
| 3 | Texas | 7,841 | 5.91% | 28 | South Carolina | 1,493 | 1.13% |
| 4 | Florida | 6,905 | 5.21% | 29 | Oklahoma | 1,192 | 0.90% |
| 5 | Pennsylvania | 6,659 | 5.02% | 30 | Kansas | 1,053 | 0.79% |
| 6 | Illinois | 5,801 | 4.37% | 31 | Iowa | 1,041 | 0.79% |
| 7 | Ohio | 5,468 | 4.12% | 32 | Mississippi | 990 | 0.75% |
| 8 | New Jersey | 4,611 | 3.48% | 33 | Arkansas | 907 | 0.68% |
| 9 | Michigan | 4,385 | 3.31% | 34 | West Virginia | 844 | 0.64% |
| 10 | Massachusetts | 4,184 | 3.16% | 35 | Utah | 837 | 0.63% |
| 11 | Maryland | 3,476 | 2.62% | 36 | Nebraska | 679 | 0.51% |
| 12 | Virginia | 3,212 | 2.42% | 37 | New Mexico | 655 | 0.49% |
| 13 | North Carolina | 3,202 | 2.41% | 38 | Hawaii | 631 | 0.48% |
| 14 | Georgia | 3,121 | 2.35% | 39 | Rhode Island | 600 | 0.45% |
| 15 | Tennessee | 2,679 | 2.02% | 40 | New Hampshire | 554 | 0.42% |
| 16 | Missouri | 2,600 | 1.96% | 41 | Maine | 521 | 0.39% |
| 17 | Louisiana | 2,529 | 1.91% | 42 | Nevada | 472 | 0.36% |
| 18 | Connecticut | 2,296 | 1.73% | 43 | Idaho | 341 | 0.26% |
| 19 | Washington | 2,254 | 1.70% | 44 | Vermont | 336 | 0.25% |
| 20 | Wisconsin | 2,141 | 1.61% | 45 | Delaware | 328 | 0.25% |
| 21 | Minnesota | 2,135 | 1.61% | 46 | Montana | 327 | 0.25% |
| 22 | Indiana | 2,091 | 1.58% | 47 | North Dakota | 266 | 0.20% |
| 23 | Arizona | 1,796 | 1.35% | 48 | South Dakota | 227 | 0.17% |
| 24 | Alabama | 1,787 | 1.35% | 49 | Alaska | 178 | 0.13% |
| 25 | Colorado | 1,661 | 1.25% | 50 | Wyoming | 168 | 0.13% |
| | | | | | District of Columbia | 877 | 0.66% |

Source: American Medical Association

*"Physician Characteristics and Distribution in the U.S." 1992 edition (Copyright, reprinted with permission)*

*As of January 1, 1990. Total includes 1,409 physicians in U.S. territories and possessions not shown separately. Surgical Specialties include Colon and Rectal, General, Neurological, Obstetrics & Gynecology, Ophthalmology, Orthopedic, Otolaryngology, Plastic, Thoracic and Urological surgeries.

# Nonfederal Physicians in Surgical Specialties per 100,000 Population in 1990

## National Rate = 53.32 Surgical Specialties Physicians per 100,000 Population*

| RANK | STATE | RATE | RANK | STATE | RATE |
|------|-------|------|------|-------|------|
| 1 | Maryland | 72.70 | 26 | Georgia | 48.18 |
| 2 | New York | 72.22 | 27 | Michigan | 47.17 |
| 3 | Connecticut | 69.85 | 28 | West Virginia | 47.06 |
| 4 | Massachusetts | 69.54 | 29 | Washington | 46.31 |
| 5 | Louisiana | 59.93 | 30 | Texas | 46.16 |
| 6 | Rhode Island | 59.79 | 31 | Alabama | 44.23 |
| 7 | Vermont | 59.71 | 32 | Wisconsin | 43.77 |
| 8 | New Jersey | 59.65 | 33 | New Mexico | 43.23 |
| 9 | Hawaii | 56.94 | 34 | Kentucky | 43.20 |
| 10 | California | 56.26 | 35 | Nebraska | 43.02 |
| 11 | Pennsylvania | 56.04 | 36 | South Carolina | 42.82 |
| 12 | Tennessee | 54.93 | 37 | Kansas | 42.50 |
| 13 | Oregon | 53.41 | 38 | Maine | 42.43 |
| 14 | Florida | 53.37 | 39 | North Dakota | 41.64 |
| 15 | Virginia | 51.91 | 40 | Montana | 40.92 |
| 16 | Missouri | 50.81 | 41 | Nevada | 39.27 |
| 17 | Illinois | 50.75 | 42 | Arkansas | 38.58 |
| 18 | Colorado | 50.42 | 43 | Mississippi | 38.47 |
| 19 | Ohio | 50.41 | 44 | Oklahoma | 37.89 |
| 20 | New Hampshire | 49.94 | 45 | Indiana | 37.72 |
| 21 | Delaware | 49.24 | 46 | Iowa | 37.49 |
| 22 | Arizona | 49.00 | 47 | Wyoming | 37.04 |
| 23 | Minnesota | 48.80 | 48 | Idaho | 33.87 |
| 24 | Utah | 48.58 | 49 | South Dakota | 32.61 |
| 25 | North Carolina | 48.31 | 50 | Alaska | 32.36 |

District of Columbia 144.50

Source: American Medical Association

"Physician Characteristics and Distribution in the U.S." 1992 Edition (Copyright, reprinted with permission)

*Calculated by the editors using 1990 Census resident population figures. As of January 1, 1990. National rate includes physicians in the U.S. territories and possessions not shown separately. Surgical Specialties include Colon and Rectal, General, Neurological, Obstetrics & Gynecology, Ophthalmology, Orthopedic, Otolaryngology, Plastic, Thoracic and Urological surgeries.

# Nonfederal Physicians in General Surgery in 1990

## National Total = 37,003 General Surgeons*

| RANK | STATE | SURGEONS | % | RANK | STATE | SURGEONS | % |
|------|-------|----------|-----|------|-------|----------|-----|
| 1 | California | 4,105 | 11.09% | 26 | Colorado | 422 | 1.14% |
| 2 | New York | 3,995 | 10.80% | 27 | South Carolina | 415 | 1.12% |
| 3 | Texas | 2,078 | 5.62% | 28 | Oregon | 399 | 1.08% |
| 4 | Pennsylvania | 1,995 | 5.39% | 29 | Kansas | 344 | 0.93% |
| 5 | Florida | 1,739 | 4.70% | 30 | Iowa | 322 | 0.87% |
| 6 | Illinois | 1,681 | 4.54% | 31 | Oklahoma | 292 | 0.79% |
| 7 | Ohio | 1,646 | 4.45% | 32 | West Virginia | 280 | 0.76% |
| 8 | Michigan | 1,341 | 3.62% | 33 | Mississippi | 278 | 0.75% |
| 9 | Massachusetts | 1,319 | 3.56% | 34 | Arkansas | 259 | 0.70% |
| 10 | New Jersey | 1,297 | 3.51% | 35 | Nebraska | 209 | 0.56% |
| 11 | Maryland | 926 | 2.50% | 36 | Rhode Island | 204 | 0.55% |
| 12 | Georgia | 852 | 2.30% | 37 | Utah | 201 | 0.54% |
| 13 | North Carolina | 850 | 2.30% | 38 | New Mexico | 165 | 0.45% |
| 14 | Virginia | 832 | 2.25% | 39 | Hawaii | 163 | 0.44% |
| 15 | Tennessee | 819 | 2.21% | 39 | Maine | 163 | 0.44% |
| 16 | Missouri | 745 | 2.01% | 41 | New Hampshire | 160 | 0.43% |
| 17 | Louisiana | 651 | 1.76% | 42 | Nevada | 126 | 0.34% |
| 18 | Connecticut | 621 | 1.68% | 43 | Vermont | 105 | 0.28% |
| 19 | Minnesota | 599 | 1.62% | 44 | Delaware | 95 | 0.26% |
| 20 | Indiana | 597 | 1.61% | 45 | Montana | 86 | 0.23% |
| 21 | Wisconsin | 575 | 1.55% | 46 | Idaho | 85 | 0.23% |
| 22 | Washington | 563 | 1.52% | 47 | North Dakota | 80 | 0.22% |
| 23 | Alabama | 531 | 1.44% | 48 | South Dakota | 74 | 0.20% |
| 24 | Kentucky | 488 | 1.32% | 49 | Wyoming | 44 | 0.12% |
| 25 | Arizona | 476 | 1.29% | 50 | Alaska | 42 | 0.11% |
|  |  |  |  |  | District of Columbia | 283 | 0.76% |

Source: American Medical Association

"Physician Characteristics and Distribution in the U.S." 1992 edition (Copyright, reprinted with permission)

*As of January 1, 1990. Total includes 388 physicians in U.S. territories and possessions not shown separately. General Surgery includes Abdominal, Cardiovascular, Hand, Head and Neck, Pediatric, Traumatic and Vascular surgeries.

# Nonfederal Physicians in General Surgery per 100,000 Population in 1990

## National Rate = 14.88 General Surgeons per 100,000 Population*

| RANK | STATE | RATE | RANK | STATE | RATE |
|------|-------|------|------|-------|------|
| 1 | New York | 22.21 | 26 | Kentucky | 13.24 |
| 2 | Massachusetts | 21.92 | 26 | Nebraska | 13.24 |
| 3 | Rhode Island | 20.33 | 28 | Georgia | 13.15 |
| 4 | Maryland | 19.37 | 29 | Alabama | 13.14 |
| 5 | Connecticut | 18.89 | 30 | Arizona | 12.99 |
| 6 | Vermont | 18.66 | 31 | North Carolina | 12.82 |
| 7 | Pennsylvania | 16.79 | 32 | Colorado | 12.81 |
| 7 | Tennessee | 16.79 | 33 | North Dakota | 12.52 |
| 9 | New Jersey | 16.78 | 34 | Texas | 12.23 |
| 10 | West Virginia | 15.61 | 35 | South Carolina | 11.90 |
| 11 | Louisiana | 15.43 | 36 | Wisconsin | 11.75 |
| 12 | Ohio | 15.17 | 37 | Utah | 11.67 |
| 13 | Hawaii | 14.71 | 38 | Iowa | 11.60 |
| 13 | Illinois | 14.71 | 39 | Washington | 11.57 |
| 15 | Missouri | 14.56 | 40 | Arkansas | 11.02 |
| 16 | Michigan | 14.43 | 41 | New Mexico | 10.89 |
| 17 | New Hampshire | 14.42 | 42 | Mississippi | 10.80 |
| 18 | Delaware | 14.26 | 43 | Indiana | 10.77 |
| 19 | Oregon | 14.04 | 44 | Montana | 10.76 |
| 20 | Kansas | 13.88 | 45 | South Dakota | 10.63 |
| 21 | California | 13.79 | 46 | Nevada | 10.48 |
| 22 | Minnesota | 13.69 | 47 | Wyoming | 9.70 |
| 23 | Virginia | 13.45 | 48 | Oklahoma | 9.28 |
| 24 | Florida | 13.44 | 49 | Idaho | 8.44 |
| 25 | Maine | 13.27 | 50 | Alaska | 7.64 |

District of Columbia          46.63

Source: American Medical Association

*"Physician Characteristics and Distribution in the U.S." 1992 Edition (Copyright, reprinted with permission)*

*Calculated by the editors using 1990 Census resident population figures. As of January 1, 1990. National rate includes physicians in the U.S. territories and possessions not shown separately. General Surgery includes Abdominal, Cardiovascular, Hand, Head and Neck, Pediatric, Traumatic and Vascular surgeries.*

## Nonfederal Physicians in Obstetrics & Gynecology in 1990

## National Total = 32,956 Obstetricians and Gynecologists*

| RANK | STATE | OBGYNs | % | RANK | STATE | OBGYNs | % |
|---|---|---|---|---|---|---|---|
| 1 | California | 4,256 | 12.91% | 26 | South Carolina | 384 | 1.17% |
| 2 | New York | 3,265 | 9.91% | 27 | Kentucky | 363 | 1.10% |
| 3 | Texas | 2,019 | 6.13% | 28 | Oregon | 347 | 1.05% |
| 4 | Florida | 1,576 | 4.78% | 29 | Oklahoma | 292 | 0.89% |
| 5 | Pennsylvania | 1,551 | 4.71% | 30 | Mississippi | 253 | 0.77% |
| 6 | Illinois | 1,542 | 4.68% | 31 | Kansas | 230 | 0.70% |
| 7 | Ohio | 1,290 | 3.91% | 32 | Arkansas | 204 | 0.62% |
| 8 | New Jersey | 1,225 | 3.72% | 33 | Utah | 200 | 0.61% |
| 9 | Michigan | 1,149 | 3.49% | 34 | Hawaii | 192 | 0.58% |
| 10 | Maryland | 987 | 2.99% | 35 | Iowa | 185 | 0.56% |
| 11 | Massachusetts | 940 | 2.85% | 36 | West Virginia | 174 | 0.53% |
| 12 | Georgia | 862 | 2.62% | 37 | New Mexico | 165 | 0.50% |
| 13 | Virginia | 853 | 2.59% | 38 | Nebraska | 143 | 0.43% |
| 14 | North Carolina | 844 | 2.56% | 39 | Rhode Island | 142 | 0.43% |
| 15 | Missouri | 644 | 1.95% | 40 | New Hampshire | 127 | 0.39% |
| 16 | Louisiana | 633 | 1.92% | 41 | Nevada | 121 | 0.37% |
| 17 | Tennessee | 627 | 1.90% | 42 | Maine | 118 | 0.36% |
| 18 | Connecticut | 612 | 1.86% | 43 | Delaware | 88 | 0.27% |
| 19 | Washington | 513 | 1.56% | 44 | Vermont | 77 | 0.23% |
| 20 | Indiana | 466 | 1.41% | 45 | Idaho | 67 | 0.20% |
| 21 | Arizona | 463 | 1.40% | 46 | Montana | 66 | 0.20% |
| 22 | Wisconsin | 460 | 1.40% | 47 | North Dakota | 54 | 0.16% |
| 23 | Alabama | 439 | 1.33% | 48 | Alaska | 45 | 0.14% |
| 24 | Minnesota | 427 | 1.30% | 49 | South Dakota | 44 | 0.13% |
| 25 | Colorado | 423 | 1.28% | 50 | Wyoming | 38 | 0.12% |
| | | | | | District of Columbia | 257 | 0.78% |

*Source: American Medical Association*

*"Physician Characteristics and Distribution in the U.S." 1992 edition (Copyright, reprinted with permission)*

*As of January 1, 1990. Total includes 515 physicians in U.S. territories and possessions not shown separately. Obstetrics & Gynecology includes Gynecology and Oncology, Maternal and Fetal Medicine and Reproductive Endocrinology.*

# Nonfederal Physicians in Obstetrics & Gynecology per 100,000 Population in 1990

## National Rate = 13.25 Obstetricians and Gynecologists per 100,000 Population*

| RANK | STATE | RATE | | RANK | STATE | RATE |
|---|---|---|---|---|---|---|
| 1 | Maryland | 20.64 | | 26 | Utah | 11.61 |
| 2 | Connecticut | 18.62 | | 27 | New Hampshire | 11.45 |
| 3 | New York | 18.15 | | 28 | South Carolina | 11.01 |
| 4 | Hawaii | 17.32 | | 29 | New Mexico | 10.89 |
| 5 | New Jersey | 15.85 | | 30 | Alabama | 10.86 |
| 6 | Massachusetts | 15.62 | | 31 | Washington | 10.54 |
| 7 | Louisiana | 15.00 | | 32 | Nevada | 10.07 |
| 8 | California | 14.30 | | 33 | Kentucky | 9.85 |
| 9 | Rhode Island | 14.15 | | 34 | Mississippi | 9.83 |
| 10 | Virginia | 13.79 | | 35 | Minnesota | 9.76 |
| 11 | Vermont | 13.68 | | 36 | West Virginia | 9.70 |
| 12 | Illinois | 13.49 | | 37 | Maine | 9.61 |
| 13 | Georgia | 13.31 | | 38 | Wisconsin | 9.40 |
| 14 | Delaware | 13.21 | | 39 | Kansas | 9.28 |
| 15 | Pennsylvania | 13.05 | | 39 | Oklahoma | 9.28 |
| 16 | Tennessee | 12.86 | | 41 | Nebraska | 9.06 |
| 17 | Colorado | 12.84 | | 42 | Arkansas | 8.68 |
| 18 | North Carolina | 12.73 | | 43 | North Dakota | 8.45 |
| 19 | Arizona | 12.63 | | 44 | Indiana | 8.41 |
| 20 | Missouri | 12.59 | | 45 | Wyoming | 8.38 |
| 21 | Michigan | 12.36 | | 46 | Montana | 8.26 |
| 22 | Oregon | 12.21 | | 47 | Alaska | 8.18 |
| 23 | Florida | 12.18 | | 48 | Idaho | 6.66 |
| 24 | Ohio | 11.89 | | 48 | Iowa | 6.66 |
| 24 | Texas | 11.89 | | 50 | South Dakota | 6.32 |

District of Columbia     42.35

*Source: American Medical Association*

*"Physician Characteristics and Distribution in the U.S." 1992 Edition (Copyright, reprinted with permission)*

*\*Calculated by the editors using 1990 Census resident population figures. As of January 1, 1990. National rate includes physicians in the U.S. territories and possessions not shown separately. Obstetrics & Gynecology includes Gynecology and Oncology, Maternal and Fetal Medicine and Reproductive Endocrinology.*

# Nonfederal Physicians in Ophthalmology in 1990

## National Total = 15,716 Ophthalmologists*

| RANK | STATE | PHYSICIANS | % | | RANK | STATE | PHYSICIANS | % |
|------|-------|-----------|-----|---|------|-------|-----------|-----|
| 1 | California | 1,993 | 12.68% | | 26 | Alabama | 175 | 1.11% |
| 2 | New York | 1,655 | 10.53% | | 27 | Kentucky | 169 | 1.08% |
| 3 | Florida | 941 | 5.99% | | 28 | South Carolina | 165 | 1.05% |
| 4 | Texas | 889 | 5.66% | | 29 | Iowa | 153 | 0.97% |
| 5 | Pennsylvania | 831 | 5.29% | | 30 | Oklahoma | 141 | 0.90% |
| 6 | Illinois | 659 | 4.19% | | 31 | Kansas | 125 | 0.80% |
| 7 | Ohio | 574 | 3.65% | | 32 | Arkansas | 121 | 0.77% |
| 8 | New Jersey | 547 | 3.48% | | 32 | Mississippi | 121 | 0.77% |
| 9 | Massachusetts | 507 | 3.23% | | 34 | Utah | 100 | 0.64% |
| 10 | Michigan | 488 | 3.11% | | 35 | West Virginia | 86 | 0.55% |
| 11 | Maryland | 426 | 2.71% | | 36 | Nebraska | 78 | 0.50% |
| 12 | North Carolina | 347 | 2.21% | | 37 | Hawaii | 72 | 0.46% |
| 12 | Virginia | 347 | 2.21% | | 38 | New Mexico | 70 | 0.45% |
| 14 | Louisiana | 330 | 2.10% | | 39 | New Hampshire | 59 | 0.38% |
| 15 | Georgia | 316 | 2.01% | | 40 | Maine | 58 | 0.37% |
| 16 | Missouri | 300 | 1.91% | | 41 | Rhode Island | 56 | 0.36% |
| 17 | Wisconsin | 295 | 1.88% | | 42 | Idaho | 49 | 0.31% |
| 18 | Connecticut | 284 | 1.81% | | 43 | Nevada | 44 | 0.28% |
| 19 | Minnesota | 276 | 1.76% | | 44 | Montana | 42 | 0.27% |
| 20 | Washington | 272 | 1.73% | | 45 | Delaware | 34 | 0.22% |
| 21 | Tennessee | 262 | 1.67% | | 46 | Vermont | 32 | 0.20% |
| 22 | Indiana | 244 | 1.55% | | 47 | North Dakota | 30 | 0.19% |
| 23 | Arizona | 225 | 1.43% | | 48 | South Dakota | 28 | 0.18% |
| 24 | Colorado | 216 | 1.37% | | 49 | Alaska | 21 | 0.13% |
| 25 | Oregon | 198 | 1.26% | | 50 | Wyoming | 19 | 0.12% |
| | | | | | | District of Columbia | 91 | 0.58% |

Source: American Medical Association

*"Physician Characteristics and Distribution in the U.S." 1992 edition (Copyright, reprinted with permission)*

*As of January 1, 1990. Total includes 18 physicians in U.S. territories and possessions not shown separately.*

# Nonfederal Physicians in Ophthalmology per 100,000 Population in 1990

## National Rate = 6.32 Ophthalmologists per 100,000 Population*

| RANK | STATE | RATE | RANK | STATE | RATE |
|---|---|---|---|---|---|
| 1 | New York | 9.20 | 26 | Ohio | 5.29 |
| 2 | Maryland | 8.91 | 27 | Montana | 5.26 |
| 3 | Connecticut | 8.64 | 28 | Michigan | 5.25 |
| 4 | Massachusetts | 8.43 | 29 | North Carolina | 5.23 |
| 5 | Louisiana | 7.82 | 29 | Texas | 5.23 |
| 6 | Florida | 7.27 | 31 | Arkansas | 5.15 |
| 7 | New Jersey | 7.08 | 32 | Delaware | 5.10 |
| 8 | Pennsylvania | 6.99 | 33 | Kansas | 5.05 |
| 9 | Oregon | 6.97 | 34 | Nebraska | 4.94 |
| 10 | California | 6.70 | 35 | Georgia | 4.88 |
| 11 | Colorado | 6.56 | 36 | Idaho | 4.87 |
| 12 | Hawaii | 6.50 | 37 | West Virginia | 4.80 |
| 13 | Minnesota | 6.31 | 38 | South Carolina | 4.73 |
| 14 | Arizona | 6.14 | 39 | Maine | 4.72 |
| 15 | Wisconsin | 6.03 | 40 | Mississippi | 4.70 |
| 16 | Missouri | 5.86 | 40 | North Dakota | 4.70 |
| 17 | Utah | 5.80 | 42 | New Mexico | 4.62 |
| 18 | Illinois | 5.77 | 43 | Kentucky | 4.59 |
| 19 | Vermont | 5.69 | 44 | Oklahoma | 4.48 |
| 20 | Virginia | 5.61 | 45 | Indiana | 4.40 |
| 21 | Washington | 5.59 | 46 | Alabama | 4.33 |
| 22 | Rhode Island | 5.58 | 47 | Wyoming | 4.19 |
| 23 | Iowa | 5.51 | 48 | South Dakota | 4.02 |
| 24 | Tennessee | 5.37 | 49 | Alaska | 3.82 |
| 25 | New Hampshire | 5.32 | 50 | Nevada | 3.66 |

District of Columbia        14.99

Source: American Medical Association

"Physician Characteristics and Distribution in the U.S." 1992 edition (Copyright, reprinted with permission)

*Calculated by the editors using 1990 Census resident population figures. As of January 1, 1990. National rate includes physicians in U.S. territories and possessions not shown separately.

# Nonfederal Physicians in Plastic Surgery in 1990

## National Total = 4,512 Plastic Surgeons*

| RANK | STATE | SURGEONS | % | RANK | STATE | SURGEONS | % |
|------|-------|----------|-----|------|-------|----------|-----|
| 1 | California | 724 | 16.05% | 26 | Alabama | 46 | 1.02% |
| 2 | New York | 459 | 10.17% | 27 | Utah | 44 | 0.98% |
| 3 | Florida | 325 | 7.20% | 28 | Oregon | 40 | 0.89% |
| 4 | Texas | 297 | 6.58% | 29 | South Carolina | 36 | 0.80% |
| 5 | Pennsylvania | 189 | 4.19% | 30 | Oklahoma | 33 | 0.73% |
| 6 | Illinois | 175 | 3.88% | 31 | Kansas | 31 | 0.69% |
| 7 | Ohio | 172 | 3.81% | 32 | Hawaii | 23 | 0.51% |
| 8 | New Jersey | 160 | 3.55% | 32 | Nevada | 23 | 0.51% |
| 9 | Michigan | 142 | 3.15% | 34 | New Mexico | 21 | 0.47% |
| 10 | Massachusetts | 133 | 2.95% | 35 | Arkansas | 19 | 0.42% |
| 11 | Virginia | 116 | 2.57% | 35 | Mississippi | 19 | 0.42% |
| 12 | Maryland | 114 | 2.53% | 35 | West Virginia | 19 | 0.42% |
| 13 | Georgia | 100 | 2.22% | 38 | Iowa | 18 | 0.40% |
| 14 | Missouri | 99 | 2.19% | 39 | New Hampshire | 17 | 0.38% |
| 15 | North Carolina | 98 | 2.17% | 39 | Rhode Island | 17 | 0.38% |
| 16 | Tennessee | 97 | 2.15% | 41 | Nebraska | 15 | 0.33% |
| 17 | Arizona | 86 | 1.91% | 42 | Idaho | 13 | 0.29% |
| 18 | Washington | 80 | 1.77% | 43 | Delaware | 10 | 0.22% |
| 19 | Louisiana | 69 | 1.53% | 43 | Maine | 10 | 0.22% |
| 20 | Colorado | 64 | 1.42% | 45 | Montana | 7 | 0.16% |
| 21 | Wisconsin | 62 | 1.37% | 46 | Alaska | 6 | 0.13% |
| 22 | Connecticut | 57 | 1.26% | 46 | North Dakota | 6 | 0.13% |
| 23 | Indiana | 56 | 1.24% | 48 | South Dakota | 5 | 0.11% |
| 24 | Kentucky | 52 | 1.15% | 48 | Vermont | 5 | 0.11% |
| 25 | Minnesota | 50 | 1.11% | 50 | Wyoming | 3 | 0.07% |
| | | | | | District of Columbia | 26 | 0.58% |

Source: American Medical Association

*Source: American Medical Association*

*"Physician Characteristics and Distribution in the U.S." 1992 edition (Copyright, reprinted with permission)*

*As of January 1, 1990. Total includes 24 physicians in U.S. territories and possessions not shown separately.*

# Nonfederal Physicians in Plastic Surgery per 100,000 Population in 1990

## National Rate = 1.81 Plastic Surgeons per 100,000 Population*

| RANK | STATE | RATE | | RANK | STATE | RATE |
|------|-------|------|---|------|-------|------|
| 1 | New York | 2.55 | | 26 | Delaware | 1.50 |
| 1 | Utah | 2.55 | | 27 | North Carolina | 1.48 |
| 3 | Florida | 2.51 | | 28 | Kentucky | 1.41 |
| 4 | California | 2.43 | | 28 | Oregon | 1.41 |
| 5 | Maryland | 2.38 | | 30 | New Mexico | 1.39 |
| 6 | Arizona | 2.35 | | 31 | Idaho | 1.29 |
| 7 | Massachusetts | 2.21 | | 32 | Wisconsin | 1.27 |
| 8 | Hawaii | 2.08 | | 33 | Kansas | 1.25 |
| 9 | New Jersey | 2.07 | | 34 | Alabama | 1.14 |
| 10 | Tennessee | 1.99 | | 34 | Minnesota | 1.14 |
| 11 | Colorado | 1.94 | | 36 | Alaska | 1.09 |
| 12 | Missouri | 1.93 | | 37 | West Virginia | 1.06 |
| 13 | Nevada | 1.91 | | 38 | Oklahoma | 1.05 |
| 14 | Virginia | 1.87 | | 39 | South Carolina | 1.03 |
| 15 | Texas | 1.75 | | 40 | Indiana | 1.01 |
| 16 | Connecticut | 1.73 | | 41 | Nebraska | 0.95 |
| 17 | Rhode Island | 1.69 | | 42 | North Dakota | 0.94 |
| 18 | Louisiana | 1.64 | | 43 | Vermont | 0.89 |
| 18 | Washington | 1.64 | | 44 | Montana | 0.88 |
| 20 | Ohio | 1.59 | | 45 | Arkansas | 0.81 |
| 20 | Pennsylvania | 1.59 | | 45 | Maine | 0.81 |
| 22 | Georgia | 1.54 | | 47 | Mississippi | 0.74 |
| 23 | Illinois | 1.53 | | 48 | South Dakota | 0.72 |
| 23 | Michigan | 1.53 | | 49 | Wyoming | 0.66 |
| 23 | New Hampshire | 1.53 | | 50 | Iowa | 0.65 |

District of Columbia     4.28

Source: American Medical Association

"Physician Characteristics and Distribution in the U.S." 1992 edition (Copyright, reprinted with permission)

*Calculated by the editors using 1990 Census resident population figures. As of January 1, 1990. National rate includes physicians in U.S. territories and possessions not shown separately.

# Nonfederal Physicians in Other Specialties in 1990

## National Total = 152,052 Physicians*

| RANK | STATE | PHYSICIANS | % | RANK | STATE | PHYSICIANS | % |
|---|---|---|---|---|---|---|---|
| 1 | California | 20,340 | 13.38% | 26 | Oregon | 1,633 | 1.07% |
| 2 | New York | 16,497 | 10.85% | 27 | Alabama | 1,551 | 1.02% |
| 3 | Pennsylvania | 8,395 | 5.52% | 28 | South Carolina | 1,461 | 0.96% |
| 4 | Texas | 8,207 | 5.40% | 29 | Kansas | 1,272 | 0.84% |
| 5 | Florida | 6,932 | 4.56% | 30 | Oklahoma | 1,261 | 0.83% |
| 6 | Illinois | 6,888 | 4.53% | 31 | Iowa | 1,100 | 0.72% |
| 7 | Massachusetts | 6,255 | 4.11% | 32 | Utah | 949 | 0.62% |
| 8 | Ohio | 5,993 | 3.94% | 33 | Arkansas | 854 | 0.56% |
| 9 | New Jersey | 5,029 | 3.31% | 34 | New Mexico | 817 | 0.54% |
| 10 | Michigan | 5,015 | 3.30% | 35 | Mississippi | 814 | 0.54% |
| 11 | Maryland | 4,796 | 3.15% | 36 | West Virginia | 798 | 0.52% |
| 12 | Virginia | 3,598 | 2.37% | 37 | Hawaii | 721 | 0.47% |
| 13 | North Carolina | 3,289 | 2.16% | 38 | Nebraska | 655 | 0.43% |
| 14 | Georgia | 3,169 | 2.08% | 39 | New Hampshire | 634 | 0.42% |
| 15 | Connecticut | 3,057 | 2.01% | 40 | Rhode Island | 618 | 0.41% |
| 16 | Washington | 2,867 | 1.89% | 41 | Maine | 566 | 0.37% |
| 17 | Missouri | 2,763 | 1.82% | 42 | Nevada | 493 | 0.32% |
| 18 | Wisconsin | 2,578 | 1.70% | 43 | Delaware | 414 | 0.27% |
| 19 | Tennessee | 2,509 | 1.65% | 44 | Vermont | 412 | 0.27% |
| 20 | Minnesota | 2,426 | 1.60% | 45 | Montana | 324 | 0.21% |
| 21 | Indiana | 2,410 | 1.58% | 46 | Idaho | 290 | 0.19% |
| 22 | Louisiana | 2,108 | 1.39% | 47 | North Dakota | 280 | 0.18% |
| 23 | Colorado | 2,013 | 1.32% | 48 | South Dakota | 226 | 0.15% |
| 24 | Arizona | 1,996 | 1.31% | 49 | Alaska | 190 | 0.12% |
| 25 | Kentucky | 1,669 | 1.10% | 50 | Wyoming | 155 | 0.10% |
|  |  |  |  |  | District of Columbia | 1,159 | 0.76% |

Source: American Medical Association

*"Physician Characteristics and Distribution in the U.S." 1992 edition (Copyright, reprinted with permission)*

*As of January 1, 1990. Total includes 412 physicians in U.S. territories and possessions not shown separately. Other Specialties include Aerospace Medicine, Anesthesiology, Child Psychiatry, Diagnostic Radiology, Emergency Medicine, Forensic Pathology, Nuclear Medicine, Occupational Medicine, Neurology, Psychiatry, Public Health, Anatomic/Clinical Pathology, Radiology, Radiation Oncology and other specialties.*

# Nonfederal Physicians in Other Specialties per 100,000 Population in 1990

## National Rate = 61.14 Physicians in Other Specialties per 100,000 Population*

| RANK | STATE | RATE | RANK | STATE | RATE |
|---|---|---|---|---|---|
| 1 | Massachusetts | 103.97 | 26 | Wisconsin | 52.70 |
| 2 | Maryland | 100.30 | 27 | Tennessee | 51.44 |
| 3 | Connecticut | 93.00 | 28 | Kansas | 51.34 |
| 4 | New York | 91.70 | 29 | Louisiana | 49.95 |
| 5 | Vermont | 73.21 | 30 | North Carolina | 49.62 |
| 6 | Pennsylvania | 70.66 | 31 | Georgia | 48.92 |
| 7 | California | 68.35 | 32 | Texas | 48.31 |
| 8 | Hawaii | 65.06 | 33 | Maine | 46.09 |
| 8 | New Jersey | 65.06 | 34 | Kentucky | 45.29 |
| 10 | Delaware | 62.15 | 35 | West Virginia | 44.49 |
| 11 | Rhode Island | 61.59 | 36 | North Dakota | 43.83 |
| 12 | Colorado | 61.10 | 37 | Indiana | 43.47 |
| 13 | Illinois | 60.26 | 38 | South Carolina | 41.90 |
| 14 | Washington | 58.91 | 39 | Nebraska | 41.50 |
| 15 | Virginia | 58.15 | 40 | Nevada | 41.02 |
| 16 | Oregon | 57.45 | 41 | Montana | 40.55 |
| 17 | New Hampshire | 57.16 | 42 | Oklahoma | 40.09 |
| 18 | Minnesota | 55.45 | 43 | Iowa | 39.61 |
| 19 | Ohio | 55.25 | 44 | Alabama | 38.39 |
| 20 | Utah | 55.08 | 45 | Arkansas | 36.33 |
| 21 | Arizona | 54.46 | 46 | Alaska | 34.54 |
| 22 | Missouri | 54.00 | 47 | Wyoming | 34.17 |
| 23 | Michigan | 53.95 | 48 | South Dakota | 32.47 |
| 24 | New Mexico | 53.92 | 49 | Mississippi | 31.63 |
| 25 | Florida | 53.58 | 50 | Idaho | 28.81 |

District of Columbia     190.97

Source: American Medical Association

"Physician Characteristics and Distribution in the U.S." 1992 edition (Copyright, reprinted with permission)

*Calculated by the editors using 1990 Census resident population figures. As of January 1, 1990. National rate includes physicians in U.S. territories and possessions not shown separately. Other Specialties include Anesthesiology, Diagnostic Radiology, Emergency Medicine, Neurology, Psychiatry, Anatomic/Clinical Pathology , Radiology and other specialties.

# Nonfederal Physicians in Anesthesiology in 1990

## National Total = 25,297 Anesthesiologists*

| RANK | STATE | PHYSICIANS | % |
|------|-------|-----------|---|
| 1 | California | 3,469 | 13.71% |
| 2 | New York | 2,352 | 9.30% |
| 3 | Texas | 1,705 | 6.74% |
| 4 | Florida | 1,339 | 5.29% |
| 5 | Pennsylvania | 1,240 | 4.90% |
| 6 | Illinois | 1,207 | 4.77% |
| 7 | Ohio | 1,061 | 4.19% |
| 8 | Massachusetts | 914 | 3.61% |
| 9 | New Jersey | 912 | 3.61% |
| 10 | Maryland | 663 | 2.62% |
| 11 | Michigan | 627 | 2.48% |
| 12 | Georgia | 588 | 2.32% |
| 13 | Washington | 586 | 2.32% |
| 14 | Virginia | 566 | 2.24% |
| 15 | Indiana | 508 | 2.01% |
| 16 | Wisconsin | 490 | 1.94% |
| 17 | North Carolina | 466 | 1.84% |
| 18 | Tennessee | 451 | 1.78% |
| 19 | Connecticut | 450 | 1.78% |
| 20 | Missouri | 435 | 1.72% |
| 21 | Arizona | 428 | 1.69% |
| 22 | Minnesota | 388 | 1.53% |
| 23 | Louisiana | 362 | 1.43% |
| 24 | Kentucky | 317 | 1.25% |
| 25 | Colorado | 316 | 1.25% |

| RANK | STATE | PHYSICIANS | % |
|------|-------|-----------|---|
| 26 | Oregon | 314 | 1.24% |
| 27 | Alabama | 292 | 1.15% |
| 28 | South Carolina | 244 | 0.96% |
| 29 | Utah | 233 | 0.92% |
| 30 | Iowa | 230 | 0.91% |
| 31 | Oklahoma | 223 | 0.88% |
| 32 | Kansas | 213 | 0.84% |
| 33 | Arkansas | 148 | 0.59% |
| 34 | Mississippi | 143 | 0.57% |
| 35 | New Mexico | 132 | 0.52% |
| 36 | Nebraska | 113 | 0.45% |
| 37 | Nevada | 106 | 0.42% |
| 37 | West Virginia | 106 | 0.42% |
| 39 | Hawaii | 96 | 0.38% |
| 39 | Maine | 96 | 0.38% |
| 41 | New Hampshire | 92 | 0.36% |
| 42 | Montana | 76 | 0.30% |
| 43 | Rhode Island | 70 | 0.28% |
| 44 | Vermont | 58 | 0.23% |
| 45 | Delaware | 44 | 0.17% |
| 46 | Idaho | 42 | 0.17% |
| 47 | North Dakota | 37 | 0.15% |
| 48 | Wyoming | 32 | 0.13% |
| 49 | Alaska | 26 | 0.10% |
| 50 | South Dakota | 23 | 0.09% |
| | District of Columbia | 94 | 0.37% |

Source: American Medical Association

*"Physician Characteristics and Distribution in the U.S." 1992 edition (Copyright, reprinted with permission)*

*As of January 1, 1990. Total includes 31 physicians in U.S. territories and possessions not shown separately.*

# Nonfederal Physicians in Anesthesiology per 100,000 Population in 1990

## National Rate = 10.17 Anesthesiologists per 100,000 Population*

| RANK | STATE | RATE | RANK | STATE | RATE |
|------|-------|------|------|-------|------|
| 1 | Massachusetts | 15.19 | 26 | New Mexico | 8.71 |
| 2 | Maryland | 13.87 | 27 | Hawaii | 8.66 |
| 3 | Connecticut | 13.69 | 28 | Kansas | 8.60 |
| 4 | Utah | 13.52 | 28 | Kentucky | 8.60 |
| 5 | New York | 13.07 | 30 | Louisiana | 8.58 |
| 6 | Washington | 12.04 | 31 | Missouri | 8.50 |
| 7 | New Jersey | 11.80 | 32 | New Hampshire | 8.29 |
| 8 | Arizona | 11.68 | 33 | Iowa | 8.28 |
| 9 | California | 11.66 | 34 | Maine | 7.82 |
| 10 | Oregon | 11.05 | 35 | Alabama | 7.23 |
| 11 | Illinois | 10.56 | 36 | Nebraska | 7.16 |
| 12 | Pennsylvania | 10.44 | 37 | Oklahoma | 7.09 |
| 13 | Florida | 10.35 | 38 | Wyoming | 7.05 |
| 14 | Vermont | 10.31 | 39 | North Carolina | 7.03 |
| 15 | Texas | 10.04 | 40 | South Carolina | 7.00 |
| 16 | Wisconsin | 10.02 | 41 | Rhode Island | 6.98 |
| 17 | Ohio | 9.78 | 42 | Michigan | 6.75 |
| 18 | Colorado | 9.59 | 43 | Delaware | 6.60 |
| 19 | Montana | 9.51 | 44 | Arkansas | 6.30 |
| 20 | Tennessee | 9.25 | 45 | West Virginia | 5.91 |
| 21 | Indiana | 9.16 | 46 | North Dakota | 5.79 |
| 22 | Virginia | 9.15 | 47 | Mississippi | 5.56 |
| 23 | Georgia | 9.08 | 48 | Alaska | 4.73 |
| 24 | Minnesota | 8.87 | 49 | Idaho | 4.17 |
| 25 | Nevada | 8.82 | 50 | South Dakota | 3.30 |

District of Columbia    15.49

Source: American Medical Association

"Physician Characteristics and Distribution in the U.S." 1992 edition (Copyright, reprinted with permission)

*Calculated by the editors using 1990 Census resident population figures. As of January 1, 1990. National rate includes physicians in U.S. territories and possessions not shown separately.

# Nonfederal Physicians in Psychiatry in 1990

## National Total = 33,347 Psychiatrists*

| RANK | STATE | PSYCHIATRISTS | % |
|------|-------|---------------|-----|
| 1 | New York | 5,329 | 15.98% |
| 2 | California | 4,683 | 14.04% |
| 3 | Massachusetts | 1,781 | 5.34% |
| 4 | Pennsylvania | 1,753 | 5.26% |
| 5 | Texas | 1,515 | 4.54% |
| 6 | Illinois | 1,314 | 3.94% |
| 7 | Florida | 1,171 | 3.51% |
| 8 | Maryland | 1,156 | 3.47% |
| 9 | New Jersey | 1,154 | 3.46% |
| 10 | Ohio | 1,040 | 3.12% |
| 11 | Michigan | 1,028 | 3.08% |
| 12 | Connecticut | 941 | 2.82% |
| 13 | Virginia | 780 | 2.34% |
| 14 | North Carolina | 719 | 2.16% |
| 15 | Georgia | 620 | 1.86% |
| 16 | Washington | 521 | 1.56% |
| 17 | Colorado | 509 | 1.53% |
| 18 | Missouri | 502 | 1.51% |
| 19 | Wisconsin | 462 | 1.39% |
| 20 | Louisiana | 394 | 1.18% |
| 21 | Tennessee | 385 | 1.15% |
| 22 | Minnesota | 382 | 1.15% |
| 23 | Arizona | 361 | 1.08% |
| 24 | Indiana | 344 | 1.03% |
| 25 | South Carolina | 328 | 0.98% |

| RANK | STATE | PSYCHIATRISTS | % |
|------|-------|---------------|-----|
| 26 | Oregon | 321 | 0.96% |
| 27 | Kansas | 309 | 0.93% |
| 28 | Kentucky | 291 | 0.87% |
| 29 | Oklahoma | 250 | 0.75% |
| 30 | Alabama | 222 | 0.67% |
| 31 | New Mexico | 193 | 0.58% |
| 32 | Iowa | 178 | 0.53% |
| 33 | New Hampshire | 169 | 0.51% |
| 34 | Hawaii | 163 | 0.49% |
| 35 | Rhode Island | 147 | 0.44% |
| 36 | Utah | 146 | 0.44% |
| 37 | Arkansas | 142 | 0.43% |
| 38 | Maine | 134 | 0.40% |
| 39 | West Virginia | 131 | 0.39% |
| 40 | Vermont | 115 | 0.34% |
| 41 | Mississippi | 112 | 0.34% |
| 41 | Nebraska | 112 | 0.34% |
| 43 | Delaware | 83 | 0.25% |
| 44 | Nevada | 65 | 0.19% |
| 45 | North Dakota | 51 | 0.15% |
| 46 | Idaho | 48 | 0.14% |
| 47 | Alaska | 43 | 0.13% |
| 47 | Montana | 43 | 0.13% |
| 49 | South Dakota | 35 | 0.10% |
| 50 | Wyoming | 19 | 0.06% |
| | District of Columbia | 379 | 1.14% |

Source: American Medical Association

*"Physician Characteristics and Distribution in the U.S." 1992 edition (Copyright, reprinted with permission)

*As of January 1, 1990. Total includes 274 physicians in U.S. territories and possessions not shown separately. Psychiatry includes psychoanalysis.

414

# Nonfederal Physicians in Psychiatry per 100,000 Population in 1990

## National Rate = 13.41 Psychiatrists per 100,000 Population*

| RANK | STATE | RATE | RANK | STATE | RATE |
|------|-------|------|------|-------|------|
| 1 | New York | 29.62 | 26 | Georgia | 9.57 |
| 2 | Massachusetts | 29.60 | 27 | Wisconsin | 9.44 |
| 3 | Connecticut | 28.63 | 28 | South Carolina | 9.41 |
| 4 | Maryland | 24.18 | 29 | Louisiana | 9.34 |
| 5 | Vermont | 20.44 | 30 | Florida | 9.05 |
| 6 | California | 15.74 | 31 | Texas | 8.92 |
| 7 | Colorado | 15.45 | 32 | Minnesota | 8.73 |
| 8 | New Hampshire | 15.24 | 33 | Utah | 8.47 |
| 9 | New Jersey | 14.93 | 34 | North Dakota | 7.98 |
| 10 | Pennsylvania | 14.75 | 35 | Oklahoma | 7.95 |
| 11 | Hawaii | 14.71 | 36 | Kentucky | 7.90 |
| 12 | Rhode Island | 14.65 | 37 | Tennessee | 7.89 |
| 13 | New Mexico | 12.74 | 38 | Alaska | 7.82 |
| 14 | Virginia | 12.61 | 39 | West Virginia | 7.30 |
| 15 | Kansas | 12.47 | 40 | Nebraska | 7.10 |
| 16 | Delaware | 12.46 | 41 | Iowa | 6.41 |
| 17 | Illinois | 11.50 | 42 | Indiana | 6.20 |
| 18 | Oregon | 11.29 | 43 | Arkansas | 6.04 |
| 19 | Michigan | 11.06 | 44 | Alabama | 5.49 |
| 20 | Maine | 10.91 | 45 | Nevada | 5.41 |
| 21 | North Carolina | 10.85 | 46 | Montana | 5.38 |
| 22 | Washington | 10.71 | 47 | South Dakota | 5.03 |
| 23 | Arizona | 9.85 | 48 | Idaho | 4.77 |
| 24 | Missouri | 9.81 | 49 | Mississippi | 4.35 |
| 25 | Ohio | 9.59 | 50 | Wyoming | 4.19 |
|  |  |  |  | District of Columbia | 62.45 |

Source: American Medical Association
    "Physician Characteristics and Distribution in the U.S." 1992 edition (Copyright, reprinted with permission)
*Calculated by the editors using 1990 Census resident population figures. As of January 1, 1990. National rate includes physicians in U.S. territories and possessions not shown separately. Psychiatry includes Psychoanalysis.

# Nonfederal International Medical School Graduates Practicing in 1990

## National Total = 126,760 Physicians*

| RANK | STATE | PHYSICIANS | % | RANK | STATE | PHYSICIANS | % |
|---|---|---|---|---|---|---|---|
| 1 | New York | 22,788 | 17.98% | 26 | Kansas | 710 | 0.56% |
| 2 | California | 14,038 | 11.07% | 26 | Rhode Island | 710 | 0.56% |
| 3 | Florida | 9,849 | 7.77% | 28 | Oklahoma | 632 | 0.50% |
| 4 | New Jersey | 8,740 | 6.89% | 29 | Iowa | 631 | 0.50% |
| 5 | Illinois | 8,653 | 6.83% | 30 | Alabama | 623 | 0.49% |
| 6 | Pennsylvania | 5,960 | 4.70% | 31 | Colorado | 433 | 0.34% |
| 7 | Texas | 5,875 | 4.63% | 32 | Hawaii | 430 | 0.34% |
| 8 | Ohio | 5,750 | 4.54% | 33 | South Carolina | 398 | 0.31% |
| 9 | Michigan | 4,994 | 3.94% | 34 | Oregon | 394 | 0.31% |
| 10 | Maryland | 4,491 | 3.54% | 35 | Delaware | 389 | 0.31% |
| 11 | Massachusetts | 3,512 | 2.77% | 36 | New Mexico | 360 | 0.28% |
| 12 | Virginia | 2,485 | 1.96% | 37 | New Hampshire | 338 | 0.27% |
| 13 | Connecticut | 2,344 | 1.85% | 38 | Maine | 264 | 0.21% |
| 14 | Missouri | 1,947 | 1.54% | 39 | Nevada | 263 | 0.21% |
| 15 | Georgia | 1,732 | 1.37% | 40 | Mississippi | 237 | 0.19% |
| 16 | Indiana | 1,461 | 1.15% | 41 | Nebraska | 219 | 0.17% |
| 17 | Wisconsin | 1,432 | 1.13% | 42 | North Dakota | 205 | 0.16% |
| 18 | Arizona | 1,105 | 0.87% | 43 | Arkansas | 199 | 0.16% |
| 19 | Tennessee | 1,099 | 0.87% | 44 | Utah | 167 | 0.13% |
| 20 | West Virginia | 1,089 | 0.86% | 45 | Vermont | 105 | 0.08% |
| 21 | North Carolina | 1,073 | 0.85% | 46 | South Dakota | 96 | 0.08% |
| 22 | Louisiana | 988 | 0.78% | 47 | Montana | 63 | 0.05% |
| 23 | Washington | 964 | 0.76% | 48 | Alaska | 52 | 0.04% |
| 24 | Minnesota | 942 | 0.74% | 49 | Idaho | 42 | 0.03% |
| 25 | Kentucky | 904 | 0.71% | 50 | Wyoming | 39 | 0.03% |
| | | | | | District of Columbia | 616 | 0.49% |
| | | | | | Puerto Rico | 3,820 | 3.01% |

Source: American Medical Association

"Physician Characteristics and Distribution in the U.S." 1992 edition (Copyright, reprinted with permission)

*As of January 1, 1990.

# Nonfederal International Medical School Graduates per 100,000 Population Practicing in 1990

## National Rate = 50.97 Physicians per 100,000 Population*

| RANK | STATE | RATE | | RANK | STATE | RATE |
|------|-------|------|---|------|-------|------|
| 1 | New York | 126.67 | | 26 | Kentucky | 24.53 |
| 2 | New Jersey | 113.06 | | 27 | New Mexico | 23.76 |
| 3 | Maryland | 93.93 | | 28 | Louisiana | 23.41 |
| 4 | Florida | 76.13 | | 29 | Iowa | 22.72 |
| 5 | Illinois | 75.70 | | 30 | Tennessee | 22.53 |
| 6 | Connecticut | 71.31 | | 31 | Nevada | 21.88 |
| 7 | Rhode Island | 70.75 | | 32 | Minnesota | 21.53 |
| 8 | West Virginia | 60.72 | | 33 | Maine | 21.50 |
| 9 | Delaware | 58.39 | | 34 | Oklahoma | 20.09 |
| 10 | Massachusetts | 58.37 | | 35 | Washington | 19.81 |
| 11 | Michigan | 53.73 | | 36 | Vermont | 18.66 |
| 12 | Ohio | 53.01 | | 37 | North Carolina | 16.19 |
| 13 | Pennsylvania | 50.16 | | 38 | Alabama | 15.42 |
| 14 | California | 47.17 | | 39 | Nebraska | 13.87 |
| 15 | Virginia | 40.16 | | 40 | Oregon | 13.86 |
| 16 | Hawaii | 38.80 | | 41 | South Dakota | 13.79 |
| 17 | Missouri | 38.05 | | 42 | Colorado | 13.14 |
| 18 | Texas | 34.59 | | 43 | South Carolina | 11.41 |
| 19 | North Dakota | 32.09 | | 44 | Utah | 9.69 |
| 20 | New Hampshire | 30.47 | | 45 | Alaska | 9.45 |
| 21 | Arizona | 30.15 | | 46 | Mississippi | 9.21 |
| 22 | Wisconsin | 29.27 | | 47 | Wyoming | 8.60 |
| 23 | Kansas | 28.66 | | 48 | Arkansas | 8.47 |
| 24 | Georgia | 26.74 | | 49 | Montana | 7.88 |
| 25 | Indiana | 26.35 | | 50 | Idaho | 4.17 |
| | | | | | District of Columbia | 101.50 |
| | | | | | Puerto Rico | 108.46 |

Source: American Medical Association

"Physician Characteristics and Distribution in the U.S." 1992 edition (Copyright, reprinted with permission)

*Calculated by the editors using 1990 Census resident population figures. As of January 1, 1990.

## International Medical School Graduates as a Percent of All Nonfederal Physicians in 1990

### National Rate = 21.4% of Nonfederal Physicians are International Medical School Graduates*

| RANK | STATE | PERCENT | RANK | STATE | PERCENT |
|---|---|---|---|---|---|
| 1 | New Jersey | 42.5 | 25 | New Hampshire | 13.5 |
| 2 | New York | 37.5 | 27 | Arizona | 13.4 |
| 3 | Illinois | 32.5 | 28 | Iowa | 13.3 |
| 4 | West Virginia | 32.1 | 29 | Oklahoma | 12.4 |
| 5 | Florida | 31.3 | 30 | New Mexico | 11.6 |
| 6 | Maryland | 26.9 | 31 | Louisiana | 11.4 |
| 7 | Delaware | 26.8 | 32 | Tennessee | 10.6 |
| 7 | Michigan | 26.8 | 33 | Maine | 10.5 |
| 9 | Rhode Island | 25.9 | 34 | Minnesota | 9.0 |
| 10 | Ohio | 24.7 | 35 | Alabama | 8.9 |
| 11 | Connecticut | 21.9 | 36 | South Dakota | 8.8 |
| 12 | Pennsylvania | 19.3 | 37 | Washington | 8.5 |
| 13 | Texas | 18.6 | 38 | North Carolina | 8.0 |
| 14 | Missouri | 18.1 | 39 | Nebraska | 7.4 |
| 15 | Virginia | 18.0 | 40 | Alaska | 6.7 |
| 16 | California | 17.9 | 41 | South Carolina | 6.5 |
| 17 | North Dakota | 17.2 | 42 | Vermont | 6.4 |
| 18 | Massachusetts | 16.4 | 43 | Mississippi | 6.3 |
| 19 | Hawaii | 15.3 | 44 | Oregon | 6.0 |
| 19 | Indiana | 15.3 | 45 | Colorado | 5.7 |
| 21 | Kansas | 14.6 | 46 | Wyoming | 5.3 |
| 22 | Georgia | 14.5 | 47 | Arkansas | 5.0 |
| 23 | Wisconsin | 14.3 | 48 | Utah | 4.9 |
| 24 | Nevada | 13.7 | 49 | Montana | 4.3 |
| 25 | Kentucky | 13.5 | 50 | Idaho | 2.9 |

| | | |
|---|---|---|
| District of Columbia | | 15.7 |
| Puerto Rico | | 54.7 |

Source: American Medical Association

"Physician Characteristics and Distribution in the U.S." 1992 edition (Copyright, reprinted with permission)

*Calculated by the editors. As of January 1, 1990.

# Counties Without an Active Physician in Patient Care in 1990

## National Total = 126 Counties*

| RANK | STATE | COUNTIES | % | RANK | STATE | COUNTIES | % |
|------|-------|----------|-----|------|-------|----------|-----|
| 1 | Texas | 19 | 15.08% | 25 | Alaska | 0 | 0.00% |
| 2 | Nebraska | 17 | 13.49% | 25 | Arizona | 0 | 0.00% |
| 3 | South Dakota | 15 | 11.90% | 25 | Connecticut | 0 | 0.00% |
| 4 | Georgia | 12 | 9.52% | 25 | Delaware | 0 | 0.00% |
| 5 | North Dakota | 11 | 8.73% | 25 | Florida | 0 | 0.00% |
| 6 | Missouri | 10 | 7.94% | 25 | Hawaii | 0 | 0.00% |
| 7 | Montana | 8 | 6.35% | 25 | Louisiana | 0 | 0.00% |
| 8 | Colorado | 5 | 3.97% | 25 | Maine | 0 | 0.00% |
| 9 | Idaho | 4 | 3.17% | 25 | Maryland | 0 | 0.00% |
| 9 | Kansas | 4 | 3.17% | 25 | Massachusetts | 0 | 0.00% |
| 11 | Oregon | 3 | 2.38% | 25 | Michigan | 0 | 0.00% |
| 11 | Utah | 3 | 2.38% | 25 | Minnesota | 0 | 0.00% |
| 13 | Kentucky | 2 | 1.59% | 25 | New Hampshire | 0 | 0.00% |
| 13 | Mississippi | 2 | 1.59% | 25 | New Jersey | 0 | 0.00% |
| 13 | Nevada | 2 | 1.59% | 25 | New York | 0 | 0.00% |
| 16 | Arkansas | 1 | 0.79% | 25 | North Carolina | 0 | 0.00% |
| 16 | California | 1 | 0.79% | 25 | Oklahoma | 0 | 0.00% |
| 16 | Illinois | 1 | 0.79% | 25 | Pennsylvania | 0 | 0.00% |
| 16 | Indiana | 1 | 0.79% | 25 | Rhode Island | 0 | 0.00% |
| 16 | Iowa | 1 | 0.79% | 25 | South Carolina | 0 | 0.00% |
| 16 | New Mexico | 1 | 0.79% | 25 | Vermont | 0 | 0.00% |
| 16 | Ohio | 1 | 0.79% | 25 | Washington | 0 | 0.00% |
| 16 | Tennessee | 1 | 0.79% | 25 | West Virginia | 0 | 0.00% |
| 16 | Virginia | 1 | 0.79% | 25 | Wisconsin | 0 | 0.00% |
| 25 | Alabama | 0 | 0.00% | 25 | Wyoming | 0 | 0.00% |

Source: American Medical Association

"Physician Characteristics and Distribution in the U.S." 1992 edition (Copyright, reprinted with permission)

*As of January 1, 1990. Patient care excludes those physicians in administrative, teaching and research positions.

# Osteopathic Physicians in 1992

## National Total = 33,511 Osteopathic Physicians*

| RANK | STATE | OSTEOPATHS | % | RANK | STATE | OSTEOPATHS | % |
|---|---|---|---|---|---|---|---|
| 1 | Michigan | 4,210 | 12.56% | 26 | Maryland | 180 | 0.54% |
| 2 | Pennsylvania | 4,085 | 12.19% | 27 | Nevada | 166 | 0.50% |
| 3 | Ohio | 2,758 | 8.23% | 27 | New Mexico | 166 | 0.50% |
| 4 | Florida | 2,178 | 6.50% | 29 | Minnesota | 155 | 0.46% |
| 5 | Texas | 1,995 | 5.95% | 30 | Rhode Island | 152 | 0.45% |
| 6 | New Jersey | 1,962 | 5.85% | 31 | Delaware | 148 | 0.44% |
| 7 | New York | 1,593 | 4.75% | 32 | Kentucky | 130 | 0.39% |
| 8 | Missouri | 1,565 | 4.67% | 33 | Alabama | 122 | 0.36% |
| 9 | California | 1,365 | 4.07% | 34 | Arkansas | 107 | 0.32% |
| 10 | Illinois | 1,290 | 3.85% | 35 | North Carolina | 106 | 0.32% |
| 11 | Oklahoma | 980 | 2.92% | 36 | Connecticut | 105 | 0.31% |
| 12 | Arizona | 852 | 2.54% | 37 | Mississippi | 97 | 0.29% |
| 13 | Iowa | 815 | 2.43% | 38 | South Carolina | 96 | 0.29% |
| 14 | Colorado | 523 | 1.56% | 39 | Louisiana | 68 | 0.20% |
| 15 | Kansas | 451 | 1.35% | 40 | Idaho | 65 | 0.19% |
| 16 | Washington | 413 | 1.23% | 41 | Hawaii | 58 | 0.17% |
| 17 | Indiana | 393 | 1.17% | 42 | Montana | 52 | 0.16% |
| 18 | Maine | 389 | 1.16% | 43 | Nebraska | 50 | 0.15% |
| 19 | West Virginia | 340 | 1.01% | 44 | Utah | 49 | 0.15% |
| 19 | Wisconsin | 340 | 1.01% | 45 | Alaska | 46 | 0.14% |
| 21 | Oregon | 335 | 1.00% | 46 | New Hampshire | 45 | 0.13% |
| 22 | Georgia | 331 | 0.99% | 47 | Vermont | 44 | 0.13% |
| 23 | Massachusetts | 267 | 0.80% | 48 | South Dakota | 42 | 0.13% |
| 24 | Virginia | 233 | 0.70% | 49 | Wyoming | 27 | 0.08% |
| 25 | Tennessee | 191 | 0.57% | 50 | North Dakota | 21 | 0.06% |
| | | | | | District of Columbia | 18 | 0.05% |

*Source: American Osteopathic Association*
*unpublished data (October 13, 1992)*

*Active, retired and disabled osteopaths. Total includes 1,342 osteopathic physicians not shown separately (1,127 in military service, 125 in U.S. Public Health Service and 90 in U.S. territories or foreign countries).*

# Active Osteopathic Physicians in 1991

## National Total = 31,108 Active Osteopathic Physicians*

| RANK | STATE | OSTEOPATHS | % | RANK | STATE | OSTEOPATHS | % |
|------|-------|-----------|-----|------|-------|-----------|-----|
| 1 | Michigan | 3,949 | 12.69% | 26 | Maryland | 170 | 0.55% |
| 2 | Pennsylvania | 3,883 | 12.48% | 27 | Nevada | 151 | 0.49% |
| 3 | Ohio | 2,615 | 8.41% | 28 | Minnesota | 142 | 0.46% |
| 4 | New Jersey | 1,888 | 6.07% | 29 | Rhode Island | 140 | 0.45% |
| 5 | Texas | 1,857 | 5.97% | 30 | Delaware | 139 | 0.45% |
| 6 | Florida | 1,827 | 5.87% | 31 | New Mexico | 137 | 0.44% |
| 7 | New York | 1,532 | 4.92% | 32 | Kentucky | 122 | 0.39% |
| 8 | Missouri | 1,394 | 4.48% | 33 | Alabama | 120 | 0.39% |
| 9 | California | 1,293 | 4.16% | 34 | Connecticut | 98 | 0.32% |
| 10 | Illinois | 1,250 | 4.02% | 35 | Arkansas | 97 | 0.31% |
| 11 | Oklahoma | 913 | 2.93% | 36 | Mississippi | 93 | 0.30% |
| 12 | Iowa | 740 | 2.38% | 37 | North Carolina | 87 | 0.28% |
| 13 | Arizona | 722 | 2.32% | 38 | South Carolina | 86 | 0.28% |
| 14 | Colorado | 478 | 1.54% | 39 | Louisiana | 66 | 0.21% |
| 15 | Kansas | 404 | 1.30% | 40 | Idaho | 55 | 0.18% |
| 16 | Washington | 374 | 1.20% | 41 | Hawaii | 52 | 0.17% |
| 17 | Indiana | 372 | 1.20% | 42 | Montana | 47 | 0.15% |
| 18 | Maine | 346 | 1.11% | 43 | Alaska | 46 | 0.15% |
| 19 | West Virginia | 323 | 1.04% | 43 | Utah | 46 | 0.15% |
| 20 | Wisconsin | 308 | 0.99% | 45 | Nebraska | 44 | 0.14% |
| 21 | Georgia | 305 | 0.98% | 46 | New Hampshire | 35 | 0.11% |
| 22 | Oregon | 285 | 0.92% | 46 | Vermont | 35 | 0.11% |
| 23 | Massachusetts | 238 | 0.77% | 48 | South Dakota | 34 | 0.11% |
| 24 | Virginia | 217 | 0.70% | 49 | Wyoming | 25 | 0.08% |
| 25 | Tennessee | 176 | 0.57% | 50 | North Dakota | 19 | 0.06% |
| | | | | | District of Columbia | 17 | 0.05% |

*Source: American Osteopathic Association*

*unpublished data (October 13, 1992)*

*\*Total includes 1,316 osteopathic physicians not shown separately (1,127 in military service, 125 in U.S. Public Health Service and 64 in U.S. territories or foreign countries).*

# Active Osteopathic Physicians per 100,000 Population in 1992

## National Rate = 12.34 Osteopaths per 100,000 Population*

| RANK | STATE | RATE | RANK | STATE | RATE |
|------|-------|------|------|-------|------|
| 1 | Michigan | 42.15 | 26 | Vermont | 6.17 |
| 2 | Pennsylvania | 32.46 | 27 | Montana | 5.82 |
| 3 | Oklahoma | 28.76 | 28 | Wyoming | 5.43 |
| 4 | Maine | 28.02 | 29 | Idaho | 5.29 |
| 5 | Missouri | 27.03 | 30 | South Dakota | 4.84 |
| 6 | Iowa | 26.48 | 31 | Georgia | 4.61 |
| 7 | New Jersey | 24.33 | 32 | Hawaii | 4.58 |
| 8 | Ohio | 23.91 | 33 | California | 4.26 |
| 9 | Delaware | 20.44 | 34 | Arkansas | 4.09 |
| 10 | Arizona | 19.25 | 35 | Massachusetts | 3.97 |
| 11 | West Virginia | 17.93 | 36 | Mississippi | 3.59 |
| 12 | Kansas | 16.19 | 37 | Tennessee | 3.55 |
| 13 | Colorado | 14.15 | 38 | Maryland | 3.50 |
| 14 | Rhode Island | 13.94 | 39 | Virginia | 3.45 |
| 15 | Florida | 13.76 | 40 | Kentucky | 3.29 |
| 16 | Nevada | 11.76 | 41 | Minnesota | 3.20 |
| 17 | Illinois | 10.83 | 42 | New Hampshire | 3.17 |
| 18 | Texas | 10.70 | 43 | North Dakota | 2.99 |
| 19 | Oregon | 9.75 | 44 | Connecticut | 2.98 |
| 20 | New Mexico | 8.85 | 45 | Alabama | 2.93 |
| 21 | New York | 8.48 | 46 | Nebraska | 2.76 |
| 22 | Alaska | 8.07 | 47 | Utah | 2.60 |
| 23 | Washington | 7.45 | 48 | South Carolina | 2.42 |
| 24 | Indiana | 6.63 | 49 | Louisiana | 1.55 |
| 25 | Wisconsin | 6.22 | 50 | North Carolina | 1.29 |
| | | | | District of Columbia | 2.84 |

*Source: American Osteopathic Association*

*unpublished data (October 13, 1992)*

*\*Calculated by the editors using 1991 Census resident population figures. National rate includes 1,316 osteopathic physicians not shown separately (1,127 in military service, 125 in U.S. Public Health Service and 64 in U.S. territories or foreign country).*

# Active Civilian Dentists in 1990

## National Total = 145,500 Active Civilian Dentists*

| RANK | STATE | DENTISTS | % | RANK | STATE | DENTISTS | % |
|---|---|---|---|---|---|---|---|
| 1 | California | 17,680 | 12.15% | 26 | Arizona | 1,790 | 1.23% |
| 2 | New York | 14,200 | 9.76% | 27 | Alabama | 1,700 | 1.17% |
| 3 | Texas | 8,140 | 5.59% | 28 | Iowa | 1,610 | 1.11% |
| 4 | Pennsylvania | 7,500 | 5.15% | 29 | Oklahoma | 1,580 | 1.09% |
| 5 | Illinois | 7,310 | 5.02% | 30 | South Carolina | 1,410 | 0.97% |
| 6 | Florida | 6,230 | 4.28% | 31 | Kansas | 1,280 | 0.88% |
| 7 | Ohio | 6,110 | 4.20% | 32 | Utah | 1,150 | 0.79% |
| 8 | Michigan | 5,860 | 4.03% | 33 | Nebraska | 1,030 | 0.71% |
| 9 | New Jersey | 5,740 | 3.95% | 34 | Mississippi | 990 | 0.68% |
| 10 | Massachusetts | 4,470 | 3.07% | 35 | Arkansas | 970 | 0.67% |
| 11 | Virginia | 3,210 | 2.21% | 36 | Hawaii | 850 | 0.58% |
| 11 | Wisconsin | 3,210 | 2.21% | 36 | West Virginia | 850 | 0.58% |
| 13 | Maryland | 3,170 | 2.18% | 38 | New Mexico | 700 | 0.48% |
| 14 | Washington | 3,150 | 2.16% | 39 | New Hampshire | 650 | 0.45% |
| 15 | Georgia | 2,950 | 2.03% | 40 | Maine | 580 | 0.40% |
| 16 | Minnesota | 2,930 | 2.01% | 41 | Rhode Island | 560 | 0.38% |
| 17 | Missouri | 2,790 | 1.92% | 42 | Idaho | 550 | 0.38% |
| 18 | North Carolina | 2,730 | 1.88% | 43 | Montana | 520 | 0.36% |
| 19 | Indiana | 2,710 | 1.86% | 44 | Nevada | 500 | 0.34% |
| 20 | Tennessee | 2,660 | 1.83% | 45 | South Dakota | 350 | 0.24% |
| 21 | Connecticut | 2,640 | 1.81% | 46 | Alaska | 340 | 0.23% |
| 22 | Colorado | 2,320 | 1.59% | 47 | North Dakota | 320 | 0.22% |
| 23 | Louisiana | 2,050 | 1.41% | 47 | Vermont | 320 | 0.22% |
| 24 | Kentucky | 2,020 | 1.39% | 49 | Delaware | 290 | 0.20% |
| 25 | Oregon | 1,970 | 1.35% | 50 | Wyoming | 260 | 0.18% |
| | | | | | District of Columbia | 600 | 0.41% |

Source: U.S. Department of Health and Human Services, Division of Associated and Dental Health Professions
Unpublished data

*As of December 31, 1990.

# Active Civilian Dentists per 100,000 Population in 1990

## National Rate = 58.5 Active Civilian Dentists per 100,000 Population*

| RANK | STATE | RATE | | RANK | STATE | RATE |
|------|-------|------|---|------|-------|------|
| 1 | Connecticut | 80.3 | | 26 | Kentucky | 54.8 |
| 2 | New York | 78.9 | | 27 | Idaho | 54.6 |
| 3 | Hawaii | 76.7 | | 28 | Missouri | 54.5 |
| 4 | Massachusetts | 74.3 | | 28 | Tennessee | 54.5 |
| 4 | New Jersey | 74.3 | | 30 | Virginia | 51.9 |
| 6 | Colorado | 70.4 | | 31 | Kansas | 51.7 |
| 7 | Oregon | 69.3 | | 32 | South Dakota | 50.3 |
| 8 | Minnesota | 67.0 | | 33 | Oklahoma | 50.2 |
| 9 | Utah | 66.7 | | 34 | North Dakota | 50.1 |
| 10 | Maryland | 66.3 | | 35 | Indiana | 48.9 |
| 11 | Wisconsin | 65.6 | | 36 | Arizona | 48.8 |
| 12 | Nebraska | 65.3 | | 37 | Louisiana | 48.6 |
| 13 | Montana | 65.1 | | 38 | Florida | 48.2 |
| 14 | Washington | 64.7 | | 39 | Texas | 47.9 |
| 15 | Illinois | 64.0 | | 40 | West Virginia | 47.4 |
| 16 | Pennsylvania | 63.1 | | 41 | Maine | 47.2 |
| 17 | Michigan | 63.0 | | 42 | New Mexico | 46.2 |
| 18 | Alaska | 61.8 | | 43 | Georgia | 45.5 |
| 19 | California | 59.4 | | 44 | Delaware | 43.5 |
| 20 | New Hampshire | 58.6 | | 45 | Alabama | 42.1 |
| 21 | Iowa | 58.0 | | 46 | Nevada | 41.6 |
| 22 | Wyoming | 57.3 | | 47 | Arkansas | 41.3 |
| 23 | Vermont | 56.9 | | 48 | North Carolina | 41.2 |
| 24 | Ohio | 56.3 | | 49 | South Carolina | 40.4 |
| 25 | Rhode Island | 55.8 | | 50 | Mississippi | 38.5 |
| | | | | | District of Columbia | 98.9 |

*Source: U.S. Department of Health and Human Services, Division of Associated and Dental Health Professions*
*Unpublished data*

*Calculated by the editors using 1990 Census resident population figures. As of December 31, 1990.*

# Doctors of Chiropractic in 1989

## National Total = 47,833 Doctors of Chiropractic*

| RANK | STATE | CHIROPRACTORS | % | RANK | STATE | CHIROPRACTORS | % |
|---|---|---|---|---|---|---|---|
| 1 | California | 8,025 | 16.78% | 26 | Connecticut | 423 | 0.88% |
| 2 | New York | 3,800 | 7.94% | 27 | Louisiana | 419 | 0.88% |
| 3 | Florida | 3,222 | 6.74% | 28 | Alabama | 391 | 0.82% |
| 4 | New Jersey | 2,369 | 4.95% | 28 | South Carolina | 391 | 0.82% |
| 5 | Pennsylvania | 2,229 | 4.66% | 30 | Maryland | 384 | 0.80% |
| 6 | Michigan* | 2,223 | 4.65% | 31 | Virginia | 346 | 0.72% |
| 7 | Illinois | 1,889 | 3.95% | 32 | Arkansas | 298 | 0.62% |
| 8 | Texas | 1,808 | 3.78% | 33 | New Mexico | 293 | 0.61% |
| 9 | Georgia* | 1,650 | 3.45% | 34 | Hawaii | 267 | 0.56% |
| 10 | Minnesota | 1,648 | 3.45% | 35 | Utah | 247 | 0.52% |
| 11 | Missouri | 1,295 | 2.71% | 36 | New Hampshire | 230 | 0.48% |
| 12 | Washington | 1,076 | 2.25% | 37 | Mississippi | 206 | 0.43% |
| 13 | Ohio | 1,045 | 2.18% | 38 | Nevada | 190 | 0.40% |
| 14 | Oregon | 1,010 | 2.11% | 39 | Nebraska | 180 | 0.38% |
| 15 | Arizona | 967 | 2.02% | 40 | Idaho | 176 | 0.37% |
| 16 | Massachusetts | 895 | 1.87% | 41 | Montana | 171 | 0.36% |
| 17 | Wisconsin | 894 | 1.87% | 42 | South Dakota | 155 | 0.32% |
| 18 | North Carolina | 861 | 1.80% | 43 | Maine | 154 | 0.32% |
| 19 | Colorado | 860 | 1.80% | 44 | Rhode Island* | 149 | 0.31% |
| 20 | Iowa | 744 | 1.56% | 45 | West Virginia | 134 | 0.28% |
| 21 | Indiana | 595 | 1.24% | 46 | North Dakota | 120 | 0.25% |
| 22 | Kansas | 562 | 1.17% | 47 | Alaska | 104 | 0.22% |
| 23 | Oklahoma | 550 | 1.15% | 48 | Vermont | 91 | 0.19% |
| 24 | Kentucky | 458 | 0.96% | 49 | Delaware | 83 | 0.17% |
| 25 | Tennessee | 443 | 0.93% | 50 | Wyoming | 80 | 0.17% |
| | | | | | District of Columbia* | 75 | 0.16% |

Source: International Chiropractors Association

"U.S. Distribution of Doctors of Chiropractic" (Reprinted with permission)

*Denotes total active licenses. May include non-resident licenses.

# Doctors of Chiropractic per 100,000 Population in 1989

## National Rate = 19 Doctors of Chiropractic per 100,000 Population

| RANK | STATE | RATE | | RANK | STATE | RATE |
|------|-------|------|---|------|-------|------|
| 1 | Minnesota | 39 | | 26 | Oklahoma | 17 |
| 2 | Oregon | 37 | | 26 | Vermont | 17 |
| 3 | New Jersey | 31 | | 28 | Illinois | 16 |
| 4 | California | 30 | | 28 | Wyoming | 16 |
| 5 | Arizona | 29 | | 30 | Massachusetts | 15 |
| 6 | Georgia | 27 | | 30 | Rhode Island | 15 |
| 7 | Colorado | 26 | | 30 | Utah | 15 |
| 7 | Iowa | 26 | | 33 | Connecticut | 13 |
| 9 | Florida | 25 | | 33 | Delaware | 13 |
| 9 | Hawaii | 25 | | 33 | Maine | 13 |
| 9 | Missouri | 25 | | 33 | North Carolina | 13 |
| 12 | Michigan | 24 | | 37 | Arkansas | 12 |
| 12 | Washington | 24 | | 37 | Kentucky | 12 |
| 14 | Kansas | 23 | | 39 | Indiana | 11 |
| 15 | New Hampshire | 22 | | 39 | Nebraska | 11 |
| 15 | South Dakota | 22 | | 39 | South Carolina | 11 |
| 17 | Montana | 21 | | 39 | Texas | 11 |
| 17 | New York | 21 | | 43 | Alabama | 10 |
| 19 | Alaska | 20 | | 43 | Ohio | 10 |
| 19 | New Mexico | 20 | | 45 | Louisiana | 9 |
| 21 | Nevada | 19 | | 45 | Tennessee | 9 |
| 21 | Pennsylvania | 19 | | 47 | Maryland | 8 |
| 21 | Wisconsin | 19 | | 47 | Mississippi | 8 |
| 24 | Idaho | 18 | | 49 | West Virginia | 7 |
| 24 | North Dakota | 18 | | 50 | Virginia | 6 |
| | | | | | District of Columbia | 12 |

Source: International Chiropractors Association
   "U.S. Distribution of Doctors of Chiropractic" (Reprinted with permission)

426

# Podiatric Physicians in 1991

## National Total = 12,786 Podiatric Physicians*

| RANK | STATE | PODIATRISTS | % | RANK | STATE | PODIATRISTS | % |
|------|-------|-------------|-----|------|-------|-------------|-----|
| 1 | New York | 1,896 | 14.83% | 26 | Oregon | 85 | 0.66% |
| 2 | California | 1,610 | 12.59% | 27 | Kansas | 77 | 0.60% |
| 3 | Pennsylvania | 1,124 | 8.79% | 28 | Oklahoma | 73 | 0.57% |
| 4 | Illinois | 947 | 7.41% | 29 | Louisiana | 68 | 0.53% |
| 5 | New Jersey | 753 | 5.89% | 30 | Rhode Island | 66 | 0.52% |
| 6 | Florida | 717 | 5.61% | 31 | Kentucky | 63 | 0.49% |
| 7 | Ohio | 634 | 4.96% | 32 | New Mexico | 56 | 0.44% |
| 8 | Michigan | 562 | 4.40% | 33 | South Carolina | 53 | 0.41% |
| 9 | Texas | 503 | 3.93% | 34 | Maine | 52 | 0.41% |
| 10 | Massachusetts | 420 | 3.28% | 35 | Alabama | 49 | 0.38% |
| 11 | Maryland | 272 | 2.13% | 35 | New Hampshire | 49 | 0.38% |
| 12 | Indiana | 269 | 2.10% | 37 | West Virginia | 45 | 0.35% |
| 13 | Connecticut | 244 | 1.91% | 38 | Nebraska | 41 | 0.32% |
| 14 | Virginia | 239 | 1.87% | 39 | Nevada | 36 | 0.28% |
| 15 | Washington | 176 | 1.38% | 40 | Arkansas | 33 | 0.26% |
| 16 | Wisconsin | 173 | 1.35% | 40 | Delaware | 33 | 0.26% |
| 17 | Arizona | 161 | 1.26% | 42 | Idaho | 28 | 0.22% |
| 18 | North Carolina | 155 | 1.21% | 42 | Montana | 28 | 0.22% |
| 19 | Missouri | 144 | 1.13% | 44 | Mississippi | 26 | 0.20% |
| 20 | Georgia | 132 | 1.03% | 45 | South Dakota | 18 | 0.14% |
| 21 | Colorado | 118 | 0.92% | 46 | Hawaii | 15 | 0.12% |
| 22 | Tennessee | 114 | 0.89% | 47 | Vermont | 14 | 0.11% |
| 23 | Iowa | 109 | 0.85% | 47 | Wyoming | 14 | 0.11% |
| 24 | Minnesota | 106 | 0.83% | 49 | North Dakota | 12 | 0.09% |
| 25 | Utah | 94 | 0.74% | 50 | Alaska | 7 | 0.05% |
|  |  |  |  |  | District of Columbia | 73 | 0.57% |

Source: Morgan Quitno Corporation

*Calculated by the editors using American Podiatric Medical Association, Inc. "Podiatric Physicians per 100,000 Population in 1991" and Census 1991 population figures.

# Podiatric Physicians per 100,000 Population in 1991

## National Rate = 5.0 Podiatrists per 100,000 Population

| RANK | STATE | RATE | RANK | STATE | RATE |
|------|-------|------|------|-------|------|
| 1 | New York | 10.5 | 26 | Kansas | 3.1 |
| 2 | New Jersey | 9.7 | 27 | Wyoming | 3.0 |
| 3 | Pennsylvania | 9.4 | 28 | Oregon | 2.9 |
| 4 | Illinois | 8.2 | 28 | Texas | 2.9 |
| 5 | Connecticut | 7.4 | 30 | Missouri | 2.8 |
| 6 | Massachusetts | 7.0 | 30 | Nevada | 2.8 |
| 7 | Rhode Island | 6.6 | 32 | Idaho | 2.7 |
| 8 | Michigan | 6.0 | 33 | Nebraska | 2.6 |
| 9 | Ohio | 5.8 | 33 | South Dakota | 2.6 |
| 10 | Maryland | 5.6 | 35 | Vermont | 2.5 |
| 11 | Florida | 5.4 | 35 | West Virginia | 2.5 |
| 12 | California | 5.3 | 37 | Minnesota | 2.4 |
| 12 | Utah | 5.3 | 38 | North Carolina | 2.3 |
| 14 | Delaware | 4.9 | 38 | Oklahoma | 2.3 |
| 15 | Indiana | 4.8 | 38 | Tennessee | 2.3 |
| 16 | New Hampshire | 4.4 | 41 | Georgia | 2.0 |
| 17 | Arizona | 4.3 | 42 | North Dakota | 1.9 |
| 18 | Maine | 4.2 | 43 | Kentucky | 1.7 |
| 19 | Iowa | 3.9 | 44 | Louisiana | 1.6 |
| 20 | Virginia | 3.8 | 45 | South Carolina | 1.5 |
| 21 | New Mexico | 3.6 | 46 | Arkansas | 1.4 |
| 22 | Colorado | 3.5 | 47 | Hawaii | 1.3 |
| 22 | Montana | 3.5 | 48 | Alabama | 1.2 |
| 22 | Washington | 3.5 | 48 | Alaska | 1.2 |
| 22 | Wisconsin | 3.5 | 50 | Mississippi | 1.0 |

District of Columbia 12.2

*Source: American Podiatric Medical Association, Inc.*
*"Podiatric Physicians per 100,000 Population, 1991"*

# Registered Nurses in 1991

## National Total = 1,758,000 Registered Nurses*

| RANK | STATE | NURSES | % |
|---|---|---|---|
| 1 | California | 179,000 | 10.18% |
| 2 | New York | 148,600 | 8.45% |
| 3 | Pennsylvania | 105,600 | 6.01% |
| 4 | Florida | 89,100 | 5.07% |
| 5 | Texas | 87,800 | 4.99% |
| 6 | Illinois | 85,900 | 4.89% |
| 7 | Ohio | 85,200 | 4.85% |
| 8 | Massachusetts | 70,600 | 4.02% |
| 9 | Michigan | 66,400 | 3.78% |
| 10 | New Jersey | 54,600 | 3.11% |
| 11 | North Carolina | 45,200 | 2.57% |
| 12 | Missouri | 41,600 | 2.37% |
| 13 | Indiana | 40,900 | 2.33% |
| 14 | Washington | 39,400 | 2.24% |
| 15 | Georgia | 38,500 | 2.19% |
| 16 | Virginia | 36,400 | 2.07% |
| 17 | Minnesota | 35,900 | 2.04% |
| 17 | Wisconsin | 35,900 | 2.04% |
| 19 | Maryland | 35,700 | 2.03% |
| 20 | Tennessee | 30,600 | 1.74% |
| 21 | Connecticut | 27,800 | 1.58% |
| 22 | Alabama | 24,900 | 1.42% |
| 23 | Arizona | 24,800 | 1.41% |
| 24 | Iowa | 24,300 | 1.38% |
| 25 | Colorado | 24,100 | 1.37% |

| RANK | STATE | NURSES | % |
|---|---|---|---|
| 26 | Oregon | 22,000 | 1.25% |
| 27 | Kansas | 19,900 | 1.13% |
| 28 | Louisiana | 19,300 | 1.10% |
| 29 | Kentucky | 18,600 | 1.06% |
| 30 | South Carolina | 17,200 | 0.98% |
| 31 | Oklahoma | 15,700 | 0.89% |
| 32 | Arkansas | 13,500 | 0.77% |
| 33 | Mississippi | 13,000 | 0.74% |
| 33 | Nebraska | 13,000 | 0.74% |
| 35 | West Virginia | 11,800 | 0.67% |
| 36 | Maine | 10,900 | 0.62% |
| 37 | New Hampshire | 10,300 | 0.59% |
| 38 | Nevada | 10,000 | 0.57% |
| 39 | Rhode Island | 9,700 | 0.55% |
| 40 | Utah | 9,100 | 0.52% |
| 41 | New Mexico | 7,600 | 0.43% |
| 42 | Delaware | 6,500 | 0.37% |
| 43 | South Dakota | 6,400 | 0.36% |
| 44 | Hawaii | 6,300 | 0.36% |
| 45 | North Dakota | 6,200 | 0.35% |
| 46 | Idaho | 5,800 | 0.33% |
| 47 | Vermont | 5,600 | 0.32% |
| 48 | Montana | 5,400 | 0.31% |
| 49 | Wyoming | 3,000 | 0.17% |
| 50 | Alaska | 2,400 | 0.14% |
| | District of Columbia | 10,500 | 0.60% |

Source: U.S. Department of Health and Human Services, Bureau of Health Professionals, Division of Nursing*

"Estimated Supply of Registered Nurses by Education Preparation and Geographic Area: December 1991"

*Estimated as of December 1991.

# Registered Nurses per 100,000 Population in 1991

## National Rate = 697 Registered Nurses per 100,000 Population*

| RANK | STATE | RATE | | RANK | STATE | RATE |
|---|---|---|---|---|---|---|
| 1 | Massachusetts | 1,177 | | 26 | Michigan | 709 |
| 2 | Vermont | 988 | | 27 | New Jersey | 704 |
| 3 | North Dakota | 976 | | 28 | Florida | 671 |
| 4 | Rhode Island | 966 | | 28 | North Carolina | 671 |
| 5 | Delaware | 956 | | 30 | Montana | 668 |
| 6 | New Hampshire | 932 | | 31 | Arizona | 661 |
| 7 | South Dakota | 910 | | 32 | West Virginia | 655 |
| 8 | Maine | 883 | | 33 | Wyoming | 652 |
| 8 | Pennsylvania | 883 | | 34 | Tennessee | 618 |
| 10 | Iowa | 869 | | 35 | Alabama | 609 |
| 11 | Connecticut | 845 | | 36 | California | 589 |
| 12 | New York | 823 | | 37 | Georgia | 581 |
| 13 | Nebraska | 816 | | 38 | Virginia | 579 |
| 14 | Minnesota | 810 | | 39 | Arkansas | 569 |
| 15 | Missouri | 807 | | 40 | Idaho | 558 |
| 16 | Kansas | 798 | | 41 | Hawaii | 555 |
| 17 | Washington | 785 | | 42 | Utah | 514 |
| 18 | Nevada | 779 | | 43 | Texas | 506 |
| 18 | Ohio | 779 | | 44 | Mississippi | 502 |
| 20 | Oregon | 753 | | 45 | Kentucky | 501 |
| 21 | Illinois | 744 | | 46 | Oklahoma | 494 |
| 22 | Maryland | 735 | | 47 | New Mexico | 491 |
| 23 | Indiana | 729 | | 48 | South Carolina | 483 |
| 24 | Wisconsin | 725 | | 49 | Louisiana | 454 |
| 25 | Colorado | 714 | | 50 | Alaska | 421 |

| District of Columbia | 1,756 |
|---|---|

Source: U.S. Department of Health and Human Services, Bureau of Health Professionals, Division of Nursing
"Estimated Supply of Registered Nurses by Educational Preparation and Geographic Area: December 1991" (Issued July 1992)
*Estimated as of December 1991.

# Personnel in Hospitals in 1990

## National Total = 4,063,288 Personnel*

| RANK | STATE | PERSONNEL | % | RANK | STATE | PERSONNEL | % |
|------|-------|-----------|---|------|-------|-----------|---|
| 1 | California | 371,490 | 9.14% | 26 | South Carolina | 49,443 | 1.22% |
| 2 | New York | 370,282 | 9.11% | 27 | Iowa | 49,425 | 1.22% |
| 3 | Texas | 248,940 | 6.13% | 28 | Colorado | 49,298 | 1.21% |
| 4 | Pennsylvania | 241,826 | 5.95% | 29 | Arizona | 45,514 | 1.12% |
| 5 | Florida | 201,474 | 4.96% | 30 | Kansas | 44,605 | 1.10% |
| 6 | Illinois | 198,088 | 4.88% | 31 | Mississippi | 42,311 | 1.04% |
| 7 | Ohio | 190,507 | 4.69% | 32 | Arkansas | 38,380 | 0.94% |
| 8 | Michigan | 148,843 | 3.66% | 33 | Oregon | 37,737 | 0.93% |
| 9 | New Jersey | 126,809 | 3.12% | 34 | West Virginia | 31,679 | 0.78% |
| 10 | Massachusetts | 125,258 | 3.08% | 35 | Nebraska | 29,117 | 0.72% |
| 11 | Georgia | 110,906 | 2.73% | 36 | New Mexico | 22,127 | 0.54% |
| 12 | North Carolina | 106,467 | 2.62% | 37 | Utah | 20,743 | 0.51% |
| 13 | Missouri | 102,631 | 2.53% | 38 | Maine | 20,474 | 0.50% |
| 14 | Tennessee | 92,472 | 2.28% | 39 | Rhode Island | 18,441 | 0.45% |
| 15 | Indiana | 92,438 | 2.27% | 40 | New Hampshire | 16,879 | 0.42% |
| 16 | Virginia | 92,432 | 2.27% | 41 | Hawaii | 16,435 | 0.40% |
| 17 | Maryland | 77,205 | 1.90% | 42 | Nevada | 14,004 | 0.34% |
| 18 | Louisiana | 73,316 | 1.80% | 43 | South Dakota | 13,878 | 0.34% |
| 19 | Wisconsin | 71,737 | 1.77% | 44 | North Dakota | 12,861 | 0.32% |
| 20 | Alabama | 68,488 | 1.69% | 45 | Montana | 12,335 | 0.30% |
| 21 | Minnesota | 64,886 | 1.60% | 46 | Delaware | 11,893 | 0.29% |
| 22 | Washington | 60,003 | 1.48% | 47 | Idaho | 11,630 | 0.29% |
| 23 | Kentucky | 58,419 | 1.44% | 48 | Vermont | 7,900 | 0.19% |
| 24 | Connecticut | 55,521 | 1.37% | 49 | Alaska | 7,349 | 0.18% |
| 25 | Oklahoma | 50,381 | 1.24% | 50 | Wyoming | 6,990 | 0.17% |
| | | | | | District of Columbia | 31,021 | 0.76% |

Source: American Hospital Association
"Hospital Statistics: A Comprehensive Summary of U.S. Hospitals 1991–1992" (Copyright, reprinted with permission)
*Full-time equivalent.

431

# Pharmacists in 1991–1992

## National Total = 249,979 Licensed Pharmacists*

| RANK | STATE | PHARMACISTS | % | RANK | STATE | PHARMACISTS | % |
|---|---|---|---|---|---|---|---|
| 1 | California | 23,581 | 9.43% | 26 | Oklahoma | 3,975 | 1.59% |
| 2 | New York | 17,226 | 6.89% | 27 | Connecticut | 3,800 | 1.52% |
| 3 | Florida | 13,979 | 5.59% | 28 | Kansas | 3,077 | 1.23% |
| 4 | Maryland | 12,800 | 5.12% | 29 | Oregon | 3,075 | 1.23% |
| 5 | Illinois | 11,834 | 4.73% | 30 | Mississippi | 2,940 | 1.18% |
| 6 | Ohio | 11,350 | 4.54% | 31 | Arkansas | 2,788 | 1.12% |
| 7 | Pennsylvania | 10,912 | 4.37% | 32 | West Virginia | 2,011 | 0.80% |
| 8 | New Jersey | 10,233 | 4.09% | 33 | Utah | 1,987 | 0.79% |
| 9 | Michigan | 9,311 | 3.72% | 34 | North Dakota | 1,984 | 0.79% |
| 10 | Massachusetts | 7,987 | 3.20% | 35 | Nebraska | 1,464 | 0.59% |
| 11 | Georgia | 7,800 | 3.12% | 36 | New Hampshire | 1,387 | 0.55% |
| 12 | North Carolina | 6,828 | 2.73% | 37 | Rhode Island | 1,376 | 0.55% |
| 13 | Virginia | 6,234 | 2.49% | 38 | Idaho | 1,311 | 0.52% |
| 14 | Missouri | 5,965 | 2.39% | 39 | Montana | 1,114 | 0.45% |
| 15 | Tennessee | 5,949 | 2.38% | 40 | Hawaii | 1,068 | 0.43% |
| 16 | Washington | 5,240 | 2.10% | 40 | New Mexico | 1,068 | 0.43% |
| 17 | Louisiana | 5,200 | 2.08% | 42 | Maine | 1,028 | 0.41% |
| 18 | Wisconsin | 5,102 | 2.04% | 43 | Wyoming | 997 | 0.40% |
| 19 | Minnesota | 4,927 | 1.97% | 44 | Vermont | 967 | 0.39% |
| 20 | Alabama | 4,900 | 1.96% | 45 | Nevada | 923 | 0.37% |
| 21 | Colorado | 4,500 | 1.80% | 46 | Delaware | 802 | 0.32% |
| 22 | Arizona | 4,404 | 1.76% | 47 | Texas | 756 | 0.30% |
| 23 | Kentucky | 4,204 | 1.68% | 48 | South Dakota | 650 | 0.26% |
| 24 | South Carolina | 4,175 | 1.67% | 49 | Alaska | 376 | 0.15% |
| 25 | Iowa | 4,081 | 1.63% | 50 | Indiana | 333 | 0.13% |

Source: Morgan Quitno Corporation
    unpublished data

*Data gathered by the editors from state licensing agencies. Some data are estimates. Most include out-of-state licenses. National total does not include the District of Columbia.

# VII. PHYSICAL FITNESS

# Alcohol Consumption in Gallons in 1989

## National Total = 6,655,781,000 Gallons of Alcohol Consumed*

| RANK | STATE | GALLONS | % | RANK | STATE | GALLONS | % |
|---|---|---|---|---|---|---|---|
| 1 | California | 820,233,000 | 12.32% | 26 | Connecticut | 80,114,000 | 1.20% |
| 2 | Texas | 513,221,000 | 7.71% | 27 | Kentucky | 78,155,000 | 1.17% |
| 3 | New York | 436,180,000 | 6.55% | 28 | Oregon | 75,461,000 | 1.13% |
| 4 | Florida | 405,913,000 | 6.10% | 29 | Iowa | 69,923,000 | 1.05% |
| 5 | Illinois | 330,281,000 | 4.96% | 30 | Oklahoma | 65,258,000 | 0.98% |
| 6 | Pennsylvania | 323,316,000 | 4.86% | 31 | Mississippi | 61,299,000 | 0.92% |
| 7 | Ohio | 286,414,000 | 4.30% | 32 | Kansas | 53,324,000 | 0.80% |
| 8 | Michigan | 242,031,000 | 3.64% | 33 | Nevada | 52,197,000 | 0.78% |
| 9 | New Jersey | 197,693,000 | 2.97% | 34 | Arkansas | 50,242,000 | 0.75% |
| 10 | Massachusetts | 166,270,000 | 2.50% | 35 | New Mexico | 46,934,000 | 0.71% |
| 11 | Wisconsin | 165,003,000 | 2.48% | 36 | New Hampshire | 44,614,000 | 0.67% |
| 12 | Virginia | 154,329,000 | 2.32% | 37 | Nebraska | 42,651,000 | 0.64% |
| 13 | Georgia | 153,632,000 | 2.31% | 38 | West Virginia | 40,178,000 | 0.60% |
| 14 | North Carolina | 153,032,000 | 2.30% | 39 | Hawaii | 34,737,000 | 0.52% |
| 15 | Missouri | 136,359,000 | 2.05% | 40 | Maine | 32,061,000 | 0.48% |
| 16 | Indiana | 133,917,000 | 2.01% | 41 | Rhode Island | 29,419,000 | 0.44% |
| 17 | Washington | 124,816,000 | 1.88% | 42 | Montana | 24,444,000 | 0.37% |
| 18 | Maryland | 120,957,000 | 1.82% | 43 | Utah | 24,281,000 | 0.36% |
| 19 | Louisiana | 118,836,000 | 1.79% | 44 | Idaho | 24,072,000 | 0.36% |
| 20 | Arizona | 116,507,000 | 1.75% | 45 | Delaware | 19,830,000 | 0.30% |
| 21 | Tennessee | 114,041,000 | 1.71% | 46 | North Dakota | 17,510,000 | 0.26% |
| 22 | Minnesota | 112,671,000 | 1.69% | 47 | Vermont | 17,509,000 | 0.26% |
| 23 | South Carolina | 95,347,000 | 1.43% | 48 | South Dakota | 17,049,000 | 0.26% |
| 24 | Colorado | 94,275,000 | 1.42% | 49 | Alaska | 16,185,000 | 0.24% |
| 25 | Alabama | 88,992,000 | 1.34% | 50 | Wyoming | 12,273,000 | 0.18% |
|  |  |  |  |  | District of Columbia | 21,790,000 | 0.33% |

Source: U.S. Department of Health and Human Services, National Institute on Alcohol Abuse and Alcoholism
"Apparent Per Capita Alcohol Consumption: National, State and Regional Trends, 1977-1989" (Surveillance Report #20, December 1991)
*Calculated by the editors by summing total beer, wine and spirit consumption. Reflects volume consumed, not alcohol content.

# Per Capita Alcohol Consumption in 1989

## National Per Capita = 34.84 Gallons of Alcohol Consumed per Population 16 and Older in 1989*

| RANK | STATE | GALLONS | RANK | STATE | GALLONS |
|------|-------|---------|------|-------|---------|
| 1 | Nevada | 60.69 | 26 | Michigan | 34.05 |
| 2 | New Hampshire | 52.00 | 27 | Washington | 34.02 |
| 3 | Wisconsin | 44.06 | 28 | Pennsylvania | 33.94 |
| 4 | Arizona | 43.60 | 29 | Minnesota | 33.74 |
| 5 | Alaska | 43.05 | 30 | Maine | 33.64 |
| 6 | New Mexico | 41.91 | 31 | Maryland | 33.07 |
| 7 | Texas | 40.91 | 32 | Idaho | 32.44 |
| 8 | Hawaii | 40.72 | 33 | New Jersey | 32.35 |
| 9 | Florida | 40.14 | 34 | Virginia | 32.27 |
| 10 | Montana | 40.07 | 35 | Georgia | 31.73 |
| 11 | Vermont | 39.70 | 36 | Iowa | 31.65 |
| 12 | Delaware | 37.99 | 37 | South Dakota | 31.63 |
| 13 | California | 37.15 | 38 | Mississippi | 31.61 |
| 14 | Colorado | 37.12 | 39 | Connecticut | 31.25 |
| 15 | Rhode Island | 37.10 | 40 | Indiana | 31.14 |
| 16 | Illinois | 36.69 | 41 | New York | 31.00 |
| 16 | Louisiana | 36.69 | 42 | North Carolina | 29.88 |
| 18 | South Carolina | 35.75 | 43 | Tennessee | 29.76 |
| 19 | Massachusetts | 35.18 | 44 | Alabama | 28.34 |
| 20 | North Dakota | 35.09 | 45 | Kansas | 27.77 |
| 21 | Wyoming | 34.87 | 46 | West Virginia | 27.67 |
| 22 | Nebraska | 34.62 | 47 | Arkansas | 27.44 |
| 23 | Oregon | 34.35 | 48 | Kentucky | 27.19 |
| 24 | Missouri | 34.11 | 49 | Oklahoma | 26.48 |
| 25 | Ohio | 34.07 | 50 | Utah | 21.47 |
| | | | | District of Columbia | 45.59 |

Source: U.S. Department of Health and Human Services, National Institute on Alcohol Abuse and Alcoholism

*"Apparent Per Capita Alcohol Consumption: National, State and Regional Trends, 1977-1989"* (Surveillance Report #20, December 1991)

*Calculated by the editors using 1989 Census resident population figures and by summing total beer, wine and spirit consumption. Reflects volume consumed, not alcohol content.

# Beer Consumption in Gallons in 1989

## National Total = 5,767,750,000 Gallons of Beer Consumed

| RANK | STATE | GALLONS | % | RANK | STATE | GALLONS | % |
|---|---|---|---|---|---|---|---|
| 1 | California | 664,432,000 | 11.52% | 26 | Kentucky | 71,336,000 | 1.24% |
| 2 | Texas | 468,126,000 | 8.12% | 27 | Connecticut | 64,158,000 | 1.11% |
| 3 | New York | 359,860,000 | 6.24% | 28 | Iowa | 63,940,000 | 1.11% |
| 4 | Florida | 349,367,000 | 6.06% | 29 | Oregon | 63,514,000 | 1.10% |
| 5 | Pennsylvania | 296,136,000 | 5.13% | 30 | Oklahoma | 59,395,000 | 1.03% |
| 6 | Illinois | 286,154,000 | 4.96% | 31 | Mississippi | 56,647,000 | 0.98% |
| 7 | Ohio | 260,695,000 | 4.52% | 32 | Kansas | 48,725,000 | 0.84% |
| 8 | Michigan | 210,798,000 | 3.65% | 33 | Arkansas | 45,736,000 | 0.79% |
| 9 | New Jersey | 158,485,000 | 2.75% | 34 | Nevada | 43,018,000 | 0.75% |
| 10 | Wisconsin | 146,865,000 | 2.55% | 35 | New Mexico | 42,497,000 | 0.74% |
| 11 | Massachusetts | 136,583,000 | 2.37% | 36 | Nebraska | 38,809,000 | 0.67% |
| 12 | Virginia | 134,680,000 | 2.34% | 37 | West Virginia | 37,567,000 | 0.65% |
| 13 | North Carolina | 133,314,000 | 2.31% | 38 | New Hampshire | 36,858,000 | 0.64% |
| 14 | Georgia | 132,593,000 | 2.30% | 39 | Hawaii | 30,138,000 | 0.52% |
| 15 | Missouri | 122,308,000 | 2.12% | 40 | Maine | 27,434,000 | 0.48% |
| 16 | Indiana | 120,376,000 | 2.09% | 41 | Rhode Island | 24,783,000 | 0.43% |
| 17 | Louisiana | 106,895,000 | 1.85% | 42 | Montana | 21,916,000 | 0.38% |
| 18 | Washington | 104,217,000 | 1.81% | 43 | Utah | 21,680,000 | 0.38% |
| 19 | Tennessee | 104,120,000 | 1.81% | 44 | Idaho | 21,195,000 | 0.37% |
| 20 | Arizona | 103,057,000 | 1.79% | 45 | Delaware | 16,769,000 | 0.29% |
| 21 | Maryland | 101,930,000 | 1.77% | 46 | North Dakota | 15,777,000 | 0.27% |
| 22 | Minnesota | 98,078,000 | 1.70% | 47 | South Dakota | 15,473,000 | 0.27% |
| 23 | South Carolina | 84,388,000 | 1.46% | 48 | Vermont | 14,720,000 | 0.26% |
| 24 | Colorado | 81,418,000 | 1.41% | 49 | Alaska | 13,624,000 | 0.24% |
| 25 | Alabama | 79,990,000 | 1.39% | 50 | Wyoming | 10,936,000 | 0.19% |
|  |  |  |  |  | District of Columbia | 16,238,000 | 0.28% |

Source: U.S. Department of Health and Human Services, National Institute on Alcohol Abuse and Alcoholism
"Apparent Per Capita Alcohol Consumption: National, State and Regional Trends, 1977-1989" (Surveillance Report #20, December 1991)

# Per Capita Beer Consumption in 1989

## National Per Capita = 30.19 Gallons of Beer Consumed per Population 16 and Older in 1989*

| RANK | STATE | GALLONS | RANK | STATE | GALLONS |
|------|-------|---------|------|-------|---------|
| 1 | Nevada | 50.02 | 26 | Minnesota | 29.37 |
| 2 | New Hampshire | 42.96 | 27 | Mississippi | 29.21 |
| 3 | Wisconsin | 39.22 | 28 | Iowa | 28.95 |
| 4 | Arizona | 38.57 | 29 | Oregon | 28.91 |
| 5 | New Mexico | 37.94 | 30 | Massachusetts | 28.90 |
| 6 | Texas | 37.32 | 31 | Maine | 28.79 |
| 7 | Alaska | 36.23 | 32 | South Dakota | 28.71 |
| 8 | Montana | 35.93 | 33 | Idaho | 28.56 |
| 9 | Hawaii | 35.33 | 34 | Washington | 28.40 |
| 10 | Florida | 34.55 | 35 | Virginia | 28.16 |
| 11 | Vermont | 33.38 | 36 | Indiana | 27.99 |
| 12 | Louisiana | 33.00 | 37 | Maryland | 27.86 |
| 13 | Delaware | 32.12 | 38 | Georgia | 27.38 |
| 14 | Colorado | 32.05 | 39 | Tennessee | 27.17 |
| 15 | Illinois | 31.78 | 40 | North Carolina | 26.03 |
| 16 | South Carolina | 31.64 | 41 | New Jersey | 25.93 |
| 17 | North Dakota | 31.62 | 42 | West Virginia | 25.87 |
| 18 | Nebraska | 31.50 | 43 | New York | 25.57 |
| 19 | Rhode Island | 31.25 | 44 | Alabama | 25.47 |
| 20 | Pennsylvania | 31.09 | 45 | Kansas | 25.38 |
| 21 | Wyoming | 31.07 | 46 | Connecticut | 25.02 |
| 22 | Ohio | 31.01 | 47 | Arkansas | 24.98 |
| 23 | Missouri | 30.59 | 48 | Kentucky | 24.82 |
| 24 | California | 30.09 | 49 | Oklahoma | 24.11 |
| 25 | Michigan | 29.66 | 50 | Utah | 19.17 |
| | | | | District of Columbia | 33.97 |

Source: U.S. Department of Health and Human Services, National Institute on Alcohol Abuse and Alcoholism
   "Apparent Per Capita Alcohol Consumption: National, State and Regional Trends, 1977–1989" (Surveillance Report #20, December 1991)
*Calculated by the editors using 1989 Census resident population figures.

# Wine Consumption in Gallons in 1989

## National Total = 516,689,000 Gallons of Wine Consumed

| RANK | STATE | GALLONS | % | RANK | STATE | GALLONS | % |
|---|---|---|---|---|---|---|---|
| 1 | California | 107,760,000 | 20.86% | 26 | Nevada | 5,039,000 | 0.98% |
| 2 | New York | 47,336,000 | 9.16% | 27 | Alabama | 4,267,000 | 0.83% |
| 3 | Florida | 31,189,000 | 6.04% | 28 | Tennessee | 4,248,000 | 0.82% |
| 4 | Texas | 26,733,000 | 5.17% | 29 | New Hampshire | 3,452,000 | 0.67% |
| 5 | Illinois | 25,448,000 | 4.93% | 30 | Iowa | 3,208,000 | 0.62% |
| 6 | New Jersey | 24,550,000 | 4.75% | 31 | Rhode Island | 2,915,000 | 0.56% |
| 7 | Massachusetts | 17,659,000 | 3.42% | 32 | Hawaii | 2,910,000 | 0.56% |
| 8 | Michigan | 16,879,000 | 3.27% | 33 | Kentucky | 2,727,000 | 0.53% |
| 9 | Ohio | 15,030,000 | 2.91% | 34 | New Mexico | 2,606,000 | 0.50% |
| 10 | Pennsylvania | 13,827,000 | 2.68% | 35 | Oklahoma | 2,601,000 | 0.50% |
| 11 | Washington | 13,670,000 | 2.65% | 36 | Maine | 2,587,000 | 0.50% |
| 12 | Virginia | 11,879,000 | 2.30% | 37 | Kansas | 1,995,000 | 0.39% |
| 13 | North Carolina | 11,230,000 | 2.17% | 38 | Nebraska | 1,914,000 | 0.37% |
| 14 | Maryland | 9,986,000 | 1.93% | 39 | Arkansas | 1,857,000 | 0.36% |
| 15 | Connecticut | 9,632,000 | 1.86% | 40 | Idaho | 1,828,000 | 0.35% |
| 16 | Georgia | 9,492,000 | 1.84% | 41 | Vermont | 1,818,000 | 0.35% |
| 17 | Wisconsin | 9,198,000 | 1.78% | 42 | Delaware | 1,584,000 | 0.31% |
| 18 | Oregon | 8,133,000 | 1.57% | 43 | Mississippi | 1,451,000 | 0.28% |
| 19 | Arizona | 7,717,000 | 1.49% | 44 | Montana | 1,417,000 | 0.27% |
| 20 | Colorado | 7,524,000 | 1.46% | 45 | Alaska | 1,389,000 | 0.27% |
| 21 | Minnesota | 7,168,000 | 1.39% | 46 | Utah | 1,237,000 | 0.24% |
| 22 | Missouri | 7,147,000 | 1.38% | 47 | West Virginia | 1,234,000 | 0.24% |
| 23 | Indiana | 6,668,000 | 1.29% | 48 | North Dakota | 683,000 | 0.13% |
| 24 | Louisiana | 6,082,000 | 1.18% | 49 | South Dakota | 629,000 | 0.12% |
| 25 | South Carolina | 5,192,000 | 1.00% | 50 | Wyoming | 611,000 | 0.12% |
| | | | | | District of Columbia | 3,352,000 | 0.65% |

Source: U.S. Department of Health and Human Services, National Institute on Alcohol Abuse and Alcoholism
"Apparent Per Capita Alcohol Consumption: National, State and Regional Trends, 1977–1989" (Surveillance Report #20, December 1991)

# Per Capita Wine Consumption in 1989

## National Per Capita = 2.70 Gallons of Wine Consumed per Population 16 and Older in 1989*

| RANK | STATE | GALLONS | | RANK | STATE | GALLONS |
|------|-------|---------|---|------|-------|---------|
| 1 | Nevada | 5.86 | | 26 | Montana | 2.32 |
| 2 | California | 4.88 | | 27 | North Carolina | 2.19 |
| 3 | Vermont | 4.12 | | 28 | Minnesota | 2.15 |
| 4 | New Hampshire | 4.02 | | 29 | Texas | 2.13 |
| 4 | New Jersey | 4.02 | | 30 | Georgia | 1.96 |
| 6 | Connecticut | 3.76 | | 31 | South Carolina | 1.95 |
| 7 | Massachusetts | 3.74 | | 32 | Louisiana | 1.88 |
| 8 | Washington | 3.73 | | 33 | Missouri | 1.79 |
| 9 | Oregon | 3.70 | | 33 | Ohio | 1.79 |
| 10 | Alaska | 3.69 | | 35 | Wyoming | 1.74 |
| 11 | Rhode Island | 3.68 | | 36 | Indiana | 1.55 |
| 12 | Hawaii | 3.41 | | 36 | Nebraska | 1.55 |
| 13 | New York | 3.36 | | 38 | Iowa | 1.45 |
| 14 | Florida | 3.08 | | 38 | Pennsylvania | 1.45 |
| 15 | Delaware | 3.03 | | 40 | North Dakota | 1.37 |
| 16 | Colorado | 2.96 | | 41 | Alabama | 1.36 |
| 17 | Arizona | 2.89 | | 42 | South Dakota | 1.17 |
| 18 | Illinois | 2.83 | | 43 | Tennessee | 1.11 |
| 19 | Maryland | 2.73 | | 44 | Utah | 1.09 |
| 20 | Maine | 2.71 | | 45 | Oklahoma | 1.06 |
| 21 | Virginia | 2.48 | | 46 | Kansas | 1.04 |
| 22 | Idaho | 2.46 | | 47 | Arkansas | 1.01 |
| 22 | Wisconsin | 2.46 | | 48 | Kentucky | 0.95 |
| 24 | Michigan | 2.37 | | 49 | West Virginia | 0.85 |
| 25 | New Mexico | 2.33 | | 50 | Mississippi | 0.75 |

District of Columbia       7.01

Source: U.S. Department of Health and Human Services, National Institute on Alcohol Abuse and Alcoholism

    "Apparent Per Capita Alcohol Consumption: National, State and Regional Trends, 1977-1989" (Surveillance Report #20, December 1991)

   *Calculated by the editors using 1989 Census resident population figures.

# Spirits Consumption in Gallons in 1989

## National Total = 371,342,000 Gallons of Spirits Consumed

| RANK | STATE | GALLONS | % | RANK | STATE | GALLONS | % |
|------|-------|---------|---|------|-------|---------|---|
| 1 | California | 48,041,000 | 12.94% | 26 | Alabama | 4,735,000 | 1.28% |
| 2 | New York | 28,984,000 | 7.81% | 27 | New Hampshire | 4,304,000 | 1.16% |
| 3 | Florida | 25,357,000 | 6.83% | 28 | Nevada | 4,140,000 | 1.11% |
| 4 | Illinois | 18,679,000 | 5.03% | 29 | Kentucky | 4,092,000 | 1.10% |
| 5 | Texas | 18,362,000 | 4.94% | 30 | Oregon | 3,814,000 | 1.03% |
| 6 | New Jersey | 14,658,000 | 3.95% | 31 | Oklahoma | 3,262,000 | 0.88% |
| 7 | Michigan | 14,354,000 | 3.87% | 32 | Mississippi | 3,201,000 | 0.86% |
| 8 | Pennsylvania | 13,353,000 | 3.60% | 33 | Iowa | 2,775,000 | 0.75% |
| 9 | Massachusetts | 12,028,000 | 3.24% | 34 | Arkansas | 2,649,000 | 0.71% |
| 10 | Georgia | 11,547,000 | 3.11% | 35 | Kansas | 2,604,000 | 0.70% |
| 11 | Ohio | 10,689,000 | 2.88% | 36 | Maine | 2,040,000 | 0.55% |
| 12 | Maryland | 9,041,000 | 2.43% | 37 | Nebraska | 1,928,000 | 0.52% |
| 13 | Wisconsin | 8,940,000 | 2.41% | 38 | New Mexico | 1,831,000 | 0.49% |
| 14 | North Carolina | 8,488,000 | 2.29% | 39 | Rhode Island | 1,721,000 | 0.46% |
| 15 | Virginia | 7,770,000 | 2.09% | 40 | Hawaii | 1,689,000 | 0.45% |
| 16 | Minnesota | 7,425,000 | 2.00% | 41 | Delaware | 1,477,000 | 0.40% |
| 17 | Washington | 6,929,000 | 1.87% | 42 | West Virginia | 1,377,000 | 0.37% |
| 18 | Missouri | 6,904,000 | 1.86% | 43 | Utah | 1,364,000 | 0.37% |
| 19 | Indiana | 6,873,000 | 1.85% | 44 | Alaska | 1,172,000 | 0.32% |
| 20 | Connecticut | 6,324,000 | 1.70% | 45 | Montana | 1,111,000 | 0.30% |
| 21 | Louisiana | 5,859,000 | 1.58% | 46 | North Dakota | 1,050,000 | 0.28% |
| 22 | South Carolina | 5,767,000 | 1.55% | 47 | Idaho | 1,049,000 | 0.28% |
| 23 | Arizona | 5,733,000 | 1.54% | 48 | Vermont | 971,000 | 0.26% |
| 24 | Tennessee | 5,673,000 | 1.53% | 49 | South Dakota | 947,000 | 0.26% |
| 25 | Colorado | 5,333,000 | 1.44% | 50 | Wyoming | 726,000 | 0.20% |
| | | | | | District of Columbia | 2,200,000 | 0.59% |

Source: U.S. Department of Health and Human Services, National Institute on Alcohol Abuse and Alcoholism
"Apparent Per Capita Alcohol Consumption: National, State and Regional Trends, 1977-1989" (Surveillance Report #20, December 1991)

# Per Capita Spirits Consumption in 1989

## National Per Capita = 1.94 Gallons of Spirits Consumed per Population 16 and Older in 1989*

| RANK | STATE | GALLONS | RANK | STATE | GALLONS |
|---|---|---|---|---|---|
| 1 | New Hampshire | 5.02 | 26 | Washington | 1.89 |
| 2 | Nevada | 4.81 | 27 | Montana | 1.82 |
| 3 | Alaska | 3.12 | 28 | Louisiana | 1.81 |
| 4 | Delaware | 2.83 | 29 | South Dakota | 1.76 |
| 5 | Massachusetts | 2.55 | 30 | Oregon | 1.74 |
| 6 | Florida | 2.51 | 31 | Missouri | 1.73 |
| 7 | Connecticut | 2.47 | 32 | North Carolina | 1.66 |
| 7 | Maryland | 2.47 | 33 | Mississippi | 1.65 |
| 9 | New Jersey | 2.40 | 34 | New Mexico | 1.63 |
| 10 | Wisconsin | 2.39 | 35 | Virginia | 1.62 |
| 11 | Georgia | 2.38 | 36 | Indiana | 1.60 |
| 12 | Minnesota | 2.22 | 37 | Nebraska | 1.56 |
| 13 | Vermont | 2.20 | 38 | Alabama | 1.51 |
| 14 | California | 2.18 | 39 | Tennessee | 1.48 |
| 15 | Rhode Island | 2.17 | 40 | Texas | 1.46 |
| 16 | South Carolina | 2.16 | 41 | Arkansas | 1.45 |
| 17 | Arizona | 2.15 | 42 | Kentucky | 1.42 |
| 18 | Maine | 2.14 | 43 | Idaho | 1.41 |
| 19 | Colorado | 2.10 | 44 | Pennsylvania | 1.40 |
| 19 | North Dakota | 2.10 | 45 | Kansas | 1.36 |
| 21 | Illinois | 2.07 | 46 | Oklahoma | 1.32 |
| 22 | New York | 2.06 | 47 | Ohio | 1.27 |
| 22 | Wyoming | 2.06 | 48 | Iowa | 1.26 |
| 24 | Michigan | 2.02 | 49 | Utah | 1.21 |
| 25 | Hawaii | 1.98 | 50 | West Virginia | 0.95 |
| | | | | District of Columbia | 4.60 |

*Source: U.S. Department of Health and Human Services, National Institute on Alcohol Abuse and Alcoholism*

*"Apparent Per Capita Alcohol Consumption: National, State and Regional Trends, 1977–1989" (Surveillance Report #20, December 1991)*

*Calculated by the editors using 1989 Census resident population figures.*

# Percent of Adult Population Abstainers from Alcohol in 1989

## National Median = 46.4%*

| RANK | STATE | PERCENT | RANK | STATE | PERCENT |
|---|---|---|---|---|---|
| 1 | West Virginia | 69.7 | 26 | Oregon | 44.6 |
| 2 | Alabama | 69.4 | 27 | Pennsylvania | 44.2 |
| 3 | Tennessee | 68.9 | 28 | South Dakota | 43.6 |
| 4 | Utah | 68.8 | 29 | Arizona | 43.2 |
| 5 | Kentucky | 65.4 | 30 | California | 42.3 |
| 6 | Oklahoma | 63.6 | 31 | Montana | 41.9 |
| 7 | North Carolina | 62.0 | 32 | North Dakota | 41.8 |
| 8 | Georgia | 61.9 | 32 | Washington | 41.8 |
| 9 | South Carolina | 61.4 | 34 | Rhode Island | 40.3 |
| 10 | Indiana | 53.5 | 35 | Minnesota | 38.4 |
| 11 | Missouri | 53.2 | 36 | Massachusetts | 32.1 |
| 12 | Idaho | 52.6 | 36 | New Hampshire | 32.1 |
| 13 | New York | 51.5 | 38 | Connecticut | 31.5 |
| 14 | Maine | 50.2 | 39 | Wisconsin | 30.1 |
| 15 | Ohio | 49.9 | – | Alaska** | N/A |
| 16 | Nebraska | 48.4 | – | Arkansas** | N/A |
| 17 | Texas | 48.1 | – | Colorado** | N/A |
| 18 | New Mexico | 47.5 | – | Delaware** | N/A |
| 19 | Hawaii | 47.1 | – | Kansas** | N/A |
| 20 | Virginia | 46.4 | – | Louisiana** | N/A |
| 21 | Illinois | 46.3 | – | Mississippi** | N/A |
| 22 | Iowa | 46.0 | – | Nevada** | N/A |
| 22 | Maryland | 46.0 | – | New Jersey** | N/A |
| 24 | Florida | 45.5 | – | Vermont** | N/A |
| 25 | Michigan | 44.8 | – | Wyoming** | N/A |

District of Columbia     61.3

Source: U.S. Department of Health and Human Services, National Institute on Alcohol Abuse and Alcoholism

*"Apparent Per Capita Alcohol Consumption: National, State and Regional Trends, 1977-1989"* (Surveillance Report #20, December 1991)

*Based on estimates of abstention among population age 18 and older from the Behavioral Risk Factors Survey of the Centers for Disease Control.

**Did not participate in survey.

# Percent of Adults Who Are Binge Drinkers in 1990

## National Median = 15.2% of Adults Are Binge Drinkers*

| RANK | STATE | PERCENT BINGE DRINKERS | RANK | STATE | PERCENT BINGE DRINKERS |
|---|---|---|---|---|---|
| 1 | Wisconsin | 26.8 | 26 | Iowa | 13.3 |
| 2 | Vermont | 21.1 | 27 | Florida | 13.2 |
| 3 | Minnesota | 21.0 | 28 | Indiana | 12.8 |
| 4 | Hawaii | 19.4 | 29 | Oregon | 12.0 |
| 5 | Montana | 18.8 | 30 | New York | 11.8 |
| 5 | Texas | 18.8 | 31 | Oklahoma | 10.7 |
| 7 | Massachusetts | 18.3 | 32 | Mississippi | 10.6 |
| 8 | Pennsylvania | 18.1 | 33 | Utah | 10.5 |
| 9 | Rhode Island | 17.9 | 34 | Maine | 10.3 |
| 10 | Michigan | 17.7 | 35 | South Carolina | 10.2 |
| 10 | Washington | 17.7 | 36 | Alabama | 10.0 |
| 12 | California | 17.3 | 37 | Idaho | 9.8 |
| 13 | Colorado | 17.2 | 38 | Kentucky | 9.5 |
| 13 | North Dakota | 17.2 | 39 | West Virginia | 9.4 |
| 15 | Nebraska | 17.1 | 40 | Ohio | 9.3 |
| 16 | Connecticut | 16.5 | 41 | North Carolina | 9.1 |
| 17 | Illinois | 16.3 | 42 | Georgia | 8.8 |
| 18 | Virginia | 16.1 | 43 | Maryland | 7.9 |
| 19 | South Dakota | 15.8 | 44 | Tennessee | 6.3 |
| 20 | New Hampshire | 15.7 | – | Alaska** | N/A |
| 21 | Louisiana | 15.6 | – | Arkansas** | N/A |
| 22 | Missouri | 15.5 | – | Kansas** | N/A |
| 23 | Delaware | 15.2 | – | Nevada** | N/A |
| 23 | New Mexico | 15.2 | – | New Jersey** | N/A |
| 25 | Arizona | 14.4 | – | Wyoming** | N/A |

District of Columbia          5.5

Source: U.S. Department of Health and Human Services, Centers for Disease Control
   "Behavioral Risk Factor Surveillance, 1986-1990" (Morbidity and Mortality Weekly Report, December 1991)
*Persons 18 and Older reporting consumption of five or more alcoholic drinks on one or more occasions during the past month.
**Not available.

## Percent of Men 18 to 34 Years Old Who Are Binge Drinkers in 1990

## National Median = 35.2% Of Men 18 to 34 Years Old Are Binge Drinkers*

| RANK | STATE | PERCENT BINGE DRINKERS | RANK | STATE | PERCENT BINGE DRINKERS |
|---|---|---|---|---|---|
| 1 | Wisconsin | 61.1 | 25 | Illinois | 33.3 |
| 2 | Vermont | 47.8 | 27 | Kentucky | 31.0 |
| 3 | Massachusetts | 47.3 | 28 | Iowa | 30.8 |
| 4 | Nebraska | 46.2 | 28 | Mississippi | 30.8 |
| 5 | Minnesota | 46.0 | 30 | New York | 30.0 |
| 6 | Pennsylvania | 45.1 | 31 | West Virginia | 28.4 |
| 7 | Rhode Island | 45.0 | 32 | South Carolina | 28.1 |
| 8 | Hawaii | 42.8 | 33 | North Carolina | 27.2 |
| 9 | Michigan | 41.3 | 34 | Alabama | 27.0 |
| 10 | Delaware | 41.0 | 35 | Louisiana | 26.9 |
| 10 | Virginia | 41.0 | 35 | Maine | 26.9 |
| 12 | Texas | 40.9 | 35 | Oregon | 26.9 |
| 13 | Montana | 40.6 | 38 | Utah | 25.0 |
| 14 | New Mexico | 40.2 | 39 | Ohio | 23.3 |
| 15 | Missouri | 39.6 | 40 | Idaho | 23.0 |
| 16 | South Dakota | 39.0 | 41 | Oklahoma | 22.8 |
| 17 | Washington | 38.7 | 42 | Georgia | 22.7 |
| 18 | North Dakota | 38.1 | 43 | Maryland | 21.6 |
| 19 | New Hampshire | 37.3 | 44 | Tennessee | 17.0 |
| 20 | California | 37.0 | – | Alaska** | N/A |
| 21 | Colorado | 36.7 | – | Arkansas** | N/A |
| 22 | Connecticut | 35.3 | – | Kansas** | N/A |
| 23 | Florida | 35.2 | – | Nevada** | N/A |
| 24 | Indiana | 34.2 | – | New Jersey** | N/A |
| 25 | Arizona | 33.3 | – | Wyoming** | N/A |

District of Columbia                 13.8

Source: U.S. Department of Health and Human Services, Centers for Disease Control
   "Behavioral Risk Factor Surveillance, 1986–1990" (Morbidity and Mortality Weekly Report, December 1991)
*Persons 18 and Older reporting consumption of five or more alcoholic drinks on one or more occasions during the past month.
**Not available.

# Percent of Adults Who Drink and Drive in 1990

## National Median = 2.9% of Adults Drink and Drive in 1990*

| RANK | STATE | PERCENT DRINK AND DRIVE | RANK | STATE | PERCENT DRINK AND DRIVE |
|---|---|---|---|---|---|
| 1 | Wisconsin | 5.9 | 26 | Rhode Island | 2.3 |
| 2 | Nebraska | 5.0 | 27 | Oklahoma | 2.2 |
| 3 | Texas | 4.8 | 28 | Florida | 2.1 |
| 4 | Vermont | 4.2 | 29 | New Hampshire | 2.0 |
| 5 | North Dakota | 4.0 | 30 | Delaware | 1.9 |
| 6 | Hawaii | 3.9 | 30 | South Carolina | 1.9 |
| 6 | Montana | 3.9 | 32 | Alabama | 1.8 |
| 8 | Illinois | 3.8 | 32 | Oregon | 1.8 |
| 9 | Virginia | 3.6 | 34 | Mississippi | 1.6 |
| 10 | Louisiana | 3.5 | 35 | Georgia | 1.5 |
| 10 | South Dakota | 3.5 | 35 | North Carolina | 1.5 |
| 12 | Arizona | 3.4 | 37 | Idaho | 1.3 |
| 12 | California | 3.4 | 37 | Utah | 1.3 |
| 12 | Connecticut | 3.4 | 39 | New York | 1.2 |
| 12 | Pennsylvania | 3.4 | 39 | Tennessee | 1.2 |
| 16 | Michigan | 3.3 | 41 | Kentucky | 0.9 |
| 16 | Minnesota | 3.3 | 41 | Maryland | 0.9 |
| 16 | Missouri | 3.3 | 41 | West Virginia | 0.9 |
| 19 | New Mexico | 3.1 | 44 | Maine | 0.7 |
| 20 | Indiana | 3.0 | – | Alaska** | N/A |
| 20 | Ohio | 3.0 | – | Arkansas** | N/A |
| 22 | Colorado | 2.9 | – | Kansas** | N/A |
| 22 | Washington | 2.9 | – | Nevada** | N/A |
| 24 | Iowa | 2.7 | – | New Jersey** | N/A |
| 24 | Massachusetts | 2.7 | – | Wyoming** | N/A |
| | | | | District of Columbia | 1.5 |

Source: U.S. Department of Health and Human Services, Centers for Disease Control

   "Behavioral Risk Factor Surveillance, 1986–1990" (Morbidity and Mortality Weekly Report, December 1991)

*Persons 18 and older who report driving after having too much to drink one or more times in the past month.

**Not available.

444

# Percent of Men 18 to 34 Years Old Who Drink and Drive in 1990

## National Median = 7.8% of Men 18 to 34 Years Old Drink and Drive*

| RANK | STATE | PERCENT DRINK AND DRIVE | RANK | STATE | PERCENT DRINK AND DRIVE |
|------|-------|-------------------------|------|-------|-------------------------|
| 1 | Nebraska | 16.8 | 26 | Colorado | 6.8 |
| 2 | Wisconsin | 15.0 | 27 | Mississippi | 6.5 |
| 3 | Texas | 13.2 | 28 | Oklahoma | 6.3 |
| 4 | Vermont | 11.8 | 29 | North Carolina | 6.1 |
| 5 | South Dakota | 9.8 | 30 | Delaware | 5.6 |
| 6 | Arizona | 9.6 | 31 | Alabama | 5.2 |
| 7 | Connecticut | 9.4 | 32 | Florida | 5.1 |
| 7 | Indiana | 9.4 | 33 | New Hampshire | 5.0 |
| 9 | Massachusetts | 9.1 | 34 | Oregon | 4.9 |
| 9 | Michigan | 9.1 | 35 | South Carolina | 3.8 |
| 9 | North Dakota | 9.1 | 35 | Tennessee | 3.8 |
| 9 | Virginia | 9.1 | 37 | New York | 3.3 |
| 13 | Iowa | 9.0 | 38 | Kentucky | 3.1 |
| 13 | Missouri | 9.0 | 39 | Utah | 2.9 |
| 13 | New Mexico | 9.0 | 40 | West Virginia | 2.8 |
| 16 | Montana | 8.8 | 41 | Georgia | 2.6 |
| 17 | Washington | 8.3 | 42 | Maryland | 2.5 |
| 18 | Louisiana | 8.2 | 43 | Idaho | 2.0 |
| 19 | California | 8.1 | 44 | Maine | 1.2 |
| 19 | Pennsylvania | 8.1 | – | Alaska** | N/A |
| 19 | Rhode Island | 8.1 | – | Arkansas** | N/A |
| 22 | Hawaii | 7.9 | – | Kansas** | N/A |
| 23 | Minnesota | 7.8 | – | Nevada** | N/A |
| 24 | Illinois | 7.5 | – | New Jersey** | N/A |
| 25 | Ohio | 7.3 | – | Wyoming** | N/A |

District of Columbia      2.2

Source: U.S. Department of Health and Human Services, Centers for Disease Control
   "Behavioral Risk Factor Surveillance, 1986–1990" (Morbidity and Mortality Weekly Report, December 1991)
*Men who report driving after having too much to drink one or more times in the past month.
**Not available.

# Percent of Safety Belt Nonuse by Adults in 1990

## National Median = 25.9% of Adults Do Not Use Safety Belts*

| RANK | STATE | SAFETY BELT NONUSE | RANK | STATE | SAFETY BELT NONUSE |
|------|-------|--------------------|------|-------|--------------------|
| 1 | North Dakota | 59.6 | 26 | Louisiana | 24.2 |
| 2 | South Dakota | 57.3 | 27 | Ohio | 23.9 |
| 3 | Nebraska | 50.9 | 28 | Iowa | 23.7 |
| 4 | Rhode Island | 48.7 | 29 | Minnesota | 23.5 |
| 5 | Mississippi | 48.2 | 30 | Georgia | 23.1 |
| 6 | Massachusetts | 46.3 | 31 | Connecticut | 22.5 |
| 7 | Kentucky | 46.1 | 32 | Michigan | 21.0 |
| 7 | West Virginia | 46.1 | 33 | New York | 20.2 |
| 9 | Maine | 41.1 | 34 | Florida | 19.9 |
| 10 | New Hampshire | 40.1 | 35 | Colorado | 17.2 |
| 11 | Alabama | 39.4 | 36 | Virginia | 16.2 |
| 12 | Vermont | 33.9 | 37 | North Carolina | 15.7 |
| 13 | Oregon | 33.4 | 38 | Washington | 15.5 |
| 14 | Delaware | 31.4 | 39 | Texas | 14.9 |
| 15 | Utah | 30.5 | 40 | South Carolina | 14.1 |
| 16 | Arizona | 30.0 | 41 | Maryland | 13.2 |
| 17 | Idaho | 29.2 | 42 | California | 12.8 |
| 18 | Illinois | 28.8 | 43 | New Mexico | 12.2 |
| 18 | Wisconsin | 28.8 | 44 | Hawaii | 4.9 |
| 20 | Montana | 28.2 | – | Alaska** | N/A |
| 21 | Indiana | 27.7 | – | Arkansas** | N/A |
| 22 | Missouri | 27.3 | – | Kansas** | N/A |
| 23 | Oklahoma | 25.9 | – | Nevada** | N/A |
| 24 | Pennsylvania | 25.7 | – | New Jersey** | N/A |
| 24 | Tennessee | 25.7 | – | Wyoming** | N/A |

District of Columbia    25.8

Source: U.S. Department of Health and Human Services, Centers for Disease Control
      "Behavioral Risk Factor Surveillance, 1986–1990" (Morbidity and Mortality Weekly Report, December 1991)
*Persons 18 years and older who report sometimes, seldom or never using safety belts.
**Not available.

# Percent of Adults Who Smoke in 1990

## National Median = 22.7% of Adults 18 and Older Smoke*

| RANK | STATE | PERCENT SMOKERS | RANK | STATE | PERCENT SMOKERS |
|---|---|---|---|---|---|
| 1 | Kentucky | 29.1 | 26 | Alabama | 22.4 |
| 1 | Michigan | 29.1 | 27 | New Mexico | 22.3 |
| 3 | North Carolina | 28.0 | 27 | Washington | 22.3 |
| 4 | Maine | 26.9 | 29 | Connecticut | 22.2 |
| 5 | Tennessee | 26.7 | 30 | Maryland | 22.0 |
| 6 | Indiana | 26.6 | 30 | New Hampshire | 22.0 |
| 6 | Oklahoma | 26.6 | 32 | Oregon | 21.9 |
| 6 | West Virginia | 26.6 | 33 | Iowa | 21.7 |
| 9 | Missouri | 26.2 | 34 | Vermont | 21.6 |
| 10 | Ohio | 26.1 | 35 | Minnesota | 21.4 |
| 11 | Rhode Island | 25.7 | 36 | Colorado | 21.3 |
| 12 | Louisiana | 24.9 | 37 | Hawaii | 21.1 |
| 12 | South Carolina | 24.9 | 38 | Arizona | 20.7 |
| 14 | Wisconsin | 24.7 | 38 | South Dakota | 20.7 |
| 15 | Illinois | 24.2 | 40 | Idaho | 20.4 |
| 16 | Mississippi | 24.1 | 41 | North Dakota | 20.3 |
| 17 | Georgia | 24.0 | 42 | California | 19.7 |
| 18 | Florida | 23.6 | 43 | Montana | 19.4 |
| 18 | Pennsylvania | 23.6 | 44 | Utah | 16.8 |
| 20 | Massachusetts | 23.5 | – | Alaska** | N/A |
| 21 | Delaware | 23.3 | – | Arkansas** | N/A |
| 22 | Texas | 22.9 | – | Kansas** | N/A |
| 23 | Nebraska | 22.7 | – | Nevada** | N/A |
| 24 | Virginia | 22.6 | – | New Jersey** | N/A |
| 25 | New York | 22.5 | – | Wyoming** | N/A |

District of Columbia     19.4

Source: U.S. Department of Health and Human Services, Centers for Disease Control
    "Behavioral Risk Factor Surveillance, 1986–1990" (Morbidity and Mortality Weekly Report, December 1991)
*Persons who have ever smoked 100 cigarettes and currently smoke regularly.
**Not available.

# Percent of Low Education Adults Who Smoke in 1990

## National Median = 28.7% of Low Education Adults 18 and Older Smoke*

| RANK | STATE | PERCENT SMOKERS | RANK | STATE | PERCENT SMOKERS |
|------|-------|-----------------|------|-------|-----------------|
| 1 | Michigan | 34.3 | 26 | South Carolina | 28.1 |
| 2 | Kentucky | 32.9 | 27 | Connecticut | 27.9 |
| 3 | Maine | 32.5 | 28 | New Mexico | 27.8 |
| 4 | Illinois | 32.2 | 29 | Hawaii | 27.4 |
| 5 | Indiana | 31.9 | 30 | Nebraska | 27.3 |
| 6 | Louisiana | 31.8 | 31 | Minnesota | 27.2 |
| 7 | Rhode Island | 31.3 | 32 | Texas | 27.0 |
| 7 | Tennessee | 31.3 | 33 | Colorado | 26.9 |
| 9 | Oklahoma | 31.2 | 34 | New York | 26.4 |
| 10 | Massachusetts | 30.8 | 35 | Oregon | 26.3 |
| 10 | West Virginia | 30.8 | 36 | Idaho | 25.9 |
| 12 | Virginia | 30.6 | 37 | Utah | 25.6 |
| 13 | Georgia | 30.5 | 38 | Alabama | 25.4 |
| 14 | North Carolina | 30.4 | 39 | California | 25.0 |
| 15 | Missouri | 30.2 | 39 | Florida | 25.0 |
| 16 | Ohio | 30.1 | 41 | Montana | 24.0 |
| 17 | Wisconsin | 29.8 | 42 | North Dakota | 23.9 |
| 18 | Maryland | 29.6 | 43 | South Dakota | 22.6 |
| 19 | Washington | 29.2 | 44 | Arizona | 22.2 |
| 20 | Pennsylvania | 29.0 | – | Alaska** | N/A |
| 21 | Vermont | 28.9 | – | Arkansas** | N/A |
| 22 | Mississippi | 28.7 | – | Kansas** | N/A |
| 22 | New Hampshire | 28.7 | – | Nevada** | N/A |
| 24 | Iowa | 28.6 | – | New Jersey** | N/A |
| 25 | Delaware | 28.3 | – | Wyoming** | N/A |

District of Columbia     21.4

Source: U.S. Department of Health and Human Services, Centers for Disease Control
    *Behavioral Risk Factor Surveillance, 1986-1990"* (Morbidity and Mortality Weekly Report, December 1991)
*Persons with high school education or less who have ever smoked 100 cigarettes and currently smoke regularly.
**Not available.

# Percent of Adults Overweight in 1990

## National Median = 22.7% of Adults 18 and Older Are Overweight*

| RANK | STATE | PERCENT OVERWEIGHT | RANK | STATE | PERCENT OVERWEIGHT |
|------|-------|-------------------|------|-------|-------------------|
| 1 | Michigan | 26.4 | 26 | Texas | 22.0 |
| 2 | Mississippi | 26.3 | 27 | Idaho | 21.6 |
| 3 | Indiana | 26.0 | 27 | New Mexico | 21.6 |
| 4 | Delaware | 25.5 | 27 | Oregon | 21.6 |
| 5 | South Carolina | 25.1 | 30 | New Hampshire | 21.4 |
| 6 | West Virginia | 24.8 | 31 | Minnesota | 21.1 |
| 7 | Iowa | 24.6 | 32 | California | 20.9 |
| 7 | Pennsylvania | 24.6 | 33 | Arizona | 20.8 |
| 9 | North Carolina | 24.3 | 33 | Illinois | 20.8 |
| 10 | Florida | 24.2 | 35 | Georgia | 20.3 |
| 10 | Louisiana | 24.2 | 35 | Montana | 20.3 |
| 12 | Alabama | 24.0 | 37 | New York | 20.1 |
| 13 | Maine | 23.6 | 37 | Vermont | 20.1 |
| 14 | Nebraska | 23.5 | 39 | Virginia | 19.5 |
| 14 | Tennessee | 23.5 | 40 | Utah | 19.4 |
| 16 | Kentucky | 23.4 | 41 | Washington | 19.0 |
| 17 | Wisconsin | 23.3 | 42 | Massachusetts | 18.9 |
| 18 | Maryland | 23.0 | 43 | Hawaii | 17.7 |
| 18 | Oklahoma | 23.0 | 44 | Colorado | 16.3 |
| 20 | Missouri | 22.9 | – | Alaska** | N/A |
| 21 | Connecticut | 22.7 | – | Arkansas** | N/A |
| 21 | North Dakota | 22.7 | – | Kansas** | N/A |
| 23 | Ohio | 22.6 | – | Nevada** | N/A |
| 23 | South Dakota | 22.6 | – | New Jersey** | N/A |
| 25 | Rhode Island | 22.3 | – | Wyoming** | N/A |

District of Columbia 27.4

Source: U.S. Department of Health and Human Services, Centers for Disease Control

    *"Behavioral Risk Factor Surveillance, 1986–1990"* (Morbidity and Mortality Weekly Report, December 1991)

*Overweight is defined as men with a body mass index of 27.8 or greater and women with an index of 27.3 or greater.

**Not available.

# Percent of Low–Income Adult Women Overweight in 1990

## National Median = 26.6% of Low–Income Adult Women 18 and Older Are Overweight*

| RANK | STATE | PERCENT OVERWEIGHT | RANK | STATE | PERCENT OVERWEIGHT |
|---|---|---|---|---|---|
| 1 | Florida | 34.6 | 26 | Virginia | 25.8 |
| 2 | Connecticut | 33.7 | 27 | South Dakota | 25.7 |
| 3 | Oklahoma | 32.6 | 27 | Utah | 25.7 |
| 4 | Alabama | 32.0 | 29 | New Mexico | 25.4 |
| 5 | Delaware | 31.8 | 30 | New Hampshire | 24.9 |
| 6 | Kentucky | 31.7 | 31 | Arizona | 24.8 |
| 7 | Michigan | 31.6 | 32 | California | 24.5 |
| 8 | Maryland | 31.4 | 33 | Louisiana | 24.3 |
| 9 | South Carolina | 31.3 | 33 | Vermont | 24.3 |
| 10 | North Carolina | 31.2 | 35 | Oregon | 23.2 |
| 11 | Georgia | 30.7 | 36 | Colorado | 23.1 |
| 12 | Mississippi | 30.4 | 36 | Wisconsin | 23.1 |
| 12 | Pennsylvania | 30.4 | 38 | New York | 22.9 |
| 14 | Tennessee | 30.2 | 39 | Washington | 22.7 |
| 15 | Maine | 29.8 | 40 | North Dakota | 22.0 |
| 16 | Missouri | 28.7 | 41 | Minnesota | 21.3 |
| 17 | West Virginia | 27.8 | 42 | Massachusetts | 21.0 |
| 18 | Ohio | 27.5 | 43 | Hawaii | 19.0 |
| 19 | Rhode Island | 27.4 | 44 | Montana | 18.4 |
| 19 | Texas | 27.4 | – | Alaska** | N/A |
| 21 | Nebraska | 26.7 | – | Arkansas** | N/A |
| 22 | Illinois | 26.6 | – | Kansas** | N/A |
| 23 | Iowa | 26.4 | – | Nevada** | N/A |
| 24 | Indiana | 26.2 | – | New Jersey** | N/A |
| 25 | Idaho | 26.0 | – | Wyoming** | N/A |

District of Columbia    37.5

Source: U.S. Department of Health and Human Services, Centers for Disease Control

"Behavioral Risk Factor Surveillance, 1986-1990" (Morbidity and Mortality Weekly Report, December 1991)

*Women with family incomes of $20,000 or less. Overweight is defined as women with a body mass index of 27.3 or greater.

**Not available.

# Percent of Adults with No Leisure–Time Physical Activity in 1990

## National Median = 28.7% of Adults 18 and Older Inactive*

| RANK | STATE | PERCENT INACTIVE | RANK | STATE | PERCENT INACTIVE |
|------|-------|------------------|------|-------|------------------|
| 1 | Kentucky | 41.8 | 25 | Indiana | 27.4 |
| 2 | Oklahoma | 41.1 | 27 | Pennsylvania | 27.0 |
| 3 | North Carolina | 40.4 | 28 | North Dakota | 26.9 |
| 4 | West Virginia | 39.5 | 29 | Rhode Island | 26.2 |
| 5 | Mississippi | 39.2 | 30 | Virginia | 26.1 |
| 6 | Tennessee | 38.5 | 31 | Connecticut | 25.5 |
| 7 | Georgia | 37.0 | 32 | Minnesota | 24.9 |
| 8 | Maine | 36.3 | 32 | Nebraska | 24.9 |
| 9 | Iowa | 33.8 | 32 | Vermont | 24.9 |
| 10 | South Carolina | 33.7 | 35 | Wisconsin | 24.6 |
| 11 | Alabama | 33.6 | 36 | California | 24.4 |
| 12 | Ohio | 33.2 | 37 | Massachusetts | 23.3 |
| 13 | Missouri | 32.6 | 38 | Utah | 23.2 |
| 13 | New York | 32.6 | 39 | Oregon | 21.5 |
| 15 | Michigan | 32.4 | 40 | Arizona | 20.7 |
| 16 | Florida | 32.1 | 41 | Washington | 19.9 |
| 17 | Illinois | 32.0 | 42 | New Hampshire | 19.6 |
| 18 | Hawaii | 31.6 | 43 | Colorado | 19.4 |
| 19 | Maryland | 30.4 | 44 | Montana | 18.0 |
| 20 | South Dakota | 29.0 | – | Alaska** | N/A |
| 21 | Louisiana | 28.7 | – | Arkansas** | N/A |
| 21 | Texas | 28.7 | – | Kansas** | N/A |
| 23 | New Mexico | 28.0 | – | Nevada** | N/A |
| 24 | Idaho | 27.8 | – | New Jersey** | N/A |
| 25 | Delaware | 27.4 | – | Wyoming** | N/A |

District of Columbia      51.9

Source: U.S. Department of Health and Human Services, Centers for Disease Control
"Behavioral Risk Factor Surveillance, 1986-1990" (Morbidity and Mortality Weekly Report, December 1991)
*Persons who report no exercise, recreation, or physical activities (other than regular job duties) during the previous month.
**Not available.

# Percent of Adults 65 and Older with No Leisure–Time Physical Activity in 1990

## National Median = 40.1% of Adults 65 and Older Inactive*

| RANK | STATE | PERCENT INACTIVE | RANK | STATE | PERCENT INACTIVE |
|---|---|---|---|---|---|
| 1 | Kentucky | 55.3 | 26 | Texas | 38.0 |
| 1 | West Virginia | 55.3 | 26 | Vermont | 38.0 |
| 3 | Maine | 53.4 | 28 | Rhode Island | 37.7 |
| 4 | Tennessee | 52.1 | 29 | New Mexico | 37.2 |
| 5 | Georgia | 51.2 | 30 | Nebraska | 36.9 |
| 6 | Mississippi | 50.7 | 31 | Connecticut | 36.8 |
| 7 | North Carolina | 50.6 | 32 | Minnesota | 36.4 |
| 8 | Oklahoma | 47.3 | 33 | Massachusetts | 36.3 |
| 8 | South Carolina | 47.3 | 34 | Wisconsin | 36.0 |
| 10 | Michigan | 46.6 | 35 | Indiana | 35.6 |
| 11 | Iowa | 46.4 | 36 | Montana | 33.4 |
| 12 | Ohio | 46.3 | 37 | Utah | 31.6 |
| 13 | Illinois | 44.6 | 38 | Colorado | 30.4 |
| 14 | Louisiana | 44.3 | 39 | California | 30.0 |
| 15 | North Dakota | 43.7 | 40 | Hawaii | 28.9 |
| 16 | Alabama | 43.6 | 40 | New Hampshire | 28.9 |
| 17 | Maryland | 43.5 | 42 | Oregon | 28.8 |
| 18 | Virginia | 41.3 | 43 | Washington | 27.9 |
| 19 | Idaho | 40.8 | 44 | Arizona | 23.4 |
| 20 | New York | 40.6 | – | Alaska** | N/A |
| 21 | South Dakota | 40.2 | – | Arkansas** | N/A |
| 22 | Pennsylvania | 40.1 | – | Kansas** | N/A |
| 23 | Delaware | 39.3 | – | Nevada** | N/A |
| 24 | Florida | 39.2 | – | New Jersey** | N/A |
| 25 | Missouri | 38.8 | – | Wyoming** | N/A |

District of Columbia          62.1

Source: U.S. Department of Health and Human Services, Centers for Disease Control
   "Behavioral Risk Factor Surveillance, 1986–1990" (Morbidity and Mortality Weekly Report, December 1991)
*Persons who report no exercise, recreation, or physical activities (other than regular job duties) during the previous month.
**Not available.

# Percent of Low Income Adults with No Leisure-Time Physical Activity in 1990

## National Median = 36.9% of Low Income Adults 18 and Older Inactive*

| RANK | STATE | PERCENT INACTIVE | RANK | STATE | PERCENT INACTIVE |
|---|---|---|---|---|---|
| 1 | Kentucky | 51.1 | 26 | California | 34.9 |
| 2 | Oklahoma | 50.6 | 27 | Illinois | 34.0 |
| 3 | West Virginia | 48.8 | 27 | Indiana | 34.0 |
| 4 | Tennessee | 48.7 | 29 | Hawaii | 33.3 |
| 5 | North Carolina | 47.1 | 30 | Minnesota | 32.6 |
| 6 | Maine | 46.1 | 31 | New Mexico | 31.9 |
| 7 | Georgia | 45.8 | 32 | Nebraska | 31.7 |
| 8 | New York | 45.3 | 32 | Rhode Island | 31.7 |
| 9 | South Carolina | 44.7 | 34 | Massachusetts | 31.5 |
| 10 | Mississippi | 44.6 | 35 | Idaho | 31.4 |
| 11 | Maryland | 43.7 | 36 | North Dakota | 31.0 |
| 12 | Michigan | 43.1 | 37 | New Hampshire | 30.0 |
| 13 | Florida | 42.3 | 38 | Wisconsin | 29.0 |
| 14 | Iowa | 42.1 | 39 | Utah | 27.0 |
| 15 | Texas | 40.3 | 40 | Montana | 26.5 |
| 16 | Missouri | 39.9 | 41 | Oregon | 26.2 |
| 17 | Delaware | 39.8 | 42 | Colorado | 26.0 |
| 18 | Alabama | 39.3 | 43 | Arizona | 25.7 |
| 19 | Connecticut | 38.8 | 44 | Washington | 24.5 |
| 19 | Virginia | 38.8 | – | Alaska** | N/A |
| 21 | Ohio | 38.1 | – | Arkansas** | N/A |
| 22 | Louisiana | 36.9 | – | Kansas** | N/A |
| 22 | Vermont | 36.9 | – | Nevada** | N/A |
| 24 | South Dakota | 36.0 | – | New Jersey** | N/A |
| 25 | Pennsylvania | 35.7 | – | Wyoming** | N/A |

District of Columbia          61.1

Source: U.S. Department of Health and Human Services, Centers for Disease Control

"Behavioral Risk Factor Surveillance, 1986–1990" (Morbidity and Mortality Weekly Report, December 1991)

*Persons with family incomes of $20,000 or less who report no exercise, recreation, or physical activities (other than regular job duties) during the previous month.

**Not available.

# Percent of Adults with Sedentary Lifestyles in 1990

## National Median = 58.5% of Adults 18 and Older are Sedentary*

| RANK | STATE | PERCENT SEDENTARY | RANK | STATE | PERCENT SEDENTARY |
|---|---|---|---|---|---|
| 1 | South Carolina | 69.7 | 26 | Minnesota | 55.3 |
| 2 | Ohio | 69.3 | 27 | Pennsylvania | 54.9 |
| 3 | Kentucky | 69.1 | 28 | Florida | 54.8 |
| 4 | West Virginia | 67.8 | 29 | Rhode Island | 54.7 |
| 5 | Mississippi | 66.4 | 30 | Delaware | 54.1 |
| 6 | Oklahoma | 66.3 | 31 | California | 53.7 |
| 7 | New York | 63.2 | 32 | Wisconsin | 53.6 |
| 8 | Hawaii | 62.4 | 33 | Texas | 53.5 |
| 9 | Georgia | 62.3 | 34 | Connecticut | 52.0 |
| 10 | Maryland | 61.6 | 34 | Montana | 52.0 |
| 11 | Indiana | 61.3 | 36 | Washington | 51.9 |
| 12 | Missouri | 61.2 | 37 | Arizona | 51.4 |
| 13 | Tennessee | 61.0 | 38 | New Mexico | 51.0 |
| 14 | North Carolina | 60.7 | 38 | Vermont | 51.0 |
| 15 | Iowa | 60.6 | 40 | Massachusetts | 49.8 |
| 16 | Alabama | 60.3 | 41 | Oregon | 48.9 |
| 16 | Illinois | 60.3 | 42 | Utah | 48.8 |
| 18 | Maine | 59.8 | 43 | New Hampshire | 46.9 |
| 19 | Michigan | 59.3 | 44 | Colorado | 44.5 |
| 20 | Virginia | 59.1 | – | Alaska** | N/A |
| 21 | Idaho | 58.7 | – | Arkansas** | N/A |
| 22 | Louisiana | 58.5 | – | Kansas** | N/A |
| 23 | South Dakota | 56.9 | – | Nevada** | N/A |
| 24 | North Dakota | 56.4 | – | New Jersey** | N/A |
| 25 | Nebraska | 55.4 | – | Wyoming** | N/A |

District of Columbia     73.3

Source: U.S. Department of Health and Human Services, Centers for Disease Control
   "Behavioral Risk Factor Surveillance, 1986-1990" (Morbidity and Mortality Weekly Report, December 1991)
*Persons who report fewer than three, 20-minute sessions of leisure-time physical activity per week.
**Not available.

# Percent of Adults 65 and Older with Sedentary Lifestyles in 1990

## National Median = 63.9% of Adults 65 and Older are Sedentary*

| RANK | STATE | PERCENT SEDENTARY | | RANK | STATE | PERCENT SEDENTARY |
|------|-------|-------------------|---|------|-------|-------------------|
| 1 | South Carolina | 78.3 | | 26 | South Dakota | 62.0 |
| 2 | Kentucky | 78.2 | | 27 | Rhode Island | 60.6 |
| 3 | West Virginia | 78.1 | | 28 | Massachusetts | 60.1 |
| 4 | Mississippi | 77.6 | | 29 | Minnesota | 59.6 |
| 5 | Ohio | 76.8 | | 30 | Montana | 59.0 |
| 6 | New York | 71.3 | | 31 | Connecticut | 58.9 |
| 7 | Maryland | 71.2 | | 32 | Hawaii | 58.0 |
| 8 | Virginia | 70.4 | | 33 | Texas | 57.0 |
| 9 | Maine | 70.1 | | 34 | Washington | 56.6 |
| 10 | Michigan | 69.6 | | 35 | New Hampshire | 55.9 |
| 11 | Illinois | 69.2 | | 36 | Vermont | 55.8 |
| 12 | North Carolina | 68.9 | | 37 | Wisconsin | 55.6 |
| 13 | Indiana | 67.6 | | 38 | Florida | 55.1 |
| 14 | Oklahoma | 67.5 | | 39 | New Mexico | 55.0 |
| 15 | Georgia | 67.2 | | 40 | California | 54.1 |
| 16 | Iowa | 66.9 | | 41 | Oregon | 52.8 |
| 17 | Alabama | 66.2 | | 42 | Utah | 48.1 |
| 18 | North Dakota | 65.3 | | 43 | Arizona | 47.4 |
| 19 | Louisiana | 65.1 | | 44 | Colorado | 46.8 |
| 19 | Tennessee | 65.1 | | – | Alaska** | N/A |
| 21 | Missouri | 64.2 | | – | Arkansas** | N/A |
| 22 | Idaho | 63.9 | | – | Kansas** | N/A |
| 23 | Delaware | 63.6 | | – | Nevada** | N/A |
| 24 | Pennsylvania | 63.1 | | – | New Jersey** | N/A |
| 25 | Nebraska | 62.7 | | – | Wyoming** | N/A |

District of Columbia     76.2

Source: U.S. Department of Health and Human Services, Centers for Disease Control
    "Behavioral Risk Factor Surveillance, 1986-1990" (Morbidity and Mortality Weekly Report, December 1991)
*Persons reporting fewer than three, 20-minute sessions of leisure-time physical activity per week.
**Not available.

# Percent of Low Income Adults with Sedentary Lifestyles in 1990

## National Median = 62.8% of Low Income Adults 18 and Older are Sedentary*

| RANK | STATE | PERCENT SEDENTARY | RANK | STATE | PERCENT SEDENTARY |
|------|-------|-------------------|------|-------|-------------------|
| 1 | South Carolina | 75.9 | 26 | California | 62.1 |
| 2 | Kentucky | 74.4 | 26 | Hawaii | 62.1 |
| 3 | West Virginia | 73.2 | 28 | Nebraska | 61.6 |
| 4 | Oklahoma | 73.1 | 29 | North Dakota | 61.0 |
| 5 | Ohio | 70.7 | 30 | Illinois | 60.8 |
| 6 | Maine | 70.4 | 31 | Minnesota | 60.6 |
| 7 | Indiana | 69.7 | 32 | Pennsylvania | 60.5 |
| 7 | Mississippi | 69.7 | 33 | Montana | 59.3 |
| 9 | New York | 69.3 | 34 | Rhode Island | 58.5 |
| 10 | Tennessee | 67.8 | 35 | Wisconsin | 57.6 |
| 11 | Michigan | 67.4 | 36 | Vermont | 56.4 |
| 11 | North Carolina | 67.4 | 37 | New Mexico | 56.3 |
| 13 | Iowa | 67.3 | 38 | Washington | 55.1 |
| 14 | Georgia | 66.6 | 39 | Massachusetts | 55.0 |
| 15 | Virginia | 65.9 | 40 | New Hampshire | 54.5 |
| 16 | Alabama | 65.7 | 41 | Oregon | 53.0 |
| 17 | Maryland | 65.2 | 42 | Utah | 52.4 |
| 18 | Missouri | 65.1 | 43 | Arizona | 52.3 |
| 19 | Florida | 64.4 | 44 | Colorado | 48.7 |
| 20 | Louisiana | 64.1 | – | Alaska** | N/A |
| 21 | Delaware | 63.0 | – | Arkansas** | N/A |
| 22 | Connecticut | 62.8 | – | Kansas** | N/A |
| 23 | South Dakota | 62.7 | – | Nevada** | N/A |
| 24 | Texas | 62.4 | – | New Jersey** | N/A |
| 25 | Idaho | 62.2 | – | Wyoming** | N/A |

District of Columbia  78.5

Source: U.S. Department of Health and Human Services, Centers for Disease Control
   "Behavioral Risk Factor Surveillance, 1986-1990" (Morbidity and Mortality Weekly Report, December 1991)
*Persons with family income of $20,000 or less who report fewer than three, 20-minute sessions of leisure-time physical activity per week
**Not available.

456

# VIII. APPENDIX
## Population Charts

# Resident State Population in 1991

## National Total = 252,177,000*

| RANK | STATE | POPULATION | % | RANK | STATE | POPULATION | % |
|---|---|---|---|---|---|---|---|
| 1 | California | 30,380,000 | 12.05% | 26 | Colorado | 3,377,000 | 1.34% |
| 2 | New York | 18,058,000 | 7.16% | 27 | Connecticut | 3,291,000 | 1.31% |
| 3 | Texas | 17,349,000 | 6.88% | 28 | Oklahoma | 3,175,000 | 1.26% |
| 4 | Florida | 13,277,000 | 5.26% | 29 | Oregon | 2,922,000 | 1.16% |
| 5 | Pennsylvania | 11,961,000 | 4.74% | 30 | Iowa | 2,795,000 | 1.11% |
| 6 | Illinois | 11,543,000 | 4.58% | 31 | Mississippi | 2,592,000 | 1.03% |
| 7 | Ohio | 10,939,000 | 4.34% | 32 | Kansas | 2,495,000 | 0.99% |
| 8 | Michigan | 9,368,000 | 3.71% | 33 | Arkansas | 2,372,000 | 0.94% |
| 9 | New Jersey | 7,760,000 | 3.08% | 34 | West Virginia | 1,801,000 | 0.71% |
| 10 | North Carolina | 6,737,000 | 2.67% | 35 | Utah | 1,770,000 | 0.70% |
| 11 | Georgia | 6,623,000 | 2.63% | 36 | Nebraska | 1,593,000 | 0.63% |
| 12 | Virginia | 6,286,000 | 2.49% | 37 | New Mexico | 1,548,000 | 0.61% |
| 13 | Massachusetts | 5,996,000 | 2.38% | 38 | Nevada | 1,284,000 | 0.51% |
| 14 | Indiana | 5,610,000 | 2.22% | 39 | Maine | 1,235,000 | 0.49% |
| 15 | Missouri | 5,158,000 | 2.05% | 40 | Hawaii | 1,135,000 | 0.45% |
| 16 | Washington | 5,018,000 | 1.99% | 41 | New Hampshire | 1,105,000 | 0.44% |
| 17 | Wisconsin | 4,955,000 | 1.96% | 42 | Idaho | 1,039,000 | 0.41% |
| 18 | Tennessee | 4,953,000 | 1.96% | 43 | Rhode Island | 1,004,000 | 0.40% |
| 19 | Maryland | 4,860,000 | 1.93% | 44 | Montana | 808,000 | 0.32% |
| 20 | Minnesota | 4,432,000 | 1.76% | 45 | South Dakota | 703,000 | 0.28% |
| 21 | Louisiana | 4,252,000 | 1.69% | 46 | Delaware | 680,000 | 0.27% |
| 22 | Alabama | 4,089,000 | 1.62% | 47 | North Dakota | 635,000 | 0.25% |
| 23 | Arizona | 3,750,000 | 1.49% | 48 | Alaska | 570,000 | 0.23% |
| 24 | Kentucky | 3,713,000 | 1.47% | 49 | Vermont | 567,000 | 0.22% |
| 25 | South Carolina | 3,560,000 | 1.41% | 50 | Wyoming | 460,000 | 0.18% |
| | | | | | District of Columbia | 598,000 | 0.24% |

Source: U.S. Bureau of the Census

   Press Release CB 91-346 (December 30, 1991)

*Estimate as of July 1, 1991.

# Resident State Population in 1990

## National Total = 248,709,873

| RANK | STATE | POPULATION | % | RANK | STATE | POPULATION | % |
|---|---|---|---|---|---|---|---|
| 1 | California | 29,760,021 | 11.97% | 26 | Colorado | 3,294,394 | 1.32% |
| 2 | New York | 17,990,455 | 7.23% | 27 | Connecticut | 3,287,116 | 1.32% |
| 3 | Texas | 16,986,510 | 6.83% | 28 | Oklahoma | 3,145,585 | 1.26% |
| 4 | Florida | 12,937,926 | 5.20% | 29 | Oregon | 2,842,321 | 1.14% |
| 5 | Pennsylvania | 11,881,632 | 4.78% | 30 | Iowa | 2,776,755 | 1.12% |
| 6 | Illinois | 11,430,602 | 4.60% | 31 | Mississippi | 2,573,216 | 1.03% |
| 7 | Ohio | 10,847,115 | 4.36% | 32 | Kansas | 2,477,574 | 1.00% |
| 8 | Michigan | 9,295,297 | 3.74% | 33 | Arkansas | 2,350,725 | 0.95% |
| 9 | New Jersey | 7,730,188 | 3.11% | 34 | West Virginia | 1,793,477 | 0.72% |
| 10 | North Carolina | 6,628,637 | 2.67% | 35 | Utah | 1,722,850 | 0.69% |
| 11 | Georgia | 6,478,216 | 2.60% | 36 | Nebraska | 1,578,385 | 0.63% |
| 12 | Virginia | 6,187,358 | 2.49% | 37 | New Mexico | 1,515,069 | 0.61% |
| 13 | Massachusetts | 6,016,425 | 2.42% | 38 | Maine | 1,227,928 | 0.49% |
| 14 | Indiana | 5,544,159 | 2.23% | 39 | Nevada | 1,201,833 | 0.48% |
| 15 | Missouri | 5,117,073 | 2.06% | 40 | New Hampshire | 1,109,252 | 0.45% |
| 16 | Wisconsin | 4,891,769 | 1.97% | 41 | Hawaii | 1,108,229 | 0.45% |
| 17 | Tennessee | 4,877,185 | 1.96% | 42 | Idaho | 1,006,749 | 0.40% |
| 18 | Washington | 4,866,692 | 1.96% | 43 | Rhode Island | 1,003,464 | 0.40% |
| 19 | Maryland | 4,781,468 | 1.92% | 44 | Montana | 799,065 | 0.32% |
| 20 | Minnesota | 4,375,099 | 1.76% | 45 | South Dakota | 696,004 | 0.28% |
| 21 | Louisiana | 4,219,973 | 1.70% | 46 | Delaware | 666,168 | 0.27% |
| 22 | Alabama | 4,040,587 | 1.62% | 47 | North Dakota | 638,800 | 0.26% |
| 23 | Kentucky | 3,685,296 | 1.48% | 48 | Vermont | 562,758 | 0.23% |
| 24 | Arizona | 3,665,228 | 1.47% | 49 | Alaska | 550,043 | 0.22% |
| 25 | South Carolina | 3,486,703 | 1.40% | 50 | Wyoming | 453,588 | 0.18% |
| | | | | | District of Columbia | 606,900 | 0.24% |

Source: U.S. Bureau of the Census
Press Release CB 91-100 (March 11, 1991)

# Resident State Population in 1989

## National Total = 248,243,000

| RANK | STATE | POPULATION | % | | RANK | STATE | POPULATION | % |
|---|---|---|---|---|---|---|---|---|
| 1 | California | 29,063,000 | 11.71% | | 26 | Colorado | 3,317,000 | 1.34% |
| 2 | New York | 17,950,000 | 7.23% | | 27 | Connecticut | 3,239,000 | 1.30% |
| 3 | Texas | 16,991,000 | 6.84% | | 28 | Oklahoma | 3,224,000 | 1.30% |
| 4 | Florida | 12,671,000 | 5.10% | | 29 | Iowa | 2,840,000 | 1.14% |
| 5 | Pennsylvania | 12,040,000 | 4.85% | | 30 | Oregon | 2,820,000 | 1.14% |
| 6 | Illinois | 11,658,000 | 4.70% | | 31 | Mississippi | 2,621,000 | 1.06% |
| 7 | Ohio | 10,907,000 | 4.39% | | 32 | Kansas | 2,513,000 | 1.01% |
| 8 | Michigan | 9,273,000 | 3.74% | | 33 | Arkansas | 2,406,000 | 0.97% |
| 9 | New Jersey | 7,736,000 | 3.12% | | 34 | West Virginia | 1,857,000 | 0.75% |
| 10 | North Carolina | 6,571,000 | 2.65% | | 35 | Utah | 1,707,000 | 0.69% |
| 11 | Georgia | 6,436,000 | 2.59% | | 36 | Nebraska | 1,611,000 | 0.65% |
| 12 | Virginia | 6,098,000 | 2.46% | | 37 | New Mexico | 1,528,000 | 0.62% |
| 13 | Massachusetts | 5,913,000 | 2.38% | | 38 | Maine | 1,222,000 | 0.49% |
| 14 | Indiana | 5,593,000 | 2.25% | | 39 | Hawaii | 1,112,000 | 0.45% |
| 15 | Missouri | 5,159,000 | 2.08% | | 40 | Nevada | 1,111,000 | 0.45% |
| 16 | Tennessee | 4,940,000 | 1.99% | | 41 | New Hampshire | 1,107,000 | 0.45% |
| 17 | Wisconsin | 4,867,000 | 1.96% | | 42 | Idaho | 1,014,000 | 0.41% |
| 18 | Washington | 4,761,000 | 1.92% | | 43 | Rhode Island | 998,000 | 0.40% |
| 19 | Maryland | 4,694,000 | 1.89% | | 44 | Montana | 806,000 | 0.32% |
| 20 | Louisiana | 4,382,000 | 1.77% | | 45 | South Dakota | 715,000 | 0.29% |
| 21 | Minnesota | 4,353,000 | 1.75% | | 46 | Delaware | 673,000 | 0.27% |
| 22 | Alabama | 4,118,000 | 1.66% | | 47 | North Dakota | 660,000 | 0.27% |
| 23 | Kentucky | 3,727,000 | 1.50% | | 48 | Vermont | 567,000 | 0.23% |
| 24 | Arizona | 3,556,000 | 1.43% | | 49 | Alaska | 527,000 | 0.21% |
| 25 | South Carolina | 3,512,000 | 1.41% | | 50 | Wyoming | 475,000 | 0.19% |
| | | | | | | District of Columbia | 604,000 | 0.24% |

Source: U.S. Bureau of the Census
"Federal Expenditures by State for FY 1989" (March 1990)

## Male Population in 1990

## National Total = 121,239,418 Males

| RANK | STATE | MALES | % |
|------|-------|-------|---|
| 1 | California | 14,897,627 | 12.29% |
| 2 | New York | 8,625,673 | 7.11% |
| 3 | Texas | 8,365,963 | 6.90% |
| 4 | Florida | 6,261,719 | 5.16% |
| 5 | Pennsylvania | 5,694,265 | 4.70% |
| 6 | Illinois | 5,552,233 | 4.58% |
| 7 | Ohio | 5,226,340 | 4.31% |
| 8 | Michigan | 4,512,781 | 3.72% |
| 9 | New Jersey | 3,735,685 | 3.08% |
| 10 | North Carolina | 3,214,290 | 2.65% |
| 11 | Georgia | 3,144,503 | 2.59% |
| 12 | Virginia | 3,033,974 | 2.50% |
| 13 | Massachusetts | 2,888,745 | 2.38% |
| 14 | Indiana | 2,688,281 | 2.22% |
| 15 | Missouri | 2,464,315 | 2.03% |
| 16 | Washington | 2,413,747 | 1.99% |
| 17 | Wisconsin | 2,392,935 | 1.97% |
| 18 | Tennessee | 2,348,928 | 1.94% |
| 19 | Maryland | 2,318,671 | 1.91% |
| 20 | Minnesota | 2,145,183 | 1.77% |
| 21 | Louisiana | 2,031,386 | 1.68% |
| 22 | Alabama | 1,936,162 | 1.60% |
| 23 | Arizona | 1,810,691 | 1.49% |
| 24 | Kentucky | 1,785,235 | 1.47% |
| 25 | South Carolina | 1,688,510 | 1.39% |

| RANK | STATE | MALES | % |
|------|-------|-------|---|
| 26 | Colorado | 1,631,295 | 1.35% |
| 27 | Connecticut | 1,592,873 | 1.31% |
| 28 | Oklahoma | 1,530,819 | 1.26% |
| 29 | Oregon | 1,397,073 | 1.15% |
| 30 | Iowa | 1,344,802 | 1.11% |
| 31 | Mississippi | 1,230,617 | 1.02% |
| 32 | Kansas | 1,214,645 | 1.00% |
| 33 | Arkansas | 1,133,076 | 0.93% |
| 34 | West Virginia | 861,536 | 0.71% |
| 35 | Utah | 855,759 | 0.71% |
| 36 | Nebraska | 769,439 | 0.63% |
| 37 | New Mexico | 745,253 | 0.61% |
| 38 | Nevada | 611,880 | 0.50% |
| 39 | Maine | 597,850 | 0.49% |
| 40 | Hawaii | 563,891 | 0.47% |
| 41 | New Hampshire | 543,544 | 0.45% |
| 42 | Idaho | 500,956 | 0.41% |
| 43 | Rhode Island | 481,496 | 0.40% |
| 44 | Montana | 395,769 | 0.33% |
| 45 | South Dakota | 342,498 | 0.28% |
| 46 | Delaware | 322,968 | 0.27% |
| 47 | North Dakota | 318,201 | 0.26% |
| 48 | Alaska | 289,867 | 0.24% |
| 49 | Vermont | 275,492 | 0.23% |
| 50 | Wyoming | 227,007 | 0.19% |
|  | District of Columbia | 282,970 | 0.23% |

Source: U.S. Bureau of the Census
Press Release CB 91–217 (June 11, 1991)

# Female Population in 1990

## National Total = 127,470,455 Females

| RANK | STATE | FEMALES | % | | RANK | STATE | FEMALES | % |
|---|---|---|---|---|---|---|---|---|
| 1 | California | 14,862,394 | 11.66% | | 26 | Connecticut | 1,694,243 | 1.33% |
| 2 | New York | 9,364,782 | 7.35% | | 27 | Colorado | 1,663,099 | 1.30% |
| 3 | Texas | 8,620,547 | 6.76% | | 28 | Oklahoma | 1,614,766 | 1.27% |
| 4 | Florida | 6,676,207 | 5.24% | | 29 | Oregon | 1,445,248 | 1.13% |
| 5 | Pennsylvania | 6,187,378 | 4.85% | | 30 | Iowa | 1,431,953 | 1.12% |
| 6 | Illinois | 5,878,369 | 4.61% | | 31 | Mississippi | 1,342,599 | 1.05% |
| 7 | Ohio | 5,620,775 | 4.41% | | 32 | Kansas | 1,262,929 | 0.99% |
| 8 | Michigan | 4,782,516 | 3.75% | | 33 | Arkansas | 1,217,649 | 0.96% |
| 9 | New Jersey | 3,994,503 | 3.13% | | 34 | West Virginia | 931,941 | 0.73% |
| 10 | North Carolina | 3,414,347 | 2.68% | | 35 | Utah | 867,091 | 0.68% |
| 11 | Georgia | 3,333,713 | 2.62% | | 36 | Nebraska | 808,946 | 0.63% |
| 12 | Virginia | 3,153,384 | 2.47% | | 37 | New Mexico | 769,816 | 0.60% |
| 13 | Massachusetts | 3,127,680 | 2.45% | | 38 | Maine | 630,078 | 0.49% |
| 14 | Indiana | 2,855,878 | 2.24% | | 39 | Nevada | 589,953 | 0.46% |
| 15 | Missouri | 2,652,758 | 2.08% | | 40 | New Hampshire | 565,708 | 0.44% |
| 16 | Tennessee | 2,528,257 | 1.98% | | 41 | Hawaii | 544,338 | 0.43% |
| 17 | Wisconsin | 2,498,834 | 1.96% | | 42 | Rhode Island | 521,968 | 0.41% |
| 18 | Maryland | 2,462,797 | 1.93% | | 43 | Idaho | 505,793 | 0.40% |
| 19 | Washington | 2,452,945 | 1.92% | | 44 | Montana | 403,296 | 0.32% |
| 20 | Minnesota | 2,229,916 | 1.75% | | 45 | South Dakota | 353,506 | 0.28% |
| 21 | Louisiana | 2,188,587 | 1.72% | | 46 | Delaware | 343,200 | 0.27% |
| 22 | Alabama | 2,104,425 | 1.65% | | 47 | North Dakota | 320,599 | 0.25% |
| 23 | Kentucky | 1,900,061 | 1.49% | | 48 | Vermont | 287,266 | 0.23% |
| 24 | Arizona | 1,854,537 | 1.45% | | 49 | Alaska | 260,176 | 0.20% |
| 25 | South Carolina | 1,798,193 | 1.41% | | 50 | Wyoming | 226,581 | 0.18% |
| | | | | | | District of Columbia | 323,930 | 0.25% |

*Source: U.S. Bureau of the Census*
   *Press Release CB 91-217 (June 11, 1991)*

# White Population in 1990

## National Total = 199,686,070 White Persons

| RANK | STATE | WHITES | % | RANK | STATE | WHITES | % |
|------|-------|--------|---|------|-------|--------|---|
| 1 | California | 20,524,327 | 10.28% | 26 | Louisiana | 2,839,138 | 1.42% |
| 2 | New York | 13,385,255 | 6.70% | 27 | Iowa | 2,683,090 | 1.34% |
| 3 | Texas | 12,774,762 | 6.40% | 28 | Oregon | 2,636,787 | 1.32% |
| 4 | Florida | 10,749,285 | 5.38% | 29 | Oklahoma | 2,583,512 | 1.29% |
| 5 | Pennsylvania | 10,520,201 | 5.27% | 30 | South Carolina | 2,406,974 | 1.21% |
| 6 | Ohio | 9,521,756 | 4.77% | 31 | Kansas | 2,231,986 | 1.12% |
| 7 | Illinois | 8,952,978 | 4.48% | 32 | Arkansas | 1,944,744 | 0.97% |
| 8 | Michigan | 7,756,086 | 3.88% | 33 | West Virginia | 1,725,523 | 0.86% |
| 9 | New Jersey | 6,130,465 | 3.07% | 34 | Mississippi | 1,633,461 | 0.82% |
| 10 | Massachusetts | 5,405,374 | 2.71% | 35 | Utah | 1,615,845 | 0.81% |
| 11 | Indiana | 5,020,700 | 2.51% | 36 | Nebraska | 1,480,558 | 0.74% |
| 12 | North Carolina | 5,008,491 | 2.51% | 37 | Maine | 1,208,360 | 0.61% |
| 13 | Virginia | 4,791,739 | 2.40% | 38 | New Mexico | 1,146,028 | 0.57% |
| 14 | Georgia | 4,600,148 | 2.30% | 39 | New Hampshire | 1,087,433 | 0.54% |
| 15 | Wisconsin | 4,512,523 | 2.26% | 40 | Nevada | 1,012,695 | 0.51% |
| 16 | Missouri | 4,486,228 | 2.25% | 41 | Idaho | 950,451 | 0.48% |
| 17 | Washington | 4,308,937 | 2.16% | 42 | Rhode Island | 917,375 | 0.46% |
| 18 | Minnesota | 4,130,395 | 2.07% | 43 | Montana | 741,111 | 0.37% |
| 19 | Tennessee | 4,048,068 | 2.03% | 44 | South Dakota | 637,515 | 0.32% |
| 20 | Maryland | 3,393,964 | 1.70% | 45 | North Dakota | 604,142 | 0.30% |
| 21 | Kentucky | 3,391,832 | 1.70% | 46 | Vermont | 555,088 | 0.28% |
| 22 | Alabama | 2,975,797 | 1.49% | 47 | Delaware | 535,094 | 0.27% |
| 23 | Arizona | 2,963,186 | 1.48% | 48 | Wyoming | 427,061 | 0.21% |
| 24 | Colorado | 2,905,474 | 1.46% | 49 | Alaska | 415,492 | 0.21% |
| 25 | Connecticut | 2,859,353 | 1.43% | 50 | Hawaii | 369,616 | 0.19% |
| | | | | | District of Columbia | 179,667 | 0.09% |

Source: U.S. Bureau of the Census
Press Release CB 91-100 (March 11, 1991)

# Black Population in 1990

## National Total = 29,986,060 Black Persons

| RANK | STATE | BLACKS | % | RANK | STATE | BLACKS | % |
|---|---|---|---|---|---|---|---|
| 1 | New York | 2,859,055 | 9.53% | 26 | Oklahoma | 233,801 | 0.78% |
| 2 | California | 2,208,801 | 7.37% | 27 | Washington | 149,801 | 0.50% |
| 3 | Texas | 2,021,632 | 6.74% | 28 | Kansas | 143,076 | 0.48% |
| 4 | Florida | 1,759,534 | 5.87% | 29 | Colorado | 133,146 | 0.44% |
| 5 | Georgia | 1,746,565 | 5.82% | 30 | Delaware | 112,460 | 0.38% |
| 6 | Illinois | 1,694,273 | 5.65% | 31 | Arizona | 110,524 | 0.37% |
| 7 | North Carolina | 1,456,323 | 4.86% | 32 | Minnesota | 94,944 | 0.32% |
| 8 | Louisiana | 1,299,281 | 4.33% | 33 | Nevada | 78,771 | 0.26% |
| 9 | Michigan | 1,291,706 | 4.31% | 34 | Nebraska | 57,404 | 0.19% |
| 10 | Maryland | 1,189,899 | 3.97% | 35 | West Virginia | 56,295 | 0.19% |
| 11 | Virginia | 1,162,994 | 3.88% | 36 | Iowa | 48,090 | 0.16% |
| 12 | Ohio | 1,154,826 | 3.85% | 37 | Oregon | 46,178 | 0.15% |
| 13 | Pennsylvania | 1,089,795 | 3.63% | 38 | Rhode Island | 38,861 | 0.13% |
| 14 | South Carolina | 1,039,884 | 3.47% | 39 | New Mexico | 30,210 | 0.10% |
| 15 | New Jersey | 1,036,825 | 3.46% | 40 | Hawaii | 27,195 | 0.09% |
| 16 | Alabama | 1,020,705 | 3.40% | 41 | Alaska | 22,451 | 0.07% |
| 17 | Mississippi | 915,057 | 3.05% | 42 | Utah | 11,576 | 0.04% |
| 18 | Tennessee | 778,035 | 2.59% | 43 | New Hampshire | 7,198 | 0.02% |
| 19 | Missouri | 548,208 | 1.83% | 44 | Maine | 5,138 | 0.02% |
| 20 | Indiana | 432,092 | 1.44% | 45 | Wyoming | 3,606 | 0.01% |
| 21 | Arkansas | 373,912 | 1.25% | 46 | North Dakota | 3,524 | 0.01% |
| 22 | Massachusetts | 300,130 | 1.00% | 47 | Idaho | 3,370 | 0.01% |
| 23 | Connecticut | 274,269 | 0.91% | 48 | South Dakota | 3,258 | 0.01% |
| 24 | Kentucky | 262,907 | 0.88% | 49 | Montana | 2,381 | 0.01% |
| 25 | Wisconsin | 244,539 | 0.82% | 50 | Vermont | 1,951 | 0.01% |
|  |  |  |  |  | District of Columbia | 399,604 | 1.33% |

Source: U.S. Bureau of the Census
*Source: U.S. Bureau of the Census*

   *Press Release CB 91-100 (March 11, 1991)*

# Projected Resident State Population in 2000

## National Total = 267,747,000

| RANK | STATE | POPULATION | % | RANK | STATE | POPULATION | % |
|------|-------|-----------|------|------|-------|-----------|------|
| 1 | California | 33,500,000 | 12.51% | 26 | Kentucky | 3,733,000 | 1.39% |
| 2 | Texas | 20,211,000 | 7.55% | 27 | Connecticut | 3,445,000 | 1.29% |
| 3 | New York | 17,986,000 | 6.72% | 28 | Oklahoma | 3,376,000 | 1.26% |
| 4 | Florida | 15,415,000 | 5.76% | 29 | Mississippi | 2,877,000 | 1.07% |
| 5 | Illinois | 11,580,000 | 4.32% | 29 | Oregon | 2,877,000 | 1.07% |
| 6 | Pennsylvania | 11,503,000 | 4.30% | 31 | Iowa | 2,549,000 | 0.95% |
| 7 | Ohio | 10,629,000 | 3.97% | 32 | Arkansas | 2,529,000 | 0.94% |
| 8 | Michigan | 9,250,000 | 3.45% | 32 | Kansas | 2,529,000 | 0.94% |
| 9 | New Jersey | 8,546,000 | 3.19% | 34 | Utah | 1,991,000 | 0.74% |
| 10 | Georgia | 7,957,000 | 2.97% | 35 | New Mexico | 1,968,000 | 0.74% |
| 11 | North Carolina | 7,483,000 | 2.79% | 36 | West Virginia | 1,722,000 | 0.64% |
| 12 | Virginia | 6,877,000 | 2.57% | 37 | Nebraska | 1,556,000 | 0.58% |
| 13 | Massachusetts | 6,087,000 | 2.27% | 38 | Hawaii | 1,345,000 | 0.50% |
| 14 | Indiana | 5,502,000 | 2.05% | 39 | New Hampshire | 1,333,000 | 0.50% |
| 15 | Missouri | 5,383,000 | 2.01% | 40 | Nevada | 1,303,000 | 0.49% |
| 16 | Maryland | 5,274,000 | 1.97% | 41 | Maine | 1,271,000 | 0.47% |
| 17 | Tennessee | 5,266,000 | 1.97% | 42 | Rhode Island | 1,049,000 | 0.39% |
| 18 | Washington | 4,991,000 | 1.86% | 43 | Idaho | 1,047,000 | 0.39% |
| 19 | Wisconsin | 4,784,000 | 1.79% | 44 | Montana | 794,000 | 0.30% |
| 20 | Arizona | 4,618,000 | 1.72% | 45 | Delaware | 734,000 | 0.27% |
| 21 | Louisiana | 4,516,000 | 1.69% | 46 | South Dakota | 714,000 | 0.27% |
| 22 | Minnesota | 4,490,000 | 1.68% | 47 | Alaska | 687,000 | 0.26% |
| 23 | Alabama | 4,410,000 | 1.65% | 48 | North Dakota | 629,000 | 0.23% |
| 24 | South Carolina | 3,906,000 | 1.46% | 49 | Vermont | 591,000 | 0.22% |
| 25 | Colorado | 3,813,000 | 1.42% | 50 | Wyoming | 489,000 | 0.18% |
| | | | | | District of Columbia | 634,000 | 0.24% |

Source: U.S. Bureau of the Census
"Current Population Reports" (series P-25, No. 1017)

# IX. SOURCES

**American Cancer Society, Inc.**
1599 Clifton Road, NE
Atlanta, GA  30329-4251
800-227-2345

**American Hospital Association**
840 North Lake Shore Drive
Chicago, IL  60611
312-280-6000

**American Managed Care & Review Assn.**
1227 25th Street, NW
Washington, DC  20037
202-728-0506

**American Medical Association**
P.O. Box 10623
Chicago, IL  60610
312-464-5000

**American Osteopathic Association**
142 East Ontario Street
Chicago, IL  60611
312-280-5800

**American Podiatric Medical Association**
9312 Old Georgetown Road
Bethesda, MD  20814
301-571-9200

**Bureau of the Census**
3 Silver Hill and Suitland Roads
Suitland, MD  20746
301-763-4040

**Bureau of Health Professions**
U.S. Department of Health and Human Services
5600 Fishers Lane
Rockville, MD  20857
301-443-8890 (medicine division)
301-443-8586 (nursing division)
301-443-6853 (dental division)

**Families USA Foundation**
1334 G Street, NW
Washington, DC  20005
202-628-3030

**Group Health Association of America**
1129 20th Street, NW  Suite 600
Washington, DC  20036
202-778-3200

**Health Care Financing Administration**
U.S. Department of Health and Human Services
6325 Security Boulevard
Baltimore, MD  21207
410-966-7843 (publications)
202-690-6113 (public affairs)

**Health Insurance Association of America**
1025 Connecticut Avenue, NW
Washington, DC  20036-3998
202-223-7780

**International Chiropractors Association**
1110 North Glebe Road, Suite 1000
Arlington, VA  22201
703-528-5000

**Medical Economics Publishing Company**
5 Paragon Drive
Montvale, NJ  07645-1742
201-358-7300

**National Center for Health Statistics**
U.S. Department of Health and Human Services
6525 Belcrest Road
Hyattsville, MD  20782
301-436-8951 (vital statistics division)

**National Institute on Alcohol Abuse**
U.S. Department of Health and Human Services
5600 Fishers Lane
Rockville, MD  20857
301-443-3885

**Public Health Service**
U.S. Department of Health and Human Services
200 Independence Avenue, SW
Washington, DC  20201
202-690-6867 (Public Information)

# X. INDEX

# X. INDEX (continued)

# X. INDEX (continued)

**Births and Reproductive Health**

**Deaths**

**Facilities**

**Finance**

**Incidence of Disease**

**Personnel**

**Physical Fitness**

# THUMB INDEX

## HOW TO USE THIS INDEX

Place left thumb on the outer edge of this page. To locate the desired entry, fold back the remaining page edges and align the index edge mark with the appropriate page edge mark.